THE CANCER PREVENTION DIET

OTHER BOOKS BY MICHIO KUSHI AND ALEX JACK

Diet for a Strong Heart

One Peaceful World

Macrobiotic Diet (with Aveline Kushi)

The Book of Macrobiotics

Food Governs Your Destiny (with Aveline Kushi)

The Gospel of Peace

The Macrobiotic Path to Total Health

THE CANCER PREVENTION DIET

The Macrobiotic Approach to
Preventing and Relieving Cancer

*Revised and Updated
25th Anniversary Edition*

MICHIO KUSHI
and ALEX JACK

ST. MARTIN'S GRIFFIN

New York

In Memory of George Ohsawa
and Aveline Kushi

Authors' Note

It is advisable for the reader to seek the guidance of a physician and appropriate
nutritionist before implementing the approach to health suggested by this book.
It is essential that any reader who has any reason to suspect cancer or illness contact a
physician promptly. Neither this nor any other book should be used as a substitute for
professional medical care or treatment.

Design by Patrice Sheridan

Chapters 8 and 9, "The Role of the Emotions in the Development of Cancer" and
"Woman and Cancer" by Anna Böhm, are used with her permission.

LIBRARY OF CONGRESS CATALOGING-IN-PUBLICATION DATA

Kushi, Michio.
    The cancer prevention diet : the macrobiotic approach to preventing and relieving
cancer / by Michio Kushi with Alex Jack.—Rev. and updated ed.
        p.   cm.
    Includes index.
    ISBN-13: 978-0-312-56106-2
    ISBN-10: 0-312-56106-7
    1. Cancer—Diet therapy.   2. Cancer—Prevention.   3. Macrobiotic diet.   I. Jack, Alex,
1945- II. Title.
    RC271.D52K86 2009
    616.99'40654—dc22   2009010690

Revised and Updated 25th Anniversary Edition: August 2009

10   9   8   7   6   5   4   3   2   1

CONTENTS

NOTE TO THE READER

Please visit www.TheCancerPreventionDiet.com for a wealth of additional information. Here you will find chapters on AIDS-related cancer, radiation and environmentally related cancer, scores of additional scientific, medical, and nutritional studies, new case histories, a comprehensive listing of macrobiotic foods, and information on how to arrange a personal consultation or obtain a personalized menu plan. This book, among others, may be purchased on the Web site, which will be constantly updated with new material and resource information. Contact Alex Jack at shenwa26@yahoo.com.

PREFACE

Every year the death toll from cancer continues to rise. In a world beset by worsening medical, food, energy, financial, and environmental crises, cancer remains one of the gravest threats to personal and planetary health. In the United States and other developed societies, nearly one in two men and one in three women will get cancer in his or her lifetime. Twenty-five years ago, when the first edition of this book appeared, its dietary and lifestyle approach was considered revolutionary. The Food and Drug Administration, the National Cancer Institute, and the American Cancer Society held that diet had little, if anything, to do with the origin or treatment of this affliction. The idea that cancer could be prevented and, in some cases, relieved by a balanced, natural way of eating was considered dangerous and unproven.

The dietary premise is now almost universally accepted. The specific approach introduced in this book has been studied by researchers and medical doctors around the world. Scientists at Harvard University, the University of Minnesota, the University of South Carolina, the National Tumor Institute in Milan, and many other universities and institutions have substantiated its benefits. These findings have been published in *Cancer Research; Cancer, Epidemiology, Biology, and Prevention; Journal of the American College of Nutrition; International Journal of Biological Markers; Integrative Cancer Therapies;* and other peer-reviewed medical journals. The American Cancer Society reversed course and endorsed aspects of our approach, the Centers for Disease Control has funded a study, and an expert panel of the National

Cancer Institute endorsed clinical trials after reviewing several medically documented recoveries drawn from a series of seventy-seven "Best Cases" collected by researchers for the National Institutes of Health. Hundreds of other successful cancer recovery stories using this method have appeared in the mainstream press, alternative media, on television and radio, and on the Internet.

Even though oncology today remains largely focused on chemotherapy, radiation, and other extreme methods of treatment, modern medicine has confirmed the anti-tumor properties of many of the foods recommended in this book. Medical centers are integrating this basic approach into their practice. Across the country, insurance providers, hospitals, and clinics are beginning to focus on prevention, starting with balanced nutrition. Whole grains, fresh vegetables, soy products such as tofu, and other natural and organic foods are now offered at over two thousand hospitals in the United States to patients with cancer, heart disease, and other disorders. For example, Baystate, the largest hospital in New England, located in Springfield, Massachusetts, has converted its food service into a heart healthy regimen, offering veggie burgers, fresh vegetables, fruit, and other wholesome fare to the thousands of patients and family support members it serves every day.

Remarkable progress has also been made in organic agriculture. Since the last edition of this book, the U.S. government has established a national organic certification program. Today the vast majority of fresh organic produce and other chemically-free or GM-free foods are sold in supermarkets. Before, they were found primarily in small natural foods stores and a few large chains such as Whole Foods that catered to upscale shoppers. Wal-Mart, Stop & Shop, Safeway, and every other large food distributor now offers organic food, and it is the largest growing segment of the industry.

New dietary trends commonly have a macrobiotic influence. *Macrobiotic* comes from the traditional Greek words for "great" or "long life," and is the approach underlying this book. Many people associate macrobiotics exclusively with Oriental philosophy and medicine. While several leading macrobiotic educators came out of Japan or were influenced by the teachings of George Ohsawa, the leading proponent of macrobiotics until his death in the 1960s, macrobiotics is universal in scope and embraces all cultures, traditions, religions, and cuisines.

An ironic example of this is shown in the reaction of a large Japanese publisher when the first edition of *The Cancer Prevention Diet* came out in the early 1980s. The editors contacted us and said they wanted to translate the book into Japanese and make it available to the Japanese public but wanted permission to change one section. We thought the conservative publishing Tokyo house was concerned about our strong critique of modern medicine and wanted to tone it down. As it turned out, that was not the issue. They wanted permission to change the menus and recipes in the book to include foods and preparations with which the Japanese were familiar!

Life is so amusing. For the Japanese, our approach was far too Western!

In Japan and some other Asian societies, they have very little diversity and scope of food compared to America or Europe. In Japan, people eat rice (mostly white), some buckwheat (in the form of soba noodles), and wheat in the form of noodles, bread, and baked goods, but many other grains are lacking. Similarly, they enjoy aduki, black beans, and soybeans, but the wide range of beans we have in the United States is missing. Similarly, there are few leafy greens in Japan (for example, no kale or collards), and many other foods we take for granted in the West are not widely available or consumed. The use of seasoning is also very different in Japan. While miso, shoyu (soy sauce), and several other key seasonings and condiments originated in the East, the Japanese tend to consume far more than Americans or Europeans. The reason for this is primarily environmental. The Japanese live on a small island, and their animal food consists mostly of fish and seafood. America and Europe are vast continents, and the main animal foods are beef, pork, and chicken, plus an array of dairy products (all high in sodium). The end result is that Westerners tend to use far less salt and related seasonings than Asians. (Guidelines for tropical and semipolar countries differ even further, as described in Appendix I.)

Large fundamental changes take time. In the last quarter century, macrobiotics has spread rapidly in Japan. Many people think it was popular there to begin with because so many of the foods we recommend came from that country. While it is true that the Japanese reverence rice, miso, and tofu, macrobiotics was regarded there the way most Americans view the Amish. They respect their sincerity and dedication, but find them wholly impractical for today's modern world. At a large macrobiotic cooking seminar for professional chefs in Osaka, Aveline Kushi found that they were bored when she taught them how to cook healthy Japanese-style dishes. When she switched to French- and German-style macrobiotic cuisine, including many delicious pastries and desserts that did not use dairy products or sugar, they were thrilled. Macrobiotics today in Japan and around the world retains a core of local, regional, and national elements but is rapidly becoming a fusion of healthful international cuisines. In the early twenty-first century, macrobiotics spread through the Arabic world thanks primarily to Miriam Nour, a journalist known as "the Oprah of the Middle East," who had a daily TV program that reached millions of viewers. Many Muslims embraced macrobiotics not only because they were suffering from cancer and other chronic diseases but also because it respected traditional foods, values, and customs. Students of Islam felt that the Koran was essentially macrobiotic, a sentiment echoed by Christians and Jews who found similar dietary and lifestyle teachings in their scriptures. Macrobiotics has the potential for unifying the planet beyond ideology, race, gender, and other differences. At one recent macrobiotic conference, people from several dozen countries taught one another songs. Soon a large Arabic contingent was singing in Hebrew, and the Israelis were chanting in Arabic! From postwar Japan, devastated by the atomic bombing of

Hiroshima and Nagasaki, macrobiotics has spiraled across the planet and is a force for world peace and harmony.

Over thousands of years humanity has sought a unifying principle. The principles governing the flow of energy and the attraction of opposites are known traditionally in the East as yin and yang, the primary forces of heaven and earth that create, sustain, and animate all things. Twenty-five years ago, yin and yang were esoteric concepts, further distancing some Western readers from reading and benefiting from our text. Today, yin and yang are universal terms, appearing regularly in global headlines, in articles, and in pop songs, and used widely in ordinary daily conversation. Understanding and applying yin and yang takes patient study and practice, and throughout this book we have attempted to describe and use these terms in a clear, accessible way.

Very gradually, macrobiotics was introduced to mainstream society by what was originally called *alternative medicine*. Within about ten years, more people were going to alternative practitioners than to medical doctors, giving rise to *complementary medicine*. (For example, the U.S. National Institutes of Health's small Office of Alternative Medicine changed into a much larger Center for Complementary and Alternative Medicine.) This meant that a holistic approach could supplement the conventional medical approach. Today, the courtship of these twin disciplines has further evolved into *integrative medicine* in which holistic and conventional approaches are combined or blended. In the future, energetic approaches based on nutrition, direct healing (for example, laying on of hands), and positive thinking and balancing the emotions will predominate. The conventional medical approach will be reserved for extremely difficult or emergency cases. In this way, medicine will come full circle. As we note in an early chapter on the history of macrobiotics, Hippocrates, the father of medicine, originally coined the term *makrobios,* and there is a long history of macrobiotics prior to its modern Japanese revival. Hippocrates' principal teaching—"Let food be thy medicine and thy medicine be food"—was eventually displaced by biochemistry and other branches of modern analytic science. Now the planet is returning to a sound diet as the foundation of personal health and happiness and as a key to solving the interrelated food, energy, climate, financial, and environmental crises.

WHAT'S NEW

Everything changes. This is the law of the infinite universe and the essence of yin and yang. All the statistics, research, and other supporting material in this new edition have been updated to reflect current societal trends and medical findings. The glossary, bibliography, resource section, and other material in the back of the book have been revised and updated, and new appendices have been added. For space considerations we have had to limit the summary of scientific and medical studies supporting our dietary and lifestyle guidelines. When this book first appeared a quarter century ago, it was controversial and needed that kind of official validation. Now, science and medicine are clearly moving in the same direction, and this immense body of research, while supportive, is no longer essential. We have retained references to all the original medical studies on macrobiotics in this book and added many new ones, as well as several key nutritional or environmental studies under each type of cancer. For a comprehensive overview of research, including the hundreds of studies mentioned in previous editions and many new findings, please visit www.makropedia.com, a new macrobiotic-oriented Web site. Moreover, our own approach to health and healing, including cancer, continues to evolve year by year, decade to decade, in the course of thousands of consultations. During this time we have counseled many thousands of individuals with cancer and supporting partners and family members who come each year for personal guidance and direction. In follow-up visits, through letters and faxes, on the telephone and Internet, and at seminars and conferences, their progress has been monitored, in some cases over the course of years and decades.

To take into account ever-changing atmospheric, environmental, and social conditions, many adjustments in dietary recommendations, including about one hundred new special dishes and drinks, compresses, and other home care, are incorporated in this new edition. These changes, as we explain in the chapters that follow, have largely been in response to the accelerating environmental, energy, and food quality crises. Global warming, pollution, GMOs (genetically modified organisms), cellular technology, and the decline in food quality (including an estimated loss of 25 to 50 percent of nutrients in most common fruits and vegetables) have necessitated major changes in macrobiotic cooking, health care, and healing. For example, as the world becomes warmer, technology further intrudes into our lives (in everything from the Internet to cell phones and iPods). As the pace of life speeds up, people become more active, tense, and hardened in their thinking and behavior. To help offset this yangizing trend in which life is heavier, busier, and more stressful, daily food needs to be lighter and more relaxing. Hence, pressure-cooked brown rice and other grains, a cornerstone of macrobiotic cooking, is giving way to proportionately more boiled and steamed grains. Couscous, bulgur, oatmeal, and other cracked grains are also used more than in the past to impart lighter energy. Fresh salad, fresh fruit, juice, oil, sweets, and other lighter, fresher foods are eaten more frequently than before. The menus and recipes in this edition reflect this trend.

THE EMOTIONS AND HEALTH AND SICKNESS

One of the major changes in this edition of the book is more emphasis on the mental, emotional, and spiritual aspects of healing. Emotions are a very important factor as a cause of cancer and sickness. Our body is constantly being composed of, and sustained by, Ki (also known as Chi) energy, or what were traditionally called the forces of heaven and earth, running through the meridians. That stream is going toward the inside where it creates energy centers known as *chakras* (from the Sanskrit word for *wheel*) and eventually differentiates into billions and trillions of streams ending in invisible cells.

Acupuncture, moxibustion, Ayerveda, and other Asian methods of healing are based on this subtle energy flow, although it remains largely unknown to modern medicine and science. Properly, the incoming energy creates a network of meridians, chakras, and invisible cells that can be called our spiritual and mental body. By attracting energy from food and the environment, it also creates the cells themselves, as well as tissues, organs, and other structures that make up our physical body. The food that we take in—originally in the form of blood in the mother's womb—is metabolized and goes through the bloodstream via the capillaries to the invisible cells, and then each cell becomes visible through physicalization. Our spiritual and mental body is thus made primarily by large cosmic and atmospheric forces spiraling into our organism, while our physical body is produced largely from within by the metabolized energy of food and drink spiraling out.

Naturally, according to this model, it follows that disorders have spiritual, mental, and emotional components as well as physical and social ones. They are influenced by large cosmic, environmental, and global influences; smaller regional and community social and cultural factors; family and interpersonal relationships; and dietary and lifestyle practices. The dietary approach to health and sickness is the foundation in most traditional societies and cultures because we eat two to three or more times a day every day of our lives. It is the central factor over which human beings have the most control. Most of the time we have a choice of the quality and quantity of the food we take in as well as the style of eating (fresh home-cooked, canned and processed, or dining out), the time of day we eat (regular or irregular hours), the manner in which we eat (orderly or chaotic), and other factors (such as thorough or little chewing).

Natural cycles, including the seasons, the climate, and the weather, are much more difficult if not impossible to control. Similarly, constantly changing personal, family, community, and natural events can be influenced to only a modest extent. We can change the world, but only if we begin by changing ourselves. Thoughts and emotions, which are shaped and influenced by all these factors as well as the foods we take in, can also be controlled to a large extent. Meditation, visualization, positive thinking, prayer, music and sound, psychological approaches, counseling, and spiritual practices can all be used to unify mind, body, and spirit; maintain good health; and prevent and relieve disease. For example, in traditional Chinese medicine, the lungs are the seat of happiness or sadness, a feeling of wholeness or fragmentation, security or insecurity. If we eat foods that strengthen the lungs, such as broccoli, cauliflower, and root vegetables, we can strengthen these organs. Breathing exercises, affirmations that center on the lungs, singing happy songs, and other practices can further strengthen the lungs and the positive feelings and sentiments associated with them. The emotions can be suppressed as well as created and nurtured. This is also a major contributor to disease, especially cancer, an affliction characterized by the accumulation and withholding of excess energy in various forms. Macrobiotics needs a more developed feminine perspective beyond the cultivation of the arts and the preparation of menus, recipes, and remedies. To help address this important dimension, new chapters have been added on the role of the emotions in the development of cancer and on woman and cancer. This material has been composed by Anna Böhm, who was born in Germany, grew up in a pioneer macrobiotic community in France, earned master's degrees in clinical psychology and psychoanalysis, and is working as a psychologist in Vienna. She is well-versed in the philosophies of the East and West, macrobiotic health care, and mind-body approaches.

Prior editions of this book minimized the vital complementary role that conventional medicine can play in the healing process. In the old days of the cold war that existed between holistic and mainstream therapies, both sides tended to ignore or criticize the other. Not only has détente thawed this hostility, but also warm, mutual relations are developing today. Each side is recognizing the pluses and minuses of the other and starting to integrate. To reflect these changes, we have added a new chapter on combining macrobiotics with other modalities, including modern medicine, alternative and complementary medicines, and traditional medicines from other cultures. This chapter also has a section on selecting a macrobiotic counselor, medical doctor, or other health professional, and it looks at about twenty-five of the leading alternative approaches to cancer, ranging from vitamins and supplements to herbs, colonics, laetrile, and others.

Unfortunately, we have had to include a new chapter on thyroid cancer. Twenty-five years ago this was a rare malignancy, and we mentioned it briefly. Since then thyroid cancer has spread rapidly, especially among women, and is the seventh leading cause of cancer death in females. The thyroid governs several hormones, which in turn are related to the emotions. The rise of this malignancy would appear to be connected not only with increased consumption of foods that harm the thyroid, but also with the suppression of feelings in the throat chakra. This energy center in the neck governs the voice box for speaking, singing, and other verbal expression. Neglect, abuse, guilt, and other factors can contribute to restricting this area. Since woman is governed more by rising yin energy from the earth than man, she has a greater natural tendency to talk, sing, dance, and express herself verbally and through music and sound. If this is thwarted by tight, contractive foods or by negative relationships in which she does not feel free to communicate, she may become ill and suffer in this region. Chapters on AIDS-related cancers and radiation-related cancers have been eliminated from this edition, because they have substantially diminished in society and are largely dealt with under individual chapters for lymphoma, leukemia, skin cancer, and other malignancies.

Respect, admiration, and gratitude are due to many friends, associates, students, and clients for their contributions to this book and to our other projects and activities. We are especially thankful to the many individuals whose case histories are presented in this volume for sharing their experience and inspiring others. Our agent, Susan Lee Cohen, shepherded this book through every step of the way, and we are grateful for her guidance and wise counsel. To Julie Coopersmith, our agent for the first two editions, we appreciate her unflagging support and encouragement. To St. Martin's Press, our publisher for more than twenty-five years, we are thankful for its steadfast loyalty and support in keeping this volume in print. Over the years, *The Cancer Prevention Diet* has been translated into many languages around the world, and we appreciate the hard work of the translators, editors, and publishers who have made this possible. We would especially like to acknowledge the lifelong dedication to macrobiotics of Mauricio Waroquiers, the pioneer Latin American publisher, who recently passed away just after completing the Spanish translation of our book, *The Macrobiotic Path to Total Health: A Complete Guide to Naturally Preventing and Relieving More Than 200 Chronic Conditions and Disorders*.

Very deep appreciation also goes to our families, our associates, and our many friends throughout the world for their love, encouragement, and support. I would particularly like to acknowledge the loving assistance and wise counsel of Midori, my new wife. (Please note that occasionally the text is written in the first person, illustrating a personal observation by me.) Alex would like to express his heartfelt gratitude to his family, especially Esther, Gale, Mariya, Vladimir, Lucy, Hanz, and Isaiah, for their patience and support; to Anna Böhm for her insightful material on emotions and women's health; and to Hiroko Ara for her encouragement and support. Shizuko Yamamoto, Adelbert and Wieke Nelissen, Nadine Barner, Jane and Lino Stanchich, Mitsuko Mikami, Edward Esko, Woodward and Florence Johnson, John and Jeanette Kozinski, Jane Teas, Kezia Snyder, Jarka Adamcova, Najla Fathi, and many other teachers, friends, and associates also assisted in various ways.

In today's fast-changing world, almost no family remains untouched by cancer, including my family (as described in Appendix II). But through sound dietary practice, positive lifestyle changes, mental and emotional development, and spiritual practices, cancer can largely be prevented and, in many cases, relieved. *Makrobios* means "long life," and we hope we are still active on the planet in 2033 to prepare a fiftieth anniversary edition of this book (or its digital paperless equivalent). But whatever changes take place in the next quarter century—and the forecasts range from dire and cataclysmic to utopian and paradisiacal—we are confident that the laws of yin and yang will still govern and the basic approach presented here will still apply. We hope that our successors, whether in the macrobiotic community, the integrative medical profession, or among ordinary planetary citizens, will build upon our experience. We trust they will correct our mistakes, come up with new insights and practical applications, and contribute to creating a world of enduring health and peace.

Someday cancer will cease to exist. In an age dominated by the Internet and cell phones, the technology is now available to spread essential information and life-preserving knowledge instantaneously around the planet. (For current macrobiotic resources on the Internet, please see Resources at the end of this book.) Whether you are an individual with cancer, a family member or friend of someone with cancer, a medical or holistic professional, or a general reader, we invite you to embark with us on a voyage of discovery and appreciation in the pages that follow. We invite you to try the macrobiotic way for yourself, begin to experience its limitless benefits and blessings, and share it with others.

—MICHIO KUSHI and ALEX JACK
January 23, 2009

PART 1

Preventing Cancer Naturally

1

Cancer, Diet, and Macrobiotics

Nearly sixty years ago, when I first came to the United States, the expected rate of people who would get cancer in their lifetime was about one out of eight. Today this rate has risen to nearly one in two men and one in three women (see Table 1). This year more than 559,000 Americans will die of cancer, and another 1,445,000 new cases will be detected. After decades of increasing mortality rates, the number of deaths from cancer has declined slightly for the first time, reflecting changes in dietary practice, less smoking, and better medical treatment. Altogether, more than 100 million Americans now living will eventually get the disease. Along with cardiovascular disease and medical error, cancer is one of the three major causes of death in modern society.

While the mortality rate from some cancers—for example, stomach, cervix, and rectum—has declined in the United States, it has steeply risen for others, notably lung, melanoma, prostate, multiple myloma, and brain tumors (see Table 2).

Despite ever more sophisticated methods of diagnosis and treatment, the consensus is that the War on Cancer declared in 1971 is being lost. "My overall assessment is that the national cancer program must be judged a qualified failure," Dr. John Bailer, who served on the staff of the National Cancer Institute for twenty years and was editor of the *New England Journal of Medicine,* contends. "The five-year survival statistics of the American Cancer Society are very misleading. They now count things that are not cancer,

TABLE 1.   CANCER INCIDENCE IN THE UNITED STATES

	1900	1962	1971*	1992	2000
New cases	25,000	520,000	635,000	1,100,000	1,220,100
Selected sites					
Breast	no data	63,000	69,600	175,900	184,200
Lung	no data	45,000	80,000	178,000	179,400
Colorectal	no data	72,000	75,000	157,500	93,800
Prostate	no data	31,000	35,000	122,000	180,400
Uterus	no data	no data	no data	46,000	48,900
Persons affected	1 in 25	1 in 6	1 in 5	1 in 3	1 in 2 (men) 1 in 3 (women)

*The year President Nixon declared war on cancer.

Source: U.S. Vital Statistics and American Cancer Society.

TABLE 2.   NEW CASES OF CANCER EACH YEAR*

Men		Women	
Prostate	218,890	Breast	178,480
Lung	114,760	Colon and rectum	57,050
Colon and rectum	55,290	Lung	98,620
Bladder	50,040	Uterus	50,230
Lymphoma	38,670	Lymphoma	32,710
Melanoma	33,910	Melanoma	26,030
Kidney	31,590	Ovary	22,430
Leukemia	24,800	Thyroid	25,480
Oral	24,180	Kidney	19,600
Pancreas	18,830	Pancreas	18,340
Stomach	13,000	Bladder	17,120
Larynx	8,960	Leukemia	19,440
All Sites	766,860	All sites	678,060

*Excluding skin cancer and carcinoma *in situ.*

Source: American Cancer Society, 2007.

and, because we are able to diagnose at an earlier stage of the disease, patients falsely appear to live longer. Our whole cancer research in the past twenty years has been a total failure. More people over thirty are dying from cancer than ever before . . . More women with mild or benign diseases are being included in statistics and reported as being 'cured.' When government officials point to survival figures and say they are winning the war against cancer they are using those survival rates improperly."

The United States is not unique in losing the battle against cancer. In fact, among the nations of the world, it ranks in the middle. Twenty-three of the fifty countries recently surveyed had higher mortality rates than the United States for cancer among men, and sixteen had higher rates among women. Hungary, Czechoslovakia, and Luxembourg had the highest death rates for men, while Denmark, Scotland, and Hungary had the highest for women.

Clearly, cancer is one of the great levelers of the modern age. It strikes high and low, rich and poor, male and female, young and old, black and white, Westerner and Easterner, Democrat and Republican, Muslim and Jew, saint and sinner. There is hardly a family today untouched.

Despite the optimistic reports of the National Cancer Institute and American Cancer Society, the nation has yet to develop a solid campaign of primary prevention. The focus remains on diagnosis and screening (which are often harmful and cancer-causing in themselves) and on treatment with drugs, surgery, and radiation, which have also been implicated in increasing the risk of the disease.

According to the International Agency for Research in Cancer, "Eighty to 90 percent of human cancer is determined environmentally and thus theoretically avoidable. These include the modern diet high in animal products and low in whole grains, fresh fruits, and vegetables; excessive exposure to sunlight, workplace hazards, pollution, toxic products; artificial electromagnetic radiation; and exposure to medical procedures and pharmaceuticals." "Despite the general recognition that 85 percent of all cancers is caused by environmental influences," Hans Ruesch, a medical historian, notes, "less than 10 percent of the National Cancer Institute budget is given to environmental causes. And despite the recognition that the majority of environmental causes are linked to nutrition, less than 1 percent of the NCI budget is devoted to nutrition studies."

"In our culture, treating disease is enormously profitable," Dr. Robert Sharpe points out. The market in cancer therapies in the United States, Europe, and Japan makes tens of billions of dollars profit annually and is growing at over 10 percent each year. "Preventing the disease benefits no one except the patient. Just as the drug industry thrives on the 'pill for every ill' mentality, so many of the leading medical charities are financially sustained by the dream of a miracle cure, just around the corner."

OTHER HEALTH TRENDS

Other chronic and degenerative illnesses are also on the rise. In the last twenty-five years, AIDS has spread around the world, affecting tens of millions of people. Though primarily an immune-deficiency disorder, AIDS is related to cancer, and many AIDS patients come down with Kaposi's sarcoma (a form of skin cancer), lymphoma, and other malignancies.

One of the most dramatic increases in recent decades has been in the area of sexual disorders. According to the British Medical Association, the number of new cases of venereal disease has risen 1,700 percent since 1957. In the United States, syphilis rose one-third between 2007 and 2008. Around the world, herpes and other sexually transmitted diseases (STDs) have assumed epidemic proportions. This year it was widely reported in the United States that one in four teenage girls had an STD. Infertility is also on the rise. Over the last sixty-five years, average sperm counts in American males have dropped dramatically. An analysis of data collected from 1938 to 1990 by the National Institutes of Health indicates that sperm densities in the United States have exhibited an average annual decrease of 1.5 million sperm per milliliter of collected sample, or about 1.5 percent per year. Those in European countries have declined at about twice that rate (3.1 percent per year). Another study of otherwise healthy college males showed that 23 percent were functionally sterile. The number of cesarean sections has doubled in the last ten years, accounting for 30 percent of all births. The risk of death for C-sections is also about four times higher than for vaginal births even if there is no medical emergency. Women are also about three times as liable to suffer severe complications or experience difficulties during subsequent births.

Moreover, more than 550,000 American women, many of childbearing age, currently have their ovaries or uteruses surgically removed each year, primarily because of cancer or the fear of cancer. Many of these are prophylactic operations in completely healthy women who have been told that their risk of developing cancer will be reduced. By age sixty-five, a majority of American women have lost their wombs. Similar trends are now spreading worldwide. According to many medical experts, more than 90 percent of hysterectomies are unnecessary, and about 40 percent of the time, the ovaries are also needlessly removed during this procedure.

In the last few years, obesity has been declared the world's number one health problem by the World Health Organization. It is an underlying condition not only for heart disease, stroke, diabetes, and many other ills, but also for many cancers, including breast cancer, colon cancer, and cancer of the esophagus, thyroid, kidney, uterus, and gall bladder. In the United States, about two out of three adults are overweight or obese, and one of every three children falls into one of these brackets.

A host of new diseases has developed to challenge medical science and global health. Avian flu, SARS, and other acute respiratory diseases have killed hundreds of people, threatening to turn into worldwide pandemics. Meanwhile, old illnesses are coming back in more virulent form. New varieties of multiple-drug resistant pneumonia and staph and other common infections have been reported for which there is no medical relief available. Overprescription of antibiotics, antivirals, and other pharmaceuticals has enabled new, more deadly strains of microbes to evolve. Malaria, once believed to have been eradicated by modern medicine, has also proved invulnerable to many drugs and is spreading, with 2.7 million deaths annually. Tuberculosis, also once believed to have been conquered by new wonder drugs after

World War II, has returned in new, virulent forms and causes an estimated 521,000 deaths globally each year.

Even the common cold, despite a much publicized medical campaign begun under President John F. Kennedy, remains largely immune to effective treatment. In fact, few major sicknesses, if any, can really be cured by modern methods. In some cases pain and other discomfort can be relieved and the symptoms temporarily diminished or controlled, but, fundamentally, illness cannot be cured. Prescription drugs, over-the-counter medications, and a host of treatments and procedures, including surgery and radiation, offer at best temporarily relief and, at worst, push the imbalance deeper into the body where it manifests in more serious form later.

Altogether, disease accounts for about 80 percent of all deaths worldwide. The rest are caused primarily by accident—often resulting from physical or mental decline—and social violence, including war, crime, and abuse and neglect of children, spouses, and the elderly. In the United States, more people have died in recent decades from homicide than have died on the battlefronts of foreign wars. Violence and terrorism are also on the rise in other parts of the world.

Like the human family, the planet as a whole is in urgent need of healing. The natural environment is being destroyed by the unchecked spread—metastases—of technology, development, and urbanization. Tropical rain forests and millions of species of plants and animals are vanishing. Desertification is spreading as topsoil becomes depleted and crops will no longer grow in soil saturated with harmful chemicals. The world's nonrenewable resources are rapidly being depleted, radioactive wastes are accumulating, the air is contaminated by industrial and household pollutants, and the ozone shield that protects the planet from harmful ultraviolet radiation is thinning. The ubiquity of artificial electromagnetic radiation—from nuclear energy to microwave cooking, from hospital X-rays to Wi-Fi Internet connections, from satellites orbiting in space to cell phones—is creating a global field of ionizing and nonionizing particles whose effects on health and human evolution may not show up for generations. Climate change is now widely recognized as the major threat to the planet, including the continuation of our species. Unless we dramatically change our way of life, global warming threatens to melt the polar ice caps, raise sea levels, and lead to the extinction of millions of species. The Intergovernmental Panel on Climate Change (IPCC) predicts widespread crop failure, massive hunger and starvation, and the spread of epidemic disease (including different types of cancer) by the end of the century unless we go on a strict carbon diet and substantially reduce greenhouse gas emissions.

Given these and many other trends, we can see that modern civilization as a whole is on the verge of self-destruction as a result of deep-seated chronic biological and spiritual degeneration. This includes virtually the entire world, both the industrialized and emerging countries. The time left to reverse direction and recover personal and planetary health is very short—practically speaking, about twenty-five years before the collapse becomes irreversible.

The problem of cancer cannot be viewed in isolation from these other trends. It is related to the overall decline of modern society, including the energy crisis, the environmental crisis, the world food crisis, the population crisis, the financial crisis, and many others. It offers us the chance to rethink our present understanding of health and sickness, of sustainable and unsustainable growth. It provides the opportunity to reexamine the basic premises of our way of life and to work together as members of a common planetary family to build a world of enduring health and peace.

CANCER TREATMENT IN THE TWENTIETH CENTURY

With the rise of the petrochemical industry in the United States and Western Europe in the early part of the twentieth century, surgery and pharmacology consolidated their triumph over other approaches to medicine. The spread of chemical agriculture and factory farming revolutionized patterns of food consumption in the industrialized world. Nutrition became relegated to the back Bunsen burner as genetics, biochemistry, and radiation techniques dominated medical research.

Despite the general neglect of dietary concerns, a host of international population studies emerged during the middle part of the century linking cancer with high fat intake, refined carbohydrates, chemical additives, and other nutritional variables. Building on the earlier reports of the colonial medical doctors and anthropologists, epidemiologists concluded that cultures and subcultures eating a traditional diet of whole grains, cooked vegetables, and fresh seasonal fruit remained largely cancer-free.

One of the clearest warnings was sounded by Frederick L. Hoffman, LL.D., cancer specialist and consulting statistician for the Prudential Life Insurance Company. In his 1937 volume, *Cancer and Diet,* he stated as follows:

I have come to the essential conclusion that there has been a decided increase in the cancer death rate and progressively so during the last century ending with 1930. From this I reflect that the profound changes in dietary habits and nutritional condition of the population taking place during the intervening years have been world wide and due to the rapid and almost universal introduction of modified food products, conserved or preserved, refrigerated or sterilized, colored or modified, aside from positive adulteration by the addition of injurious mineral substances close to being of a poisonous nature. To a diminishing extent food is being consumed in its natural state, at least by urban populations everywhere, and to a lesser degree also among persons in rural communities.

In the 1940s and 1950s, laboratory studies on mice and other animals began to confirm these findings. Also, several European countries experienced a significant drop in cancer mortality rates during World Wars I and II when meat, dairy food, and eggs became scarce and local populations were forced to survive on brown bread, oats and barley meal, and homegrown produce.

Following World War II, frozen and enriched foods became more widely available; many tropical and subtropical foods such as oranges, grapefruits, and pineapples found their way to the daily breakfast table; and soft drinks, ice cream, candy bars, pizza, hamburgers, french fries, potato chips, and other fast foods became a way of life. As cancer rates climbed, the medical profession stepped up its technological arsenal. In 1971 President Nixon formally declared war on the disease and commissioned the National Cancer Institute (NCI) to eradicate it. However, this mobilization largely excluded dietary means.

In twenty-five hundred years, since cancer was first described in ancient Greece, medicine had come full circle. In *Epidemics,* Book I, Hippocrates cited factors for the physician to consider in making diagnoses and recommending treatment. At the head of the list comes "what food is given to him [the patient] and who gives it," followed by conditions of the climate and local environment, and the patient's customs, mode of life, pursuits, age, speech, mannerisms, silences, thoughts, sleeping patterns, and dreams. Last on the list is physical symptoms. The priorities of modern medicine were just reversed. In 1973, according to a Harvard School of Public Health study, only 4 percent of the nation's medical schools had an independent course in nutrition. Today the number has risen to about 66 percent, or two out of every three schools. A recent article on integrating alternative and complementary medicine into the medical school curricula published in the *Journal of the American Medical Association* strongly recommended that all medical students be introduced to macrobiotic food because it was the leading special diet for cancer patients.

A RETURN TO WHOLE FOODS

In nature, just as day follows night and valleys turn into mountains, societies regenerate after a long period of decay. In the modern world, the turning point came in the 1960s and 1970s when awareness of the deficiencies of the contemporary way of life and eating generated the natural foods and holistic health movements. Vegetarian and health foods had long been available, but their quality was often low and they appealed only to a tiny market. Suddenly, the postwar generation, which had become active in integrating southern lunch counters and preserving the rice fields of Vietnam from destruction by bombs and chemical reagents, became conscious of the food they ate and organized Food Days to consider the impact of modern agriculture on world hunger, energy conservation, and the quality of the environment.

By 1976 the concern for healthy food echoed through the halls of Congress. In its historic report, *Dietary Goals for the United States,* the Senate Select Committee on Nutrition and Human Needs listed cancer as one of the six major degenerative diseases associated with improper nutrition. The report sent shock waves through the American food industry and medical profession. The cattle- and hog-growers' associations, the poultry and egg producers, and the refined salt institute condemned the report.

However, at the highest national level, the door had been opened for a return to healthy food. Within the next five years dozens of medical and scientific associations corroborated the link between diet and degenerative disease. In his 1979 report, *Healthy People: Health Promotion and Disease Prevention,* the U.S. Surgeon General stated: "People should consume . . . less saturated fat and cholesterol, . . . less red meat, . . . [and] more complex carbohydrates such as whole grains, cereals, fruits and vegetables." The American Heart Association, the American Diabetes Association, the American Society for Clinical Nutrition, and the U.S. Department of Agriculture issued similar statements. In 1981 a panel of the American Association for the Advancement of Science reported on the social impact of a change to a whole-grain diet. The scientists declared that changes in our eating habits could have significant beneficial effects on everything from land, water, fuel, and mineral use to the cost of living, unemployment, and the balance of international trade, as well as reduce coronary heart disease by 88 percent and cancer by 50 percent.

In 1982 the National Academy of Sciences issued a 472-page report, *Diet, Nutrition, and Cancer,* calling upon the general public to reduce substantially the consumption of foods high in saturated and unsaturated fat and increase the daily intake of whole grains, vegetables, and fruit. The panel reviewed hundreds of current medical studies, associating long-term eating patterns with the development of most common cancers, including those of the colon, stomach, breast, lung, esophagus, ovary, and prostate. The thirteen-member scientific committee suggested that diet could be responsible for 30 to 40 percent of cancers in men and 60 percent in women. The flood of interest and activity in the relation between diet and cancer in the last ten years has been recounted in the preface to this newly revised edition.

LAUNCHING A HEALTH REVOLUTION

While, along with George Ohsawa and early macrobiotic pioneers, we had been promoting natural foods and a dietary approach to cancer, heart disease, and other ills since the 1950s, the role of the macrobiotic community in helping to launch the health revolution of the 1970s and 1980s is not widely known. In 1972 my wife, Aveline, invited Sadayo Kita, one of the leading Noh actors in Japan, to come to the United States to perform under the auspices of the East West Foundation (EWF), a cultural and educational foundation that we founded to promote international friendship and world peace. Mr. Kita's public performances in Boston and New York were so successful that he returned on a regular basis. In connection with the EWF's Noh program, I had the opportunity to meet Edwin Reischauer, one of the world's leading scholars of Far Eastern culture. Professor Reischauer, who passed away in 1990, was born and grew up in Japan. He spoke fluent Japanese and served as ambassador to Japan under Presidents John F. Kennedy and Lyndon B. Johnson in the 1960s and, after returning to Harvard, headed up the East Asian Studies program. In 1973 my wife and I met with Professor Reischauer at the Seventh Inn, a macrobiotic restaurant in Boston. While our meeting, and others between Reischauer and my associates, focused largely on the meeting of East and West, the dialogue often turned to a discussion of macrobiotics in the United States and the relation of diet and health.

In *The Japanese,* published several years later by Harvard University Press, Professor Reischauer addressed the role that diet played in modern Japanese culture and history: "The traditional Japanese diet of rice, vegetables, and fish, which contrasts with the heavy consumption of meat and fat in the West, would be almost a perfect health diet if the Japanese did not insist on polishing their rice. This diet may account in part for the low incidence of heart disease as compared with Americans."

Noting the increase in size and weight of Japanese children following World War II, he went on: "Since World War II, Japanese children have increased several inches in height and many pounds in weight. Part of the increased height may be attributed to the straightening of legs, as Japanese sit less on the floor and more on chairs, but, like the weight, it may be chiefly due to a richer diet, which now includes dairy products and more meat and bread. Young Japanese today are quite visibly a bigger breed than their ancestors, and fat children, which were formerly never encountered, have become a commonplace sight."

Another of our friends at Harvard, Edward Kass, M.D., was one of the nation's leading researchers on cardiovascular disease. As director of Channing Laboratories, Dr. Kass oversaw research, beginning in 1973 and extending on and off for more than a decade, on macrobiotic people living in Boston. With Frank Sacks, M.D., of Harvard Medical School; William Castelli, M.D., director of the Framingham Heart Study; and other colleagues, Dr. Kass reported on the protective health benefits of the macrobiotic dietary approach, particularly in lowering cholesterol and high blood pressure. These studies were published in the *American Journal of Epidemiology,* the

New England Journal of Medicine, the *Journal of the American Medical Association, Atherosclerosis,* and other professional journals and were the turning point in the medical profession's recognition of the relation of diet to heart disease. Popular publications such as *Vogue,* the *Boston Globe,* and the *New York Times* also ran articles featuring this research, and the notion that diet was connected to heart disease and thus could be prevented—and possibly relieved—spread throughout society.

Meanwhile, in 1976 the *East West Journal (EWJ)*, a monthly magazine that my associates and I had started several years earlier, began publishing special issues devoted to cancer and diet. The editors, Sherman Goldman and Alex Jack, introduced case histories of individuals with cancer who had recovered using a macrobiotic diet, as well as theoretical articles by me and a series of investigative reports on the NCI, the American Cancer Society, and the pharmaceutical industry by journalist Peter Barry Chowka. The *EWJ* issues received national attention and helped to focus public attention on what was being done—or not being done—to end the cancer epidemic.

In 1976 the Senate Select Committee on Nutrition and Human Needs in Washington, D.C., responding to this grassroots movement to address causes rather than symptoms of disease, began to hold hearings and take scientific testimony linking diet with heart disease, cancer, and other degenerative diseases. One of the star witnesses was Dr. Gio B. Gori of the NCI. In his testimony (and subsequent candid interview with *EWJ* for which he got in trouble with his superiors), he suggested that diet was possibly the most important factor in the development of cancer and that more research should be focused in this direction. In Boston, meanwhile, the EWF, under the guidance of Edward Esko and Stephen Uprichard, published the first book-length report on macrobiotics and cancer, titled *A Dietary Approach to Cancer According to the Principles of Macrobiotics.* Through the EWF we also began to contact and in some cases meet with government policymakers, medical researchers, and scientists throughout the world in order to let them know about our approach, including many researchers who appeared before the dietary goals hearings or later became part of the National Academy of Sciences panel that compiled the landmark report, *Diet, Nutrition, and Cancer.*

Among the scientists we met with were Mark Hegsted, M.D., of the Department of Nutrition at the Harvard School of Public Health, who was one of the key witnesses before the Senate dietary goals hearings, and Dr. Gori of the NCI. At one meeting at Boston City Hospital, I introduced Dr. Kass to Jean Kohler, a professor of music at Ball State University in Muncie, Indiana. Professor Kohler had developed pancreatic cancer in 1973 and completely recovered his health after adopting a macrobiotic diet. Medical documentation, based on tests performed by the Indiana University Medical Center in Indianapolis, was very persuasive, as was the fact that Jean Kohler was still alive. About 90 percent of all pancreatic patients die within the first year, and the disease is considered almost invariably terminal. Now almost five years had passed since his original diagnosis.

Dr. Kass became very interested in Professor Kohler's case and suggested ways that future research could be carried out. He recommended that a group of twenty-five patients with the same type of cancer begin to eat macrobiotically under the supervision of the EWF and that after a period of time their status be compared to that of a control group with the same type of cancer eating the standard modern diet. Afterward, Dr. Kass introduced me to Dr. Emil Frei, the director of the Dana Farber Cancer Center in Boston, one of the leading cancer research institutes in the world. My associates and I introduced several macrobiotic case histories and discussed with Dr. Frei the possibility of conducting future research on the macrobiotic approach. He seemed very open-minded to our suggestions and said he felt the subject warranted further study.

In March 1977 the EWF sponsored its first conference on a nutritional approach to cancer at Pine Manor College, outside of Boston. Many medical doctors and researchers attended the gathering, including Dr. Robert Mendelsohn, one of the nation's best-known pediatricians and author of a popular newspaper column, "The People's Doctor." The Pine Manor conference brought together for the first time leading scientific and medical researchers, leading teachers of the international macrobiotic community, and ordinary men and women from many walks of life who had recovered from cancer following adoption of a macrobiotic diet. An active public program followed, with annual diet and cancer conferences, public symposiums, and television and radio interviews with EWF staff in New York, Boston, Philadelphia, Baltimore, Miami, Atlanta, Dallas, and other big cities.

In the summer of 1977, influenced by the Senate's report, *Dietary Goals for the United States,* which came out earlier in the year, President Jimmy Carter ordered an official review of governmental food policy. In September, along with Dr. Mendelsohn and several staff members of the EWF and *EWJ,* I met with members of the president's domestic policy staff at the White House. We presented the advisers with a series of food policy recommendations and warned that unless the nation changed its national food policy, a wave of epidemic diseases would threaten the survival of the nation within the next generation. In subsequent meetings with the president's advisers in the areas of health and consumer affairs, as well as with members of the U.S. Department of Agriculture, my associates presented further information and policy recommendations. (Some of the research on those who were on macrobiotic diets was cited by the U.S. Surgeon General in his report, *Healthy People,* in 1979.)

At a personal as well as a professional level, macrobiotics began to have an impact on key government policymakers. When President Carter's sister, Jean Stapleton, was diagnosed with pancreatic cancer, she came to us for advice. In 1985 the NCI reported that radiation therapy and chemotherapy were ineffective and in some cases produced toxic side effects as follow-ups to surgery in the treatment of cancer: "Except possibly in selected patients with cancer of the stomach, there has been no demonstrated im-provement in the survival of patients with the ten most common cancers when radiation therapy, chemotherapy, or both have been added to surgical resection." The ten most common cancers are lung, colorectal, breast, prostate, uterus, bladder, pancreas, stomach, skin, and kidney. Shortly after the report was published, the author, Dr. Steven A. Rosenberg, the NCI's chief of surgery, operated on President Ronald Reagan's colon cancer, and instead of chemotherapy or radiation treatment, he put the president on a modified whole-grain diet.

Macrobiotic food was prepared at United Nations functions by Laura Masini, who had recovered from breast cancer with the help of macrobiotics and who served as hostess for her brother, Vernon Walters, the U.S. ambas-sador, who was a bachelor. In Washington, Blande Keith, wife of a former Republican congressman from Massachusetts, was influential in introducing macrobiotics to the family and staff of other government officials. Over the years many governors, senators, congressmen, and heads of state have come to me for advice, especially when cancer struck themselves or their families.

As a result of the EWF and *EWJ*'s pioneering activities, the awareness of diet and health began to spread throughout the United States. Articles on our approach appeared in the *Saturday Evening Post, Life* magazine, and other publications, as well as on radio and television. The health revolution of the late 1970s and 1980s was the successor to the natural foods movement of the 1960s.

Leading scientific and medical associations began to take a serious in-terest in studying the relation between diet and degenerative disease and for the first time issued dietary guidelines to protect against cancer and other degenerative diseases. In the early 1980s, the U.S. government released the Food Guide Pyramid, calling on the American people to consume a majority of their food in the form of grains, vegetables, fruits, and other plant-quality foods. The pyramid replaced the Four Food Groups, the nutritional paradigm that had governed up until then based on the primacy of meat and dairy products.

Macrobiotic dietary principles also continued to influence scientific and medical research. In the early 1980s, researchers at the New England Med-ical Center in Boston reported that macrobiotic and vegetarian women are less likely to develop breast cancer. The scientists found that macrobiotic and vegetarian women process estrogen differently from other women and eliminate it more quickly from their body. The study involved forty-five pre- and postmenopausal women, about half of whom were macrobiotic and vegetarian and half nonvegetarian.

The women consumed about the same number of total calories. Although the vegetarian women took in only one-third as much animal protein and animal fat, they excreted two to three times as much estrogen. High levels of estrogen have been associated with the development of breast cancer. "The difference in estrogen metabolism may explain the lower incidence of breast cancer in vegetarian women," the study published in *Cancer Research* reported.

In the late 1980s, researchers at Boston University under the direction of Dr. Robert Lerman and Dr. Donald Miller made an effort to review individuals who had visited me for counseling from 1981 to 1984. Sixty-eight percent of those who responded to questionnaires reported that they had benefited from macrobiotics, 24 percent reported no effects, and 4 percent observed detrimental effects. Fifty-nine percent felt that their tolerance to chemotherapy or radiation treatment had improved. Overall, health improvement was noted by 82 percent, improved emotional well-being by 85 percent, and improved family-social relationships by 43 percent. Ninety percent reported that their spouses/partners supported their use of macrobiotics, and 82 percent of other family members were supportive. In contrast, only 25 percent reported that their doctors actively supported their macrobiotic approach. Opposition was observed by 19 percent, and 50 percent experienced indifference. Six percent did not notify their physicians of their change in dietary practice. Because diagnoses were not confirmed by medical records or other objective documentation, the response rate was low (17.9 percent), and due to lack of funding to investigate further, the Boston University study could be regarded only as tentative.

In the mid-1990s, the National Institutes of Health funded a rigorous Best Case series of macrobiotic cancer recoveries with researchers at the University of Minnesota and the Kushi Institute. The Best Case series was later continued by scientists at Harvard University and the University of South Carolina. My associate, Christiane Akbar, an MIT-trained scientist who recovered from inoperable breast cancer with the help of macrobiotics over ten years earlier, spearheaded much of the final logistics for this project, including obtaining the original biopsies and before and after medical records for scores of patients. Ultimately, 77 medically well-documented cases were compiled of individuals who had recovered from cancer while observing a macrobiotic way of eating. These included cancers of the prostate (20 cases), breast (12 cases), malignant melanoma (8), lymphoma (8), leukemia (6), astrocytoma (5), colorectal (4), endometrium (3), ovary (3), pancreas (3), kidney (2), liver (1), small cell lung (1), multiple myeloma (1), nose plasmacytoma (1), parotic gland (1), sarcoma (1), and small intestine (1).

The U.S. government's National Cancer Institute (NCI) and Cancer Advisory Panel on Complementary and Alternative Medicine (CAPCAM) held a meeting in 2002 to review selected cases from the macrobiotic Best Case series and unanimously recommended that research funds be made available for further study of the macrobiotic approach to cancer, including possibly a prospective study.

In his newsletter on cancer research, Dr. Ralph Moss, a cancer expert and member of the CAPCAM committee, described the enthusiasm the macrobiotic presentation made on the panel:

> The session brought forth strong testimony that sometimes the adoption of a macrobiotic diet is followed by the dramatic regression of advanced cancers. A nurse told how, in 1995, she was diagnosed with lung cancer that had spread all over her body. She received no effective conventional therapy, and reluctantly went on the macrobiotics diet. . . . What makes this case so extraordinary is that her progress was monitored weekly by a sympathetic physician colleague. The shrinkage, and finally the disappearance, of her tumors was documented millimeter by millimeter! She has now been disease-free for over five years.
>
> After this week's meeting I could definitely say there is real gold in macrobiotics. . . . What is needed now is a serious clinical study in patients, using all the resources the NIH can muster. The Kushi Institute deserves credit for having taken these first steps toward documenting its methods and results. An influential government panel is at last listening.

Other researchers came to similar conclusions. In a review of current evidence on the efficacy and safety of selected complementary and alternative medical (CAM) therapies that are commonly used by patients with cancer, researchers at Harvard Medical School, the National Institutes of Health, and other institutions concluded in an article published in the *Annals of Internal Medicine,*

> Several CAM therapies offer potential benefits for patients with cancer. Others, however, seem to be ineffective, and may present risks for direct adverse effects or interactions with conventional treatments. Therefore, it is important for physicians to communicate openly with patients about CAM use. Current evidence, although limited, suggests that physicians may reasonably accept some CAM therapies as adjuncts to conventional care and discourage others. As more data are gathered, the evidence-based recommendation of some CAM therapies and the evidence-based rejection of others will become more definite.

Reviewing "the opinions of respected authorities, based on clinical evidence, descriptive studies, or reports of expert committees," the researchers recommended that "it seems reasonable to accept macrobiotics as an adjunct to conventional treatment" for most types of cancer.

Cancer researchers at M. D. Anderson Cancer Center at the University of Texas in Houston posted a historical overview of macrobiotics as a therapy for cancer patients and the general public on their Web site in early 2003, saying:

> The macrobiotic diet is part of a way of life that attempts to achieve balance by applying the oriental principles of yin and yang to the selection of foods. Grains and vegetables are considered to be the ideal center of a diet that also includes beans, fish, fowl, fruits, seeds, nuts and condiments. While no foods are actually forbidden, some may be limited in a therapeutic context.

The M. D. Anderson site reviews the Office of Technology Assessment (OTA) study that found macrobiotics to be among the most popular alternative cancer approaches; the study of the macrobiotic approach to pancreatic cancer at Tulane University; and the book *Cancer Free: 30 Who Triumphed Over Cancer Naturally,* which included prostate cancer (3 cases), melanoma (6), uterus (3), breast (5), stomach, leukemia, and pancreas (2 each), colon (2), astrocytoma, urethra, lung, brain, thyroid, leukemia (CML), bile duct, Hodgkin's disease, and ovarian (1 each); a Best Case series of six medically documented cases: pancreatic cancer metastasized to the liver, malignant melanoma, malignant astrocyoma, endometrial stromal sarcoma, adenocarcinoma of the colon, and abdominal leiomyosarcoma; and other retrospective cohort studies, Best Case series, and case reports. According to one study, 63 percent of cancer patients who received some form of dietary therapy received or were exposed to the macrobiotic diet.

The above-mentioned studies and others showing the benefits of the macrobiotic approach to pancreatic cancer, breast cancer, prostate cancer, and other malignancies will be described in full detail later in this book. During this period I continued to lecture and present at scientific and medical conferences around the world. On June 10, 1999, I testified on "The Dietary Causes of Cancer" before the House of Representatives Government Reform Committee in Washington, D.C. On March 1–2, 2001, I made a presentation to the Asian Therapies for Cancer Conference in the nation's capital, and on March 27, 2001, I made a further presentation before the White House Commission on Complementary and Alternative Medicine Policy Public Hearing on CAM in Self-Care and Wellness on Capitol Hill.

As the new century approached, the major cancer societies were beginning to take positive notice of macrobiotics. In a statement on alternative therapies, the American Cancer Society stated, "Today's most popular anticancer diet is probably macrobiotics." While no diet has yet been shown to be able to reverse existing tumors, the ACS further observed:

Like other fat-reducing diets, macrobiotics may help prevent some cancers. It may reduce the risk of developing cancers that appear related to higher fat intake, such as colon cancer and possibly some breast cancers. The macrobiotic diet, like other fat-free diets, can lower blood pressure and perhaps reduce the chance of heart disease.

Taking part in a macrobiotics program may provide some sense of balance with nature and harmony with the total universe and as such promote a sense of calmness and reduced stress.

In further recommendations to cancer survivors about diet and exercise in 2003, the American Cancer Society declared that the macrobiotic way of eating could be beneficial.

The macrobiotic diet and lifestyle is not primarily aimed at cancer survivors, yet many persons first encounter this diet in the context of cancer. This diet is based on whole grains, vegetables, sea vegetables, beans, fermented soy products, fruit, nuts, seeds, soups, small amounts of fish, and teas. Individualized diets are based on whether a cancer is classified yin or yang. Macrobiotic diets may be used as an adjuvant to conventional treatment with careful planning to ensure nutritional variety and adequacy.

Recognizing that "a healthy diet can substantially reduce one's lifetime risk of developing cancer," the American Cancer Society's most recent dietary guidelines released in 2006 called for people to "consume a healthy diet with an emphasis on plant sources." The organization's four major dietary recommendations advise as follows: (1) Choose foods and beverages in amounts that help achieve and maintain a healthy weight. (2) Eat five or more servings of a variety of vegetables and fruits each day. (3) Choose whole grains in preference to processed (refined) grains. (4) Limit consumption of processed and red meats.

The principal author of the ACS report was my son, Lawrence Kushi, Sc.D., a lifelong macrobiotic practitioner and chief investigator for the National Institutes of Health (NIH) Best Cases study of macrobiotics and cancer mentioned above. Dr. Kushi is currently associate director for etiology and prevention research at Kaiser Permanente, Oakland, California, one of the nation's leading health care providers.

The new ACS guidelines call for choosing whole grain rice, bread, pasta, and cereals in preference to processed grains and sugars; selecting fish, poultry, or beans as an alternative to beef, pork, and lamb; selecting leaner cuts of meat and eating smaller portions; and avoiding frying and charbroiling of animal food.

"The scientific study of nutrition and cancer is highly complex, and many important questions remain unanswered," the report states, presenting a more sophisticated energetic approach to nutrition and diet than most current medical studies.

For example, it is not presently completely understood how energy imbalance or how single or combined nutrients or foods affect one's risk of specific cancers. In addition, many dietary factors and lifestyle practices tend to correlate with each other; for example, people who consume a diet high in vegetables and fruits also tend to eat less meat and be more physically active. Foods and nutrients may have additive or synergistic effects on health and need to be considered in the context of the total diet.

Grains such as wheat, rice, oats, and barley, and the foods made from them, are an important part of an overall healthful diet. Whole grain foods, which are those made from the entire grain seed, are relatively low in caloric density and can contribute to maintaining energy balance. In addition, whole grains are higher in fiber, certain vitamins, and minerals than processed (refined) flour products. Some of these vitamins and minerals have been associated with lower risk of cancer.

[In respect to meat, the report notes,] Many epidemiologic studies have examined the association between cancer and the consumption of red meats (defined as beef, pork, or lamb) and processed meats (cold cuts, bacon, hot dogs, etc.). Current evidence supports an increased risk of cancers of the colon and/or rectum and prostate. More limited evidence exists for other sites. Studies that have examined red meat and processed meat separately suggest that risks associated with processed meat may be slightly greater than red meat, but the consumption of both should be limited.

The report goes on to say that soy-derived foods are an excellent source of protein and a good alternative to meat.

Soy contains several phytochemicals, some of which have weak estrogenic activity and appear to protect against hormone-dependent cancers in animal studies.

Making a distinction between traditional soy products and soy supplements, the report continues:

Presently, there are limited data to support a potentially beneficial effect of soy supplements on reducing cancer risk. Furthermore, adverse effects of high doses of soy supplements on the risk of estrogen-responsive cancers, such as breast or endometrial cancer, are possible. Breast cancer survivors should consume only moderate amounts of soy foods as part of a healthy plant-based diet, and they should not intentionally ingest very high levels of soy products in their diet or more concentrated sources of soy, such as soy-containing pills, powders, or supplements containing isolated or concentrated isoflavones.

In respect to sugar, the ACS report states,

Sugar increases caloric intake without providing any of the nutrients that reduce cancer risk. By promoting obesity and elevating insulin levels, high sugar intake may indirectly increase cancer risk. White (refined) sugar is no different from brown (unrefined) sugar or honey with regard to these effects on body weight or insulin. Limiting foods such as cakes, candy, cookies, and sweetened cereals, as well as high-sugar beverages such as soda, can help reduce sugar intake.*

The American Medical Association also reversed course and began to support alternative and complementary therapies. As early as 1987, in a review of special diets, the nation's leading medical association noted:

In the macrobiotic diets foods fall into two main groups, known as yin and yang (based on an Eastern principle of opposites), depending on where they have been grown, their texture, color, and composition. The general principle behind this diet is that foods biologically furthermost away from us are better for us. Cereals, therefore, form the basis of the diet and fish is preferred to meat. Although fresh foods free of additives are preferred, no food is actually prohibited, in the belief that a craving for any food may reflect a genuine bodily need. In general, the macrobiotic diet is a healthful way of eating.[1]

In 1998, the AMA reported that two-thirds of medical schools in the United States offered courses in holistic approaches. Among the key recommendations offered in the *Journal of the American Medical Association* (*JAMA*) was that the new medical school curricula include an experiential

---

*For further information, please see Lawrence H. Kushi et al., "American Cancer Society Guidelines on Nutrition and Physical Activity for Cancer Prevention: Reducing the Risk of Cancer with Healthy Food Choices and Physical Activity," *Calif.: A Cancer Journal for Clinicians* 2006; 56:254–281. The article is available online at http://caonline.amcancersoc.org/cgi/content/full/56/2/254.

component. As noted above, macrobiotics was singled out as one of the principal modalities that young medical school students should be familiar with: "Experiencing acupuncture or therapeutic massage or tasting a macrobiotic meal adds a dimension to the learning experience that a lecture or simple demonstration cannot. The deeper understanding that results should provide a better basis for responsibly advising patients."[2]

America's embrace of macrobiotics climaxed when the Smithsonian Institution honored the macrobiotic community with a gala event opening the Michio Kushi Family Collection on the History of Macrobiotics and Alternative and Complementary Health Practice at the National Museum of American History in Washington, D.C., on June 8, 1999.

The day featured speeches by Dr. T. Colin Campbell (director of the China Health Study), Congressman Dennis Kucinich (who introduced a resolution that was unanimously passed by the House of Representatives honoring macrobiotics), and William Dufty (author of *Sugar Blues*); the dedication of the exhibit (including Aveline Kushi's pressure cooker, macrobiotic quality foods, and the first two editions of *The Cancer Prevention Diet*); and a buffet reception prepared by the Ritz-Carlton Hotel featuring brown rice stir-fried with vegetables, lentil vegetable stew with tofu, and poppyseed cake with maple tofu cream. Periodically, the Smithsonian puts macrobiotic food, literature, and other items on display, holds symposia on diet and health, and honors the contribution that the macrobiotic way of life has made to America and the planet.

From this brief overview it is clear that the major scientific and medical organizations have come to adopt many of the basic principles of macrobiotics. The fear and hostility that characterized their response a generation ago to holistic dietary approaches have generally been replaced by openness and warmth. Today, physicians, nurses, and other health care professionals often work side by side with macrobiotic teachers and counselors to bring the best possible integrative methods to individuals and families dealing with cancer, heart disease, and other chronic ills.

THE MACROBIOTIC APPROACH

It is important to understand that macrobiotics is not just a diet in the modern sense of the term, but a way of life encompassing all dimensions of living. From such diverse phenomena as the size and shape of distant galaxies to the movements of subatomic particles, from the periodic rise and fall of civilizations to the patterns of our own individual lives, macrobiotic philosophy offers a unifying principle to understand the order of the universe as a whole.

Translated literally, *macro* is the Greek word for "great" or "long" and *bios* is the word for "life." Macrobiotics means the way of life according to the greatest or longest possible view. The earliest recorded usage of the term is found in the writings of Hippocrates. In the essay *Airs, Waters, and Places,* the Father of Western medicine introduces the word to describe a group of young men who are healthy and relatively long-lived. Other classical writers, including Herodotus, Aristotle, Galen, and Lucian, also used the term, and the concept came to signify living in harmony with nature, eating a simple balanced diet, and living to an active old age. In the popular imagination, macrobiotics became particularly associated with the Ethiopians of Africa, who were said to live 120 years or more, the biblical patriarchs, and the Chinese sages. In *Pantagruel and Gargantua,* the sixteenth-century French humanist Rabelais mentions a fabulous Isle of the Macreons where his adventurers meet a sage named Macrobius who guides them along their way. In 1797 the German physician and philosopher Christoph W. Hufeland, M.D., wrote an influential book on diet and health titled *Macrobiotics or the Art of Prolonging Life.*

In the Near-East and Far East, the macrobiotic spirit also guided and shaped civilization. Dietary common sense and principles of natural healing underlie the Bible, the I Ching, the Tao Te Ching, the Bhagavad Gita, the Kojiki, the Koran, and many other scriptures and epics. Down through the centuries, as we have seen, cultural movements surfaced in Asia to extol the benefits of the traditional way of eating and to caution against increasingly artificial ways.

In the late nineteenth and early twentieth centuries, macrobiotics experienced a revival originating in Japan. Two educators, Sagen Ishitsuka, M.D., and Yukikazu Sakurazawa, cured themselves of serious illnesses by changing from the modern refined diet then sweeping Japan to a simple diet of brown rice, miso soup, sea vegetables, and other traditional foods. After restoring their health, they went on to integrate traditional Oriental medicine and philosophy with Vedanta, original Jewish and Christian teachings, and holistic perspectives in modern science and medicine. When Sakurazawa went to Paris in the 1920s, he adopted George Ohsawa as his pen name and called his teachings *macrobiotics.*

Thus macrobiotics today is a unique synthesis of Eastern and Western influences. It is the way of life according to the largest possible view, the infinite order of the universe. The practice of macrobiotics is the understanding and practical application of this order to our lifestyle, including the selection, preparation, and manner of eating of our daily food, as well as the orientation of consciousness. Macrobiotics does not offer a single diet for everyone but a dietary principle that takes into account differing climatic and geographical considerations; varying ages, sexes, and levels of activity; and ever-changing personal needs. Macrobiotics also embraces the variety and richness of all the world's cultures and heritages.

Broadly speaking, dietary practice according to macrobiotics is the way of eating that flourished from before the time of Homer to the Renaissance.

It is the diet that Buddha ate under the tree of enlightenment and that Jesus shared with his disciples at the Last Supper. It is the diet that helped Moses free his people from bondage and that sustained the Pilgrims upon their arrival in the New World. Most of all macrobiotics is the way of life followed by ordinary men and women throughout history: farmers, shepherds, fishermen, merchants, traders, artisans, weavers, scribes, monks, bards. From the earliest campfires in the Ice Age to the latest space launches in the Atomic Age, countless mothers, fathers, daughters, sons, babies, and grandparents have shared nourishing food together and saved the seeds to plant the following spring.

To the eye of Heaven, our era is but a day. The spread of cancer and the proliferation of nuclear weapons are only passing shadows in humanity's prolonged adolescence. One day future generations will look back at the cult of modern civilization and regard its unnatural food and artificial way of life as a fad that flared up and extinguished itself in the relatively short span of four hundred years. Under many names and forms, macrobiotics will continue, as long as human life continues to exist, as its most fundamental and intuitive wisdom. It offers a key to restoring our health, a vision for regenerating the world, and a compass for charting our endless voyage toward freedom and enduring peace.

2

Cancer and Modern Civilization

Over the last half century, modern medical science has mounted a tremendous campaign to solve the problems of cancer and other degenerative illnesses. To date, however, this large-scale effort has produced no lasting, comprehensive solutions.

In the field of cancer research, for example, modern medicine has pioneered such techniques as surgery, radiation therapy, laser therapy, chemotherapy, hormone therapy, and others. But these treatments are successful in achieving only temporary relief of symptoms, at best. In the majority of cases they fail to prevent the disease from recurring because they do not address the root cause or origin of the problem.

We believe that this biological decline is not irreversible but that to prevent such a catastrophe from occurring we must begin to approach such problems as cancer with a new orientation. Specifically, we must begin to seek out the most basic causes and to implement the most basic solutions rather than continue the present approach of treating each problem separately in terms of its symptoms alone. The problem of degenerative disease affects us all in one way or another in all domains of modern life. Therefore, the responsibility for finding and implementing solutions should not be left only to those within the medical and scientific communities. We believe that the recovery of global health will emerge only through a cooperative effort involving people at all levels of society.

The epidemic of degenerative disease, the decline of traditional human values, and the decomposition of society itself are all clear indications that something is deeply wrong with the modern orientation of life. At present we tend to value the development of civilization in terms of our advancing material prosperity. At the same time we tend to undervalue the development of human consciousness, intuition, and spiritual development. But this viewpoint is out of proportion with the very nature of existence. The world of matter itself is a small, fragmentary, and almost infinitesimal manifestation when compared to the vast currents of moving space and energy that envelop it and out of which it has come into physical existence.

Not only is the material world infinitesimally small by comparison, but also, as modern quantum physics has demonstrated, the more we analyze and take it apart, the more we discover that it actually has no concrete substance. The search for an ultimate unit of matter, which began with Democritus's assumption that reality could be divided into atoms and space, has ended in the twentieth century with the discovery that subatomic particles are nothing but charged matrixes of moving energy. Albert Einstein's formulation that $E = MC^2$ signifies that matter is not solid material at all but waves of energy or vibration.

However, our limited senses easily delude us into believing that things have a fixed or unchanging quality, in spite of the fact that all the cells, tissues, skin, and organs that comprise the human body are continuously changing. The red blood cells in the bloodstream live about 120 days. In order to maintain a relatively constant number of these cells, an astounding 200 million new cells are created every minute, while an equal number of old cells are continuously destroyed. The entire body regenerates itself about every seven years. As a result, what we think of as today's "self" is very different from yesterday's "self" and tomorrow's "self." This is obvious to parents who have watched their children grow. However, our development does not stop when we reach physical maturity: Our consciousness and judgment also change and develop during the entire period of life.

ENLARGING OUR PERSPECTIVE

In reality, there is nothing static, fixed, or permanent. Yet modern people frequently adopt an unchanging and inflexible attitude and as a result experience repeated frustration and disappointment when faced with the ephemerality of life. Today's culture, which overemphasizes competition and material acquisition, is based primarily on consumer values, and the successful production of consumer goods depends largely on mass marketing. In order to succeed, a product must stimulate or gratify our physical senses. Of itself, sensory satisfaction is not necessarily destructive; we are all entitled to satisfy our basic senses. However, trouble arises when sensory gratification becomes a society's driving motive. This causes a society to degenerate since the realm of the senses is extremely limited in comparison to our comprehensive native capacities, including emotion, intellect, imagination, understanding, compassion, insight, aspiration, and inspiration.

In the past, most people appreciated the simple, natural taste and texture of brown bread, brown rice, and other whole natural foods. Now, in order to stimulate the senses, whole wheat bread has been replaced by soft, often sugary white bread, while brown rice is usually refined and polished into nutritionally deficient white rice.

At the same time a food industry has developed to enhance sensory appeal by adding artificial colorings, flavorings, and texture agents to our daily foods. Over the last fifty years this trend has extended to many items necessary for daily living, including clothing, cosmetics, housing materials, furniture, sleeping materials, and kitchenware. As many people have discovered, however, the application of technology to the production of synthetic consumer goods often results in lower quality, poorer service, less material satisfaction, and it is ultimately hazardous to our health. All in all we have created a totally artificial way of life and have moved further and further from our origins in the natural world. By orienting our way of life against nature, we are separating ourselves from our evolutionary environment and threatening to weaken and destroy ourselves as a species that is naturally evolving on this planet.

Cancer is only one result of this total orientation. Instead of considering the larger environmental, social, and dietary causes of cancer, however, most research up to now has been oriented in the opposite direction, viewing the disease mainly as an isolated cellular disorder. Most therapies focus only on removing or destroying the cancerous tumor while ignoring the overall bodily conditions that caused it to develop.

Cancer originates long before the formation of a malignant growth and is rooted in the quality of the external factors that we select and consume in our day-to-day life. When a cancerous symptom is finally discovered, however, this external origin is overlooked, and the disease is considered cured if the symptom or tumor has been removed or destroyed. But because the cause has not been changed, the cancer will often return in either the same form or some other form and location. This is usually met by another round of treatment that again ignores the cause. This type of approach represents an often futile attempt to control the disease by suppressing its symptoms.

In order to control cancer, we need to see beyond the immediate symptoms and consider larger factors such as the patient's overall blood quality, the types of food that have contributed to create that blood quality, and the mentality and way of life that have led the patient to consume those particular foods. It is also important to see beyond the individual patient and into the realm of society at large. Factors such as the trends of the food industry, the quality of modern agriculture, and our increasingly unnatural and sedentary way of life also apply.

For the past fifty years I have been seriously studying this larger problem with many people. The first conclusion my associates and I reached was that if cancer is to be cured, it must first be understood. If it is to be understood, dualism must be outgrown in favor of a unified perspective. From this more holistic perspective we can see that no enemy or conflict really exists. On the contrary, all factors proceed in a very harmonious manner, coexisting and supporting one another.

THE BENEFICIAL NATURE OF DISEASE

In our experience, cancer is only the final stage in a sequence of events in an illness through which individuals in the modern world tend to pass because we fail to appreciate the beneficial nature of disease symptoms. A healthy system can deal with a limited amount of excess nutrients or toxic materials taken in the form of daily food. This imbalance can be naturally eliminated through daily activity, sweat, urination, or other means. If we overconsume or increase the amount of toxins over a long period of time, however, the body begins to fall back on more serious measures for elimination: fever, skin disease, and other superficial symptoms. Such sickness is a natural adjustment, the result of the wisdom of the body trying to keep us in natural balance.

Many people are alarmed by those symptoms and think there is something unnatural or undesirable about them, so they try to suppress or control those natural manifestations with pills, cough syrups, or other medications that separate them from the natural workings of their own bodies. If minor ailments are treated in this symptomatic way with no adjustment in what we consume, the excess held in the body eventually begins to accumulate in the form of fatty-acid deposits and chronically troublesome mucus, and manifests in vaginal discharges, ovarian cysts, kidney stones, or other troublesome conditions. In this state the body is still able at least to localize the excess and toxins that we continue to take in. By gathering the unwanted material in local areas, the rest of the body is maintained in a relatively clean and functioning condition. That process of localization is part of our natural healing power, saving us from total breakdown. But the modern view looks on those localizations as dangerous enemies to be destroyed and removed. This is comparable to the behavior of the inhabitants of a city troubled by too much waste. Instead of investigating the source of waste, the city dwellers blame the sanitation department for the accumulation of garbage in designated locations and decide to do away with the sanitation department.

As long as we continue to take in excessive nutrients, chemicals, and other factors that serve no purpose in the body, they must continue to accumulate somewhere in order to continue our normal living functions. If we don't allow them to accumulate in limited areas and form tumors, they will spread throughout the body, resulting in a total collapse of our vital functions and death by toxemia. Cancer is only the terminal stage of a long process. Cancer is the body's healthy attempt to isolate toxins ingested and accumulated through years of eating the modern unnatural diet and living in an artificial environment. Cancer is the body's last drastic effort to prolong life for a few more months or years.

Cancer is not the result of some alien factor over which we have no control. Rather, it is simply the product of our own daily behavior, including our thinking, lifestyle, and daily way of eating. We must go beyond looking at cancer at the cellular level and realize that our cells are constantly changing in quality, being nourished and rejuvenated as a result of nourishment and energy coming into them. Whatever is in the nucleus of a cell is nothing but the end result of what originally came in from the outside and formed the cell components. If the cell is abnormal, something coming in is abnormal, such as the blood, lymph, or vibrational energy, including electromagnetic waves from the environment.

The cell is only the terminal of a long organic process and cannot be isolated from its surroundings and other body functions. Instead of focusing on the cell, we need to change the blood, lymph, and environmental conditions that have created malignant cells. Instead of treating isolated organs in the body, we need to treat the source of nourishment and other factors going into those organs and change the character of those organs. The proper place to perform cancer surgery is not in the operating room after the disease has run its course, but in the kitchen and in other areas of daily life before it has developed. By removing certain foods from the pantry and refrigerator, replacing them with the proper quality and variety of foods, and applying proper cooking methods, together with correcting environmental conditions and our daily way of life, we can ensure that cancer and other degenerative illnesses do not arise.

3

Preventing Cancer Naturally

When considering two people living in the same environment, we often find that one develops cancer while the other does not. This difference must be the result of each person's own unique way of behavior, including thinking, lifestyle, and way of eating. When we bring these simple factors into a less extreme, more manageable balance, the symptoms of illness no longer appear. Accordingly, the following practices are beneficial in restoring balance to our lives.

SELF-REFLECTION

Sickness is an indication that our way of life is not in harmony with the environment. Therefore, to establish genuine health, we must rethink our basic outlook on life. In one sense, sickness results largely from thinking that life's main purpose is to give us sensory satisfaction, emotional comfort, or material prosperity. This more limited view places our happiness above that of those around us. Our daily life becomes competitive, aggressive, and demanding, on the one hand, or withdrawn, suspicious, and defensive, on the other. In either case, we continually take in more than we are able to give out.

A more natural, harmonious balance can only be established by overcoming egocentric views and adopting a more universal attitude. As a first step we can begin to offer our love and care to our parents, family, friends, and all members of society, even extending our love and sympathy to those who have hurt us in some way or whom we think of as our enemies. By taking responsibility for all aspects of our lives, we begin to see that failure and illness contribute to our overall development as much as success and well-being. In reality, difficulties and obstacles challenge us to develop our intuition, compassion, and understanding. By appreciating the gift of life in all its manifestations, we increase the universe's faith in us, and life becomes an endlessly amusing and joyful adventure. If we have cancer, for example, we accept what it has to teach us about ourselves. We never lament over our fate and blame it on an accident, karma, evil spirits, or an indifferent cosmos. We look for the source of our problems within ourselves, and when we make a mistake, we learn from it and gratefully move on.

Self-reflection involves using our higher consciousness to observe, review, examine, and judge our thoughts and behavior as well as contemplate the larger order of nature or what we might call the law of God. The more we reflect upon ourselves and the eternal order of change, the more refined and universal our awareness becomes. We begin to remember our origin, foresee our destiny, and understand what we came to accomplish on this earth. As our consciousness develops, our life manifests the spirit of endless giving just as the universe itself expands infinitely. Our motto becomes "One grain, ten thousand grains." For each seed planted in the soil, the earth returns many thousand seeds. By endlessly distributing our knowledge and insight, our understanding deepens, and we become one with the eternal order of creation.

Self-reflection may take many forms, including a short period each day in quiet meditation or prayer. Questions we might ask and areas we might seek guidance in include the following:

1. Did I eat today in harmony with my environment?
2. Did I think of my parents, relatives, teachers, and elders with love and respect?
3. Did I happily greet everyone today and express an interest in his or her life?
4. Did I contemplate the sky, the trees, and the flowers, and marvel at the wonders of nature?
5. Did I thank everyone and appreciate everything I experienced today?
6. Did I perform my tasks faithfully and thereby contribute to a more peaceful world?

RESPECT FOR THE NATURAL ENVIRONMENT

The relation between humanity and nature is like that between the embryo and the placenta. The placenta nourishes, supports, and sustains the developing embryo. It would be bizarre if the embryo were to seek to destroy this protecting organism. Likewise, it is simply a matter of common sense that we should strive to preserve the integrity of the natural environment on which we depend for life itself. Over the last century, however, we have steadily contaminated our soil, water, and air, and destroyed many of the plant and animal species on which our fragile ecology rests. Our daily way of life has also become more unnatural, relying heavily on synthetic fabrics and materials, and exposing us continually to great quantities of artificial electromagnetic radiation. These actually weaken our natural ability to resist disease.

A NATURALLY BALANCED DIET

The trillions of cells that make up the human body are created and nourished by the bloodstream. New blood cells are constantly being manufactured from the nutrients provided by our daily foods. If we eat improperly, the quality of our blood and cells, including our brain cells, and quality of thinking begin to deteriorate. Cancer, a disease characterized by the abnormal multiplication of cells, is largely the result of improper eating over a long period. For restoring a sound, healthy blood and cell quality, the following dietary principles are recommended.

Harmony with the Evolutionary Order

Nature is continually transforming one species into another. A great food chain extends from bacteria and enzymes to sea invertebrates and vertebrates, amphibians, reptiles, birds, mammals, primates, and human beings. Complementary to this line of animal evolution is a line of plant development ranging from bacteria and enzymes to sea moss and sea vegetables, primitive land vegetables, ancient vegetables, modern vegetables, fruits and nuts, and cereal grains. Whole grains evolved parallel with human beings and therefore should form the major portion of our diet. The remainder of our food should be selected from among more remote evolutionary varieties of plants and may include land and sea vegetables, fresh fruit, seeds and nuts, and soup containing fermented enzymes and bacteria representing the most primordial form of life.

In traditional cancer-free societies, this way of eating is reflected in the natural development of infants and children. After conception, the human embryo develops from a single-celled fertilized egg into a multicellular infant and is nourished entirely on its mother's blood, analogous to the ancient ocean in which biological life began. At birth, mother's milk is the principal food, and as children begin to stand, whole grains become their staple fare.

The exact proportion of plant food to animal food, with the latter being eaten primarily as a dietary supplement, also reflects our ancestors' understanding of nature's delicate balance. The ratio approximated seven parts vegetable food to about one part animal food. Modern views of geological and biological evolution have also found a similar proportion in the evolutionary period of water life, roughly 2.8 billion years, compared to the period of land life, approximately 400 million years. The structure of human teeth offers another biological clue to humanity's natural way of eating. The thirty-two teeth include twenty molars and premolars for grinding grains, legumes, and seeds; eight incisors for cutting vegetables; and four canines for tearing animal and sea food. Expressed as a ratio of teeth designed for plant use and for animal use, the figure once again is seven to one. If animal food is eaten, it is ideally selected from among species most distant from human beings in the evolutionary order, especially fish and primitive sea life such as shrimp and oysters.

The modern notion that primitive hunting societies lived chiefly on mastadons, deer, birds, and other game has recently been shown by scientists to be exaggerated. Paleolithic cultures hunted mostly for undomesticated cereals and wild grasses, and foraged for plants, berries, and roots. Animal life was taken only when necessary and consumed in small amounts. The *New York Times* science section reported in a lengthy article on the early human diet:

> Recent investigations into the dietary habits of prehistoric peoples and their primate predecessors suggest that heavy meat-eating by modern affluent societies may be exceeding the biological capacities evolution built into the human body. The result may be a host of diet-related health problems, such as diabetes, obesity, high blood pressure, coronary heart disease, and some cancers.
>
> The studies challenge the notion that human beings evolved as aggressive hunting animals who depended primarily upon meat for survival. The new view—coming from findings in such fields as archaeology, anthropology, primatology, and comparative anatomy—instead portrays early humans and their forebears more as herbivores than carnivores. According to these studies, the prehistoric table for at least the last million and a half years was probably set with three times more plant than animal foods, the reverse of what the average American currently eats (see Table 3).

Harmony with Universal Dietary Tradition and Contemporary Food Changes

According to calculations based on U.S. Department of Agriculture surveys from 1910 to 1976, the per capita consumption of wheat fell 48 percent, corn 85 percent, rye 78 percent, barley 66 percent, buckwheat 98 percent, beans and legumes 46 percent, fresh vegetables 23 percent, and fresh fruit 33 percent. Over this same period, beef intake rose 72 percent, poultry 194

TABLE 3. PALEOLITHIC AND MODERN DIETARY COMPOSITION

	Paleolithic Diet	Standard American Diet	Current Dietary Recommendations
Dietary Energy (%)			
Protein	33	12	12
Carbohydrate	46	46	58
Fat	21	42	30
Poly/Sat Lipid Ratio	1.41	0.44	1
Fiber (g)	100–150	19.7	30–60
Sodium (mg)	690	2300–6900	1000–3300
Calcium (mg)	1500–2000	740	800–1500
Ascorbic Acid (mg)	440	90	60

Source: New England Journal of Medicine, 1985.

percent, cheese 322 percent, canned vegetables 320 percent, frozen vegetables 1,650 percent, processed fruit 556 percent, ice cream 852 percent, yogurt 300 percent, corn syrup 761 percent, and soft drinks 2,638 percent. Since 1940, when per capita intake of chemical additives and preservatives was first recorded, the amount of artificial food colors added to the diet has climbed 995 percent.

The USDA further reports that total caloric intake has increased by 24.5 percent, or over 500 calories per person per day, since the 1950s. Eating out almost doubled since the 1970s, accounting for much of this increase, from providing 18 percent of total food energy consumption to 32 percent.

As the following table shows, animal food consumption is at a record high today, nearly 25 percent above average annual consumption in the 1950s. Today each American consumes an average of 7 pounds more red meat than in the 1950s, 46 pounds more poultry, and 4 pounds more fish and shellfish. Because of widespread concern about fat and cholesterol in the diet, the total amount of fat and especially saturated fat has dropped significantly since the late 1970s. The amount of fat in the U.S. food supply from animal products declined from 33 percent in the 1950s to 24 percent in 2000. Saturated fat in the diet fell from 33 percent to 26 percent during the same period.

Dairy food consumption has also shifted as consumers seek leaner products. Milk consumption is down a whopping 38 percent, and the trend is toward lower-fat milk. Cheese consumption almost tripled since the 1950s, primarily as a result of processed cheese in pizza, tacos, nachos, salad bars, bagel spreads, and other prepared foods. Added fats and oils dropped modestly in the 1990s but then soared in the new century as consumers found

TABLE 4.   MEAT CONSUMPTION 1950–2000

In 2000, Americans consumed an average 57 pounds more meat than they did annually in the 1950s, and a third fewer eggs.

| | Annual averages | | | | | |
Item	1950–59	1960–69	1970–79	1980–89	1990–99	2000
	Pounds per capita, boneless-trimmed weight					
Total meats	138.2	161.7	177.2	182.2	189.0	195.2
Red meats	106.7	122.34	129.5	121.8	112.4	113.5
Beef	52.8	69.2	80.9	71.7	63.2	64.4
Pork	45.4	46.9	45.0	47.7	47.6	47.7
Veal and lamb	8.5	6.2	3.5	2.4	1.7	1.4
Poultry	20.5	28.7	35.2	46.2	61.9	66.5
Chicken	16.4	22.7	28.4	36.3	47.9	52.9
Turkey	4.1	6.0	6.8	9.9	13.9	13.6
Fish and shellfish	10.9	10.7	12.5	14.2	14.7	15.2
	Number per capita					
Eggs	374	320	285	257	236	250

Note: Totals may not add due to rounding.
Source: USDA's Economic Research Service.

the fat-free types of foods unpalatable. The type of oils consumed have also changed, with olive and canola oil zooming from less than 4 percent in 1985 to 23 percent today because of their benefits for protecting the heart. Overall, Americans in 2000 consumed almost four times as much salad and cooking oil than in the 1950s.

Fruit and vegetable consumption has also risen sharply. Today, Americans eat 20 percent more fruit and vegetables than in the 1970s, with fresh fruit up 28 percent compared to processed fruit up 2 percent. Fresh vegetable consumption is up 26 percent, including broccoli which is up nearly a third because of its association with strong anti-cancer activity. Except for tomatoes, canned vegetable intake declined 13 percent since the 1970s. French fries soared 63 percent, and the consumption of other frozen vegetables rose 41 percent.

Cereal grain and flour consumption reached 200 pounds per capita in 2000, up from an annual intake of 155 pounds in the 1950s and 138 pounds in the 1970s when it reached historic lows. Whole grains have increased in popularity, but the average diet still falls far short of the daily recommended

TABLE 5.   DAIRY CONSUMPTION, 1950–2000

Americans are drinking less milk, eating more cheese.

Per capita annual averages

Item	Unit	1950–59	1960–69	1970–79	1980–89	1990–99	2000
All dairy products[1]	lb	703	619	548	573	571	593
Cheese[2]	lb	7.7	9.5	14.4	21.5	26.7	29.8
Cottage cheese	lb	3.9	4.6	4.9	4.1	2.9	2.6
Frozen dairy products	lb	23.0	27.5	27.8	27.4	28.8	27.8
Ice cream	lb	18.1	18.3	17.7	17.7	16.0	16.5
Low-fat ice cream	lb	2.7	6.2	7.6	7.2	7.5	7.3
Sherbet	lb	1.3	1.5	1.5	1.3	1.3	1.2
Other (including frozen yogurt)	lb	1.0	1.5	1.0	1.2	4.0	3.1
Nonfat dry milk	lb	4.9	5.9	4.1	2.4	3.1	3.4
Dry whey	lb	.2	.6	2.1	3.2	3.5	3.4
Condensed and evaporated milks	lb	21.6	15.7	9.4	7.5	7.3	5.8
Cream products	½ pt	18.1	13.3	10.1	12.8	15.7	18.6
Yogurt	½ pt	0.2	0.7	3.2	6.5	8.5	9.9
Beverage milk	gal	36.4	32.6	29.8	26.5	24.3	22.6
Whole	gal	33.5	28.8	21.7	14.3	9.1	8.1
Lower fat	gal	2.9	3.7	8.1	12.2	15.3	14.5

Note: Totals may not add due to rounding.

[1]Milk-equivalent, milk-fat basis; includes butter. Individual items are on a product-weight basis.

[2]Natural equivalent of cheese and cheese products, excludes full-skim American, cottage, pot, and baker's cheese. *Source:* USDA's Economic Research Service.

three servings. Only 7 percent of Americans meet the whole grain target of the Food Guide Pyramid.

The consumption of sweets has also reached record highs, as sucrose (from cane and beets) and corn sweeteners (especially high-fructose corn syrup) increased 43 pounds, or 39 percent, per capita over the last half century. In 2000 the average American consumed 152 pounds of caloric sweeteners annually, the equivalent after accounting for waste of 32 teaspoons of added sugars per person per day!

Despite the spread of refined and synthetic foods around the world, cooked whole grains, beans, and vegetables continue to be the principal foods in many cultures today. For example, corn tortillas and black beans are the staple foods in Central America, rice and soybean products are eaten throughout Southeast Asia, and whole and cracked wheat and chickpeas are

TABLE 6.   FAT CONSUMPTION, 1950–2000

Average consumption of added fats increased by two-thirds between 1950–59 and 2000.

	Annual averages					
Item	1950–59	1960–69	1970–79	1980–89	1990–99	2000
	Pounds per capita[1]					
Total added fats and oils	44.6	47.8	53.4	60.8	65.5	74.5
Salad and cooking oils[2]	9.8	13.9	20.2	25.0	28.2	35.2
Baking and frying fats[3]	21.4	20.7	20.5	23.6	26.2	29.0
Shortening	10.9	14.6	17.4	20.5	22.7	23.1
Lard and beef tallow[4]	10.5	6.1	3.5	3.1	4.0	6.0
Table spreads	17.0	16.5	15.9	15.3	14.0	12.8
Butter	9.0	6.6	4.7	4.6	4.4	4.6
Margarine	8.0	9.9	11.2	10.7	9.6	8.2

[1]Total added fats and oils is on a fat-content basis. Individual items are on a product-weight basis.
[2]Includes a small amount of specialty fats used mainly in confectionery products and nondairy creamers.
[3]Total may not add due to rounding.
[4]Direct use; excludes use in margarine or shortening.
Source: USDA's Economic Research Service.

staples in the Middle East. These regions enjoy the lowest cancer rates in the world.

Harmony with the Ecological Order

It is advisable to base our diet primarily on foods produced in the same general area in which we live. For example, a traditional people like the Inuit base their diet mostly on animal products, and this is appropriate in a polar climate. However, in India and other more tropical regions, a diet based almost entirely on grains and other vegetable foods is more conducive to health. When we begin to eat foods that have been imported from regions with different climatic conditions, we lose our natural immunity to diseases in our own local environment, and a condition of chronic imbalance results. In recent decades, advances in refrigeration, transportation, and other technologies have made it possible for millions of people in temperate zones to consume large quantities of pineapples, bananas, grapefruits, avocados, and other tropical and subtropical products. Similarly, people in southern latitudes are now consuming significant amounts of milk, cheese, ice cream,

TABLE 7.   FRUIT AND VEGETABLE CONSUMPTION, 1970–2000

Per capita consumption of fruit and vegetables increased by one-fifth between 1970–79 and 2000.

	Annual averages			
Item	1970–79	1980–89	1990–99	2000
	Pounds per capita, fresh-weight equivalent			
Total fruit and vegetables	587.5	622.1	688.3	707.7
Total fruit	248.7	269.0	280.1	279.4
Fresh fruit	99.4	113.1	123.7	126.8
Citrus	27.2	24.2	23.7	23.4
Noncitrus	72.2	88.9	100.0	103.3
Processed fruit	149.3	155.9	156.5	152.7
Frozen fruit, noncitrus	3.4	3.4	3.8	3.7
Dried fruit, noncitrus	9.9	12.2	11.7	10.5
Canned fruit, noncitrus	24.7	21.3	19.7	17.4
Fruit juices	110.7	118.6	120.8	120.6
Total vegetables	338.8	353.1	408.2	428.3
Fresh vegetables	147.9	157.2	181.9	201.7
Potatoes	52.5	48.5	48.8	47.2
Other	95.4	108.7	133.1	154.5
Processing vegetables	190.9	195.9	226.3	226.6
Vegetables for canning	101.1	98.9	109.4	104.7
Tomatoes	62.9	63.5	74.4	69.9
Other	38.2	35.4	35.0	34.8
Vegetables for freezing	52.1	61.0	76.8	79.7
Potatoes	36.1	42.8	54.9	57.8
Other	16.0	18.2	21.9	21.9
Dehydrated vegetables and chips	30.8	29.4	32.0	33.7
Pulses	7.0	6.5	8.1	8.6

Note: Totals may not add due to rounding.
Source: USDA's Economic Research Service.

other dairy products, and frozen foods that were originally eaten in more northerly or arctic regions. Since 1948, for example, when frozen orange juice became available, the intake of frozen citrus drinks in the United States soared 11,600 percent. The violation of ecological eating habits contributes to biological degeneration and the development of serious disease.

TABLE 8. GRAIN CONSUMPTION, 1950–2000

Annual average grain consumption was 45 percent higher in 2000 than in the 1970s.

	Annual averages					
Item	1950–59	1960–69	1970–79	1980–89	1990–99	2000
	Pounds per capita					
Total grain products[1]	155.4	142.5	138.2	157.4	190.6	199.9
Wheat flour	125.7	114.4	113.6	122.8	141.8	146.3
Corn products	15.4	13.8	11.0	17.3	24.5	28.4
Rice	5.3	7.1	7.3	11.3	17.5	19.7

[1]Includes oat products, barley products, and rye flour not shown separately.
Source: USDA's Economic Research Service.

TABLE 9. SUGAR CONSUMPTION, 1950–2000

America's sweet tooth increased 39 percent between 1950–59 and 2000 as use of corn sweeteners octupled.

	Annual averages					
Item	1950–59	1960–69	1970–79	1980–89	1990–99	2000
	Pounds per capita, dry weight					
Total caloric sweeteners	109.6	114.4	123.7	126.5	145.9	152.4
Cane and beet sugar	96.7	96.0	96.0	68.4	64.7	65.6
Corn sweeteners	11.0	14.9	26.3	56.8	79.9	85.3
High fructose corn syrup	0	0	5.5	37.3	56.6	63.8
Glucose	7.4	10.9	16.6	16.0	19.3	18.1
Dextrose	3.5	4.1	4.3	3.5	3.8	3.4
Other caloric sweeteners	2.0	1.5	1.4	1.3	1.3	1.5

Note: Totals may not add due to rounding.
[1]Edible syrups (sugarcane, sorgo, maple, and refiner's), edible molasses, and honey.
Source: USDA's Economic Research Service.

Harmony with the Changing Seasons

A habit such as eating ice cream in a heated apartment while snow is falling outside is obviously not in harmony with the seasonal order, nor is charcoal-broiling steaks in the heat of summer. It is better to adjust naturally the selection and preparation of daily foods to harmonize with the changing seasons. In colder weather, for example, we can apply longer cooking times while minimizing the intake of raw salad or fruit. In the summer, lightly cooked dishes are more appropriate while the intake of animal food and heavily cooked items can be minimized.

Harmony with Individual Differences

Personal differences need to be considered in the selection and preparation of our daily foods, with variations according to age, sex, type of activity, occupation, original physiological constitution, present condition of health, and other factors. As individuals we are constantly developing physically, mentally, and spiritually, and our day-to-day eating naturally changes to reflect this growth. The following nutritional considerations are recommended to help us select a balanced diet:

1. Water: It is preferable to use clean natural water for cooking and drinking. Spring or well water is recommended for regular use. It is best to avoid chemically treated municipal water or distilled water.

2. Carbohydrates: It is advisable to eat carbohydrates primarily in the form of polysaccharide glucose, such as that found in cereal grains, vegetables, and beans, while minimizing or avoiding the intake of monosaccharide or disaccharide sugars, such as those in fruit, honey, dairy foods, refined sugar, and other sweeteners.

3. Protein: Protein from such vegetable sources as whole grains and bean products is more easily assimilated by the body than protein from animal sources. When we examine the dietary patterns of people living in Hunza in Pakistan and Vilcabamba in Ecuador, who are noted for their health, vitality, and longevity, we find that they rely primarily on vegetable sources for protein. In a study recently published by *National Geographic,* the average daily caloric intake of a group of men in Hunza was found to be 1,923 calories, with 50 grams of protein, 35 grams of fat, and 354 grams of carbohydrate. In Vilcabamba, the average daily caloric intake was found to be 1,200 calories, with 35 to 38 grams of protein, 12 to 19 grams of fat, and 200 to 260 grams of carbohydrate. In both cases, protein was obtained principally from vegetable sources. It should be noted that cancer is virtually unknown in both these regions. In comparison, in America the average intake is 3,800 calories per day per capita, although about 1,100 of these calories are lost due to spoilage, plate waste, and cooking. Altogether, the typical person in this country consumes 109 grams of protein daily (two-thirds from animal sources).

4. Fat: It is better to avoid the hard saturated fats found in most types of meat and dairy products as well as the polyunsaturated fats found in margarine and hydrogenated cooking oils. Fat currently makes up about 40 percent of the modern diet and in medical studies is the nutrient most associated with degenerative illnesses, including heart disease and cancer. Whole grains, beans, nuts, and seeds contain fat in the ideal proportions for daily consumption. For cooking purposes, high-quality unrefined sesame, corn, or other vegetable oil is recommended for regular use. In recent years, canola oil (made from rapeseed) has become very popular and is widely used in restaurants. Rapeseed oil, however, is not traditionally used as a cooking oil. It was used industrially as a solvent, and questions have been raised by nutritionists and medical experts about its suitability for regular use. Until comprehensive studies are done of its effects on human populations, the recommendation is to avoid this product as much as possible. Also, rapeseed is one of the major North American crops that is genetically engineered. While organic canola is grown and available, it is liable to have genetically modified (GM) contamination from neighboring fields. Be mindful.

5. Salt: It is better to rely primarily on natural sea salt, which contains a variety of trace minerals, and to avoid refined table salt, which is almost 100 percent sodium chloride.

6. Vitamins: Vitamins exist naturally in whole foods and should be consumed as a part of the food together with other nutrients. Vitamin pills and other nutritional supplements became popular in recent decades to offset the deficiencies caused by modern food refining. However, when taken as a supplement to our regular food, vitamins produce a chaotic effect on our body's metabolism. In its report, *Diet, Nutrition, and Cancer,* the National Academy of Sciences warned that some vitamins were toxic in high doses and advised that it was preferable to focus on whole foods rather than individual nutrients when planning our diet.

In a temperate, four-season climate, an optimum daily diet that will help protect against cancer and other serious illnesses consists of about 40 to 50 percent whole cereal grains, 5 to 10 percent soup (especially soups made with a fermented vegetable base and sea-based minerals), 25 to 35 percent vegetables prepared in a variety of styles, and 5 to 10 percent beans and sea vegetables. Supplementary foods for occasional use include locally grown fruits, preferably cooked; fish and other seafood; and a variety of seeds and nuts. (A complete description of the Cancer Prevention Diet is presented in Chapter 5.)

AN ACTIVE DAILY LIFE

For many of us, modern life offers fewer physical and mental challenges than did life in the past. As a result, functions such as the active generation of caloric and electromagnetic energy, the circulation of blood and lymph, and the activity of the digestive, nervous, and reproductive systems often stagnate. However, a physically and mentally active life is essential for good health. The people living in Hunza and Vilcabamba remain active well into their eighties, nineties, and over a hundred. Their cultures have no concept of retirement, and their elders continue to farm, garden, teach, and walk long distances until the very end of their days. In contrast, modern life has become sedentary, soft, and comfortable. After age fifty-five or sixty-five, many people decline and die from lack of meaningful work or recreation. Regular physical and mental exercise throughout life will contribute to overall health and happiness.

4

Diet and the Development of Cancer

To understand how cancer develops, use the analogy of a tree. A tree's structure is opposite to that of the human body. For example, the leaves of a tree have a more open structure and a green color, while the cells of the human body, which correspond to the leaves of a tree, have a more closed structure and are nourished by blood, which is red in color. A tree's sustenance comes from the nutrients absorbed through the external roots. The roots of the human body lie deep in the intestines in the region where nutrients are absorbed into the blood and lymph, from which they are then distributed to all of the body's cells. If the quality of nourishment is chronically poor in the soil or in the food that is consumed, the leaves of the tree or the cells of the body eventually lose their normal functional ability and begin to deteriorate. This condition results from the repeated intake of poor nutrients and does not arise suddenly. While it is developing, many other symptoms might arise in other parts of the tree trunk and branches or in the body.

Cancer develops over a period of time out of a chronically precancerous state. In my estimation, as many as 80 to 90 percent of Americans, Europeans, Japanese, and other modern people have some type of precancerous condition. The repeated overconsumption of excessive dietary factors causes a variety of adjustment mechanisms in the body, which progressively develop toward cancer. Since the body seeks balance with the surrounding environment at all times, the normal process is for this excess to be eliminated or stored when it exceeds the body's capacity for elimination. Eventually, the overaccumulation will be stored in the form of excessive layers of fat, cholesterol, and the formation of cysts and tumors. Let us consider the gradual stages in this process, particularly in their relation to the appearance of cancer.

DISCHARGE

Normal elimination occurs through the processes of urination, bowel movement, respiration (exhaling carbon dioxide), and perspiration, in which excessive chemical compounds are broken down into simple compounds and ultimately into carbon dioxide and water for discharge from the body. Discharge also occurs through physical, mental, and emotional activity. Mental discharge occurs in the form of wave vibrations, while emotions such as anger indicate that a great amount of excess is being eliminated.

Women have several additional means through which excess is naturally discharged. These include menstruation, childbirth, and lactation. Women have a distinct advantage over men in more efficiently discharging excess and thereby maintaining a cleaner condition. They tend to adjust more harmoniously with their environment and usually live longer than men. To compensate for this disadvantage, men usually go out into society and expend energy through additional physical, mental, and social activities. All these processes take place continually throughout life. If we take in only a moderate amount of excess, they will proceed smoothly. If the quantity of excess is large, however, these natural processes are not capable of discharging it, and various abnormal processes begin.

Today, practically everyone eats and drinks excessively, which often triggers a variety of abnormal discharge mechanisms in the body such as diarrhea, excessive sweating, overly frequent bowel movements, or excessive urination. Habits such as scratching the head, tapping the feet, and frequent blinking of the eyes also represent abnormal discharges of imbalanced energy, as do strong emotions such as fear, anger, and anxiety. Periodically, excess is discharged through more acute or violent symptoms such as a fever, coughing, sneezing, shouting, screaming, trembling, and shivering, as well as wild thoughts and behavior.

Chronic discharges are the next stage in this process and often take the form of skin diseases. These are common in cases where the kidneys have lost their ability to properly cleanse the bloodstream. For example, freckles, dark spots, and similar skin markings indicate the chronic discharge of sugar and other refined carbohydrates, while white patches indicate the discharge of milk, cottage cheese, or other dairy products.

Hard, dry skin arises after the bloodstream fills with fat and oil, eventually causing blockage of the pores, hair follicles, and sweat glands. When these blockages prevent the flow of liquid toward the surface, the skin becomes dry.

Many people believe that this condition results from a lack of oil when in fact it is caused by the intake of too much fat and oil.

Skin cancers are more serious forms of skin disease. However, skin disorders are usually not very serious, since in most cases the discharge of toxins toward the surface of the body permits the internal organs and tissues to continue functioning smoothly. If our eating continues to be excessive and we cannot eliminate effectively, the body will start to accumulate this excess in other locations.

If we continue to eat poorly, we eventually exhaust the body's ability to discharge. This can be serious if an underlying layer of fat has developed under the skin, which prevents discharge toward the surface of the body. Such a condition is caused by the repeated overconsumption of milk, cheese, eggs, meat, and other fatty, oily, or greasy foods. When this stage has been reached, internal deposits of mucus or fat begin to form, initially in areas that have some direct access to the outside and in the following regions.

Sinuses

The sinuses are a frequent site of mucous accumulation, and symptoms such as allergies, hay fever, and blocked sinuses often result. Hay fever and sneezing arise when dust or pollen stimulates the discharge of this excess, while calcified stones often form deep within the sinuses. Thick, heavy deposits of mucus in the sinuses diminish our mental clarity and alertness.

Inner Ear

The accumulation of mucus and fat in the inner ear interferes with the smooth functioning of the inner-ear mechanism and can lead to frequent pain, impaired hearing, and even deafness.

Lungs

Various forms of excess often accumulate in the lungs. Aside from the obvious symptoms of coughing and chest congestion, mucus often fills the alveoli or air sacs and breathing becomes more difficult. Occasionally, a coat of mucus in the bronchi can be loosened and discharged by coughing, but once the sacs are surrounded, it becomes more firmly lodged and can remain there for years. Then, if air pollutants or cigarette smoke enters the lungs, their heavier components are attracted to and remain in this sticky environment. In severe cases, these deposits can trigger the development of lung cancer. However, the underlying cause of this condition is the accumulation of sticky fat and mucus in the alveoli and in the blood and capillaries surrounding them.

Breasts

The accumulation of excess in this region often results in a hardening of the breasts and the formation of cysts. Excess usually accumulates here in the form of mucus and deposits of fatty acid, both of which take the form of a sticky or heavy liquid. These deposits develop into cysts in the same way that water solidifies into ice, a process that is accelerated by the intake of ice cream, cold milk, soft drinks, orange juice, and other foods that produce a cooling or freezing effect. Women who have breast-fed are less likely to develop breast cysts or cancer since this reduces excess accumulation in this region.

Intestines

In many cases, excess will begin accumulating in the lower part of the body as mucous and fat deposits coating the intestinal wall. This will often cause the intestines to expand or become less flexible, resulting in a bulging abdomen. A large number of people in the United States have this problem. Young people are often very stylish and attractive. However, after the age of thirty, and particularly between the ages of thirty-five and forty, a large number of Americans lose their youthful appearance and become overweight.

Kidneys

Deposits of fat and mucus may also accumulate in the kidneys. Problems arise when these elements clog the fine network of cells in the interior of these organs, causing them to accumulate water and become chronically swollen. Since elimination is hampered, fluid that cannot be discharged is often deposited in the legs, producing periodic swelling and weakness. If someone with this condition consumes a large quantity of foods that produce a chilling effect, the deposited fat and mucus will often crystallize into kidney stones.

Reproductive Organs

In men the prostate gland is a frequent site of accumulation. As a result of continued consumption of excess or imbalanced food, the prostate often becomes enlarged and hard fat deposits or cysts often form within and around it. This is one of the principal causes of impotence. In women, excess may also accumulate within and around the sexual organs, leading to the formation of ovarian cysts, dermoid tumors, or the blockage of the fallopian tubes. In some cases, mucus or fat in the ovaries or fallopian tubes prevents the passage of the egg and sperm, resulting in an inability to conceive. Chronic vaginal discharge is one indication of accumulation in the reproductive region.

Although the symptoms that affect these inner organs may seem unrelated, they all stem from the same underlying cause. However, modern medicine often does not view them as related. For example, a person with hearing trouble or cataracts is often referred to an ear or eye specialist. Cataracts are a symptom of a variety of related problems such as mucous accumulation in the breasts, kidneys, and sexual organs.

STORAGE

In this stage, excess in various forms is stored within and around the deeper vital organs, including the heart and the liver. In the case of the circulatory system, excess often accumulates around and inside the heart as well as within the heart tissues. Accumulation may also occur both in and around the arteries. These fatty deposits, including cholesterol accumulation, replace the heart's ability to function properly and hamper the smooth passage of blood through the arteries. The end result is often a heart attack. The major causes of this problem are foods containing large amounts of hard, saturated fat. Many nutritionists and medical doctors are now aware of the relationship between the intake of saturated fats and cholesterol and cardiovascular disease, but they often overlook the effects of sugar and dairy products, both of which contribute greatly to the development of these illnesses.

Within the body, the proteins, carbohydrates, and fats that we consume often change into each other, depending on the amount of each consumed as well as the body's needs at a particular time. If we consume more of these than we need, the excess is normally discharged. However, the quantity of excess often exceeds the body's capacity to discharge it. When this happens, the excess is stored in the liver in the form of carbohydrate, in the muscles in the form of protein, or throughout the body in the form of fatty acids.

DEGENERATION OF THE BLOOD AND LYMPH

If the bloodstream is filled with fat and mucus, an excess will begin to accumulate, as we have seen, in the organs. Since the lungs and kidneys are usually affected first, their functions of filtering and cleansing the blood become less efficient. The situation leads to further deterioration of the blood quality and also affects the lymphatic system. Operations such as tonsillectomies also contribute to the deterioration of the lymphatic system since they reduce the ability of this system to cleanse itself. Such operations eventually lead to frequent swelling and lymph gland inflammation, producing a chronic deterioration of the quality of the blood, particularly the red and white blood cells.

TUMORS

When the red blood cells begin to lose their capacity to change into normal body cells, an organism cannot long survive. Poorly functioning intestines can also contribute to the degeneration of blood quality since the qualities of blood cells and plasma originate largely in the small intestine. In many cases, the villi of the small intestine are coated with fat and mucus, and the condition in the intestines is often acidic. A naturally healthy bloodstream will not be created in this type of environment.

Therefore, in order to prevent immediate collapse, the body localizes toxins at this stage in the form of a tumor. A tumor may be likened to a storage depot for the collection of degenerative cells from the bloodstream. As long as improper nourishment is taken in, the body will continue to isolate abnormal excess and toxins in specific areas, resulting in the continual growth of the cancer. When a particular location can no longer absorb the toxic excess, the body must search for another place to localize it, and so the cancer spreads. This process continues until the cancer metastasizes throughout the body and the person eventually dies.

In summary, we may conclude that symptoms such as dry skin, skin discharges, hardening of the breasts, prostate trouble, vaginal discharge, and ovarian cysts all represent potentially precancerous conditions. However, they need not develop toward cancer if we change our daily way of eating.

The Macrobiotic Cancer Prevention Diet

Following the introduction of the Food Guide Pyramid, the Mediterranean Diet Pyramid, the Asian-American Diet Pyramid, and many others, we created a macrobiotic-style graphic that we called the Great Life Pyramid (from the original Greek meaning of the term *macrobios* or "great life").

The graphic illustrates the principal categories of food that may be taken on a daily or regular basis (five to seven times a week), foods that may be taken weekly or occasionally (one to three times a week) by those in good health, and those that may be consumed monthly or less frequently. The last category, represented by foods at the top of the Great Life Pyramid, consists of animal quality foods that are not particularly suited to a temperate climate or environment and may cause health problems. They are included primarily for those in the general population who are in transition toward a macrobiotic or more plant-centered way of eating.

The Great Life Pyramid shows the relative proportion and importance of the different food groups, with whole grains as the foundation. We are very pleased that the U.S. government's Food Guide Pyramid has not only adopted grains as the foundation of a healthy way of eating but also for the first time in 2005 called on the American people to eat a majority of grain and grain products from whole grains, including brown rice, millet, whole wheat, and others.

The following dietary guidelines have been formulated with universal human dietary traditions in mind from East, West, North, and South, and they

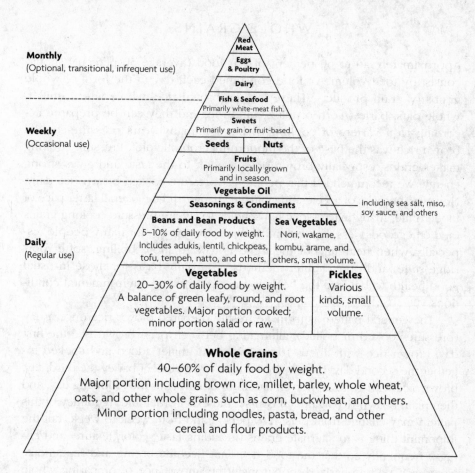

Monthly
(Optional, transitional, infrequent use)

Weekly
(Occasional use)

Daily
(Regular use)

Red Meat

Eggs & Poultry

Dairy

Fish & Seafood
Primarily white-meat fish.

Sweets
Primarily grain or fruit-based.

Seeds | **Nuts**

Fruits
Primarily locally grown
and in season.

Vegetable Oil

Seasonings & Condiments — including sea salt, miso, soy sauce, and others

Beans and Bean Products
5–10% of daily food by weight.
Includes adukis, lentil, chickpeas,
tofu, tempeh, natto, and others.

Sea Vegetables
Nori, wakame,
kombu, arame, and
others, small volume.

Vegetables
20–30% of daily food by weight.
A balance of green leafy, round, and root
vegetables. Major portion cooked;
minor portion salad or raw.

Pickles
Various
kinds, small
volume.

Whole Grains
40–60% of daily food by weight.
Major portion including brown rice, millet, barley, whole wheat,
oats, and other whole grains such as corn, buckwheat, and others.
Minor portion including noodles, pasta, bread, and other
cereal and flour products.

have been further refined over a half century of contemporary macrobiotic practice. When applied conscientiously, these guidelines create a stabilized state of overall physical and mental balance. They may therefore be followed not only for the prevention of cancer but also for the prevention of most other illnesses, including cardiovascular disease, diabetes, and many others. For those people who already have cancer or a precancerous condition, adjustments or modifications need to be made depending on the specific case, and it is advisable to do so under the supervision of a qualified macrobiotic teacher or medical professional. (See Resources for recommendations.) Specific guidelines to relieve each type of cancer are given in Part II, but keep in mind that these are generic and will usually need to be modified for each person's unique energy, condition, level of activity, and personal needs. The following recommendations are primarily for temperate latitudes, including most of the United States, Europe, Russia, China, and Japan. For guidelines in tropical, semitropical, desert, island, and other habitats, see Appendix I.

WHOLE GRAINS

Approximately 40 to 60 percent of our food (average 50 percent) should consist by total volume of food consumed each day in the form of whole grains or grain products. These include brown rice, whole wheat, millet, whole oats, barley, corn or maize, and rye, and they can be prepared according to a variety of cooking styles. For many years pressure-cooked brown rice was the base of the modern macrobiotic diet. Pressure cooking makes grains, especially brown rice, sweeter to the taste and gives strong energy. We recommended that people eat pressure-cooked brown rice daily. However, because of accelerating climate change and the overall faster pace of modern life, many macrobiotic households today are pressure-cooking grains (and other foods) less than before. It is still appropriate for many people, especially when healing, but the trend is toward more boiling, softer porridge style, and other lighter methods on a daily basis for those in usual good health to balance the heavier atmospheric and environmental conditions.

The general pattern is to make freshly prepared brown rice once a day (pressure-cooked or boiled), alternating between plain brown rice the first day, brown rice with about 10 to 20 percent millet added and cooked together the second day, brown rice with 10 to 20 percent barley the third day, brown rice with 10 to 20 percent aduki or other beans the following day, and then plain brown rice again. Of course, the exact order and frequency of this pattern may change from person to person and from week to week, but the important thing is to alternate grains (including taste, color, texture, and energy) frequently so that the food does not become boring and repetitious. Nor can it be emphasized too strongly the importance of preparing whole grains fresh each day and consuming them within a twenty-four-hour cycle. Keeping them overnight is fine, and they can be reused as porridge or made into rice balls, fried rice, or sushi at lunch. But then start fresh again the next evening. Otherwise, the energy of the rice (or other grain) will quickly diminish even though it will keep for several days without spoiling (refrigerated or in some cases in a wooden serving bowl, covered, on a counter). For day-to-day energy, vitality, and strength, freshly cooked food is essential. This is also true for healing.

In the case of wheat, whole wheat berries are rather tough and somewhat difficult to chew, so they are usually ground into flour, which is baked into bread. Bread should ideally be baked from freshly ground flour without the addition of yeast. Sourdough wheat, rye, or spelt bread from a natural foods store or bakery is suitable for occasional use several times a week if it does not include harmful sweeteners, dairy, preservatives, etc.

Other grains such as quinoa, amaranth, and teff may be taken once in a while. For cancer patients, hato mugi (also known as Job's Tears and pearl

THE MACROBIOTIC CANCER PREVENTION DIET

barley) is not recommended because it is too fatty. For people in usual good health, hato mugi may be taken occasionally and has traditionally been used to beautify the skin.

In general, the majority of grain dishes should be eaten primarily in complete or whole form rather than in cracked or processed form. However, a portion may occasionally be consumed in the form of bulgur, couscous, corn grits, polenta, or rolled oats. Again, because of the climate change crisis and the accelerating speed of modern life today, many macrobiotic households are eating more cracked or naturally processed grains. Bread and flour products tend to be more difficult to digest and, especially hard-baked flour products, tend to be mucus-producing. Next to grain in whole form or the traditionally processed grains mentioned above, chapatis, tortillas, and other traditional flat breads are most recommended. Grains may also be eaten in the form of noodles or pasta, especially Asian-style noodles (udon, somen, ramen, etc.) or Western-style spaghetti, spirals, shells, etc. Again, it is recommended that the noodles and pasta be whole grain as opposed to refined. These softly prepared flour products are much easier to digest than hard-baked ones. Note that when cooking, noodles expand, while bread and baked goods contract. Too much baked food contributes to hardening, tightening, and other contractions in the body. All things considered, noodles and pasta (which expand when cooked) are preferable to bread and baked goods (which contract when baked), but both may be enjoyed in moderation by those in usual good health.

Grain products such as mochi (pounded sweet rice) and seitan (wheat meat or wheat gluten) may be consumed a few times a week. These give dynamic energy, have a rich, satisfying taste, and are a nice supplement to grain in other forms. Just be careful of the salty liquid in which commercial seitan is packaged.

As a rule, white rice, white flour, and other refined grains and grain products are avoided. However, a small amount may be consumed infrequently by those in usual good health, especially if it is consumed at a restaurant or outside the house. Ideally, the macrobiotic kitchen is kept pure with only the highest quality foods. Consuming unhealthful foods and bingeing are best done outside the home so that one's central commitment to a healthful way of life and natural order is not lost.

SOUP

About 5 to 10 percent (one or two cups or bowls) of daily intake may be in the form of soup. Soup broth can be made with miso or shoyu (natural soy sauce), which are prepared from naturally fermented soybeans, sea salt, and grains, to which several varieties of land and sea vegetables, especially wakame or kombu (kelp), green vegetables, and occasionally shiitake mushroom, may be added during cooking. The taste of miso or shoyu should be mild, not too salty or too bland. Barley miso, rise miso, or all-soybean miso (hatcho miso), aged naturally two to three years, is recommended for regular use. Soups made with grains, beans, or vegetables can also be served from time to time. For instance, delicious seasonal varieties can be made, such as broccoli, cauliflower, or corn soup in the summer or squash or parsnip soup in the fall.

VEGETABLE DISHES

About 25 to 30 percent of our daily food should be fresh vegetable dishes, which can be prepared in a wide variety of cooking styles: sautéing, steaming, boiling, blanching, deep-frying, marinating, and pressed and boiled salads. Among root and stem vegetables, carrots, onions, daikon (white radishes), turnips, red radishes, burdock, lotus root, rutabagas, and parsnips are excellent. When preparing root vegetables, cook both the root and the leaf portions so as to achieve a proper balance of nutrients by using the whole food. Among vegetables from the ground, cabbage, cauliflower, broccoli, brussels sprouts, Chinese cabbage, acorn squash, butternut squash, buttercup squash, and pumpkin are quite nutritious and may be used daily. Among green and white leafy vegetables, watercress, kale, parsley, leeks, scallions, dandelions, collard greens, bok choy, carrot tops, daikon greens, turnip greens, and mustard greens are fine for regular use. Vegetables for occasional use include cucumbers, lettuce, string beans, celery, sprouts, yellow squash, peas, red cabbage, mushrooms (various, including shiitake), kohlrabi, and others. In general, up to one-third of vegetable intake may be eaten raw in the form of fresh salad or traditionally prepared pickles. However, it is better to avoid mayonnaise and commercial salad dressings. Vegetables that originated historically in tropical or semitropical environments, such as eggplants, potatoes, tomatoes, asparagus, spinach, sweet potatoes, yams, avocados, green and red peppers, and other varieties, tend to produce acid and should be avoided or minimized unless you live in a hot and humid climate. However, for some conditions, including some types of cancer, tropical or semitropical foods may be taken in small volume, as explained later in this book.

BEANS AND SEA VEGETABLES

From 5 to 10 percent of daily intake may be eaten in the form of cooked beans and sea vegetables. Beans for daily use are aduki (small red) beans, chickpeas, lentils, and black soybeans. Other beans may be used occasionally, two to three times a month: yellow soybeans, pinto, white, black turtle, navy, kidney, and lima beans, split peas, black-eyed peas, and others. Soybean products such as tofu, tempeh, and natto may be used daily or regularly in moderation and be considered part of the daily volume for this category. Sea vegetables are rich in minerals and should be used in small volume on a daily basis in soups, cooked with vegetables or beans, or prepared as a side dish. Wakame, kombu, and nori are usually used daily, while all other seaweeds, including arame and hijiki, may be used occasionally. These dishes may be seasoned with a moderate amount of shoyu, sea salt, or a grain-based vinegar, such as brown rice vinegar.

SUPPLEMENTARY FOODS

Persons in usually good health may wish to include some of the following additional supplementary foods in their diet.

Animal Food

A small volume of white-meat fish or seafood may be eaten a few times per week. White-meat fish such as cod and haddock contains less fat than red-meat or blue-skin varieties. Saltwater fish also usually have fewer pollutants in their systems than freshwater varieties. Whole small dried fish (iriko), which can be consumed entirely including bones, may also be used occasionally as a side dish with vegetables, in soup, or as a seasoning. Avoid or drastically limit all other animal products, including beef, lamb, pork, veal, chicken, turkey, duck, goose, wild game, and eggs. Avoid or drastically limit all dairy foods, including cheese, butter, milk, skim milk, buttermilk, yogurt, ice cream, cream, sour cream, whipped cream, margarine, and kefir.

Fruit

Fruit may be eaten several times a week as a supplement or dessert, provided the fruits grow in the local or similar climatic zone. Fresh fruits can also be consumed in moderate volume during their growing season. In temperate areas these include apples, strawberries, cherries, peaches, pears, plums, grapes, apricots, prunes, blueberries, blackberries, raspberries, cantaloupe, honeydew melon, watermelon, tangerines, oranges, and grapefruit. In these climates avoid or limit tropical or semitropical fruits such as bananas, pineapples, mangoes, papayas, figs, dates, coconut, and kiwis. In the areas in which they grow, these fruits may be eaten in modest amounts. Fruit juice is very concentrated (for example, ten apples go into one glass of apple juice), so its use should be moderate. Fresh juice is especially relaxing in warm or hot weather, and consumption of apple cider is enjoyable in the fall. Dried fruit may be eaten in moderation as long as it is from the same or a similar climatic region.

Overall, macrobiotic people have tended to eat too little fruit. Now with global warming, the increased pace of modern life, and the heavy effects of cellular technology and other electromagnetic radiation, a lighter diet is necessary, including proportionately more fruit and juice.

Snacks

Seeds and nuts that have been blanched or lightly roasted may be enjoyed occasionally as snacks. Suitable seeds and nuts include sesame seeds, sunflower seeds, pumpkin seeds, almonds, walnuts, pecans, filberts, and peanuts. It is preferable not to overconsume nuts and nut butters, because they are difficult to digest and are high in fat and oil. Other snacks may include mochi (pounded sweet rice), noodles, rice balls, vegetable sushi, rice cakes, puffed grain cereals, popcorn (homemade and unbuttered), and roasted beans and grains.

Desserts

Desserts may be eaten in moderate volume two or three times a week and may include cookies, pudding, cake, pie, and other sweet dishes prepared with natural ingredients. Often desserts can be prepared from apples, fall and winter squash, pumpkin, aduki beans, or dried fruit and other naturally sweet foods without adding a sweetener. However, for dishes that need one, recommended sweeteners include rice syrup, barley malt, amasake (a fermented sweet rice beverage), chestnuts, apple juice and cider, dried fruits such as apricots, and very occasionally maple syrup.

As a rule, avoid white sugar, brown sugar, raw sugar, turbinado sugar, molasses, honey, corn syrup, chocolate, carob, fructose, saccharine, and other concentrated or artificial sweeteners. For custards, whipped toppings, and frosting, plant-quality ingredients such as kudzu (also known as kuzu) root, agar, tofu, or tahini (toasted sesame butter) should be used instead of eggs, cream, milk, and similar animal products. A delicious sea vegetable gelatin made of agar, called kanten, can be seasoned with fruit, apple juice, and other natural sweeteners.

BEVERAGES

Recommended daily beverages include roasted bancha twig tea (also known as kukicha), roasted brown rice tea, roasted barley tea, and spring or well water. Occasional-use beverages include grain coffee (made without molasses, figs, etc.), dandelion tea, kombu tea, umeboshi tea, mu tea, carrot juice, celery juice, and sweet vegetable drink. Infrequent-use beverages include green tea, vegetable juice, fruit juice, beer, sake (hot or cool), and soy milk (with kombu). Any traditional tea that does not have an aromatic fragrance or a stimulant effect may also be used. However, coffee, black tea, and aromatic herbal teas such as peppermint, rose hips, and chamomile should be avoided. Daily foods and beverages should preferably be prepared or cooked with spring or well water.

Avoid municipal tap water that may be chlorinated or chemicalized, distilled water, cold drinks (served with ice cubes), mineral water, all bubbling (carbonated) waters, sugared and soft drinks, and hard liquor.

ADDITIONAL DIETARY SUGGESTIONS

Oil

For daily use, unrefined sesame, corn, or other vegetable oil in moderate amounts is recommended. Oil should be used in cooking and not eaten raw at the table as in salad dressings. Other unrefined vegetable oils, such as safflower, sunflower, soy, and olive, may be used occasionally. Avoid or limit all chemically processed vegetable oils, butter, lard, shortening, palm oil, coconut oil, and egg or soy margarine.

Salt

Naturally processed, mineral-rich sea salt and traditional, nonchemicalized miso and shoyu may be used as seasonings. Daily meals, however, should not have an overly salty flavor, and seasonings should generally be added during cooking and not at the table except for condiments and garnishes. Avoid commercial table salt (to which additives and sugar are usually added) and gray sea salt or other sea salt excessively high in minerals. (Free-flowing white sea salt is usually suitable.)

Other Seasonings

In addition to oil and salt, miso, and shoyu, other seasonings may be used in cooking and before serving. The seasonings are all vegetable-quality, naturally processed. Suitable for occasional use are ginger, horseradish, mirin (fermented sweet brown rice sweetener), rice vinegar, umeboshi vinegar, umeboshi plum, umeboshi paste, garlic, lemon, orange, mustard, and black or red pepper. Commercial seasonings, spices, herbs, and other sugary, hot, pungent, aromatic seasonings, including all spices and herbs, are avoided or limited.

Pickles

A small volume of homemade pickles may be eaten each day to aid in digestion. In macrobiotic food preparation, this naturally fermented type of food is made with a variety of root and round vegetables, such as daikon or radishes, turnips, carrots, cabbage, and cauliflower, and preserved in sea salt, rice or wheat bran, shoyu, umeboshi, or miso. Spices, sugar, and vinegar are avoided. Short-time fermented, lighter pickles are recommended in warmer weather or for persons who need to reduce their salt intake. Long-time fermented, saltier pickles can be eaten during colder weather or by those who wish to strengthen their condition. Different jars, crocks, and kegs can be used in pickle preparation, and aging varies from several hours to weeks or months.

Condiments

Condiments should be available on the table for daily use if desired. They allow family members to individually adjust taste and seasoning. Condiments for daily use include gomashio (toasted sesame seed salt), made usually from sixteen to eighteen parts roasted sesame seeds to one part roasted sea salt, half-ground together in a small earthenware bowl called a suribachi; roasted kombu or wakame powder, made from baking these sea vegetables in the oven until black and crushing in a suribachi and sometimes adding toasted sesame seeds and storing in a small container or jar; umeboshi plums, small salt plums that have been dried and pickled for many months with sea salt and flavored with shiso (beefsteak) leaves; tekka, a combination of carrot, burdock, and lotus root that has been finely chopped and sautéed in sesame oil and miso for many hours; shoyu, which is traditionally processed natural soy sauce; and green nori flakes. Some of these, such as gomashio and the sea vegetable powders, should be prepared fresh in the home, while others, such as umeboshi plums and tekka, are available ready-made in natural foods stores. Other condiments may be used from time to time.

Garnishes

To balance various dishes at the table and make the meal more attractive, garnishes are frequently prepared. These include grated daikon, grated radish, grated horseradish, chopped scallions, grated ginger, green mustard pâte, freshly ground pepper, lemon pieces, red pepper, and others.

WAY OF EATING

You may eat regularly two to three times per day, as much as is comfortable, provided the proportion of each category of food is generally correct and in daily consumption each mouthful is thoroughly chewed. Proper chewing is essential to digestion, and it is recommended that each mouthful of food be chewed fifty times or more or until it becomes liquid in form. Eat when you are hungry, but it is best to leave the table feeling satisfied but not full. Similarly, drink only when thirsty. Avoid eating for three hours before sleeping, because this causes stagnation in the intestines and throughout the body. Before and after each meal, express your gratitude verbally or silently to nature, the universe, or God who created the food, and reflect on the health and happiness it is dedicated to achieving. This acknowledgment may take the form of grace, prayer, chanting, or a moment of silence. Express your thanks to parents, grandparents, and past generations who nourished us and whose dreams we embody, to the vegetables or animals who gave their lives so we may live, and to the farmer, shopkeeper, and cook who contributed their energies to making the food available.

Eating less is also important. Researchers at Tufts University reported that mice on a very low calorie diet lived 29 percent longer than fully fed mice and had few tumors and other disorders. In studies designed to identify the changes that occur with aging, mice fed a diet containing 40 percent fewer calories enjoyed consistently better health and longer life. "What stunned us in this study was that every single type of tumor and nearly every kind of lesion were delayed," noted Richard Sprott, associate director for the National Institute on Aging's Biology of Aging program.

Chewing is a very important daily practice in the macrobiotic community, and medical studies are beginning to show its benefits. For example, broccoli sprouts are a rich source of compounds and enzymes that boost antioxidant status and protect against chemically induced cancer in laboratory studies. Researchers at the Johns Hopkins University School of Medicine reported that thorough chewing of fresh broccoli sprouts, rather than swallowing them whole, exposed them to more beneficial enzymes and resulted in increased excretion of toxins. In another report, an Indian cancer researcher concluded that thorough chewing lowered the risk of cancer. "The proper chewing of meals ensuring that mucus-rich saliva mixed with the food seemed to be protective factors."

OBTAINING NATURAL FOODS

In selecting your foods it is important to obtain the freshest and highest quality natural foods. Of course, growing your own grains and vegetables is ideal, and you may want to make your own miso, tofu, or seitan at home.

For many people, however, especially those living in the city, the local natural foods, health food, or grocery and produce store will be the primary source of their daily food. Farmers' markets are increasing in popularity.

Applied to food, the word *natural* means whole and unprocessed or processed by natural methods. The term *organic,* when further applied to natural foods, is understood to mean food that is grown without the use of chemical fertilizers, herbicides, pesticides, or other artificial sprays. Since it is fairly difficult to distinguish organic foods from nonorganic except by taste, you may need to rely on the reputation of the local store or the distributor. Many suppliers have been certified by an organic growers' association, which makes on-site inspections, performs lab tests on soil and product samples, and offers educational guidance to farmers and consumers.

The harmful effects of chemical farming on human health as well as on the topsoil and the environment have been well documented. As long ago as the end of the nineteenth century, Dr. Julius Hensel, a German agricultural chemist, warned that the introduction of synthetic fertilizers, insecticides, the forced fattening of livestock, and other modern practices were resulting in the degeneration of the human blood and lymph and giving rise to a host of degenerative diseases.

Organic foods are not always available, nor can they always be afforded, because of their higher price. In this case, the next best available produce should be obtained, thoroughly cleaned, and properly cooked to eliminate potentially harmful chemicals. For better health it is also wise to avoid all industrially mass-produced foods, including instant foods, canned foods, frozen foods, refined grains or flour, sprayed foods, dyed foods, irradiated foods, and all foods made with chemicals, additives, preservatives, stabilizers, emulsifiers, and artificial coloring.

Several years ago the U.S. government started certifying organic foods. This has vastly increased their popularity, and today more organic foods are sold in supermarkets than in natural foods stores. However, there is still some confusion on labeling. When the label shows "100 percent organic," the product is completely chemical-free; "organic" means that at least 95 percent of the item is made without chemicals, but a small amount of nonorganic ingredients may be included.

The introduction of genetically modified foods has further complicated the situation. In the field, GM pollen can contaminate conventional and organic produce. Corn and soy are particularly susceptible to contamination, and unfortunately a significant amount of organic products, including corn oil, polenta, tofu, and others, may be compromised. For this reason it is best to buy locally grown produce whenever available, especially from a natural foods store, CSA (community-supported agriculture) network, or farmers' market where you can talk to and get to know local growers. Overall, buying locally is much better for the environment and mitigating climate change than purchasing food that is transported across the country. In some cases, obtaining high-quality organic products from abroad is recommended, especially for healing purposes. Organic foods from Europe and Japan generally give stronger energy and are less contaminated than those grown in the United States. With the influx of organic food from China, South America, and other regions, there is growing concern that organic certification standards are not adequate or enforced. Eventually this problem will probably be resolved, but in the meantime it is advisable to be mindful of where food originates.

Another major concern is that the nutrients in food have steadily declined over the last twenty-five years (since the first edition of this book came out), primarily as a result of the environmental crisis, the use of new high-yielding hybrid seeds, and marketing methods that emphasize shelf life over freshness. In an analysis of new U.S. Department of Agriculture food composition tables several years ago, we reported a sharp decline in minerals, vitamins, and other nutrients in many common foods between 1975 and 1997 when the last comprehensive survey was published.

A random sampling of twelve garden vegetables found that calcium levels declined on average 26.5 percent, vitamin A dropped 21.4 percent, and vitamin C fell 29.9 percent. Whole grains and beans also showed sharp fluctuations. The amount of calcium and iron in millet fell 60 percent and 55.7 percent, and thiamin and riboflavin declined 42.3 percent and 23.7 percent, but niacin rose 105.2 percent. Brown rice also showed mixed results, with slight decreases in calcium and riboflavin, and mild increases in iron, thiamine, and niacin. Overall, green leafy vegetables appeared to have lost the most nutrients, while root vegetables, beans, and grains lost the least. The loss of nutrients in fruits was comparable to those of vegetables.

Our study made international headlines and was subsequently confirmed by the USDA and several other scientific studies. It also substantiates what we and many other friends, associates, and clients have observed in recent years, namely, that the food today—whether organic or conventional—is not as strong as it was twenty-five or ten years ago. Organic farming today is largely controlled by large commercial enterprises or distributors so that higher-yielding, larger, more colorful, or more tasteful hybrid strains are commonly preferred to traditional, open-pollinated varieties. As much as possible we recommend growing or purchasing these older, hardier heirloom varieties (which are usually smaller and have more imperfections). Several years ago some ancient rice was discovered at an archaeological site in Japan. Though centuries old, the seeds propagated and gave rise to a line of red, black, and other colored rice that has been distributed mostly by word of mouth among macrobiotic friends in Japan. This temple rice is much stronger than usual organic rice. Around the world there are many heirloom crops like this that need to be preserved and reintroduced. Some of the macrobiotic mail order companies in the Resources section occasionally make available rice, maize, or other ancient seeds.

STUDIES ON KEY FOODS
IN THE MACROBIOTIC DIET

Over the last generation, modern society has gradually become aware of the limits of chemical agriculture, food technology, and nutritional models of health based on meat and dairy consumption. Recent medical studies have shown that most of the foods in the macrobiotic dietary approach protect against cancer and other chronic diseases. In Part II we summarize many of these findings and classify them under specific forms of malignancies. However, as we have seen, cancer is not an isolated phenomenon but a disease of the whole body. These foods will substantially help reduce the risk of cancer in general. Briefly, let us look at the major scientific and medical findings as they apply to the basic categories of food in the Cancer Prevention Diet.

1. Whole Grains: A wide variety of epidemiological, laboratory, and case control studies show that as part of a balanced diet whole grains, high in fiber and bran, protect against many forms of cancer. The U.S. Senate's report *Dietary Goals,* the Surgeon General's reports, the National Academy of Sciences' reports, the Food Guide Pyramid, and World Health Organization studies all call for substantial increases in the daily consumption of whole grains, including brown rice, millet, barley, oats, and whole wheat. The American Cancer Society and other organizations have sponsored intervention studies on persons at high risk for cancer, emphasizing whole grains and other high-fiber foods.

    For example, in a review of case-control studies in Italy between 1983 and 1996 involving fifteen thousand people, researchers reported that a high intake of whole grain foods consistently reduced the risk of cancers of the oral cavity and pharynx, esophagus, stomach, colon, rectum, liver, gallbladder, pancreas, larynx, breast, endometrium, ovary, prostate, bladder, kidney, lymphatic system, and multiple myelomas. Reduced risk ranged from 10 to 80 percent depending on the site.

    The researchers emphasized that the protective effects were observed only with whole grains and their products in contrast to refined grains. Refined bread, pasta, or rice, they noted, are associated with elevated risk of stomach and colorectal cancer.[1]

2. Soup: A ten-year study by the National Cancer Center of Japan reported that people who ate miso soup daily were 33 percent less likely to contract stomach cancer than those who never ate miso (see Table 10). The study also found that miso was effective in preventing cancer at all other sites and helped protect against heart and

TABLE 10. RELATION OF MISO INTAKE, CANCER, AND DISEASE

| Cause of Death* | Daily | MISO SOUP CONSUMPTION | | |
		Occasionally (%)	Rarely (%)	Never (%)
Stomach cancer	Baseline	Up 18	Up 34	Up 48
Cancer at all sites	Baseline	Up 4	Up 12	Up 19
Coronary heart disease	Baseline	Up 7	Up 10	Up 43
High blood pressure	Baseline	Up 29	Up 11	Up 453
Cerebrovascular disease	Baseline	Down 11	Down 13	Up 29
Liver cirrhosis	Baseline	Up 25	Up 25	Up 57
Peptic ulcer	Baseline	Up 17	Up 41	Up 52
All causes of death	Baseline	Up 2	Up 6	Up 33

*Association of age-sex standardized rate ratio for major causes of death, 1966–78.
Source: Nutrition and Cancer, 1982.

liver disease. A recent study of atomic bomb survivors in Hiroshima and Nagasaki found that 90 percent attributed their survival from radiation sickness (a syndrome that often leads to leukemia, lymphoma, bone cancer, or thyroid cancer) to eating miso soup following the blast and exposure to potentially lethal radiation. Soy sauce (shoyu) is also used frequently in soups and other dishes in macrobiotic cooking. A study by researchers at the University of Wisconsin found that in laboratory experiments, subjects eating a soy sauce enhanced diet contracted 26 percent less stomach cancer, and the soy-supplement group averaged about one-quarter the number of tumors as the control group. Soy sauce "exhibited a pronounced anti-carcinogenic effect," the researchers concluded.

3. Vegetables: A wide range of international population studies show that regular consumption of vegetables high in beta-carotene, particularly dark green and dark yellow and orange vegetables such as broccoli, brussels sprouts, carrots, cabbage, kale, and collards, protect against cancer. The National Cancer Institute, the American Cancer Society, and other organizations have recommended daily consumption of these vegetables, which have long been emphasized in the standard macrobiotic way of eating. In addition, foods high in vitamin C have been shown to lower the risk of some malignancies. These vitamins are found in natural abundance in green leafy vegetables, some citrus fruits, and whole grains, and this is the form in which they are ideally consumed.

For example, in a review of seven cohort studies and eighty-seven case-control studies around the world, researchers in the Netherlands reported that 67 percent of the studies found that the consumption of broccoli, cabbage, and cauliflower lowered the risk of lung cancer, stomach cancer, colon cancer, and rectal cancer.[2]

Another promising food to reduce the risk of cancer is shiitake mushroom, a staple of Asian cooking that is now grown and sold widely in this country. Medical studies in the laboratory found that shiitakes had a strong antitumor effect in induced cancer and no toxic side effects. In macrobiotic cooking and home care, shiitake mushrooms, especially the dried variety, are used to help reduce and eliminate fat deposits that have accumulated in the body.

"The dietary changes now under way appear to be reducing our dependence on foods from animal sources," the National Academy of Sciences' panel commented in its comprehensive report on cancer. "It is likely that there will be continued reduction in fats from animal sources and an increasing dependence on vegetable and other plant products for protein supplies. Hence, diets may contain increasing amounts of vegetable products, some of which may be protective against cancer."

4. Beans and Bean Products: Epidemiological studies indicate that regular consumption of beans, pulses, and bean products reduces the risk of cancer. Beans have been shown to lower bile acid production by up to 30 percent. Bile acids are necessary for proper fat digestion but in excess have been associated with causing cancer, especially in the large intestine. Beans also contain fiber, which is protective in the colon and elsewhere. Soybeans and soy products, a major source of protein in the macrobiotic diet, have been singled out as especially effective in reducing tumors. Soybeans contain protease inhibitors, isoflavanoids, lignons, and other components that have been shown to help prevent the development of breast, stomach, and skin tumors.

For example, in laboratory studies, scientists reported that a hot-water extract of aduki beans (a popular Asian bean now grown in the United States) significantly reduced the number of lung tumor colonies and the invasion of melanoma cells. A previous study showed that adukis inhibited stomach cancer by 36 to 62 percent in tumor weight relative to controls.[3]

In Japan, the incidence of breast cancer is about one-fifth that in the United States. To test the hypothesis that soy foods helped protect against this disease, researchers at the University of Alabama initiated lab studies and found that subjects given miso, tempeh, natto, soy sauce, and other traditionally fermented soybean foods had fewer induced tumors, more benign tumors, and a slower growth rate of malignancy than the control group. "This date suggests that miso consumption may be a factor producing a lower breast cancer incidence in Japanese women," the researchers concluded. "Organic compounds found in fermented soybean-based foods may exert a chemoprotective effect."

It is important to note that the protective effects of soy are associated with traditional and naturally fermented soy foods, not with modern, artificially processed soy products. These latter include commercial soymilk, soy cheese, soy burgers, soy hot dogs and other meat analogues, textured soy protein, soy ice cream, and similar products. These foods are generally discouraged in the macrobiotic approach, except for infrequent use as party foods.

Traditional nonfermented soy products such as tofu and edamame may be part of a healthy cancer-prevention diet. However, for those with cancer, they may need to be limited depending on the type of cancer (especially breast cancer) or the individual's condition. The role of tofu is very controversial in modern cancer research. Some studies show that it helps protect against tumors, especially those of the stomach. But others suggest that it may increase estrogen levels and enhance the risk, especially those of the breast. Some of these negative effects may be attributed to nonorganic tofu, tofu made with inferior ingredients, tofu consumed raw, and tofu combined with sweets—all of which are nontraditional.

5. Sea Vegetables: Kombu, wakame, nori, and other edible seaweeds are a small but important part of the daily macrobiotic diet. In Japan, a macrobiotic doctor in Nagasaki who survived the atomic bombing in August 1945 put all of his surviving patients on a strict diet of brown rice, miso soup, sea vegetables, and sea salt. In contrast to many patients at other hospitals and medical centers who contracted or died from radiation sickness, all his patients and staff were saved. This experience (and others in Hiroshima) inspired scientists to study the mechanism by which certain foods protect against cancer. Beginning in the 1960s, scientists at McGill University in Montreal reported that a substance in kelp and other common sea vegetables could reduce the amount of radioactive strontium-90 absorbed through the intestine by 50 to 80 percent. Japanese scientists subsequently reported that adding seaweed to the diet resulted in the complete regression of induced sarcomas in more than half of laboratory animals tested (see Table 11). Similar experiments with

TABLE 11.   ANTITUMOR EFFECT OF SEAWEED ON SARCOMAS IN MICE

Sample	Dose (mg/kg)	Average tumor weight (g)	Inhibition ratio (%)	Complete regression	Mortality
Sargassum fulvellum	100×10	0.18	89.3	7/9	1/10
Control		1.67		0/10	0/10
Laminaria angustata	100×5	0.08	94.8	6/9	1/10
Control		1.59		0/10	0/10
Laminaria angustata var. longissima	100×5	0.21	92.3	5/9	1/10
Control		2.71		0/7	0/7
Laminaria japonica	100×5	1.40	13.6	2/9	1/10
Control		1.62		0/9	1/10

Source: Japanese Journal of Experimental Medicine, 1974.

leukemia have also shown promising results. Subjects given miso were found to be five times more resistant to radiation-induced tumors than controls.

In the last twenty-five years, there has been increasing study of the protective effects of sea vegetables on breast cancer and other tumors. At Harvard School of Public Health, feeding trials were initiated in which it was found that laboratory animals fed kombu developed induced breast cancer later than controls. "Seaweed has shown consistent antitumor activity in several in vivo animal tests," the researchers concluded. "In extrapolating these results to the Japanese population, seaweed may be an important factor in explaining the low rates of certain cancers in Japan."

A note of caution, however, is warranted. Because sea vegetables are so high in vitamins, minerals, and other nutrients and have such strong life energy, only small amounts are recommended. Also, in our experience, too many sea vegetables, especially kombu (which tends to be the strongest variety), may worsen certain tumors, especially those of the prostate, ovary, and other more contractive—or yang—types. Hence, moderation is advised and proper guidance and counseling may be needed in any given case.

STUDIES ON THE MACROBIOTIC APPROACH TO CANCER

During the last twenty-five years, more than a dozen scientific and medical studies on the macrobiotic approach to cancer have showed a variety of positive benefits:

1. Macrobiotic Diet Lessens Breast Cancer Risk

    Macrobiotic and vegetarian women are less likely to develop breast cancer, researchers at New England Medical Center in Boston reported. The scientists found that macrobiotic and vegetarian women process estrogen differently from other women and eliminate it more quickly from their body. The study involved forty-five pre- and postmenopausal women, about half of whom were macrobiotic and vegetarian and half nonvegetarian.

    The women consumed about the same number of total calories. Although the vegetarian women took in only one-third as much animal protein and animal fat, they excreted two to three times as much estrogen. High levels of estrogen have been associated with the development of breast cancer. "The difference in estrogen metabolism may explain the lower incidence of breast cancer in vegetarian women," the study concluded.[4]

2. Medical Doctor Healed of Incurable Metastatic Cancer

    In 1978, Dr. Anthony J. Sattilaro was diagnosed with terminal prostate cancer. Tests at Philadelphia's Methodist Hospital, where he was CEO, showed that it had spread to the bones, testicles, and other internal organs. One day while driving back to Philadelphia after burying his own father, who had died of cancer, Dr. Sattilaro uncharacteristically picked up two young hitchhikers. Resigned to dying before he was fifty, Dr. Sattilaro was shocked when he was told by these hitchhikers that he didn't necessarily have to die and that there was a diet that might help him recover.

    Though highly skeptical, he had nothing to lose. In Philadelphia he contacted the East West Center, met with director Denny Waxman, and changed his diet to one consisting of brown rice and other whole grains, beans and soy products, fresh vegetables from land and sea, and occasional white-meat fish. A positive, spiritual approach to life was also encouraged.

    Within just a few weeks the back pain he suffered for years eased, and after several months his tumors went away. One- and four-year follow-up scans at his own hospital confirmed that the cancer had completely disappeared. Dr. Sattilaro went on to write a bestselling book and was profiled in the *Saturday Evening Post* and *Life* magazines.

"I was the paragon cancer victim, not so much because of the specific details of my life, but because of the motives and attitudes that drove my life," he explained at a macrobiotic conference. "I had lived a life of selfishness, greed, self-centered ambition, and fear. I was bent on satisfying my own appetites and was intractable in my dealings with others. . . . Because I am an affluent American who, to some degree, has power and authority, I could easily satisfy my appetites. I had enough rope to hang myself. Yes, I believe diet was definitely the cause of my cancer."

Dr. Sattilaro remained cancer-free for seven years but gradually reverted to some of his prior eating habits. He started eating chicken and ice cream, and the tumors came back. Once again he returned to a macrobiotic way of eating, avoiding these and other extreme foods. But this time his body was not strong enough to heal, and he passed away in 1989. Although his own life ended prematurely, his recovery inspired countless others and helped change society.[5]

3. Macrobiotics Benefits Advanced Cancers

In a study of patients with advanced malignancies who followed a macrobiotic way of eating, Vivien Newbold, M.D., a Philadelphia physician, documented six cases of remission. The patients had pancreatic cancer with metastases to the liver; malignant melanoma; malignant astrocytoma; endometrial stromal sarcoma; adenocarcinoma of the colon; and inoperable intraabdominal leimyosarcoma.

A review of CT scans and other medical tests revealed no evidence of tumors after adherence to the macrobiotic diet. All the patients (except for one whose cancer came back after she discontinued macrobiotics) were reported working full-time, leading very active lives, and feeling in excellent health. The cases were all reviewed independently and the diagnoses confirmed by the pathology and radiology departments of Holy Redeemer Hospital in Meadowbrook, Pennsylvania.

The cases included Dr. Newbold's husband: "Eight months after being described as hopeless, he was feeling 'healthier than he ever felt in his life. . . . A follow-up CT scan revealed that about 70 percent of the cancer was gone.'"

In a review of her study, Congressional investigators recommended further research on the macrobiotic approach to cancer: "If cases such as Newbold's were presented in the medical literature, it might help stimulate interest among clinical investigators in conducting controlled, prospective trials of macrobiotic regimens, which could provide valid data on effectiveness." The Office of Technology Assessment's (OTA) assessment found that macrobiotics was "among the most popular unconventional approaches used by cancer patients."[6]

4. Pancreatic and Prostate Cancer Patients Live Longer on Macrobiotics
    In the first case control study of the macrobiotic approach to cancer, researchers at Tulane University reported that the one-year survival rate among patients with pancreatic cancer was significantly higher among those who modified their diet than among those who did not (seventeen months versus six months). The one-year survival rate was 54.2 percent in the macrobiotic patients versus 10 percent in the controls. All comparisons were statistically significant.

    For patients with metastatic prostate cancer, the study demonstrated that those who ate macrobiotically lived longer (177 months compared to 91 months) and enjoyed an improved quality of life. The researchers also reviewed 182 subjects with other forms of histologically confirmed primary or secondary invasive cancer who had sought macrobiotic guidance.

    > The three sets of studies presented indicate a possible association of dietary modification, involving a high fiber, vegetable and low-fat diet, with enhanced survival in primary pancreatic cancer, prostate cancer, and possibly other cancers as well, [the researchers concluded]. If this association is indeed causal, it would suggest dietary inhibition of tumor progression in humans, a phenomenon similar to that observed in animal models. However, because of the small sample sizes and the possibility of bias in the selection of cases, these findings must be interpreted with caution. Nonetheless, they raise the important question of whether dietary modification may be effective adjunctive treatment to either chemotherapy/radiation therapy and/or surgery/substitution therapy for those refusing standard treatment, or in primary management of cancers whose etiologies have nutritional links, especially when the prognosis with other forms of management is grim. . . . This exploratory analysis suggests that a strict macrobiotic diet is more likely to be effective in the long-term management of cancer than are diets that provide a variety of other foods.[7]

5. Macrobiotics and Cancer Risk Factors
    In 1983, J. P. Deslypere, M.D., a researcher at the Academic Hospital of the Ghent University in Belgium, conducted medical

tests, especially blood work, on twenty men eating macrobiotically. "In the field of cardiovascular and cancer risk factors this kind of blood is very favorable," he reported. "It's ideal, we couldn't do better, that's what we're dreaming of. It's really fantastic, like children, whose blood vessels are still completely open and whole. This is a very important matter, deserving our full attention."[8]

6. Macrobiotics and General Health
    In 1986, Dr. Peter Gruner, director of oncology at St. Mary's Hospital in Montreal, launched a study of approximately thirty individuals on macrobiotic diets to find if there were significant differences between their levels of health and that of the general population. Gruner subjected the participants, who had been practicing a macrobiotic diet for anywhere from nine months to fourteen years, to a battery of physiological tests and found them to be in excellent health.[9]

7. Macrobiotic Diet Reduces Risk of Breast Cancer in Postmenopausal Women
    In a random case control study involving 104 middle-aged women, researchers at the National Tumor Institute in Milan, Italy, reported that a macrobiotic diet could substantially reduce hormonal levels associated with a higher risk of breast cancer.
    The women in the study, aged fifty to sixty-five years, had testosterone levels that were two-thirds or more higher than average and hence put them at elevated risk for breast cancer. All had been postmenopausal for at least two years, had at least one ovary, had not taken hormonal replacement therapy for at least the previous six months, and were not diabetic. None of the women was following a vegetarian, macrobiotic, or other medically prescribed diet.
    The fifty-two women in the intervention group attended macrobiotic cooking classes twice a week for eighteen weeks and were encouraged to cook and eat macrobiotically at home, especially one soy product daily such as miso soup, tofu, or tempeh. Every week the women received whole grains and other products donated by local natural foods manufacturers. During the first month, the women were advised to make dietary changes gradually, but later no advice was given to reduce total food intake or to count calories.
    Prior to the trial, both groups of women received about 37 percent of calories from fat (mainly meat, dairy, and olive oil) and 42 percent from carbohydrate (bread and pasta). The intervention group shifted from animal to vegetable sources, reducing their meat consumption from daily to one to two times a week; dairy was halved, and butter was virtually eliminated. Soy products were consumed on average 1.7 times daily, and sea vegetables used every other day.

Brown rice and other whole grains were consumed 2.5 times per day compared to 0.5 times by controls, and intake of legumes, cruciferous vegetables, and berries were four to eight times higher.

Total cholesterol decreased from 240 to 206 mg/dl compared to 230 in the control group. The intervention group lost more weight, 8.95 pounds (4.06 kilograms) compared to 1.19 pounds (0.54 kilograms) and underwent statistically significant improvements in the five major hormonal and metabolic values associated with breast cancer risk: sex hormone-binding globulin, testosterone, estradiol, fasting insulin, and fasting glycemia. Serum sex hormone-binding globulin levels increased 25.2 percent, while testosterone and estradiol decreased 19.5 percent and 18 percent.

"We observed significant and favorable changes in hormonal indicators of breast cancer risk in a group of postmenopausal women living in northern Italy," the researchers concluded. "These results suggest that the multifactorial dietary intervention applied in this study may prevent breast cancer if continued in the long term." The scientists further noted, "Compared with the usual Western microflora, the gut of macrobiotic or vegetarian subjects may be richer in lactobacilli and bifidobacteria."[10]

8. NIH Best Cases Cancer Study

   In 1992, the National Institutes of Health awarded a grant to the University of Minnesota and the Kushi Institute to compile a Best Cases series of macrobiotic cancer case histories. After advertising in six magazines during the next two years, 233 survivors were identified and sent a Best Case screening questionnaire. One hundred twenty-six responded. Thirty-seven were eliminated due to concurrent use of chemotherapy/radiation; surgical tumor removal; inadequate diagnosis or noncancerous condition; or no clinical follow-up after initial medical therapy.

   Detailed questionnaires and medical record release forms were sent to the remaining 89, and ultimately 77 cases were reviewed. These included cancers of the prostate (20 cases), breast (12 cases), malignant melanoma (8), lymphoma (8), leukemia (6), astrocytoma (5), colorectal (4), endometrium (3), ovary (3), pancreas (3), kidney (2), liver (1), small cell lung (1), multiple myeloma (1), nose plasmacytoma (1), parotic gland (1), sarcoma (1), and small intestine (1).[11]

9. National Cancer Institute Panel Recommends Macrobiotic Studies

   The Cancer Advisory Panel on Complementary and Alternative Medicine (CAPCAM), an expert committee of the National Cancer Institute (NCI), reviewed the cases of six cancer patients who recovered from untreatable cancer with the help of macrobiotics. The cases were drawn from the Macrobiotic Best Case Series undertaken by the University of Minnesota and Kushi Institute described above.

All six persons whose cases were reviewed had been diagnosed with fourth-stage metastasized cancer and attributed their recoveries to following a macrobiotic practice. The CAPCAM review included viewing patient slides and records, hearing expert testimony from a radiologist and pathologist, and listening to an explanation on macrobiotic theory and practice. In addition, three of the six persons whose cases were being reviewed gave personal testimony and answered questions from the panelists. At the end of a daylong rigorous review, the panel of fifteen physicians and scientists voted unanimously to recommend to the NCI that governmental funding be expeditiously provided for new studies on macrobiotics and cancer, including possible clinical trials.

George W. Yu, M.D., a clinical professor of urology at George Washington University Medical Center in Washington, D.C., coordinated the systematized final preparation of medical data for the CAPCAM presentation. As a surgeon, he said that he had noticed the poor survival rate of his patients with invasive bladder cancer. The best chemotherapy results in about a 50 percent partial response and a 10 to 15 percent complete response. His investigation for an alternative approach led him to macrobiotics.

Two of the people whose cancer cases were reviewed have written autobiographies documenting their stories: *Recovery from Cancer* by Elaine Nussbaum, who had terminal uterine cancer, and *When Hope Never Dies* by Marlene McKenna, who had terminal melanoma.

In his newsletter on cancer research, Dr. Ralph Moss, a cancer expert and member of the CAPCAM committee, recounted:

> The members of the panel have displayed an extraordinary degree of expertise in their respective fields. Some are top experts in cancer treatment, diagnostic radiology, tumor pathology and statistics. . . . For the last few years, NCI has been asking alternative practitioners to submit their best cases for evaluation . . . yet surprisingly few alternative practitioners have taken up this challenge.
>
> At this week's session, one group did. This was macrobiotics, presented by the Kushi Institute of Becket, Mass. Macrobiotics is more than a diet. It is a philosophical system based on the idea of achieving a balance. . . .
>
> The session brought forth strong testimony that sometimes the adoption of a macrobiotic diet is followed by the dramatic regression of advanced cancers. A nurse told how, in 1995, she was diagnosed with lung cancer that had

spread all over her body. She received no effective conventional therapy, and reluctantly went on the macrobiotics diet. . . . What makes this case so extraordinary is that her progress was monitored weekly by a sympathetic physician colleague. The shrinkage, and finally the disappearance, of her tumors was documented millimeter by millimeter! She has now been disease-free for over five years.

After this week's meeting I could definitely say there is real gold in macrobiotics. . . . What is needed now is a serious clinical study in patients, using all the resources the NIH can muster. The Kushi Institute deserves credit for having taken these first steps toward documenting its methods and results. An influential government panel is at last listening.[12]

10. University of South Carolina Cancer Study

In a two-year grant sponsored by the Centers for Disease Control and Disease Prevention, the public health arm of the United States, cancer researchers at the School of Public Health, University of South Carolina, investigated the macrobiotic way of life. In a report, "Macrobiotics in the United States: An Assessment of Services and Activities," Sheldon and Guinat Rice interviewed 124 practitioners in forty-four locales. Fifty-one people successfully used macrobiotics to treat cancer, either alone or in combination with conventional medical therapies. Sites included brain, breast, cervical, colon, leukemia, lung, lymphoma, melanoma, multiple sites, ovarian, prostate, skin, and thyroid. Eleven of the people had been told by their doctors that they had terminal cancer for which there was no effective conventional therapy. Ten others felt alienated by the modern medicine they already received or felt that macrobiotics was more appealing. One person observed macrobiotics because of her fear of ordinary treatment and 29 people combined macrobiotics and medical therapy.

"The benefits of macrobiotics for cancer treatment included reduced or eliminated pain and other symptoms, and/or caused the cancer to regress," reported Jane Teas, Ph.D., research assistant professor at the University of South Carolina, the principal investigator. "They were all satisfied with their current health and choice of using macrobiotics to heal. It was our sense that using macrobiotics for these patients provided a sense of personal control that was lacking in conventional medical therapies. The patients accepted that their previous diet was the cause of their cancer and that by changing their diet, the cancer process could be reversed. . . . In the end, these people were alive and well an average of almost 10 years after what each person felt had been a cancer death sentence, and all these people were content with their choices."

The researchers posted a selection of recovery stories from cancer and other chronic diseases on the Internet along with a list of macrobiotic resources, including educational centers, teachers and counselors, and books and other study materials for the use of the general public.[13]

11. M. D. Anderson Review of Macrobiotics and Cancer

Cancer researchers at M. D. Anderson Cancer Center at the University of Texas in Houston posted a historical overview of macrobiotics as a therapy for cancer patients and the general public on their Web site in early 2003. "The macrobiotic diet is part of a way of life that attempts to achieve balance by applying the Oriental principles of yin and yang to the selection of foods. Grains and vegetables are considered to be the ideal center of a diet that also includes beans, fish, fruits, seeds, nuts and condiments. While no foods are actually forbidden, some may be limited in a therapeutic context." The site reviews the Office of Technology Assessment (OTA) study that found macrobiotics to be among the most popular unconventional cancer approaches; the study of the macrobiotic approach to pancreatic cancer at Tulane University; a review of the book *Cancer Free: 30 Who Triumphed Over Cancer Naturally* (New York: Japan Publications, 1991) including prostate cancer (3 cases), melanoma (6), uterus (3), breast (5), stomach, leukemia, and pancreas (2 each), colon (2), astrocytoma, urethra, lung, brain, thyroid, leukemia (CML), bile duct, Hodgkin's disease, and ovarian (1 each); a Best Case series of six medically documented cases: pancreatic metastasized to the liver, malignant melanoma; malignant astrocyoma, endometrial stromal sarcoma; adenocarcinoma of the colon, and abdominal leiomyosarcoma; and other retrospective cohort studies, Best Case series, and case reports.

According to one study (Cassileth, 1984), 63 percent of cancer patients who received some form of dietary therapy received or were exposed to the macrobiotic diet.[14]

12. Macrobiotic Diet Helps Protect Against Breast Cancer

In a follow-up to their earlier macrobiotic study, researchers at the International Agency for Research on Cancer in Lyon, France, and the National Tumor Institute in Milan, Italy, reported that forty-nine women randomly assigned to the experimental diet low in fat and high in complex carbohydrates, dietary fiber, and phytoestrogens showed a significant reduction of body weight, waist circumference, fasting serum levels of testosterone, C peptide, glucose, and insulin, and an increase of serum levels of sex hormone-binding globulin, IGFBP-1, -2, and growth hormone-binding protein compared to controls. The scientists concluded, "This comprehensive dietary intervention strategy proved to be successful in inducing changes in endogenous hormone metabolism that might eventually result in reduced breast cancer risk."[15]

13. Plant-Based Diet Protects Against Breast Cancer Risk
       In another follow-up to their original macrobiotic study, researchers at the National Tumor Institute in Milan, Italy, tested a plant-based diet low in animal fat and rich in polyunsaturated fatty acids on the production of free radicals and high calorie and fat consumption, major risk factors in breast cancer and other diseases. In a random study of 104 postmenopausal women, those assigned to the dietary intervention group ate biweekly meals together for eighteen weeks. At the end of the testing period, the intervention group showed a significant reduction of unhealthy saturated acids and an increase in beneficial polyunsaturated fatty acids. The ratio of omega-3 to omega-6 fatty acids improved 24 percent. The production of free radicals markedly decreased. "The results indicated that a plant-based diet can improve the serum fatty acid profile and decrease ROMs [reactive oxygen metabolites or free radicals] production. These results suggest that a plant-based diet may reduce the body's exposure to oxidative stress."[16]

14. Modified Macrobiotic Diet Protects from Prostate Cancer
       Researchers at Moores Cancer Center, University of California, San Diego, undertook an intervention study of patients with recurrent prostate cancer. In a six-month pilot clinical trial to investigate whether adoption of a modified macrobiotic diet, reinforced by stress management training, could attenuate the rate of further rise of PSA [prostate-specific antigen, a risk factor], fourteen patients with recurrent prostate cancer experienced a significant decrease in the rate of PSA rise. Four of ten evaluable patients experienced an absolute reduction in their PSA levels, and nine of ten had a reduction in their rates of PSA rise and improvement of their PSA doubling times. Mean PSA doubling time increased from 11.9 months to 112.3 months. "These results provide preliminary evidence that adoption of a plant-based diet, in combination with stress reduction, may attenuate disease progression and have therapeutic potential for clinical management of recurrent prostate cancer."[17]

15. Macrobiotic Approach Helps Protect Against Prostate Cancer Recurrence

In a multifaceted dietary intervention conducted by researchers at the School of Medicine, University of California, San Diego, patients and their spouses were encouraged to adopt and maintain a plant-based, modified macrobiotic diet. Median intake of whole grains increased from 1.7 servings a day to 6.9 and 5.0 at three and six months. The rate of PSA rise decreased when compared with the prestudy period after three months and went up slightly from three to six months when whole grain consumption slightly declined. "Changes in the rate of rise in PSA, an indicator of disease progression, were in the opposite direction as changes in the intake of plant-based food groups, raising the provocative possibility that PSA may have inversely tracked intake of these foods and suggesting that adoption of a plant-based diet may have therapeutic potential in the management of this condition," the scientists, led by Gordon Saxe, observed.[18]

SWITCHING TO NATURAL FOODS

Over the last decade, hundreds of thousands of people in the United States, Canada, Europe, Latin America, the Middle East, Australia, and the Far East have adopted the Cancer Prevention Diet and have found it nourishing, satisfying, and delicious. Most people find that soon after changing to whole unprocessed foods, their natural sense of taste returns. After years of eating refined foods and artifically flavored products, our taste buds begin to atrophy, and we forget the rich flavors, subtle aromas, and variety of textures offered by grains and vegetables. Changing to natural foods ultimately results

TABLE 12.   CANCER-INHIBITING SUBSTANCES IN BASIC MACROBIOTIC FOODS

Food	Cancer-Inhibiting Factors
Whole grains	Fiber, protease inhibitors, vitamin E
Beans	Fiber, protease inhibitors, vitamin E
Miso, tofu, tempeh, and other soyfoods	Isoflavones, protease inhibitors, phytosterols, saponins, phytoestrogens
Green leafy vegetables	Beta-carotene and other carotenoid pigments, chlorophyll, fiber, vitamins A, C, and E
Orange-yellow vegetables	Beta-carotene and other carotenoid pigments, fiber, vitamins A and C
Cruciferous vegetables	Indoles, dithiolthiones, glucosinolates, carotenoids

TABLE 13. CANCER, DIET, AND OTHER FACTORS

Cancer	High Risk		Low Risk
	Primary Factors	Contributing Factors	Protective Factors
Bone	Chicken, eggs, hard fat, salted and baked food	Sugar, dairy, stimulants, radiation and electro-magnetic fields, pesticides	Whole grains, beans, green and yellow vegetables, sea vegetables, shiitake mush-rooms, sea salt
Brain (inner regions)	Meat, dairy, poultry, eggs, oily fish	Sugar, oil, fruit, juices, spices, stimulants, drugs, medications, pesticides	Whole grains, beans, green and yellow vegetables, sea vegetables
Brain (outer regions)	Oil, fat, sugar, dairy, spices, soft drinks, chemicals, medi-cations, drugs	Animal food, vinyl chloride and other plastics, synthetic clothing, electro-magnetic fields	Whole grains, beans, green and yellow vegetables, sea vegetables
Breast	Milk, cheese, butter, and other dairy; fat; sugar; oil; white flour; low fiber	Meat, eggs, poultry, spices, soft drinks, drugs, medications, X-rays, mammograms, hair dyes, synthetic clothing, electro-magnetic fields	Whole grains, beans, miso, shoyu, tempeh, tofu, leafy green and white vegetables, sea vegetables, breast-feeding
Children's (leukemia, lymphoma, brain, bone, kidney)	Milk and other dairy, eggs, meat, sugar, sweets	Cold foods, spices, herbs, stimulants, tropical foods, pesticides, tonsil-lectomies, chemicals, radiation, electro-magnetic fields	Whole grains, beans, miso, shoyu, green and yellow vegetables, sea vegetables, breast-feeding
Colon and rectum	Beef, pork, lamb, and other meat; eggs; hard fats; poultry; white flour	Sugar, dairy, oil, spices, soft drinks, beer, chemicals, drugs, medications, sedentary jobs and lifestyle	Whole grains, fiber, beans and lentils, leafy green vegeta-bles, sea vegeta-bles, thorough chewing, exercise
Female reproductive (ovary, uterus, cervix)	Meat, hard fat, eggs, animal protein, dairy, oil	Sugar, white flour, fruit, juices, stimulants, chemicals, birth-control pills, medications, DES (diethylstilbestrol)	Whole grains, beans, green and yellow vegetables, shiitake mushrooms

(continued)

TABLE 13. *(continued)*

Cancer	High Risk		Low Risk
	Primary Factors	Contributing Factors	Protective Factors
Kidney and bladder	Fats, oil, meat, dairy, eggs, sugar	Fruit, juices, spices, soft drinks, stimulants, chemicals, drugs, medications, coffee, chlorinated water, artificial sweeteners, air pollution	Whole grains, lentils and beans, green and yellow vegetables, sea vegetables, spring water
Leukemia	Oil, fat, sugar, soft drinks, stimulants, chemicals	Animal food, fruit, spices, pesticides, radiation, X-rays, industrial pollutants, electromagnetic fields	Whole grains, miso, shoyu, beans, vegetables, sea vegetables, sea salt
Liver	Chicken, eggs, hard fat, cheese, animal protein, oil, white flour	Sugar, spices, dairy, alcohol, pesticides, birth-control pills, drugs, medications	Whole grains, beans, vegetables, sea vegetables, shiitake mushrooms
Lung	Meat, eggs, poultry, cheese, dairy, sugar, oil, white flour	Spices, fruit, stimulants, drugs, smoking, second-hand smoke, air pollution, asbestos	Whole grains, leafy green and yellow vegetables, beans, sea vegetables, fresh air
Lymphatic	Milk and other dairy, sugar, oil, fat, soft drinks, chemicals	Animal food, spices, pesticides, benzene, radiation, X-rays, tonsillectomies	Whole grains, pulses, beans, green and yellow vegetables, seeds, sea vegetables
Male reproductive (prostate, testicular)	Hard fats, meat, eggs, cheese, milk	Oil, dairy, sugar, white flour, fruit, coffee, chemicals, drugs, medications, surgery and radiation	Whole grains, beans, green and yellow vegetables, sea vegetables, shiitake mushrooms
Melanoma	Meat, sugar, poultry, eggs, cheese and other dairy, oil, white flour	Fruit, soft drinks, spices, stimulants, chemicals, medications, PCBs, fluorescent lights	Whole grains, beans, green and yellow vegetables, sea vegetables
Oral and upper digestive tract	Oil, fat, sugar, dairy, spices, chemicals, soft drinks, refined flour and white rice, alcohol	Animal food, especially cured meats, ham, bacon; alcohol; tobacco; radiation	Whole grains, lentils and beans, green and yellow vegetables, sea vegetables

Cancer	High Risk		Low Risk
	Primary Factors	Contributing Factors	Protective Factors
Pancreatic	Meat, eggs, poultry, cheese, fat, oil, sugar	Milk and other dairy, white flour, spices, coffee, tobacco, radiation	Whole grains, beans, green and yellow vegetables, sea vegetables, shiitake mushrooms
Skin	Fat, oil, dairy, white flour, sugar, fruit, juices, spices, soft drinks, chemicals	Animal food, sunlight, industrial pollutants, fluorescent lights, halogen lights, electromagnetic fields	Whole grains, beans, miso, shoyu, vegetables, sea vegetables
Stomach	White rice, white flour, oil, vinegar, MSG, stimulants, alcohol	Animal food, dairy, industrial pollutants	Whole grains, beans, miso, shoyu, leafy green and white vegetables, sea vegetables, ginger
Thyroid	Chicken, poultry, eggs, oily and fatty foods, chemicals, radiation, electro-magnetic fields	Meat, tuna, salmon, sugar, sweets	Whole grains, beans, miso, shoyu, natto, tempeh; kombu, wakame, kelp, and other sea vegetables; sea salt

not only in improved health but also in recovery of our appetite for life itself.

In making the transition from a refined modern diet, it is important to proceed gradually and not try to make the change all at once. Meat and poultry are relatively easy to give up, and most people discover that they have little or no desire to consume them after a few weeks. However, if cravings occur, seitan (wheat meat) or tempeh (soy meat) may be consumed more frequently in such forms as a grain- or soyburger. The wheat or soy meat tastes and looks like hamburger, and many people cannot tell the difference.

Sugar and sweets are usually more difficult to give up than meat. A gradual transition to more natural sweeteners should be made to allow the body to adjust itself to a change in blood sugar levels. First, honey or maple syrup may be substituted for sugar. When balance begins to be restored, after a period of several weeks to several months, the change to the comparatively milder rice syrup, barley malt, or other grain-based sweetener can easily be made. When full health is restored, a single mouthful of food containing sugar, honey, or maple syrup will usually trigger an instant headache or discomfort as the body's natural defense system signals the ingestion of highly imbalanced food. Modern people, however, have consumed so much sugar and sweets over the years (32 teaspoons a day, on average) that their bodies have become dulled to these effects.

For psychological reasons the third category of foods, dairy products, is the most difficult for people to give up. In many cases dairy food was the original food of infants and children for several generations of mothers who avoided breast-feeding. We all have a strong emotional attachment to the food on which we were initially raised. In the case of cow's milk and other dairy products, it often takes a long time for modern people, including otherwise nutritionally aware individuals, to overcome this unconscious dependency. Soy foods and other bean products, which have little saturated fat and no cholesterol, provide an excellent alternative to dairy products. In the natural foods kitchen, a wide variety of homemade foods that have a taste and texture similar to dairy products can be prepared for those in transition, including soy milk, soy ice cream, soy yogurt, tofu cheese, and tofu cheesecake. But be careful to avoid store-bought or commercial soy products like these because they are too lightly processed.

Depending on their condition, cancer patients and other people with serious illnesses may not have time to make this gradual transition and need to adopt a stricter, more medicinal form of the diet immediately. Information on how to accomplish this is presented in subsequent chapters of Part I and in Part II. In order to make a successful change in the way you eat, proper cooking is essential. Everyone, well or sick, is strongly encouraged to learn how to cook from qualified macrobiotic instructors. Until you have actually tasted the full range of macrobiotically prepared foods and seen how they are prepared, you may not fully appreciate the depth and scope of the diet or have a standard against which to measure your own cooking. Cooking is the supreme art, and cookbooks, including this one, can only provide general guidance. You will save yourself endless confusion and mistakes by receiving introductory cooking instruction. Once you have mastered the fundamentals, you can improvise and experiment on your own and ultimately learn to cook with only your intuitive sense of balance as your guide.

6

Yin and Yang in the Development of Cancer

Everything in the universe is eternally changing, and this change proceeds according to the infinite order of the universe. This order of the universe has been discovered, understood, and expressed at different times and places throughout human history, forming the universal and common basis for all great spiritual, philosophical, scientific, medical, and social traditions. The way to practice this universal and eternal order in daily life was taught by Lao-tzu, Confucius, Buddha, Moses, Jesus, Muhammad, and other great teachers in ancient times, and has been rediscovered, reapplied, and taught repeatedly in many lands and cultures over the past twenty centuries.

From observation of our day-to-day thought and activity, we can see that everything is in motion. Everything changes: Electrons spin around a central nucleus in the atom; the Earth rotates on its axis while orbiting the sun; the solar system is revolving around the galaxy; and galaxies are moving away from one another with enormous velocity as the universe continues to expand. Within this unceasing movement, however, an order or pattern is discernible. Opposites attract each other to achieve harmony; the similar repel each other to avoid disharmony. One tendency changes into its opposite, which will return to the previous state. Thus summer changes into winter; youth changes into old age; action changes into rest; the mountain changes into the valley; day changes into night; hate changes into love; the poor change into the rich; civilization rises and falls; life appears and disappears; land changes into ocean; matter changes into energy; space changes into time. These cycles occur everywhere throughout nature and the universe.

Several thousand years ago in China, the universal process of change was called the Tao. Understanding the dynamic nature of reality formed the basis for the *I Ching* or *Book of Changes,* which was studied by thousands of people, including Confucius and Lao-tzu. These two philosophers based their teachings on the underlying principle of yin and yang—the universal laws of harmony and relativity. Thus in most complete translations of the *I Ching,* such as the Wilhelm/Baynes edition, we find the Book of Commentaries, which was added by Confucius, in which he recorded his interpretation of the order of change. Lao-tzu wrote his own interpretation in the *Tao Te Ching,* the central verses of which read:

> *Tao gave birth to One,*
> *One gave birth to Two,*
> *Two gave birth to Three,*
> *Three gave birth to all the myriad things.*
> *All the myriad things carry the Yin on their backs*
> *and the Yang in their embrace,*
> *Deriving their vital harmony from the proper blending*
> *of the two vital Breaths.*

We find the same underlying principles in other Eastern philosophies. For instance, in Hinduism we find Brahman, or the Absolute, differentiating into Shiva and Parvati, the god and goddess whose cosmic dance animates and gives rise to all phenomena in the universe. The same concept is expressed in Shinto in the *Kojiki* or Book of Ancient Matters. In this version of the creation story, Ame-no-minakanushi, or Infinity, gives birth to Takami-musabi and Kamimusubi, or the gods of centrifugality and centripetality, and from these two deities the entire phenomenal universe arose. In Buddhism, the world of change is called *samsara* and is viewed as a revolving wheel turned by the forces of sorrow and compassion. The traditions and legends of most ancient societies, especially myths about twin brothers or brother and sister, all point to the same idea.

In the West, the unifying principle has also been expressed under a multitude of names and forms. In ancient Greece, the philosopher Empedocles held that the universe is the eternal playground of two forces, which he called Love and Strife. Although only fragments of his work survive, we find one passage that reminds us very much of the *Tao Te Ching,* which was composed about the same era:

> *I shall speak a double truth; at times*
> *one alone comes into being;*

at other times, out of one several things grow.
Double is the birth of mortal things and double
  demise . . .
They [Love and Strife] are for ever themselves,
  but running
through each other they become at times different,
  yet are for ever
and ever the same.

In the Old Testament, the rhythmic alternation of complementary energies is often expressed in terms of light and darkness and symbolized in the six-pointed Star of David, showing the balanced intersection of ascending and descending triangles. In the New Testament, we find evidence of an underlying teaching about two interrelated opposites in the story of the Sermon on the Mount, where Jesus feeds the multitude with loaves of barley bread and two small fishes. The fishes can be seen to symbolize the two fundamental energies of the universe whose understanding satisfies our spiritual hunger and confers eternal life. In the recently discovered Gospel according to Thomas, we find further elaboration upon this theme. In this text, Jesus says to his disciples, "If they ask you, 'What is the sign of your Father in you?' say to them: 'It is movement and rest.' "

In more recent times, the unifying principle has been studied and applied, directly and indirectly, by many great philosophers and scientists. In 1790 the English essayist Walking John Stewart observed, "Discover that moral and physical motion have the same double force, centripetal and centrifugal, and that, as the celestial bodies are detained in tranquil orbits . . . so moral bodies . . . move . . . in the orbit of society." In Ralph Waldo Emerson's writings, we find further development of this idea. For example, in his essay "History" he wrote: "As the air I breathe is drawn from the great repositories of nature, as the light on my book is yielded by a star a hundred millions of miles distant, as the poise of my body depends on the equilibrium of centrifugal and centripetal forces, so the hours should be instructed by the ages and the ages explained by the hours. Of the universal mind each individual man is one more incarnation."

Meanwhile, in Europe the German philosopher Hegel postulated that human affairs develop from a phase of unity, which he termed thesis, through a period of disunity, or antithesis, and on to a higher plane of reintegration, or synthesis. Hegel's principle of dialectics was, of course, later studied by Karl Marx and formed the basis of his powerful and often brilliant philosophical speculations in the sphere of politics and economics. Unfortunately, Marx's system remained largely abstract, and he did not apply dialectics to health and many other aspects of daily life.

In the twentieth century, Albert Einstein, among many other scientific thinkers, sensed the complementary antagonism between the visible world of matter and the invisible world of vibration, or energy. Based on this insight, he formulated the universal theory of relativity, in which he stated that energy is constantly changing into matter and matter is continuously becoming energy. The present generation of scientists has discovered the nondual nature of reality under the electron microscope in the double helical structure of DNA. The coiled spirals of chromosomes in the nucleus remind us of the ancient caduceus, the intertwined snake or snakes that have long served as the symbol of Hermes, the god of healing, and the medical profession.

In the social sciences, historian Arnold Toynbee based his study of civilization on the alternating movement of two forces, which he called challenge and response. In one of the early chapters of his multivolume *Study of History,* we read: "Of the various symbols in which different observers in different societies have expressed the alternation between a static condition and a dynamic activity in the rhythm of the Universe, Yin and Yang are the most apt, because they convey the measure of the rhythm directly and not through some metaphor derived from psychology or mechanics or mathematics. We will therefore use these Sinic [Chinese] symbols in this study henceforward."

By whatever name we call them, yin and yang govern all phenomena and produce either an outward or inward movement or tendency. Yin, or outward centrifugal movement, results in expansion, while yang, or inward centripetal movement, produces contraction. We can see these universal tendencies in the human body as the alternating expansion and contraction of the heart and lungs, for example, or in the stomach and intestines during the natural process of digestion. In the areas of astronomy and geophysics, these two forces are manifested as a downward, centripetal, or yang force generated inward to the center of the Earth by the sun, the stars, and far distant galaxies; and an upward, centrifugal, or yin force generated outward due to the rotation of the Earth. All phenomena on the Earth are created and maintained in balance by these two forces, which ancient people universally referred to as the forces of Heaven and Earth.

The classifications shown in Table 14 of the antagonistic and complemental tendencies, yin and yang, show practical examples of these relative forces.

CLASSIFYING FOODS INTO YIN AND YANG

As we saw in an earlier chapter, food is the mode of evolution, the way one species transforms into another. To eat is to take in the whole environment: sunlight, soil, water, and air. The classification of foods into categories of yin and yang is essential for the development of a balanced diet. Different factors in the growth and structure of foods indicate whether the food is predominantly yin or yang:

TABLE 14. EXAMPLES OF YIN AND YANG

	YIN ▼*	YANG Δ*
Attribute	Centrifugal Force	Centripetal Force
Tendency	Expansion	Contraction
Function	Diffusion	Fusion
	Dispersion	Assimilation
	Separation	Gathering
	Decomposition	Organization
Movement	More inactive, slower	More active, faster
Vibration	Shorter wave and higher frequency	Longer wave and lower frequency
Direction	Ascent and vertical	Descent and horizontal
Position	More outward and peripheral	More inward and central
Weight	Lighter	Heavier
Temperature	Colder	Hotter
Light	Darker	Brighter
Humidity	Wetter	Drier
Density	Thinner	Thicker
Size	Larger	Smaller
Shape	More expansive and fragile	More contractive and harder
Form	Longer	Shorter
Texture	Softer	Harder
Atomic particle	Electron	Proton
Elements	N, O, P, Ca, etc.	H, C, Na, As, Mg, etc.
Environment	Vibration ... Air ... Water	... Earth
Climatic effects	Tropical climate	Colder climate
Biological	More vegetable quality	More animal quality
Organ structure	More hollow and expansive	More compacted and condensed
Nerves	More peripheral, orthosympathetic	More central, parasympathetic
Attitude, emotion	More gentle, negative, defensive	More active, positive, aggressive
Work	More psychological and mental	More physical and social
Consciousness	More universal	More specific
Mental function	Dealing more with the future	Dealing more with the past
Culture	More spiritually oriented	More materially oriented

*For convenience, the symbols ▼ for Yin and Δ for Yang are used.

Yin energy creates:

Growth in a hot climate
Foods containing more water
Fruits and leaves
Growth upward, high above the ground
Sour, bitter, sharply sweet, hot, and aromatic foods

Yang energy creates:

Growth in a cold climate
Drier foods
Stems, roots, and seeds
Growth downward, below ground
Salty, plainly sweet, and pungent foods

To classify foods we must see the predominant factors, since all foods have both yin and yang qualities. One of the most accurate methods of classification is to observe the cycle of growth in food plants. During the winter, the climate is colder (yin); at this time of year the vegetal energy descends into the root system. Leaves wither and die as the sap descends to the roots and the vitality of the plant becomes more condensed. Plants used for food and grown in the late autumn and winter are drier and more concentrated. They can be kept for a long time without spoiling. Examples of these plants are carrots, parsnips, turnips, and cabbages. During the spring and early summer, the vegetal energy ascends and new greens appear as the weather becomes hotter (yang). These plants are more yin in nature. Summer vegetables are more watery and perish quickly. They provide a cooling effect, which is needed in warm months. In late summer, the vegetal energy has reached its zenith and the fruits become ripe. They are very watery and sweet and develop higher above the ground.

This yearly cycle shows the alternation between predominating yin and yang energies as the seasons turn. This same cycle can be applied to the part of the world in which a food originates. Foods that find their origin in hot tropical climates where the vegetation is lush and abundant are more yin, while foods originating in northern or colder climates are more yang. We can also generally classify plants according to color, although there are often exceptions, from the more yin colors (violet, indigo, green, and white) through the more yang colors (yellow, brown, and red). In addition, we should also consider the ratio of various chemical components such as sodium, which is yang or contractive, to potassium, which is yin or expansive, in determining the yin/yang qualities of vegetables and other foods.

In the practice of a daily diet, we need to exercise proper selection of the kinds, quality, and volume of both vegetable and animal food. With some minor exceptions, most vegetable food is more yin than animal food because of the following factors:

1. Vegetable species are fixed or stationary, growing in one place, while animal species are independently mobile, able to cover a large space by their activity.

2. Vegetable species universally manifest their structure in an expanding form, the major portion growing from the ground upward toward the sky or spreading over the ground laterally. On the other hand, animal species generally form compact and separate unities. Vegetables have more expanded forms, such as branches and leaves, growing outward, while animal bodies are formed in a more inward direction, with compact organs and cells.

3. The body temperatures of plants are cooler than those of some species of animals, and generally they inhale carbon dioxide and exhale oxygen. Animal species generally inhale oxygen and exhale carbon dioxide. Vegetables are mainly represented by the color green, chlorophyll, while animals are manifested in the color red, hemoglobin. Their chemical structures resemble each other, yet their nuclei are, respectively, magnesium in the case of chlorophyll and iron in the case of hemoglobin.

Although vegetable species are more yin than animal species, there are different degrees even among the same species, and we can distinguish which vegetables are relatively more yin and which are yang. As a general principle, when we use plant foods in the warmer season of the year or in a warmer environment, it is safer to balance these yang factors with vegetables from the yin category. Conversely, when selecting plants in the colder season of the year or in colder regions, we can offset these yin environmental factors with a diet high in vegetable food from the yang category. Food can also be made more yang by increasing the length of cooking as well as increasing other factors such as heat, pressure, and salt.

Thus we are able to classify, from yin to yang to yin, the entire scope of food as well as classify within each category. Generally speaking, animal food is extremely yang; fruits, dairy food, sugar, and spices are extremely yin; and grains, beans, and vegetables are more centered and fall in the middle of the spectrum. Within the category of extreme yang foods, we can further classify from most yang to less yang the following: salt, eggs, meat, poultry, salty cheeses, and fish. In the category of extreme yin, from less yin to most yin, we find milk and other dairy products; tropical vegetables and fruits; coffee and tea; alcohol; spices; honey, sugar, soft drinks, and other sweetened foods; all food prepared with chemicals or artificial additives;

marijuana, cocaine, and other drugs; and most medications. In the center of the spectrum, relative to each other, cereal grains are more yang, followed by beans, seeds, root vegetables, leafy round vegetables, leafy expanded vegetables, nuts, and fruits grown in a temperate climate.

Since we need to maintain a continually dynamic balance and harmony between yin and yang in order to adapt to our immediate environment, when we eat foods from one extreme we are naturally attracted to the other. For example, a diet consisting of large quantities of meats, eggs, and other animal foods, which are very yang, requires a correspondingly large intake of products in the extreme yin category such as tropical fruits, sugar, alcohol, spices, and, in some cases, drugs. However, a diet based on such extremes is very difficult to balance and often results in sickness, which is nothing but imbalance caused by excess of one of the two factors or both.

Among our foods, the cereal grains are unique. As both seed and fruit, they combine the beginning and end of the vegetal cycle and provide the most balanced food for human consumption. It is for this evolutionary reason, as well as their well-balanced nutritional contents and the great ability of cereals to combine well with other vegetables, that whole grains formed the principal food in all previous civilizations and cancer-free societies.

CLASSIFYING DISEASES INTO YIN AND YANG

The principle of yin and yang can also be used to understand the structure of the body and the origin and development of disease. In the human body, for example, the two branches of the autonomic nervous system—the orthosympathetic and parasympathetic—work in an antagonistic yet complementary manner to control the body's automatic functions. The endocrine system functions in a similar way. The pancreas, for example, secretes insulin, which controls the blood sugar level, and also secretes anti-insulin, which causes the level to rise.

Among sicknesses, some are caused by an overly expanding tendency; others result from an overly contracting tendency, while others result from an excessive combination of both. An example of a more yang sickness is a headache caused when the tissues and cells of the brain contract and press against each other, resulting in pain, while a more yin headache arises when the tissues and cells press against each other as a result of swelling or expansion. Therefore, similar symptoms can arise from opposite causes.

Cancer is characterized by a rapid increase in the number of cells and in this respect is a more expansive or yin phenomenon. However, the cause of cancer is more complex. As everyone knows, cancer can appear almost anywhere in the body. Skin, brain, liver, uterine, colon, lung, and bone cancer are just a few of the more common types. Each type has a slightly different cause. To better understand this, let us consider the difference between prostate and breast cancer, both of which are increasing in incidence. Recently, female hormones have been used to control prostate cancer temporarily. At the same time, a male hormone has been found to have a similar controlling effect with breast cancer. Suppose, however, that female hormones were given to women with breast cancer. This would cause their cancers to develop more rapidly, while male hormones would accelerate the growth of prostate cancer. Therefore, women who have taken birth-control pills containing estrogen have a higher risk of developing breast cancer.

As we can see in the above example, breast and prostate cancer have opposite causes. Since more yin female hormones help neutralize prostate cancer, we can assume that this condition is caused by an excess of yang factors. Since breast cancer can be temporarily neutralized by more yang male hormones, this disorder has an opposite, or more yin, cause. In general, there are two types of cancer, which we can classify according to cause. The first results from excess consumption of foods in the extreme yang category, including eggs, meat, fish, poultry, condensed types of dairy food such as cheese, other salty foods, and baked flour products. The second type of cancer is caused by excessive intake of foods in the extreme yin category, including soft drinks, sugar, milk and ice cream, citrus fruit, stimulants, chemicals, refined flour, spices, and foods containing chemicals and artificial additives.

In general, if the cancer appears in the deeper or lower parts of the body or involves the more compact organs, it is caused by the overconsumption of yang foods. Yin cancers usually develop at the peripheral or upper parts of the body or in the more hollow, expanded organs. However, this classification is not absolute. Although cancer arises as the result of a predominance of one factor or another, the opposite factor is also involved, though to a lesser degree. For example, cancers resulting from the overconsumption of yang foods also require an intake of extreme yin, since this provides the stimulus for tumor growth.

Thus, among the Inuit, whose diet consists largely of meat and fish, cancer was unknown until sugar and other refined products of modern civilization were introduced. The inclusion of these extremely yin items provided the necessary stimulus for their normally very yang diet to lead to the formation of a variety of malignant tumors.

Also, regions within each organ of the body have a more yin or more yang nature. For example, the stomach as a whole is classified as a yin organ because it is relatively hollow and expanded in comparison, say, to the pancreas, which is tight and compact. However, the stomach can be divided into the more expanded upper region, which secretes a strong acid (more yin), and the more compact lower region, which secretes a much weaker acid (less yin). The upper portion of the stomach known as the body is more yin, while the lower pylorus is more yang in structure. Cancers that appear in the upper stomach region result from the intake of foods such as sugar, MSG, white rice, white flour, and other extremely yin products; those tumors that develop in the pylorus result from the overconsumption of meat, eggs, fish, and other

TABLE 15.   GENERAL YIN AND YANG CLASSIFICATION OF CANCER SITES

More Yin Cancer	Combination of Both	More Yang Cancer
Brain (outer regions)	Bladder/kidney	Bone
Breast	Leukemia (some cases)	Brain (inner regions)
Esophagus	Liver	Colon
Hodgkin's disease	Lung	Ovary
Leukemia (most cases)	Lymphoma (some cases)	Pancreas
Lymphoma (most cases)	Melanoma	Prostate
Mouth (except tongue)	Spleen	Rectum
Skin	Stomach (lower)	
Stomach (upper)	Thyroid	
Testicular	Tongue	
	Uterus	

extremely yang products combined together with yin substances. Since these more yin foods are consumed widely in Japan, the people in that nation have a very high incidence of stomach cancer. Cancers of the large intestine, rectum, prostate, and ovaries, resulting from the intake of more yang foods including saturated fat, are predominant in the United States, where more red meat and other animal foods are consumed. Other cancers, such as those of the lung, kidney, bladder, and more centrally located organs, are usually caused by a combination of extreme yin and extreme yang foods, though more yang foods are the primary cause. Table 15 shows common varieties of cancer and their general classification according to yin and yang. It should be kept in mind that different parts of each organ—for example, the upper or lower part, the expanded or condensed part, the peripheral or central part, the ascending or descending part—differ respectively in their degree of yin and yang owing to various combinations of yin foods and yang foods.

To help offset the development of cancer, it is important to center the diet and avoid foods from both the extreme yin and yang categories. A more centrally balanced diet based on foods such as whole grain cereals, beans, and cooked vegetables can help protect against and relieve cancers caused by either more yin or yang factors. This does not mean, however, that the same dietary program should be adopted in every case. For a person in good health, the Cancer Prevention Diet allows a wide variety of foods and cooking styles to be selected according to several different factors, including personal needs and enjoyment. For persons with cancer or a serious precancerous condition, a stricter diet needs to be followed at first until vitality is restored, and then gradually more and more foods can be added for variety.

7

Relieving Cancer Naturally

In treating illness with dietary methods, it is important that the sickness be properly classified as predominantly yin or yang, or sometimes as a combination of both extremes. This is especially true with a life-threatening disease such as cancer. Once the determination is made, dietary recommendations can be more specifically aimed at alleviating the particular condition of excess.

Location of the tumor in the body generally determines whether a cancer is more yin or yang. In some cases, however, as we have seen, cancer in a specific organ can take either a yin or a yang form. In the case of a predominantly yang cancer, the general Cancer Prevention Diet should be followed, slightly modified so as to accentuate more yin factors. The reverse is true in the case of more yin cancers. The standard diet should be followed and partially adjusted to emphasize more yang factors. For cancers caused by both extremes, a central way of eating is recommended. In all cases, however, all overly expansive and overly contractive food should be strictly avoided since these items initially caused the cancer to appear.

By centering the diet and, if necessary, making nutritional adjustments emphasizing the complementary opposite quality, healthy balance can be restored. This commonsense method underlies traditional healing and medicine in both East and West. For example, in Hippocrates' *The Nature of Man,* we read: "Diseases caused by overeating are cured by fasting; those caused by starvation are cured by feeding up. Diseases caused by exertion are cured by rest; those caused by indolence are cured by exertion. To put it briefly: the physician should treat disease by the principle of opposition to the cause of the disease according to its form, its seasonal and age incidence, countering tenseness by relaxation, and vice versa. This will bring the patient most relief and seems to me to be the principle of healing."

In treating illness, the Hippocratic writings employ a variety of polarities and relativities to describe the organs of the body, the different foods that relieve illnesses, and varying human constitutions and conditions. These include strong/weak, fierce/tame, and elongated/hollow.

Over the last twenty-five hundred years, the unifying principle has gradually disappeared from the Western scientific and medical vocabulary as ever smaller fragments of reality have been discovered under the magnifying glass and the microscope. Diseases are no longer looked at as wholes or parts of larger systems, but are broken down into cellular components. Instead of seeing sickness as a form of healthy adjustment, modern medicine sees health and disease as deadly enemies to one another. Instead of seeing that disease develops in one of two fundamentally different directions, modern medicine categorizes sickness into thousands of unrelated subgroupings and symptoms.

A failure to understand the distinction between the general tendencies of yin and yang illnesses explains why some people experience serious side effects from certain medications and others do not. It also explains why so many nutritional therapies and popular health diets produce mixed results or fail entirely. Vitamin C, for instance, is a yin substance that can benefit people with a cold caused by overconsumption of contractive yang foods. However, vitamin C taken in supplement form rather than in daily whole foods can further weaken persons with a cold caused by intake of excessive yin because it contributes further expansive energy to their system.

Across-the-board recommendations to take vitamin X, drug Y, or food Z to prevent or relieve cancer do not take into account the two opposite forms that illness may take. Nor do they always make room for differing human constitutions and conditions and varying geographical, social, and personal factors. Modern science is justified in rejecting alternative cancer remedies that ignore these variables. On the other hand, holistic medicine is correct in questioning modern science for focusing on quantity rather than quality. Eating whole foods containing vitamin C, such as broccoli, produces a different effect on the body than taking vitamin C pills, even though the actual amount of the nutrient may be the same.

DIETARY CONSIDERATIONS

On the whole, dietary suggestions should be directed primarily toward restoring the individual's excessively yin or yang condition to one that is less extreme. Signs of an overly yin condition include passivity, negativity, and shy-

TABLE 16. SELF-EVALUATION OF
HEALTH CONDITION

Too Yin	Too Yang
Passive	Aggressive
Overly relaxed	Overactive
Depressed, sad	Angry, irritable
Negative, retreating	Attacking, intolerant
Self-pity	Self-pride
Voice too soft, timid	Voice too loud, tense
Loose muscles	Tense muscles
Moist skin	Dry skin

ness, while signs of an overly yang condition include hyperactivity, aggression, and loudness (see Table 16). Once a more natural, balanced condition has been established and stabilized, the person's body will no longer need to accumulate toxic excess in the form of cancer. If we keep this holistic view in mind, we can avoid being caught up in an endless maze of symptoms.

If there is any uncertainty about whether the cause of a cancer is more yin or yang, we can safely recommend the central Cancer Prevention Diet, which minimizes both tendencies.

Since cancer is a disease of excess, someone with cancer should be careful not to overeat. To prevent this, two important practices are advised. The first is to chew very well, at least fifty and preferably one hundred times per mouthful, until the food becomes liquefied. A person may eat as much food as he or she wants, provided it is well chewed and thoroughly mixed with saliva. Proper chewing releases an important enzyme in the mouth, which is essential for digestion.

The second point of caution is not to eat for at least three hours before going to bed. Food eaten during that time often becomes surplus and will serve to accelerate indigestion, gas, mucus and fat formation, and enhance the development of cancer. Regarding liquid intake, the individual should drink moderately and only when thirsty.

For both yin and yang cancers, all intake of fatty animal foods, including meat, eggs, poultry, and dairy food, and other oily, greasy foods (including those of vegetable quality) should be strictly avoided. A person with more yin cancer, however, may have a very small quantity of fish once or twice a week if he or she craves it. In such instances, cooking a small portion of dried fish in a soup may be appropriate. A person with yang cancer should stay away from all animal food, including fish, at least for the initial period of a few months. In both cases, nuts and nut butters should be avoided or limited because they are very oily and contain excess protein. It is also advisable for an individual with a more yin cancer to avoid or limit fruit and dessert completely. A person with a more yang cancer may occasionally have small amounts of cooked, dried, and, in some cases, fresh fruit, but only when craved.

The cooking of vegetables is slightly different for yin and yang cancers. In the case of yang cancer, one advisable method is to chop the vegetables while bringing water to a boil; add the vegetables to the boiling water for a few minutes or just one minute, then remove; a small amount of shoyu may be added for taste. Another method is to sauté the vegetables quickly for about two to three minutes on a high flame, adding a pinch of sea salt. These styles of cooking will preserve the crispness, freshness, and slightly more yin qualities of the vegetables. For yin cancer, vegetables should be cooked in a slower, longer, and more thorough manner, and shoyu or miso seasoning may be a little stronger. An emphasis on green leafy vegetables such as watercress or kale produces a slightly more yin effect; an emphasis on root vegetables such as carrots or turnips will produce a slightly more yang effect; an emphasis on round vegetables such as onions or acorn squash will result in a slightly more centered effect.

As for daily beverages, there are now several varieties of bancha tea available in natural food and health food stores, including green tea, usual bancha tea, and bancha twig tea. Bancha twig tea is also commonly known as kukicha tea. All are produced from the same tea bush. Green tea is harvested in the summer and consists of the green leaves taken from the upper parts of the bush. However, some leaves are left on the plant until fall, at which time they become harder, drier, and darker in color. These leaves are used to produce the usual bancha tea. Bancha stem tea is made from the branches and stems of the plant, which are then dry-roasted. More yin green tea contains plenty of vitamin C and can be used to help offset the toxic effects resulting from the overconsumption of animal foods, while more yang bancha stem tea contains less vitamin C but plenty of calcium and minerals. It is advisable for all cancer patients to use bancha stem tea (kukicha) as their usual beverage. However, persons with more yang cancers may occasionally use the green tea from time to time for a short duration only. Green tea is not recommended for persons with other types of cancer. Of course, dyed black tea and aromatic herbal teas, especially those that have been cultivated and processed chemically, are not recommended for use even by healthy persons.

Among some daily condiments such as gomashio (sesame salt) or umeboshi salt plums, slight adjustments in use may also need to be made depending upon the form of cancer. The specific dietary recommendations for each major form of cancer are listed in detail in Part II and recipes and sample menus are provided in Part III.

GUIDELINES FOLLOWING MEDICAL TREATMENT AND NUTRITIONAL SUPPLEMENTS

Based on medical advice, some people may choose to treat their cancer with surgery, chemotherapy, radiation treatment, hormone treatment, or vitamin or mineral supplementation, as well as observe the approach presented in this book. In other cases, some people may have had medical treatment or nutritional supplementation prior to starting macrobiotics. In such cases, the following general principles may be followed:

1. Surgery: In case of surgery, the standard dietary recommendations for each particular form of cancer listed in Part II may be followed, including the use of oil for sautéing, unyeasted whole grain bread, and cooked fruits several times a week. Since surgery is usually weakening, kombu tea can be taken following the operation three to four times a week for about three weeks and then occasionally as needed. Ume-sho-kuzu drink may also be taken two to three times a week for about three weeks and then as needed in order to develop strength. As an external application, a kombu plaster may be prepared and placed over the scar to help the healing process.

2. Chemotherapy: Chemotherapy is very yangizing. Strong drugs are used to shrink or dissolve the tumor, and the body as a whole tends to lose moisture, dry out, and contract. To balance this treatment, it is important that the dietary guidelines encompass a variety of foods, including lighter cooking. Steamed greens and boiled salad should be prepared daily or often. To normalize white blood cell counts, fish can be eaten twice a week. Carp and burdock soup (koi koku), which is very good for this purpose, can be prepared and served three times over a ten-day period: one bowl a day for three days, then repeated a week later, followed by one more series of one bowl for three days after another week. Mochi is also strengthening and may be taken two to three times a week, prepared in the usual way or added to soup. Kinpira soup is also very strengthening, especially for those who don't eat fish.

   Sweets are often craved following chemotherapy. Sweet vegetable drink may be taken daily or every other day during or following chemotherapy. Fresh carrot juice may be taken two to three times a week, and fruits can also be consumed two to three times a week, cooked, dried, or occasionally raw. Amasake and grain-based sweeteners such as barley malt or rice syrup may also be taken to satisfy a sweet craving.

3.   Radiation therapy: Radiation has a very yinnizing effect. It is espe-
     cially important to avoid raw salad and too much fruit and juice.
     Steamed greens and boiled salad may be prepared daily or often. Oil
     should be minimized during or following radiation treatment, though
     several times a week a small volume of oil may be brushed on the
     skillet in cooking, following the guidelines in the chapters that follow.
     Sweet vegetables may be eaten daily, though in small volume. For
     strength, ume-sho-kuzu drink may be prepared three times a week
     for about three weeks and then occasionally as needed.

     A kombu plaster may be placed over the irradiated part of the
     body for ten days to two weeks to facilitate healing. As an alterna-
     tive, a green chlorophyll plaster may be used instead.

4.   Hormone therapy: Hormone therapy can have either strong yin or
     yang effects depending on the treatment. Some medications such as
     tamoxifen, used to treat breast cancer in women, give strong yang
     results. Others, including some estrogen treatments given to men
     with prostate cancer, are very yin.

     There is no particular special drink, dish, or home care remedy
     recommended for counteracting the effects of hormone therapy. Gen-
     erally, it is advisable to limit hormone treatment, usually taking it
     for not longer than six months. The amount of the dose can also be
     controlled. Moderate doses produce longer, more gradual effects
     than high doses aimed at immediate relief.

5.   Supplements: Mineral supplements are usually recommended by the
     doctor according to the blood condition. If the blood is normally bal-
     anced, such supplements are not necessary. However, abnormal con-
     ditions sometimes arise in the course of illness, including anemia or
     lack of iron in the blood, prolonged or heavy bleeding, and others. In
     such cases, mineral supplements based on blood analyses and car-
     ried out under medical supervision may be needed. There is no spe-
     cial macrobiotic approach to adjusting or modifying the diet in cases
     of supplementation.

6.   Vitamins: In the event of general fatigue or lack of vitality, the condi-
     tion may temporarily be improved by use of vitamin supplements.
     However, their use should not be continued indefinitely. In general,
     we recommend that vitamins be consumed primarily in natural form
     in whole foods or (in the case of vitamin D) through outdoor activi-
     ties in the sunshine. In some cases, however, vitamin or mineral sup-
     plements may be taken over a period of one month to several months
     until the general condition improves, together with proper lifestyle
     and dietary practice. Generally, vitamins and supplements should be

of the highest quality, made from organically grown ingredients, and as a rule be all plant (or vegan) quality. Many supplements include animal products that may not be clearly labeled, or may come in capsules made of animal-based gelatin or include genetically modified ingredients. Be careful and don't hesitate to inquire about ingredients. If negative effects come, discontinue and seek another source.

8

The Role of the Emotions in the Development of Cancer

by Anna Böhm

THE ORIGIN OF THE EMOTIONS

Emotional expression is by no means solely up to the individual. It is conditioned by cultural precepts and proscriptions, as we shall see below. First, let's make clear what an emotion is. An emotion is the manifestation of change or movement in the living world. The word *emotion* comes from *agitation,* so it means to put something in motion, into movement. Physiologically, the source of the emotions is in the region of our brain called the *amygdale*. The role of the amygdale is to regulate our emotions and to control emotional memory. The activation of any emotion is related to our way of living and our way of relating to our environment. As we all know, psychologically human beings cannot live without relations to other human beings.

Emotions are first of all internal, and they generate an external reaction. Different situations and the interpretation of these contexts activate the emotions. There is a difference between "sensation" and emotion. Sensation is related directly to bodily processes such as the sensation of temperature. Sensation is also directly associated with sensorial perception. There is also a difference between emotion and "feeling," because feeling is not a reaction "to something," but the accumulation of feelings could lead to an emotion. Emotions may be understood as a change in fluctuation in one or more of five different organic systems: (1) the cognitive system, (2) the neuropsychological system, (3) the motor system, (4) the motivational system, and (5) the senso-rial system. These systems (which function according to the four humors or elements of Greek philosophy and the five stages of transformation in Chi-nese philosophy and medicine, as noted below) work in an independent and at the same time synchronistic way to respond to external or internal stimu-lations and help maintain the organism's central or primary health and well-being.

Ultimately, it is very difficult to give an exact definition for the origin of emotions, especially something so personal and private that makes human beings so funny, wonderful, crazy, and mysterious. We all know how diffi-cult it is to express our emotions—for example, voicing love, the most sub-lime human emotion, and saying the three words "I love you."

Let us take a look now at the history of the emotions and the first "thinkers" to speak about them. The earliest record of ancient thought dates back to between 4000 B.C. and 800 B.C. Psychological insight on our ances-tors' understanding of emotion comes from Homer's writing in the *Iliad* and the *Odyssey*. By this time, living was attributed to three processes. First came "Menos," the process shared by all living things. It was the source of action not only in humans and animals but also in rivers and wind. Then there was "Thymos," the locus of feelings and emotions, wishes, plans, and hopes. Thy-mos directed the vitality of Menos, which was impulsive thought, and as the "source of action" gave rise to the passions. The third was "Noos," the pro-cess of understanding, but there are no surviving concrete concepts or ex-amples. With Menos, Thymos, Noos, and Psyche (or Soul, a fundamental concept in Greek thought) we have a sophisticated motivational and intel-lectual system, and also one that differentiates between humans and other creatures.

Other schools of thought subsequently developed, including rationalism associated with Parmenides, empiricism associated with Xenophanes, ideal-ism associated with Plato, and realism associated with Aristotle. These thinkers viewed life in terms of dual energies (described variously as Form and Matter, or Body and Mind) that interacted in complementary/antagonistic ways.

The Four Humors (Hippocrates' Vision)

The history of cancer goes back twenty-five hundred years to ancient Greece, where Hippocrates first identified and described the illness. In Greek the word *karkinos*, from which our word *cancer* comes, originally meant "crab." The Father of Western Medicine evidently chose the image be-cause of the disease's crablike spread through the body.

In the ancient world, nutritional therapy formed the core of medical un-derstanding and practice. Hippocrates' writings are permeated with dietary considerations, and he frequently emphasizes the importance of wheat and barley, the two principal grains of the Hellenistic world. "I know too that the

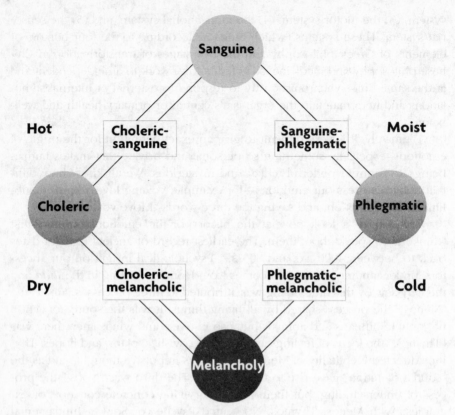

body is affected differently by bread according to the manner in which it is prepared," he explains in *Tradition in Medicine.* "It differs according as it is made from pure flour or meal with bran, whether it is prepared from winnowed or unwinnowed wheat, whether it is mixed with much water or little, whether well mixed or poorly mixed, overbaked or underbaked, and countless other points besides. The same is true of the preparation of barley meal. The influence of each process is considerable and each has a totally different effect from another. How can anyone who has not considered such matters and come to understand them possibly know anything of the diseases that afflict mankind? Each one of the substances of a man's diet acts upon his body and changes it in some way and upon these changes his whole life depends."

In treating serious illnesses in the fifth century B.C., Hippocrates stressed the importance of using dietary methods. In *The Book on Nutriment* he declares: "Let food be thy medicine and medicine thy food." The Hippocratic Oath, still taken by modern medical doctors, states in part: "I will apply dietetic measures for the benefit of the sick according to my ability and judgment; I will keep them from harm and injustice. I will neither give a deadly drug to anybody if asked for it, nor will I make a suggestion to this effect. . . . I will not use the knife." His favorite remedy was cooked whole grain barley cereal. He hailed this broth as "smooth, consistent, soothing; slippery and fairly soft; thirst-quenching and easily got rid of; doesn't produce constipation or rumbling or swell up the stomach." He described various ways that the barley meal could be modified for different illnesses, and he supplemented dietary adjustments with simple, safe compresses made of grains, vegetables, and herbs, which could be prepared in the home. In the case of cancer, he warned against surgery: "If treated, the patients die quickly; but if not treated, they hold out for a long time."

In the twenty-five hundred years since cancer was first described in ancient Greece, medicine has come full circle. In *Epidemics*, Book I, Hippocrates cited factors for the physician to consider in making diagnoses and recommending treatment. At the head of the list comes "what food is given to him [the patient] and who gives it," followed by conditions of the climate and local environment, and the patient's customs, mode of life, pursuits, age, speech, mannerisms, silences, thoughts, sleeping patterns, and dreams. Last on the list is physical symptoms.

An elder contemporary of Hippocrates, Alcmaeon of Croton, started a trend in medicine that was divorced from supernatural and irrational aspects of temple healing. He concluded that perception and the soul resided in the brain, and he recognized thinking and perceiving as separate processes. Influenced by Hippocrates, he taught that health is a matter of equilibrium, balancing forces within the body. Alcmaeon wrote works on the diagnosis of disease and on the art of healing.

Objecting to earlier medicine as overly rationalistic, Alcmaeon developed the model of the "humors." According to this view, the universe is composed of air, earth, fire, and water, and these take bodily form in the humors. The four humors were nutritive fluids or energies that included blood, black bile, yellow bile, and phlegm. The humors gave rise to psychological tendencies. Persons with strong phlegm tended to be unemotional. Those with enhanced blood were cheerful. Yellow bile in excess led to a quick temper, while black bile manifested as sadness. When the humors were not in balance, a person would become sick and remain that way until balance was restored.

The Hippocratic school adopted this view, and its therapy was directed at restoring the humoral balance, an approach with clear parallels to the yin/yang system. It was Theophrastus (the successor of Aristotle), among others, who developed a set of correspondences based on the humors, and it dominated medical practice through the neoclassical revival in Europe. Hence, the primary contribution to the influence of "emotions" on health originated with the Hippocratic humoral system.

Experiencing the Emotions

Now let's turn to the emotions themselves and their real influence on health and well-being. First, let's be clear about what kind of emotions we are talking about and their influence because they are so hard to define. Among the questions we will consider are these: Can cancer arise from the emotions and from an "imbalance" among them? If so, what kind of emotions can create cancer, and what kinds of cancer are most susceptible to emotional influence? We will answer these questions with knowledge from the psychological domain because this is the discipline that integrates Body (organism) and Mind (psyche). Psychology, in turn, finds its foundation in philosophy. Once again, this leads us back to ancient Greece and Hippocrates, who postulated that illness does not come from nature but from an inner imbalance. And that imbalance among the four bodily humors leads directly to a consideration of the emotions.

According to behaviorist John B. Watson, emotions are like hereditary reaction patterns formed directly after birth. He makes a comparison between the forger working with metal and the formation of emotional patterns. The forger can form the metal with a hammer in different ways, lightly or strongly, depending on his goal or imagination. In the same way we start to form the emotional life of our children immediately after their birth. In this comparison the forger has a big advantage because if he makes a mistake, he can reheat the metal and start over again. We don't have that opportunity in the life of our child. Every "beat," good or bad, leaves an indelible impression. The three main emotions are happiness, anxiety, and anger. These influence our decisions and command our attention, often leading to regrettable actions. In the agony of passion, for example, we can easily lose our head.

The Evolutionary History of the Emotions

The emotions have an evolutionary history. As humans developed physically, mentally, and socially, the emotions also became more and more sophisticated. Psychology, as we know it, didn't suddenly appear on the intellectual scene. It is impossible to say just when it began or who was responsible for it. Instead, we can only point to a number of currents that take us from philosophy and the natural sciences into something recognizably psychological. Often there was some misunderstanding between philosophers and the first psychological thinkers or creators. The philosophers stated unequivocally that psychology could never be a science. The activities and the contents of the mind could not be measured, and therefore an objectivity such as that achieved in physics and chemistry was out of reach. Psychology would forever remain subjective!

Psychology is the scientific study of mental processes and behavior. Psychologists observe and record how people and other animals relate to one another and to the environment. They look for patterns that will help them understand and predict behavior, and they use scientific methods to test their ideas. Through such studies, psychologists have learned much that can help people fulfill their potential as human beings and increase understanding among individuals, groups, nations, and cultures. Psychology is a broad field that explores a variety of questions about thoughts, feelings, and actions. Psychologists ask such questions as these: How do we see, hear, smell, taste, and feel? What enables us to learn, think, and remember, and why do we forget? What activities distinguish human beings from other animals? What abilities are we born with, and which must we learn? How much does the mind affect the body, and how does the body affect the mind? For example, can we change our heart rate or temperature just by thinking about doing so? What can our dreams tell us about our needs, wishes, and desires? Why do we like the people we like? Why are some people bashful and others not shy at all? What causes violence? What is mental illness, and how can it be cured?

The research findings of psychologists have greatly increased our understanding of why people behave as they do. For example, psychologists have discovered much about how personality develops and how to promote healthy development. They have some knowledge of how to help people change bad habits and how to help students learn. They understand some of the conditions that can make workers more productive. A great deal remains to be discovered. Nevertheless, insights provided by psychology can help people function better as individuals, friends, family members, and workers.

In the beginning, the main occupation of human beings was survival. In *Why Men Don't Listen and Women Can't Read Maps,* Allan and Barbara Pease summarize seven years' research, interviewing experts and presenting a comprehensive study of the profound communication differences between men and women. They tell us a kind of evolutionary story of male and female emotions, explaining from where the main differences between the sexes originated. The main role of the men was to care for the sustenance and the security of the household, while the main role of the woman was to care for the family, namely, the children and the home or originally the cave. It seems the same role partition still holds today.

Most important, the Peases show that emotions reflect the world we live in. In today's modern world, people are very focused on their emotional condition or state. In a way everything depends on the emotions or is related to them. Take health and happiness. The mass media focus on the well-being of the population, but the hidden goal is profit. Hence, we are educated from the beginning to live a life of endless consumption. The problem is that once our immediate needs are met, there are many other things we require, so we forget what we really need. Our society presents an image of happiness and affluence which changes so constantly that the little human remains lost in the knowledge of what he really wants. In psychology we say that the human being is forever unsatisfied. If humans were truly satisfied, they would be dead for all intents and purposes because they would require nothing more. The quest for satisfaction enables human beings to be active and motivated. If we always get what we want, there would be no more reason to live. Our consumer society knows this very well, so it lets us believe that we constantly need to consume objects to be happy. Many of the illnesses of modern society, such as depression, anorexia, toxic dependence, insomnia, obsessions, and many more, are what Freud called "the psychological problems of everyday life." These problems are created by society when people start thinking that if they don't have or can't afford what is expected or advertised, they are not good enough, successful enough, or "normal." Nearly every image we see inspires us to material gratification and possessing the newest, latest, most desirable products and services. In this way, we are told, we will find happiness and satisfaction. Of course, this is an artificial image. True happiness does not depend on money or excessive material comfort but on spiritual riches such as sincerity, truth, modesty, compassion, and love.

THE EMOTIONS AS A FORM OF ENERGY

Can cancer arise from the emotions or an imbalance among them? Any imbalance of mood can lead to dis-ease and eventually illness. First of all, we have to consider the emotions as a form of energy. Everything is made of energy, and some things can give us energy and others take it away. This was common knowledge in traditional cultures and societies, and is the way of thinking and the lifestyle of macrobiotic people today. The energy of food, for example, can be looked at in terms of yin and yang nutriments. If we eat too yang, we get contracted and may become impatient and angry. If we eat too yin, we may lose our focus and concentration. In this way we try to moderate our intake and remain as balanced as possible. It means always harmonizing with the situation. If you are tired, you can't ask as much of yourself as when you are active. Even reading this chapter may be difficult for some people because of the thoughts and feelings it raises. But it is hoped that it will help you understand your own emotions.

Emotions are the predominant form of human energy. They keep us alive and strongly influence our health. They are indispensable to life. Many people don't believe in the power of the emotions when it comes to illness, yet they are the first ones to call if they have emotional problems and talk about relationships and love. We don't consider the emotions when we are ill because modern education teaches us that everything we cannot see and categorize does not exist. Our fears also play a role. On the other hand, if we think in terms of limitless energy and the world of spirits and the supernatural, the world seems very large, and there is nothing we can firmly believe in. In both cases we feel insecure and lose our normal perception. We must find a way to see the world in a much wider way without feeling overwhelmed and lost. Looking at the emotions from three perspectives—those of feeling, understanding, and letting go of negative attitudes and beliefs—may help us gain insight into the nature of health and sickness.

The Nature of Feelings

Emotions are creating feelings. When we start to learn language, we also start to express our feelings in words. We can say when it hurts and where it hurts, while before we were just crying, hoping that our parents or others would understand what was the matter. But in learning language we learn also to share our thinking, our feelings, and our emotions. At the same time that we learn what is right and wrong, we learn which emotions or feelings we have the right to express and which ones are forbidden. Forbidden means that these emotions are very personal, and in giving voice to these "forbidden" feelings, we may be excluded from society. As a result, we learn that it would be better to keep them to ourselves and not tell them to others. Here the first suppression of our emotions starts and integration into the social world begins, where there are rules that we have to respect. For example, there are rules about not expressing some emotions or at least not showing them to others. The modern world in which we live is actually very cruel. At most, many of the emotions we feel so strongly can be shared with others only halfway. This creates tension and conflicts in the body. In psychology the first "emotional trauma" is called the Oedipus complex. In this phase we learn to understand the rules about expressing our positive feelings in a way that is acceptable to our society. The little boy learns that he cannot love his mother in the same way that his father does, and the daughter learns she cannot love her father the same way that her mother does. We learn to know our place in the family, assuming everything is going and functioning well. In childhood there are many situations where we start to suppress our emotions for the goal of socialization. There is a fine balance here. In order to live together, we all need to follow the same rules to some extent. However, in the modern world the focus is so outwardly directed to adjusting to society's expectations that we forget to care about our inner balance and needs.

Since we don't know what to do when we can't express ourselves, we just suppress everything (especially what society considers "forbidden") and try to find other ways to make ourselves feel good. Modern society is built on this alienation from ourselves and from our feelings. As a substitute we are brought up to consume material things that will give us pleasure and happiness. Also, recreational drug consumption, sexual relations without feeling, excessive partying, and other indulgences make us believe for a short time that we are happy and contented. Such masked pleasure only allows us to escape from our real needs. By tolerating if not encouraging such practices, society lets us believe we can find happiness, and we forget our real needs and dreams. As a result, we live in a veiled world, and from the beginning until the end of our lives we pretend to be someone else. We are afraid to show our true face, feelings, and thinking. This is what we are taught, and this is how we have to behave in order to be an accepted member of our wonderful society. One small and fleeting pleasure is followed by another just because of the fear that we have internalized and that governs social relations. If we started to express our real needs, we would no longer support a society based on endless consumption. Hence, in "everyday life," no one speaks about his or her real problems, real feelings, or what is truly on one's mind.

We are born alone in the sense that each of us is unique. No one else is exactly like us, has the same feelings, or sees things in the same way. That's what makes life so beautiful and humans so intelligent. Because of our education we only really say what we mean on rare occasions. For the most part we will die alone because we will take all the things that we learned are forbidden to say with us into the next life (if we believe in one). That is why we can say that we live in a "cruel little world"; it is because we are unable to express our true selves and unable to leave our "masked" life. We are afraid to reveal our real selves to one another. Unmasked, we could just be as we are and live together in an open-minded, easy, and simple way.

We want all the time for "others" to love us and, as a great deal of research has shown, to be accepted by the group. From an evolutionary view of love, acceptance, or membership in a group, tribe, or community, our ancestors' primary goal was to find security. And this involved continually creating objects for making life more comfortable with the aim of giving love or security to one's "family" or wife, husband, or friends. Over time we learned to be more and more "educated" and to act in a more structured way. We created more and more rules and laws to govern social behavior. And now, in our world today, we are confronted with cancer and other diseases that have spread to every country, developed and undeveloped, and to every culture and religion.

As we have seen, cancer is influenced by improper lifestyles, by pollution and other environmental factors, and especially by fast food and nutritional excess. In short, it is a disease of excessive consumption. But emotions are also a primary cause. Everything is related to them. When we eat, for example, as described in earlier chapters, our body takes in energy as well as nutrients, calories, and other material things. This energy influences our emotional behavior. At the most basic level, if we don't have a proper balance of foods, our vitality declines and we become tired. When we are tired, we easily become angry or nervous and are unable to behave nicely around others.

What we expect the most is love. This is the most precious thing a person can give. Love means much more than money. It is the real money. If you have love, you will not care about the money, and it would become secondary (though still important). If you know there is someone who really loves you, you worry less about everything else. Everyone expects this "unconditional love" from the "other," but if you don't love and accept yourself with everything you have (and perhaps don't have), you can never love someone else. You would always be expecting something you could not even give yourself. For emotional health, try to give yourself everything you expect. This does not mean squandering "objects" of consumption that society teaches us we need to be happy. Rather, it means treating yourself the way you would like to be treated by others. We have all heard this expressed as the Golden Rule: "Do unto others as you would have others do unto you." But I use it in another way. Just try to keep this sentence in your mind and reflect that you don't have to put all your negative moods on others because then you'll get them back. Interact with other people and your surroundings in a way that you receive good energy and not bad energy. If you spread good energy, you'll get it back. It is very simple, and it works. Just be happy, just accept differences between yourself and others, just accept yourself, and just accept your problems. But do not accept the belief that these things all depend on or arise from others. The totality of your life makes you what you are and how you act and react. Accept your own personal history and do not blame others for your troubles. This is the beginning of self-knowledge. By understanding each of our actions and not holding others responsible, we can strengthen our positive qualities and improve our negative ones. This is what is meant by the injunction: "Treat yourself as you would like to be treated by others."

This outlook will help us feel less confused about our feelings and our emotions. We learn to accept our loneliness and our uniqueness. Psychology teaches us that the "demand" for love comes from the child, not from the parents. Even if a child is abused by his or her parents, the child will try over and over again to gain their love. That's why abused children often never tell about their mistreatment. They unfortunately think that this abuse is their fault. We need to stop thinking that our parents are loving us. We are in love with our parents (let's hope) and need to stop expecting something that we cannot give ourselves.

Love yourself and then you can truly love all other persons. This doesn't mean that you have to love everything about yourself and then become very arrogant. It means trying to accept yourself as you are while working on those points that perhaps you don't love. For example, if you have a skin problem, you can try to care for yourself in another way. You can then start to love and accept yourself more and give more love to others. You need not instantly think, "They don't love me or consider me beautiful because of my bad skin and don't want to stay with me because I'm a monster." This kind of thinking must be stopped because it all depends on the expectations of others. Start to consider yourself more. In growing old, the best lesson is that if you don't care about yourself, no one else will do it for you.

The world today operates too much according to the principle "You give something and then you get something in return." This is sad because in trading our "freedom" for social integration, it means that the only freedom we truly enjoyed was in our first month of life when we didn't understand language and the world of rules and social expectations. Our feelings and emotional expression narrowed so that we could integrate into the civilized world. We paid a big price: the loss of our wide view of a free world. It is important for people to work together, but we don't speak enough. When you really think about what you said the whole day long, you notice that most of the time it was only "small talk." And from the person you "love" (if you have already found that person) you expect the feelings and emotions that you can't give yourself. In modern relationships, two persons are often more in war than in love. Today's world has so many relationship problems because we are all thinking just about our own satisfaction. A couple today is not walking together side by side; instead, each person is trying to possess the other. So you are lonelier than ever. The end result is that we stop giving to each other except in expectation of a return, of money or something with material value. Expectations only make us sad, angry, and imbalanced.

If you feel that you lack any emotion or feeling, then try first to give it to yourself by caring more about yourself. In finding some solutions to your problems, speak honestly to others about what you think and share your feelings and emotions. Psychologists serve as the ear for everybody who would like to speak. They are the ear and the friend with knowledge about human functioning, listening (for money) to the problems of others only because society has forbidden this expression.

We create more and more consumer objects to enable us to feel "temporarily" happy by possessing them. We create more and more medications to mask the pain of our daily lives. The headaches, depression, insomnia, and other symptoms we feel are often caused by suppressing our feelings and emotions. We hold them inside because they are forbidden to be expressed. Society today accepts only strong people, and all the normal and important weaknesses of humans have to be hidden or covered up. A weak person who cannot work causes problems for the group and is not accepted. Thus we are taught to take medications and supplements to be "artificially strong" again and always mask our weakness. The stronger we are, the higher we will rise in society. The weaker we are, the lower we will fall. Many people fall into a black hole of depression just because of the arbitrary rules of our society and because of their fear of facing their true feelings. The suppression of the weak side of human nature is also shown, for example, in nearly all the new video and computer games. They teach us to learn the way of war instead of the way of peace. All the games on the market such as Counter Strike teach our children that war, force, violence, hardness, guns, and even muscles are good. "Play with a gun, my son, and never cry." We hold our feelings inside, and then they manifest first as common and then as chronic ills. We forget that we search our whole lives for love. And there is no object, no money, and no medication that can give us the wonderful feeling that love gives us. Starting with ourselves is the easiest way. By giving love to ourselves, we can then give love to others. By caring about our own feelings, considering our emotions, and trying to keep them in balance, we learn to treat ourselves as we would like to treat the person we may love someday and who loves us. Health begins with unconditional love for ourselves.

Unconditional love for ourselves but also for others means that we will never need to expect that the person we love conforms to our childish imaginations. Love means that we would like to know the other person and see him or her as this person truly is. We should never try to change the person we love. This is not love but pretending to love. Love is developing more and more knowledge about this wonderful being and always accepting that being as he or she is. Unconditional love can transform our entire life. It enables us to expect less from others and allows us to have more energy to give ourselves and other people. By speaking and explaining what is going on inside ourselves, we will find that the reaction of others is not as horrible as we were brought up to believe. In speaking about ourselves with others, we may find that they have the same problems and views. By letting go of our old beliefs and learned behavior, even just a little, we will discover that others are happy to meet someone who shows real strength in taking off the social mask.

In this section we learned that feelings are conditioned by our education and culture. Feelings are suppressed in most cases throughout our life, even though they are one of our most important capacities. In today's society we prefer to hide our emotions instead of openly revealing them to others. This behavior creates much of the anger and hatred in our world and also the pseudo-individualization that characterizes modern society. This behavior contributes to the new illnesses we are facing, and the neglect or suppression of our feelings will not help us improve or change our lives for the better. The world today needs enormous modifications in many domains. Taking positive steps in this one little domain—changing the way we look at our feelings and emotional behavior—could help shape and influence the others.

The Understanding of Feelings/Emotions and Letting Go of Negative Attitudes and Beliefs

What is the origin of our own emotional condition? We need to know where our feelings come from, not to control them but to understand our actions and reactions better and not blame others. For example, when we are afraid to reveal what we are really thinking, our understanding "when, why, and how" fear has manifested before will enable us to feel less dread and anxiety. From a psychological view, cancer may arise as the end result of a major suppression that we couldn't handle emotionally. We suppress our feelings about the situation, and every time a similar situation develops, we react in the same way. Because of our fear, we prefer to suppress our feelings rather than confront the situation. Instead of running away, we need to work on our fear. When our bodies hold in suppressed emotions, a large amount of energy accumulates. Over time, this stagnation can lead to serious disease, including cancer. As we have seen, everything is a manifestation of energy. If the organism accepts a certain level of suppression, its energy accumulates inside and eventually has to find a way to be released. Otherwise, complete blockage arises and we cannot survive.

Our organism is very gentle with us. At the earliest stage of imbalance, it gives a sign or warning that something is wrong. Hence, we have a little illness. But continuing to remain ignorant or suppress the emotion could after some time create a little cancer. From this perspective a tumor can be the physical expression of a long-suppressed situation. It is a reflection of an emotional trauma we had and couldn't contend with. The subconscious suppresses feelings arising from situations we don't want to confront. Often the subconscious releases itself from these suppressed senses through dreams or lapses in speaking (such as "Freudian slips"). To deal with this process, we need first of all to understand our feelings and try to discover why we feel the way we do. As in psychological therapy, we can begin with the first moment in our lives when we didn't understand our reactions or the reactions of others. A very good way to visualize this is to draw a long line—a lifeline—on a piece of paper. On this line mark down all the key moments in your life when you had a traumatic situation or problem voicing your feelings or thoughts. On one side put a plus sign and on the other a minus sign. On the top, mark your actual age at the time of each event (see fictional example below):

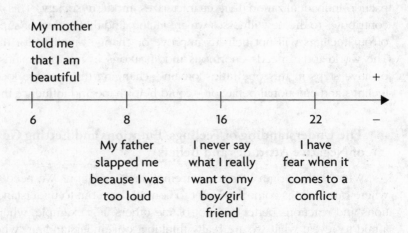

Understanding our feelings is a long and hard process. Of course, we cannot possibly understand all our emotional reactions over the course of a day or two.

As we have learned, first of all we need to understand others and their feelings, and we need to understand that in many different situations we are suppressing our emotions. Language and the actions and reactions of other people condition us to suppress our feelings. From a young age we learn the rules of society and that we are "forbidden to show" many emotions or that it is "good or bad to feel them." We learn "when, how, and to whom" we have the right to express or not express our emotions. Perhaps for some readers just reading this chapter is the first time they have considered the origin and nature of their feelings because most of the time certain feelings are suppressed or not welcome. We have to stop quietly blaming all our emotional problems on others. This only creates immense misunderstanding in the world and leads to many illnesses. Instead, we must start with understanding emotions, and then we can find resolutions to any problems that arise.

Understanding our own emotional process is very important. We must know why, for example, we feel fear or happiness in some moments or situations and how we express these feelings. To understand our feelings, we need to know which are main emotional "behavior patterns." To do this, you can write a list, noting all the following "primary emotions": jealousy, anger, revenge/hate, love/happiness, lust/desire/sex, intellectual interest/other. Then to every primary emotion join a situation from your life when you felt one of these sentiments. In this way it will become much clearer to see and to understand everything. This exercise allows you to start thinking about your emotions and about "why you feel, when you feel, and how you feel."

In the beginning it may take a long time for you to develop a little understanding about your feelings. In trying to make a list like this, many situations will be hard to remember. You will discover that there are many situations you forgot or had to forget or suppress from your memories because they were not acceptable, such as jealousy about a brother or sister. But such feelings are important to express even though, to carry through the example, you learned to suppress them because you didn't want your mother or father to be angry with you. No jealousy was allowed.

Start to remember all those moments in your life and try to understand yourself better. At the same time, don't blame yourself for those moments or blame others. Just try to recall and observe. This will help you find out which emotions you are most confronted with and which ones you had to learn to suppress. It is very important that you select from your list the strongest emotional situations. If you know your main emotional behavior—the "when and how much"—then try to think about the "why." In the above example, you may find that you are jealous of your brother or sister because you felt he or she received more attention than you did at the time.

Then if you reflect on your emotional behavior, you may see that you feel jealousy every time someone else gets more attention than you do. In the end, you have to think about "how" to handle this emotional behavior. For example, when you have developed this new self-awareness about jealousy, you will find that when you feel jealousy in the future, it has nothing to do with the current situation or the person you feel jealous about but with suppressed emotions related to your past relationship. In this case, just say to yourself, "No, I am just jealous about my sister/brother and not about this person in front of me." Try to work on your jealous feeling. Perhaps you can speak with your parents and tell them that in the past you felt neglected many times. In speaking out like this, your body will feel much lighter because you are releasing a great deal of suppressed emotional energy. This emotional behavior (as distinct from mechanical behavior) is never bad, and we should never blame ourselves for our emotions or for suppressing them. Just try to understand them and then think about "why" they are like this. Then decide whether you will keep these old emotional reaction patterns or free yourself from them.

From my psychological understanding, I think that in many cases cancer arises from one of the main emotional reactions that you have always suppressed because they were not allowed. In working to understand your feelings, you should always relate them to your life history. This is not a simple task, but in the end you will find the main "emotional behavior" easy to release. Once pulled from the subconscious into consciousness, you will be able to confront your emotional situation for real for the first time because you want to resolve it. Start with understanding all your emotional reactions. Ask "why, how, and when" they developed and then resolve them. Give understanding to yourself and let go of all bad beliefs.

To understand yourself and let go of all negative beliefs, I highly recommend *The Four Agreements* by Don Miguel Ruiz. From this book it is very easy to learn how to let go of opinions arising from our education and also from destructive emotional behavior encouraged by our environment. He describes how our beliefs and the agreements we make with ourselves and others limit our freedom and create unhappiness. The Four Agreements are (1) Be impeccable with your word, (2) Don't take anything personally, (3) Don't make assumptions, and (4) Always do your best.

This chapter is general in its scope because I noticed during my research that beliefs about the emotions are divided. Most research and treatment of cancer do not consider the emotions, as I already explained, because in the modern world we just consider the things we can see and explain. We consider material things as real, and everything we cannot count and see are unreal, including the emotions. I didn't want to comment on something that's not real. I speak only generally about the emotions, describing where they come from and the role they may play in the development of cancer, especially from an energetic "imbalance" among them. I based this on my own understanding and knowledge from psychology. Many other views should be taken into consideration about the influence of the emotions in the creation of cancer. The observations I presented in this chapter are personal views that I wanted to share with you. As we saw, macrobiotic knowledge and way of life begins with a belief in "energy." It is my strong conviction that since everything consists of energy, the emotions are very important to consider in illness. The macrobiotic way of life also rests on a foundation of the balance of energy between yin and yang. If you believe in the primary importance of energy, you can change your condition by working on the balance of your emotions. It is my hope that this chapter will help you start thinking about something that is not always visible: the all-important force we call energy. Energy creates our emotions, and the emotions create our behavior and, hence, our condition. I always keep this very important equation in mind.

The affirmations or beliefs I place my faith in include these: I am what I eat. I treat others as I would like to be treated by others. I love myself so I can love others. I do not blame others for all the things I don't like. I love this world, and I try to change little things in my own behavior. In this way perhaps the world will someday change so that people will begin to notice that many things which appear to come from elsewhere originate within themselves. We are focused on negative things these days, such as money, wealth, power, and high status. All these create strong egoism and individualism in the human character. By just changing our emotional patterns and behavior we can start to develop new goals in our world to replace the comfort and endless consumption of objects that offer only artificial happiness. Let us spend more time with our feelings.

9

Woman and Cancer

by Anna Böhm

This chapter like the last continues to focus on the influence of energy. The cancer we speak of foremost when considering the woman is breast cancer. In due course we shall examine how the emotions affect the development of breast cancer and other female malignancies. But first, let's look at woman's background and history.

In the history of woman, we notice that for the bulk of her life she was under suppression by man. Through most of history she had no major place in society or individual rights. Only in the last seventy years has woman started to assume a major role in society. Now she has the right to vote, to use contraception, to divorce, and to earn money. She may also rise to be the leader of any enterprise and can wear whatever she likes. Yes, now she officially enjoys these rights, but they are not always respected. Hence, their application spreads little by little. In many cultures and religions, woman is still suppressed by her husband or by the head of the family in the person of the father, grandfather, or brother. Especially in European and American law, she has the right to use her new "freedoms," but in many other nations she still does not. Unfortunately, even in the nations where she enjoys the freedom to be freer as a woman, she remains suppressed. Despite the hard-earned freedoms she fought for, she continues to be the object of prejudice and discrimination. Society tries all the time to characterize woman and describe how she has to behave, what she has the right to say and do, and how she should clothe herself. The truth is that in the last century and the start of this one, the social rights woman enjoyed were largely granted by man. Our society today is created mostly by man, not by humans together. Almost everything has been created and decided by man. Now woman enjoys some rights but not all, and obtaining them was a long, hard struggle. She continues to be discriminated against in many social situations and contexts.

In America, woman's suffrage won the right to vote in 1920 after a century of marching and protest. The right to divorce took longer, as did the right to marry a person of another race. But, overall, America is still about fifty years behind Europe in granting woman's rights.

The emancipation of woman proceeded very slowly. In traditional society the role of woman also defined the role of man. The place of woman was in the household, which she supervised, including the education of the children, cleaning, the kitchen and nutrition, and other household arrangements. Man carried out the social functions and had to earn the money for the family. This is the old role model in our society. Traditionally, none of the social decisions was made by the woman. But the energy of woman is very important and can change many things. All the laws are based on decisions made by man. Perhaps everything would function in another way if woman had won her emancipation and integration much earlier. Little by little, woman is acquiring a considerable place in society, even if it is still not equal.

Now that woman has achieved emancipation in many domains, we continue to characterize and define her. We still observe her sexuality and judge whether it is too free. Is she presenting herself as a sex object, or is she just exercising her freedom? We continue to fashion an image for woman about how she should behave. All of the media are aimed at influencing the way she has to be: beautiful, thin, smart, nice, and polite. Such images just drive consumption of more unnecessary goods and services in society. Woman's place is also a very important demographic question. If a country feels there are too few births, more images are shown on television of happy families with happy children. Social rights are improved, and child care becomes less expensive. Many changes in woman's place in society transpired over the last century, but she is still not as free as she would like to be. She is not as free as man because society depends on her to maintain or increase the birthrate. Contraception also gives a new freedom to woman and allows her greater control over her life. She can decide if she would like to assume the role of "mother" or not. She also has the right to work and to control her own money. She has the right to divorce and to live without a man. She has the right to say if she is mistreated by others. She has the right to educate herself to become a doctor or master of science and of all other domains. She has the right to found and run her own enterprise. She has the right to be an active socialized human being. These changes took place just during the last century. A truly independent woman has not existed for very long. She is now on her way to finding out what she can do with this newly earned freedom.

Meanwhile, society continues to implement new ways to discriminate against woman. In many parts of the world, woman still has no social rights and is under the control of man. At this time we cannot really say that woman truly enjoys equal integration into social life. She remains under scrutiny by society and is subject to suppression, influence, and control. As the Bible said, Eve tempted Adam to eat the apple. Woman enjoys the gift of bearing life. She has enormous energy and creative power. Man is just her defender and the supporter of her strong, natural, feminine energy. Man realized this quickly, and from the beginning he tried to seduce her with the argument that he is stronger. He tried to subdue and control her because, in fact, he is physically stronger than she is. Woman's history is one of subjugation. Like a slave, for most of history she has been dominated by the physically stronger sex: man. Now, with liberation, there are many new domains for her to discover. Her social life continues to be shaped and influenced by man. Now she has the right to behave under new independent roles largely created by man. Progress has been made, but not as much as it seems. There are many things we still do not know about woman's real "power" and knowledge. We don't know how woman experiences social life and how she would like society to work. There is still a long way to go before we can speak about an equal society. Even more important, a unified society created by both man and woman remains to be created.

Change follows change, and I hope that progress will continue. I hope that soon we will have female presidents. I hope that we will see the "big" decisions made by a woman. I think her leadership would be different. But humans fear this change and are not yet convinced that a woman has the capacity to do "hard and important" work. This to me is the crucial question. If we just fear and do not give woman a chance, we will never know. We have to place more value than we do now on woman's view in every important domain. We need her active participation, along with man's, in every big decision made in the fields of law, politics, and medicine. If we had granted equal rights to woman and man from the onset, the world would not be as it is today. Instead, woman continues to be suppressed because she shows her emotional side. We continue to believe that man has no right to show his emotions and that only woman has the natural "talent" and capacity to be emotional. Who was the man that said the emotions are bad? I would like to meet him. Emotions create life! Without emotions there would be no desire, no passion, and no procreation. There would also be no anger, no hate, and no sadness. That is why we need more balance in our emotions and why we have to spend more time with our feelings. We have to speak and communicate more about them and accept the fact that they exist. We need more balance in all social domains, including respect for religious differences and life standards. We need more balance in our way of eating and in our way of life. Let's start with the easiest: our own feelings. We need no money for this. Woman has the gift to remember at any time the energetic, emotional, and natural aspects of life. We need this more than ever, especially now when everything is so diffi-cult. Society teaches us to buy or die. We are conditioned to want money and live well by working in meaningless jobs and consuming meaningless things, fearing that we will pass our lives in unhappiness and want. The strongest al-ways wins. Take a gun, my son, and don't cry. There is no place for emotional behavior. These are modern society's precepts. But life started from this all-important emotional behavior. If we began to accept woman as she is, we could change this world. Instead, we are destroying it by ignoring her view. Like two little boys playing "crash the car," our largely man-made society is playing "crash the earth."

Yes, these are harsh words, but we need a fundamental change to recog-nize and respect woman's energy. Let the woman be. Don't try to classify her. Let her react after this long time of suppression. Give her just a little bit more freedom, such as man enjoys, and find out what would happen. Today the sexes are not equal because woman has to adapt to masculine-based rights and laws. This system is designed for the strong, hard man devoid of emotions—he who is so functional that society fears any change. The woman who cannot work is still expected to be as functional as a man. This is not right because woman and man are very different. We cannot expect the same from both. It is really not possible. But then let us accept her functionality. Let us stop speak-ing negatively about woman's talents, character, behavior, acting, and way of making a decision.

Man also has the right to behave as he does. Let's just see what happens when woman is given consideration and really assumes more freedom. Let us stop fearing to give woman her place, and, if you are a man, stop fearing your emotions. If you are a woman, stop behaving socially as man would like. Accept that you are a woman and that you understand the emotions. Take them into consideration. Society suppresses woman now because she has to work like man, but she cannot. If she also has a family, she has to care for the household because, for the most part, man won't. She naturally loves to take care of the family and encourage and support her children. From the beginning of humanity she is conditioned to nurture others. That is why she should also take responsibility, as well as man, for making political deci-sions. From the start, man has been conditioned to take charge of the "secu-rity" part of life. That is also important, and he could not live without it. But there has to be a balance between these two behaviors and energies. Both sexes have to walk side by side together in an equal rhythm. Don't suppress the strengths and weaknesses of either man or woman. Both are important.

From my psychological view, woman is still suppressed on her emo-tional side. With her new rights, she now has to become stronger and inte-grate herself into the social realm. This need not change her basic character, behavior, and emotions, but often it can create a big suppression of her emotional side. Breast cancer, for example, in my psychological view, is an expression of the suppression of her femininity. The breasts especially are a symbol of femininity. In the medical treatment of breast cancer, we take the breast away. In this approach we take her femininity away. This understandably leads to major psychological problems regarding her identity as a woman. I am also deeply disturbed about mammography or preventive X-rays for breast cancer. Woman is driven to distraction with all the different diagnostic tests and preventive measures for cancer of the breasts and of the female organs. This also creates a subconscious fear. The girl or young woman today is confronted with this dilemma from the beginning of her femininity. She is aware that she risks losing her breast and her femininity. This only adds to her fear about man, because he is stronger and at any time can hurt her.

I think the same nutritional and environmental factors, living conditions, and genetic considerations are important for both woman and man. But we should not forget the long suppression that woman has experienced and the fear it creates. Many of the cancers affecting woman are related to the sexual organs and are signs of her femininity. My hypothesis is that any suppression of femininity could create imbalance in the energy of a woman and create or contribute to cancer. The irony is that the treatment often involves a real loss of the "imaginary image of the woman." We take the breast away or we take the uterus away so that she is no longer a woman. There must be a better way to prevent cancer than mammography that only awakens her fear and contributes to creating the disease it is designed to prevent. We could be more accepting from birth of woman's feminine behavior and way of expressing herself as a human being. Please, lovely woman, give more attention to yourself. Let us say it right: Give more space to woman and to her energy—more space in every domain.

Woman has so much power but not the right to express that power. All her wonderful femininity is not allowed or accepted. It is hidden and considered a sign of weakness. For example, menstruation always has to be hidden. This time of the month is a very important time for the woman. Every month she has this special energy when a potential life goes out of her body. It is normal that her hormones are in flux and she is very energized. She has to take time for herself at this special time. In ancient India, woman had many visions during menstruation. She stopped working and took time to cultivate her dreams because they were in harmony with the Earth and with life. Nowadays, a woman hides her menstruation. She goes to work or she cares for the household as she ordinarily would. She takes some medication if it hurts and uses a tampon so that there is no contact with the blood. Nobody notices that she has her period. This is also what makes a woman a woman. But in our society there is no free day for her to menstruate. I propose we observe a free menstruation day. Now you may smile at this suggestion, but it is no joke. If we want a balanced society, give space to the woman. She needs a free menstruation day to observe her uniqueness as a woman. Unfortunately, we don't have this important day, and we are expected to act at this time as on any other day.

At this time of the month, woman takes a lot of medication just to continue functioning as normal. We are more stressed on these days and feel and act differently. But man is not aware of what we experience, nor does he take it into consideration. He needs to respect woman's energy. Let woman speak and give her the space to show her emotions and their central importance in the world. I don't know very many men who consider the menstruation of their female friends. I know some, and I respect them a lot because they tell me that they try to understand this special time for the woman. I know one who told me that my boss should be happy that I come to work even if I have my menstruation. I was really happy when I heard this because with these words he respected my femininity. He did not say something like "Why don't you take some medication against the pain?" or "It will pass; just stay strong." In saying this, he respected that I am a woman because he said that my boss should be happy if I come to work. This is what I mean about respect. But the woman, too, has the obligation to explain and make understandable to the man why she is as she is. This is one of the most important things humans have to learn: to explain their actions and reactions to each other more fully. If I had not explained to my friend why I was angry and in a bad mood on that day and why I didn't want to go to work, I would never have had the experience of respect toward my femininity. I spoke about my femininity. As man and woman, we have to speak about our differences more, to share our abilities more, and to accept our different ways of behavior and the different emotions we feel. We cannot expect that man will understand everything at the end and act as we want. But if woman is to be a real part of society, man has to stop believing that he can expect the same from the woman as from the man. We need to stop trying to create dependency. Neither man nor woman should be dependent on the other. They should accept and respect their differences and work together. We should work on this. Give more space to the woman. After a long time of suppression, encourage her to speak more often. Let her express herself and show what a woman really is. To release the old image of the "man-woman," let us look to the "woman's woman."

Cancer in general, for both sexes, as I explained in the last chapter, may result from some energetic (emotional) suppression and, of course, from other factors. Woman's cancer works in the same way. It can also be influenced by any suppression of feminine energy. That is why often the sexual organs are affected. In starting to consider more feminine energy and emotions, cancer can be prevented. As noted in the last chapter, if you suppress your feelings for any reason—education, a bad experience, or bad behavior on the part of others or even yourself—your suppressed feminine energy eventually has to find a way to release itself. Hence, the body creates signs of imbalance. Perhaps the first sign is a feeling of weakness and then a little cough in moments of stress. This could be followed by a chronic pain in the chest and then, over time, by cancer. It depends on the individual. Try to work on your femininity; try to express it and accept it for what it is. The feminine is not bad. It is one of the most wonderful manifestations of humanity, as is masculinity. But society accepts the expression of masculinity and not femininity. Embrace femininity. It is wonderful to be a woman. Woman often automatically believes she is of less value than man, so we have to work on this belief pattern. To change the belief of woman, we need to make her more confident about who she is!

Exercises for Woman

As I did in the last chapter, I would like to present an exercise for woman. This exercise may help her work on her suppressed feminine energy and feelings. In recent times, woman has not enjoyed the right to say what she likes and dislikes, what she really wants and what she doesn't want. With this exercise she can start to understand that she has the freedom to express herself openly and voice her true desires. The first exercise involves taking a piece of paper and writing at the top of one side "I like" and on the other side "I don't like." Then under each heading, start listing examples. For instance, in the second column under "I don't like," you could write "I often do not say what I really think," "I have no time for myself," "My mother and father never regarded me as a woman," "I don't have the money to buy all the clothes I would like"—anything that comes into your head. Include the emotional things, the consumer objects you don't possess, the beauty that perhaps you don't have, the things you have no right to do. Just jot down everything. Then remove those items you consider less important and concentrate on the main ones. Observe whether you wrote down mostly positive or negative things in both lists. If there are mostly negative things, voice them out loud. You have to hear yourself saying the things you don't like. This is very important because the negative things are coming from situations in which you didn't say what you wanted. You have to verbalize all these things. Because woman did not have the right to say these things, she doesn't like them. With this exercise you will start to realize that woman has the right to say all the things she doesn't like, what she would like to have, and what she doesn't agree with. When you speak them aloud, you start to open yourself and reverse the old patterns that reinforce the belief that woman has less value than man and has nothing to say. You also start to understand where the things you don't like come from. As noted in the chapter on emotions, we need to understand the origin and cause of negative thoughts and bad feelings. This exercise is very important in helping woman say what she wants. As a woman, say what you want and what you don't want. Stop thinking that you have to be only as your parents, brothers, boyfriends, or husband desires—a functional beautiful woman, for example. No, you have to be as you would like to be. Only you can decide your feelings about yourself.

The next exercise is very easy. Lie down, close your eyes, breathe deeply, and just say to yourself: "I like myself as a woman in this world, and I am wonderful in my being and actions. I love myself as a woman in this world, and I accept all my feminine energy. I love myself as a woman in this world, and I love all women and man." Then see all the feminine energy you possess surrounding you from head to foot, from one hand to the other, from behind to the front. Visualize yourself surrounded by all your wonderful and beautiful feminine energy and by all the energy from other feminine beings. Then breathe and create energy flowing endlessly from the inside to the outside, from your inner world to the outer world, from the outer world to the inner world. Breathe and release all your negative emotions and belief patterns. Take in strong, positive energy from the outside. Breathe and give back good energy to the outside. The most important thing in this exercise is just to relax and tell yourself that you are good. In very simple words, tell yourself to relax and be a woman.

Another important thing for all humans is to be in contact with other people. We need to share with others, and so we created language. We need to speak and exchange our thoughts with one another. As Descartes said, "I think, therefore I am." I say, "I feel, therefore I am." Working as a psychologist, I know that all human beings desire to speak with others about their feelings. If you find you do not really have someone to speak with, go to a psychologist and speak with him or her. As I said in the previous chapter, sadly, society does not really encourage speaking from the heart. We speak often about our job, the weather, and the concert we went to see. Small talk is important, but sometimes we need deep or long talks and to talk about our feelings, impressions, and thoughts. Our society doesn't allow us time to speak openly and honestly with one another. It does not encourage close friendships, and in today's crazy world, it is often hard to meet people.

Psychologists also tend to be viewed negatively. People go to the psychologist when they are ill. This is not right. Everyone needs someone to speak with. As psychologists we listen, try to understand, and help to provide self-awareness. Psychologists are not only there for mentally or emotionally ill people. We are there for everyone who needs to speak, think, and share. If you need someone to speak with and need to work on your feelings, old behavior patterns, and beliefs, find a good psychologist. Many people who do not have anyone to speak with won't see a counselor because they are afraid. As a psychologist, I assure you we will not label you as neurotic or psychotic but will accept you just the way you are.

With these concluding words, I would like to encourage you to look at your life from the perspective of the emotions. I hope that you found some things in this chapter and the previous one that resonate with your feelings and will help you. Any kind of dark or negative mood, bad condition, or illness could be shaped and influenced by the emotions and their possible suppression. Just consider this possibility, and if you get a chance, do the exercises I suggest.

Accept yourself, wonderful woman, and embrace all other women. Wonderful man, do the same. And both of you, be more accepting of the emotional influences in your lives. Take care of the balance on this Earth and among others, and have fun! Enjoy life. Stop destroying the Earth. Accept and respect more the wonderful things we cannot explain with only scientific points of view. Let us develop a larger view. Let us stop harming ourselves. Let us change and continue to grow and develop endlessly. By honoring our emotions we can prevent cancer and other serious diseases. By respecting our femininity and masculinity we can live as free human beings on this beautiful planet.

10

Exercise, Lifestyle, and the Power of the Mind

PHYSICAL ACTIVITY

In addition to dietary change, several other measures are important in cancer recovery. When we start to change our blood to a healthy quality by eating a more centrally balanced diet, we naturally become more physically active and begin to reduce our reliance on technological comforts in our environment. Our natural defense mechanism is restored, and our bodies adjust more easily to extremes of hot and cold, necessitating less dependence on central heating in winter and air-conditioning in summer. We appreciate, value, and continue to use some of the technological advances that modern civilization offers. However, we should reduce our reliance on the use of excessive mechanical or electronic conveniences that may hinder the smooth exchange of energy between ourselves and the natural environment. We especially try to avoid those features of modern life that may contribute to the development of sickness or make the recovery from sickness more difficult.

Stress Reduction

Stress has become a byword referring to all the pressures and strains of modern life, and stress reduction has become a big industry. The pace of life today is certainly faster and more contracted than in the past. However, most stress originates from the inside rather than the outside. The declining health of people today makes it more difficult to carry out normal daily activities, and they can no longer cope with life. From the macrobiotic view, the problem of stress is largely one of no longer being able to exchange energy, or discharge energy, smoothly with the environment. If we continuously take in more energy than we need, especially high-caloric, high-fat, high-protein foods, blockages develop under the skin and around the organs and tissues. We no longer sweat properly. Our lungs, kidneys, liver, intestines, and other organs of discharge become overburdened as fat, mucus, and other excess accumulates. We carry stress inside, yet complain as if it were coming from outside. Our inside condition creates continuous pressure. Then each cell begins to pool or collect high energy. An explosion finally comes, which we call cell division. We call it cancer. If we are active, we can discharge more harmoniously. The sedentary modern way of life and lack of hardship and difficulties are contributing factors to degenerative disease. Ultimately, to reduce stress we must regulate and control the basic energy coming into our bodies in the form of daily food.

Among modern foods, salty foods, hard-baked flour products, icy drinks, food that has been broiled, grilled, baked, or roasted, and some sour foods inhibit or suppress discharging. Among external conditions, cold temperature, dry air, smoking, and air pollution, especially the buildup of carbon dioxide, inhibit the discharge process. Conversely, among modern foods, sugar, fruit juice, coffee, tea, and other stimulants, alcohol, drugs, and other excessively yin products cause high dispersing energy and can lead to wild, erratic behavior. Hot temperature, high humidity, chemical pollution, electrical or microwave cooking, and exposure to artificial electromagnetic fields can also lead to rapid decomposing, disintegrating tendencies. Grains, beans, and vegetables from land and sea give more stable, balanced energy, and it is far safer to manage our health on this foundation.

Walking

To promote better circulation of the body's natural flow of energy, direct contact with the elements of nature is advisable. Walking outdoors on the grass, soil, or beach, preferably barefoot, is an excellent therapeutic measure. In my personal guidance sessions, I usually recommend that everyone take a half hour walk each day, rain or shine. This helps the body adjust to seasonal change and builds up natural immunity. A recent study published in the *Journal of the American Medical Association* noted that people who exercise moderately, including a half hour walk each day, live longer and have less risk of cancer and heart disease. Walking activates circulation, improves breathing, tones the muscles, and improves appetite. Walking increases oxygen in the blood and lymph, which stimulate cleansing and disposal of waste from body cells and tissues. Walking calms and clears the mind and helps reduce stress and tension.

Exercise

Modern life is basically sedentary, and a high percentage of people today are overweight. The average American uses the Internet three hours a day and watches TV about two hours. A sedentary lifestyle contributes to stagnation in the generation of caloric and electromagnetic energy, blood and lymph circulation, and digestive and nervous system functions. Regular exercise, including Do-in (Oriental self-massage), yoga, the martial arts, dancing, or sports, can be beneficial. A person should be as active as his or her health allows without becoming tired or overworked. Several recent scientific and medical studies have shown that people who exercise are healthier than those who are sedentary. The incidence of cardiovascular disease and other serious illnesses is often less for those who are physically active.

Daily Body Scrubbing

Scrubbing your body with a moist hot towel is a marvelous way to relieve stress, reduce tension, and energize your daily life. It also activates circulation, softens deposits of hard fat below the skin, opens the pores, and allows excess to be actively discharged to the surface rather than accumulate around deeper vital organs. For maximum effect you can scrub your body twice a day: once in the morning and again in the evening. See Chapter 36 for a recommended procedure.

ARTIFICIAL ELECTROMAGNETIC ENERGY

The discoveries and inventions of modern science and technology have contributed substantial convenience and efficiency to our daily life. However, at the same time, many technological applications are hazardous to our health and well-being. Artificial electromagnetic energy in our environment changes the atmospheric charge surrounding us, producing various effects on our physical and mental condition. We may often notice a general fatigue, mental irritability, and unnatural metabolism as the result of high-voltage lines, electrical appliances, cell phones, and other communications equipment in our vicinity. Electricity particularly affects the nervous system.

Over the last twenty years, research has begun to emerge showing that leukemia, lymphoma, brain cancer, and other tumors, as well as many other serious illnesses, are more frequent in those who live in close proximity to power lines, transformers, and electrical stations and those who use electric blankets, fluorescent lights, and other devices (see Table 17). Some modern medical tests are potentially harmful. For example, in some studies X-rays and mammograms have been associated with enhancing the risk of breast cancer. The most advanced technology, including CT scans and MRI (magnetic

TABLE 17.   MODERN APPLIANCES AND RELATIVE RISK OF DISEASE

High Risk	Medium Risk	Low Risk
Fluorescent lights	Desk lamps	Electric lights
Hair dryers, electric shavers	Washers, dryers	Irons
Computers	Televisions	Radios, stereos, MP3
Microwave ovens	Electric ovens, ranges	devices, iPods
Blenders, can openers, mixers	Dishwashers	Refrigerators
Electric blankets	Vacuum cleaners	Coffeemakers
Power lines	Fans, heaters	Disposals

Source: International Electricity Energy Exchange, *New York Times,* and other sources.

resonance imaging) scans, also exposes the patient to various kinds of radiation, and further studies will show whether they are safe or harmful.

ELECTRIC AND MICROWAVE COOKING

Cooking on an electric range or in a microwave oven may contribute to undesirable effects on our digestion and nourishment, and generally should be avoided. Electricity alternates at sixty cycles per second, emitting radiation that can cause biochemical changes and affect human health. Microwave vibrates at 2.45 million times per second, changing the molecular structure of the food. Overall, both electric and microwave cooking contribute to an overall weakening and loss of natural immunity. When people adopt a macrobiotic way of eating but do not experience an improvement in their condition, one of the first things I ask them is how they are cooking their food. In many cases, switching to gas heat produces an immediate benefit. If they are renting and their landlord will not install gas or gas service is not available, I will recommend that they get a portable gas stove—with one, two, or four burners—to prepare their food. Inexpensive propane camping stoves are fine for this purpose. Wood heat is also recommended and, in fact, gives the strongest energy and most delicious food. However, wood heat is very yangizing, is most suitable for active people working outdoors, and is not usually practical in modern urban society, so gas—which gives a calm, balanced flame and energy—is the standard in most macrobiotic homes.

COMPUTERS

Over the last twenty-five years the personal computer entered millions of households as well as many businesses, shops, schools, and other institutions.

Computers and video display terminals (VDTs) give off various kinds of artificial electromagnetic radiation, which are increasingly suspected to be harmful to human health and, like cigarette smoke, affect not only the user but also others in the immediate vicinity. An Environmental Protection Agency draft report recommended that extremely low frequency (ELF) radiation generated by ordinary personal computers be designated a possible human carcinogen. Exposure to ELF emissions has been particularly associated with leukemia, lymphoma, nervous system malignancies, and other cancers. For people with cancer we advise that computers be avoided or exposure be limited to one half hour per day.

It is widely believed that LCD or notebook computers are safer than desktop models. This is not necessarily true. Some LCD models emit less radiation, but others emit more. The only sure way to tell is to use a gauss meter to check the electromagnetic field for yourself. These are available relatively cheaply at electronic supply stores such as Radio Shack. Computer safety regulations, especially the radiation levels of monitors and guidelines for recycling toxic ingredients, have improved in recent years. However, they are far from ideal for daily health. The safest practice for people who use computers on a daily basis is to have their computer professionally shielded by an environmentally responsible company that offers this service. Costs range from about $100 to $300, but such shielding usually guarantees zero radiation and is worth the cost and peace of mind.

TELEVISION

Television, too, has potentially harmful effects, especially color television. TVs contain a cathode ray tube (CRT) that zigzags fifteen thousand times a second down the screen, projecting a big electromagnetic field. Several decades ago, as a spoof, a British epidemiologist correlated television use with cardiovascular disease in a medical journal and found an almost exact correspondence between the rise in number of TV sets in use and serious illness. Since then, various studies have come out showing that television, like computers, may have small but incremental adverse effects on our health. For those with cancer, we advise that TV be avoided or limited to a half hour a day.

CLOTHING AND PERSONAL ACCESSORIES

Synthetic clothing, such as that made of nylon, polyester, and acrylic, impedes the regular flow of energy through the body. It is therefore advisable to begin to change to more natural materials such as cotton, especially for clothing that comes into direct contact with the skin. Cotton underwear, socks, and shirts are widely available, and as we gradually replace our wardrobe, we begin to feel more comfortable in all-natural clothing. (Since a lot of cotton is genetically engineered, organic is preferred as much as possible.) Synthetic sheets, blankets, and other furnishings should be avoided if possible. Metallic accessories such as rings, pendants, and other jewelry should be kept to a minimum, though it is fine to wear a wedding ring.

BODY CARE

Commercial soaps, deodorants, and other body care products may be harmful. Safe, simple products can be made at home using all-natural ingredients (see Aveline Kushi and Wendy Esko's book, *Diet for Natural Beauty* [New York and Tokyo: Japan Publications, 1991]) or obtained at the natural foods store. Long hot baths or showers, which deplete the supply of minerals in the body, should be reduced.

AIR CIRCULATION

Free circulation of air and open sunshine should be encouraged in the home or place where the person is recovering. The addition of several green plants will also help stimulate deeper breathing and stronger metabolism. Plants are complementary to human beings. While humans breathe in oxygen and give off carbon dioxide, plants take in carbon dioxide and give off oxygen. Recent scientific studies showed that nineteen common house plants, including the peace lily, gerbera daisy, English ivy, chrysanthemum, bamboo palm, and moss cane, increased oxygen content in the house and helped eliminate harmful chemicals from the air, including benzene, formaldehyde, and trichloroethylene. Green plants may also help protect against radon, a naturally occurring gas present in the ground, surface water, and granite or other construction materials, which can accumulate indoors and has been associated with a higher risk for lung cancer.

HOME FURNISHINGS
AND BUILDING MATERIALS

Synthetic home furnishings and artificial building materials may prevent healthy relaxation and cause a variety of health problems. These include furniture, appliances, building materials, paints and varnishes, and other items in our home environment that are made of artificial materials or contain potentially harmful chemicals and toxins. As our health is restored, we may want to gradually furnish our home with rugs, draperies, and other materials made of natural fabrics, with furnishings and structural parts made of wood, glass, metal, straw, or other natural substances. However, we should not become overly concerned about our immediate environment and try to replace everything at once. This is impractical and stressful. Slow and steady change, once again, is the general rule.

OCCUPATIONAL HAZARDS

People whose daily work involves chemicals, drugs, electronics, and other potentially harmful materials or who are exposed to artificial electromagnetic fields have a higher risk of cancer than others. This includes painters, printers, carpenters, chemists, textile workers, farmers, foundry workers, computer operators, and telephone repairmen.

Table 18 summarizes a holistic approach to cancer and serious illness.

TABLE 18. A HOLISTIC APPROACH TO CANCER

Way of Life	Healthy	Unhealthy
Daily food	Whole	Processed
	Natural	Artificial
	Organic	Chemical
	Balanced	Extreme
	Seasonal	Unseasonal
	Locally grown	Transcontinental, global
	Home-cooked	Precooked
	GMO-free	GM
Environment and lifestyle	Clean	Polluted
	Orderly	Disorderly
	Active	Sedentary
	Real	Synthetic
	Renewable	Unrenewable
Emotions and mind	Peaceful	Complaining
	Grateful	Arrogant
	Flexible	Rigid
	Cooperative	Competitive
	Patient	Angry
	Steady	Erratic
	Focused	Scattered
	Communicative	Closed
	Compassionate	Unfeeling

OUTLOOK AND SPIRITUAL PRACTICE

Mental attitude is, of course, very important in maintaining our health and well-being. Everything in the universe is composed of energy, including the mind and the body. In fact, we may say that the mind is an expanded form of the body, and the body is a condensed form of the mind or spirit. Outlook and mental and spiritual practice take a variety of forms, including the following:

Developing Intuition

Deeper consciousness, or intuition, transcends ordinary levels of awareness and helps alert us to potential danger, sickness, or harm. It functions as an internal compass or inner guide that helps us make balance, or rebalance, with nature. Intuition inspires us to change our thinking and way of life, especially self-destructive habits that have guided our behavior until now. It is the basis for self-reflection and change, and emerges at times of crisis, including serious illness. Intuition is the unlearned, spontaneous awareness of the order of nature and the way to live in harmony with that changing order. It is the foundation for a long and healthy life on this planet. Intuition is the key to survival and realization and the foundation for self-reflection and change. The best way to develop our daily intuition is through our daily way of eating—eating very simply in harmony with the natural environment, being grateful for all difficulties including our sickness, and extending our love and care to everyone.

Self-Reflection

A person with cancer needs to understand that while cancer and other sicknesses are a disease of modern civilization as a whole, he or she was largely responsible for the development of the disease through his or her daily diet, environment, and lifestyle choices, way of thinking, and way of life. The person should be encouraged to reflect deeply, to examine those aspects of modern mentality that have produced the problem of cancer and a host of other unhappy situations. These reflections should include a review of the rich heritage of traditional wisdom developed by many cultures over thousands of years, an appreciation of the endless wonders of the natural world, including the body's marvelous self-protective and recuperative mechanisms, and a respect for the order of the universe that produces these phenomena.

The purpose of self-reflection is to review one's way of life, including way of eating, and take responsibility for one's condition. The purpose of self-reflection is also to resolve to take control in the future and change in a more positive direction. It is not aimed at producing guilt or guilty feelings.

Once one has recognized one's past ignorance and foolishness, one should then put it aside. There is no need to dwell on the past. The universe is very happy to hear your admission of past errors and resolution to continue now in a more healthful direction.

Prayer and Meditation

There are many prayers and meditations to calm the mind, dissolve negative thoughts and patterns of behavior, and heal the body. Several recent medical studies have shown that mental relaxation, emotional support, and awareness of being part of a larger community can improve health. Specifically, meditation helps to relax autonomic nerves, lowers blood pressure, and relieves stress on the heart and other internal organs. It can help us consciously control digestive, respiratory, and circulatory functions. In the case of cancer, meditation can help reduce tumor development in some cases by dissolving negative thoughts and images that disturb the smooth flow of healing energy in the chakras, meridians, and cells.

In Spiritual Development Training Seminars, we have taught palm healing, meditation, and other mental and physical exercises from around the world that have proved beneficial in helping people recover from sickness. It is important to understand, however, that these techniques and methods are all based on an understanding of yin and yang, or the flow of natural electromagnetic energy. When we eat, we are taking in the essence of those energies in the simplest, most balanced form. These energies can also be applied directly. However, these methods should serve as a complement to and not as a replacement for fundamental dietary change.

All of us must realize that without food there is no life; without food we cannot create healthy blood; and without healthy blood there is no cell formation, including the formation of healthy brain cells. The strength of our minds, emotions, and spirits is conditioned by the daily food we take, and these, in turn, reciprocally influence the health and vitality of our physical being. This relationship has often been misunderstood, however, and disease has been equated with sin and health with saintliness. To the eye of the universe, however, moral sanctity and religious practice do not necessarily protect from sickness or disability.

A number of years ago my wife and I returned from giving seminars in Spain and Portugal. While in Spain I saw many sick people who came to me for macrobiotic advice. One Catholic nun, about thirty-five years old, was among them. She attended my seminars, and when I saw her privately, she explained that she was suffering from breast cancer. I asked her how many nuns were in her convent, and she replied that about three hundred were living there. I then asked how many had developed cancer, and she told me that sixty nuns had developed the disease, and of these, thirty had already died. Thirteen women had entered the convent when she did, and of this original group, twelve had died from cancer; she was the only one left. In some instances, prayer may have prolonged the lives of these unfortunate women. However, only by changing the convent's daily way of eating would their lives be saved. Prayer and meditation are helpful, but if poor-quality food—the main cause of the problem—continues, there can never be complete recovery. Together, proper food plus prayer and meditation is very powerful.

Meditation offers a simple and practical method to quiet the mind, reduce stress and anxiety, and develop intuition. Please see Chapter 37 for one simple meditation that can be done at home.

Sound and Vibration

Sound and vibration carry energy. For thousands of years people have used words and music, including songs and chanting, to harmonize their inner and outer environment. In personal guidance sessions I always tell people with cancer who come to see me to sing a happy song each day. It doesn't matter what the song is as long as it is cheerful and positive. "You Are My Sunshine," "Row, Row, Row Your Boat," or practically any simple song like these will raise your spirits as well as harmonize your mental and physical condition. Of course, singing stimulates breathing, and the lungs, as we have seen, are one of the main avenues of discharge for the body as a whole. Excessive fat and mucus may accumulate or travel there, and singing will help them come out. Like everything else, sound and vibration are governed by yin and yang. Some sounds are more contractive, others more expansive. Sounds affect different organs and functions of the body differently. Some sounds energize and activate; others soothe and tranquilize. Correctly used, sound and vibration are powerful tools to help recover from sickness and maintain usual good health. Reading poetry or literature out loud for a few minutes each day is also very good exercise.

For a comprehensive look at the relationship between sound, music, and healing, see *The Mozart Effect* by Don Campbell with Alex Jack (Avon Books, 1997). Interestingly, Mozart came from a macrobiotically oriented family. His mother and father were both eating natural foods and insisted that their son be given barley and oat milk instead of dairy food while growing up. There is considerable material on the role of diet in this book, including the use of humming and toning in difficult cases where dietary approaches and compresses are not working. Traditionally, sound and music were considered the highest form of healing, as explained in *The Yellow Emperor's Classic,* the primary source text on Asian medicine and philosophy in the Far East. In the West, Apollo, the god of medicine invoked at the beginning of the Hippocratic oath, was also the god of healing. He is portrayed with his harp, and like Orpheus, David (in the Bible), and other sacred musicians, he could intuitively heal with voice and song.

Creative Imaging or Visualization

Over the last decade many people have turned to creating imaging or visualization to help recover from cancer and other serious illnesses, and research is beginning to show the effectiveness of this approach. However, as in the case of prayer and meditation, by itself the power of visualization is limited. Combined with proper diet and way of life in general, it can be very effective (see Table 19).

It is important when we visualize that we do so in a peaceful, harmonious way. Some current visualization methods are based on negative images, including the same violent, conflicting model that gives rise to the disease. For example, some people ask my opinion about visualizing armies of white blood cells with laser beams going out to do battle and zapping cancer cells. I tell them this kind of imagery is completely inappropriate for healing and reinforces the idea that we are not responsible for our health and sickness and that our body is a battlefield.

Cancer, as we have seen, is not an enemy but a friend. It does not originate outside but inside. It is not caused by evil forces that invade and attack us. It is not caused by any moral or spiritual failing or character defect. Rather, cancer is the body's own self-defense mechanism to protect itself against longtime dietary and environmental abuse. Cancer cells are localizing toxins in our body, allowing it to continue functioning until fundamental changes in diet and lifestyle are made. Cancer cells are working in harmony with all other cells, including white and red blood cells. This is an example of the process of natural attraction and harmony that is found throughout the universe. The antibodies secreted by immune cells actually complement and make a balance with cancer cells, viruses, or other potentially harmful substances. Antibodies have an

TABLE 19.   THE PHYSIOLOGICAL BENEFITS OF EXERCISE AND MEDITATION

Walking/Light Exercise	Meditation/Visualization
Stimulates circulation	Relaxes the autonomic nerves
Improves breathing	Lowers blood pressure
Tones the muscles	Relieves stress on internal organs
Increases appetite	Improves control over digestive, respiratory, and
Clears the mind	circulatory functions
Increases bowel motility	Dissolves negative thoughts and emotions and
Improves energy flow to	promotes positive feelings and images
chakras, meridians, tissues,	Improves energy flow to chakras, meridians,
and cells	tissues, and cells

opposite polarity to these cells and neutralize their extreme or excessive qualities, thus keeping the body in a state of healthy equilibrium. When we are in good health, the immune system functions efficiently, and we remain free of sickness. When our overall condition deteriorates, the immune system loses the ability to neutralize these substances, and we become sick.

Visualization should be calm and peaceful. Visualizing our blood cells doing battle with sickness creates stress and anxiety that interfere with the harmonious flow of energy throughout the body. In order to be healthy, we need to bring our view of life into alignment with natural order. Love, gratefulness, and acceptance are basic to health and to living in harmony with ourselves and others around us. During visualization, rather than struggle and combat, we should concentrate on images of overall mental and physical health, on the nourishing properties and energy (ki or electromagnetic energy) of daily food, and on the beneficial influences of the sun and moon, the stars, and the environment. At the cellular level we can imagine tumors naturally regressing as healthy blood and lymph are produced. At the family level we can imagine our families and friends supporting, nourishing, and encouraging us and eventually, guided by our example, making changes in their own way of life. Several peaceful visualizations like this are included in Chapter 37.

FACTORS THAT ENHANCE RECOVERY

Over the years I have seen thousands of people with cancer. In my view, there are several factors that influence the chances of recovery.

Gratitude

Some people are genuinely grateful for their illness and what it has to teach them. They do not complain and blame others but look within themselves for the source of their troubles. They realize that their former way of eating and living was imbalanced, and they are happy to make a fresh start and change. Such people often have a deep faith in something larger than themselves, such as God, nature, or the universe, and they experience the coming of macrobiotics into their lives as an expression of that faith. As their health improves, they grow closer to their original religious heritage, whether it is Catholicism, Judaism, Protestantism, Hinduism, or Buddhism, and their appreciation of other spiritual traditions deepens. After healing themselves, such people go on to help many others. Looking back on their illness, they often say that cancer was one of the best things that ever happened to them because of the changes it brought in their understanding of life and relations with others.

Deep Suffering

People who have experienced the full range of pain and fear and who truly want to be free from suffering readily embrace the diet. They have tried many different symptomatic approaches and been disappointed. They are now ready to give up their defensive way of life, their stubbornness, and their rigidity to find freedom and regain their health. They have developed the ability to self-reflect and embarked on a personal search for truth. When they discover the unifying principle of yin and yang, they learn how to transmute sickness into health and sorrow into joy.

Will and Determination

People who have cancer but still retain their cheerfulness, humor, and will to live also have a high likelihood of success. These people usually have very strong native constitutions inherited from their parents, grandparents, and ancestors who ate grains and vegetables as a major portion of their diet. Even though such persons have spoiled their health in later life, they have reservoirs of strength. They also have a foundation of common sense and appreciation, which they have forgotten. They only need to be reminded.

In contrast, some people who have no desire to live are introduced to macrobiotics (or to some other approach, including medical treatment), often by some well-intentioned family member or friend. Such persons, who frequently ignore the advice they are given, have a very slight chance of recovery. We can continue to extend to them our love, sympathy, and prayers, but ultimately we must respect a person's decision to die.

Love and Care of Family and Friends

With the close cooperation and support of the patient's immediate family, a successful outcome is greatly enhanced. The person's family should clearly understand the situation and begin to eat in a similar manner, while extending their love and support to the person in every possible way.

The approach offered in this book provides a clear and hopeful direction. However, it is usually up to the immediate family members to help the person implement that direction and make day-to-day decisions about what to cook, when to give a compress, and how to handle the disagreements and crises that inevitably crop up. Family members or friends taking care of the person with cancer must also constantly self-reflect and consider whether their advice is sound. As we develop as teachers and healers, we will face many difficulties and frustrations. However, as our own way of eating improves and our intuition develops, we are able to help more and more people.

Proper Dietary Practice

In some cases the macrobiotic dietary recommendations are not well understood or carefully practiced. For example, when I advise, "Eat 40 to 50 percent whole grains every day, prepare rice in a high-quality saucepan with a heavy lid, and add a pinch of sea salt," most people indicate that they understand. However, upon returning home, some might cook with plenty of salt and others with no salt. They may use too much water or not enough. Rather than buying a high-quality ceramic or cast-iron cooker for the price of less than one hospital X-ray, they use an aluminum or other cheap pot or pan with a thin lid. Still others apply the conventional wisdom that if a little is good, a lot is better, and eat 100 percent instead of 50 percent grain. As a result, their condition becomes excessively contracted, and soon they are consuming desserts, salads, fruit juice, and other excessively expansive foods to restore balance. Naturally, these practices hinder recovery.

Another mistake is to confuse the macrobiotic approach with other dietary or nutritional approaches and, "to be on the safe side," try to combine them all. Moreover, some people new to natural foods assume that everything sold in the health food store or organic section of the supermarket is safe to eat, or otherwise it wouldn't be sold there. These misconceptions must be overcome, or the way of eating will become chaotic and disorderly.

The most successful people are those who take macrobiotic cooking classes and learn from the beginning how to prepare foods properly. Without actually seeing the foods cooked by an experienced cook and tasting them for oneself, there is no standard to judge one's own cooking. So in the beginning we recommend that everyone—men and women, boys and girls, young and old—take cooking classes.

Women, and sometimes men, who are experienced cooks sometimes think they already know how to prepare natural foods and neglect to take macrobiotic cooking classes. This is a big mistake. No matter how wonderful their previous style of cooking, they must recognize that this was a major cause of their problem. People who have never cooked for themselves have less trouble adjusting. They have what is called in the Far East "Beginner's Mind." Like children, their minds are open, fresh, original, and clear. That is the kind of spirit that succeeds.

It isn't necessary to spend a great deal of time attending classes. If you are able to learn at least ten or twenty basic dishes, you can go on to develop your own cooking style. When beginning the diet, seek the advice of friends with experience who live near you. Don't hesitate to show them dishes you have prepared and ask for their advice and suggestions.

Following are some of the most common mistakes people make when beginning the macrobiotic dietary approach:

1. Using too much salt in the form of sea salt, miso, shoyu, umeboshi, and other seasonings, and using too many condiments at the table.

2. Using poor-quality salt such as gray sea salt, miso that has not aged two or three years, shoyu that contains chemicals, real or genuine tamari (which can contribute to poor digestion) instead of shoyu, umeboshi that have been treated with chemicals, etc.

3. Using too much oil or poor-quality oil, such as refined vegetable oil as opposed to unrefined vegetable oil, which retains its natural taste, aroma, and nutrients.

4. Not eating whole grain at every meal and taking too many grain products, such as oatmeal, rye flakes, bulgur, grits, etc.

5. Eating too much bread and other hard-baked flour products, including crackers, cookies, muffins, and biscuits, which easily create mucus, intestinal stagnation, and hardness. Instead of a whole bowl of popcorn, take just a handful. Instead of a whole pack of rice cakes, take just a couple.

6. Eating too many sweets and desserts, including too much barley malt and rice syrup.

7. Not eating enough greens.

8. Eating too much liquid or using poor-quality water (too high or too low in minerals) for cooking and drinking.

9. Eating in a disorderly way, eating before sleeping, and not chewing enough. Also, using an electric rather than a gas range.

10. Lack of variety in cooking, which leads to bingeing and eating out.

11. Cooking with a distracted or divided mind, such as watching TV or listening to music or surfing the Net; harboring resentment or anger over some problems at home or work; and not putting your love and positive intention into the food.

12. Neglecting to express your gratitude to the food, the farmer, the food industry, the economy, nature, the universe, and God for one's daily food and dedicating it to creating health, happiness, peace, and love for all beings.

Difficulties in recovery often have to do with one of these or other common mistakes, and when the mistake is corrected, immediate improvement is experienced.

GETTING STARTED

Once the decision has been made to reverse the cancerous condition by embracing a more balanced way of life, combining diet, physical activity, and mental or spiritual exercises, the person should forget about the sickness and live as happily, actively, and normally as possible.

More serious cases may require the use of external applications along with the proper way of eating. Food should be cooked to the normal texture and consistency, provided the person is able to chew and swallow. If the person has difficulty eating in this manner, it is advisable to mash the foods after they have been cooked. It may also be necessary to cook the food with more water than usual, to arrive at a softer, creamier consistency. Grains, vegetables, beans, and other foods can be cooked in this way and then mashed by hand in a traditional mortar called a suribachi. As a general rule, an electric blender, toaster, or other electrical device should not be used because it can create a chaotic vibration in the food. (For preparing party food for a special occasion, especially for large numbers of people, electric devices may be used in moderation, but they should be avoided in day-to-day use and especially for healing.)

Special drinks, dishes, and home care techniques include Sweet Vegetable Drink, Carrot-Daikon Drink, the Potato-Cabbage Plaster, and many others. The methods for preparing these and their proper uses are given in Part III. Most conditions can be dealt with successfully without the use of such external treatments. Only 20 to 30 percent require these special methods. These external applications are also effective for the relief of a variety of precancerous conditions, benign tumors, and cysts, including fibroid tumors, ovarian cysts, and breast cysts.

Simple, safe, and effective solutions to the problem of cancer and other degenerative diseases already exist. These methods extend back to the common roots of traditional global medicine, including home remedies and folk medicine, and are now being successfully practiced by millions of people around the world to improve their health. Our being able as a society to implement these approaches will determine whether modern civilization continues to degenerate biologically or whether we create a sound and healthy future for ourselves, our children, and all humanity.

11

Diagnosing Cancer Safely

Early detection of cancer and accurate classification into categories of yin and yang make adjusting the diet and lifestyle easier and contribute to a smoother recovery. One of the universal features of modern life is that we have lost the natural ability to diagnose and treat disease without recourse to complex, expensive, and often dangerous technology.

However, over the last several years the limits of this approach to sickness, and to cancer in particular, have become more widely recognized. Mammograms have been implicated in causing leukemia, and other diagnostic X-rays may also be hazardous. Cervical Pap smears sometimes show the presence of cancer where none exists, or vice versa. Tissue samples taken in biopsies are subject to contamination and distortion in the operating room and can be misjudged under the microscope. Surgical procedures to remove tumors have actually helped some cancers spread. Radiation therapy can damage healthy tissue and lead to acute or chronic secondary disorders. Chemotherapy can poison normal as well as malignant cells and cause a host of blood-deficiency diseases that lead to massive infection.

Hormone treatments have resulted in impotence or sterility. Anesthetics and painkillers frequently weaken the body's immune system and make healing more difficult. Today's miracle cure for cancer, such as Interferon, turns out to be tomorrow's tumor promoter. Even the chemical solution in which surgical instruments are routinely cleaned and the plastic tubing for intravenous feeding have been implicated in medical tests as cancer-causing.

Despite the most optimistic predictions and interpretation of the statistics, the casualties in the war on cancer continue to mount. As a result of this dilemma, the concept of a cure for cancer has undergone a significant change during this century. In cancer treatment, cure no longer carries the usual dictionary definition of restoration to a healthy and sound condition, but signifies only that the patient is still alive five years from the time the tumor was originally treated. *Control* is a more appropriate word than *cure,* and over the last few decades the slight increase in the control rate has reflected advances in surgery, blood transfusions, and antibiotics more than breakthroughs in actual cancer treatment.

The challenge to modern cancer therapy was underscored in an address to a panel of the American Cancer Society by Dr. Hardin Jones, a professor of medical physics at the University of California in Berkeley and an expert on statistics and the effects of surgery, drugs, and radiation. "My studies have proven conclusively that untested cancer victims actually live up to four times longer than treated individuals. For a typical type of cancer, people who refused treatment lived for an average 12½ years. Those who accepted surgery and other kinds of treatment lived an average of only three years. . . . I attribute this to the traumatic effect of surgery on the body's natural defense mechanism. The body has a natural defense against every type of cancer."

Dr. Hardin's conclusions echo Hippocrates' warning that cancer patients who are treated with incision die, but those who are not treated with the knife live a relatively long time. Three hundred years ago, on the eve of the scientific revolution, the French author Molière observed laconically, "If we leave Nature alone, she recovers gently from the disorder into which she has fallen. It is our anxiety, our impatience, which spoils all; and nearly all men die of their remedies, not of their diseases."

From reports such as Dr. Hardin Jones's, some people have concluded that modern medicine is iatrogenic (disease-causing) and will no longer see a doctor or go to a hospital under any circumstances. However, this is to overlook the many positive advances in emergency treatment and in the control and relief of pain that have developed over the decades. In general, we recommend avoiding those features of modern medicine that treat symptoms rather than underlying causes and that are potentially harmful. However, under a few special circumstances, it may be necessary to take advantage of the lifesaving apparatus and techniques afforded by hospitals. For example, if a cancer patient can no longer eat and is rapidly losing weight, it may be necessary to supply intravenous glucose injections until the body metabolism is stabilized. Meanwhile, soft grains and mashed vegetables can be prepared and given to the patient in the hospital room as his or her appetite returns. Similarly, there may be emergency situations when surgery or radiation treatment is advisable, such as obstructions in the digestive system that totally block the ingestion of food of any kind.

The crisis of faith in modern medicine's ability to cure cancer reflects a deeper loss of the awareness and judgment we all share regarding our health and well-being. Every day we hear about someone who is active and seemingly fit discovering in a routine medical examination that his body is riddled with tumors. How often we hear of someone who died of a heart attack shortly after being given a clean bill of health by his or her doctor, or we read in the newspaper about a tragic crime that has been committed by someone with a serious mental or emotional disorder that has escaped the attention of his or her family, neighbors, and coworkers. Our most sophisticated technology can reveal the chemical structure of our blood and brain tissue, but it cannot tell us very long in advance whether we are developing a serious physical, mental, or emotional ailment. It is increasingly acknowledged that cancer takes many years, perhaps decades, to develop. However, approximately 50 percent of tumors are not discovered until after they have spread from the primary site to other regions or organs of the body.

Clearly we need to supplement our health care with a medicine that is preventive in direction and humane and educational in application. The traditional medicine in China, Japan, and other countries of the Far East, as well as folk medicine and home care, can contribute greatly to filling this need.

The Yellow Emperor's Classic of Internal Medicine, Caraka Samhita, and other standard Oriental medical texts on the causes of disease stressed the relationship between an individual's health and his or her diet, activity, emotions, spiritual development, and environment. No single aspect of human life was considered separate from another aspect. The biological, psychological, and spiritual were seen as interrelated aspects of the totality. The medical practitioner was an adviser and teacher who could point out the source of a potential sickness and give practical suggestions for changes in diet and lifestyle that could eliminate the problem before visible symptoms occurred.

Modern medicine diagnoses a disease principally by observing physical symptoms. The experienced macrobiotic counselor, however, can foresee the development of sickness before pain, fever, rash, or other symptoms surface. In former times, Oriental physicians were ordinarily paid by a family as long as the family members remained in good health. In case of sickness, the doctor received no stipend because he or she should have foreseen the ailment and prevented it through proper dietary adjustments. This was the traditional test of a good healer.

DIAGNOSIS BY PHYSIOGNOMY

The principal tool of macrobiotic diagnosis is physiognomy, which the *Oxford English Dictionary* defines as "the art of judging character and disposition

from the features of the face or the form and lineaments of the body generally." The basic premise of physiognomy is that each of us represents a living
encyclopedia of our entire physical, mental, emotional, and spiritual development. The strengths and weaknesses of our parents, the environment we grew
up in, and the food we have eaten are all expressed in our present condition.
Our posture, the color of our skin, the tone of our voice, and other traits are
external manifestations of our blood quality, inner organs, nervous system,
and skeletal structure. These, in turn, are the result of our heredity, diet, environment, daily activity, thoughts, and feelings.

The secret of diagnostic skill is to recognize the signs of a particular
set of changes before they become serious—to see visual clues on the face
or in the eyes that stones are developing in the kidneys, that the heart is
expanding, or that a cancer is developing—and before these symptoms bring
pain or discomfort. This type of diagnosis depends completely on the
practitioner developing his or her own sensitivity and understanding fully
the principles that underlie the techniques, together with his or her life experience.

The study of physiognomy originally developed in the West as well as in
the East and served as an integral part of everyday life and medicine in the
ancient Hellenistic world and in Europe through the Renaissance. In the Zo-
har, a book of Jewish teachings from the Middle Ages, we read: "The character of man is revealed in the hair, the forehead, the eyes, the lips, the
features of the face, the lines of the hands, and even the ears. By these seven
the different types of men can be recognized." Leonardo da Vinci's note-
books contain numerous materials on physiognomy. For example, he compiled a reference dictionary for his own use of heads, eyes, mouths, chins,
necks, throats, shoulders, and noses on which he drew for his famous
anatomical sketches and character studies. Western literature abounds with
references to physiognomy, and until the nineteenth century many great authors drew upon their knowledge of this art for development of their char-
acters.

The general principles of physiognomy can be found in a macrobiotic
text or in Sir Walter Scott's *Ivanhoe* or Shakespeare or Dickens. However,
development of the art requires that the practitioner's own health and judgment be refined and involves much study and patience. My own practical
study of physiognomy began in the early 1950s, shortly after I arrived in the
United States and settled in New York. I used to stand on Forty-second Street
and Broadway and along Fifth Avenue observing thousands of people: their
body structure, their way of walking, their way of expression, their faces,
their behavior, and their thinking. In cafeterias and restaurants, theaters and
amusement parts, trains and subways, shops and schools, every day I observed the countless variety of human faces and forms.

Week by week, month by month, year by year it became apparent that all physical, psychological, social, and cultural manifestations of human activity depend on our environment and dietary habits. It became clear that hereditary factors are nothing but the result of the past environment in which our ancestors lived and the food they observed in their daily diet. The constitution we inherit at birth is largely influenced by the food our mothers ate during pregnancy. Leonardo da Vinci succinctly summed up this relationship in his writings on the embryo: "The mother desires a certain food and the child bears the mark of it."

During the embryonic period, all major systems of the body gather and form the entire facial structure. These include the digestive and respiratory systems, the nervous system, and the circulatory and excretory systems. As the fetus grows, the upper and lower parts of the body develop in parallel. Following birth, each area of the face correlates with an inner organ and its functions. These major correlations are discussed below.

Correlation of Inner Organs and Facial Features

The condition of the cheeks shows the condition of the chest cavity including the lungs and breasts and their functions. The tip of the nose represents the heart and its functions, while the nostrils represent the bronchi connecting the lungs. The middle part of the nose represents the stomach, and the middle to upper part of the nose the pancreas. The eyes represent the kidneys as well as the condition of the ovaries in the case of a woman and the testicles in the case of a man. Also, the left eye represents the condition of the spleen and pancreas, and the right eye the liver and gallbladder. The irises and whites of the eyes reflect the condition of the entire body. The area on the lower forehead between the eyebrows shows the condition of the liver, and the temples on both sides the condition of the spleen. The forehead as a whole represents the small intestines, and the peripheral region of the forehead represents the large intestines. The upper part of the forehead shows the condition of the bladder. The ears represent the kidneys: the left ear the left kidney, and the right ear the right kidney. The mouth as a whole shows the condition of the entire digestive tract. More specifically, the upper lip shows the stomach, and the lower lip shows the small intestines at the inner part of the lip and the large intestine at the more peripheral part of the lip. The corners of the lips show the condition of the duodenum. The area around the mouth represents the sexual organs and their functions.

Lines, spots, moles, swellings, discolorations, and other abnormalities in any of these locations indicate specific malfunctions in the corresponding inner organs as a result of improper food consumption. The markings of the hands, feet, chest, back, and all other parts of the body also offer clues to the internal physiological condition of the individual as well as mental and psychological tendencies. On the basis of these observations and other simple, safe techniques, the person's overall health can be ascertained and season-to-season, week-to-week, or day-to-day fluctuations can be monitored.

Identification of Diseased Conditions

In this way chronic ailments or precancerous conditions can be identified long before they develop, and appropriate dietary adjustments can be made. For example, developing obstructions, cysts, and tumors can be diagnosed through careful observation of the whites of the eyes, which represent the condition of the whole body. Precancerous conditions often correlate with the following markings:

1. Calcified deposits in the sinuses are frequently indicated by dark spots in the upper portion of the white of the eye.

2. Kidney stones and ovarian cysts are often indicated by dark spots in the lower white of the eye.

3. The accumulation of mucus and fat in the centrally located organs (liver, gallbladder, spleen, and pancreas) frequently appears in the form of a blue, green, or brownish shade, or white patches, in the white of the eye on either side of the iris, often indicating reduced functioning in these organs.

4. Accumulation of fat and mucus in and around the prostate is often indicated by a yellow or white coating on the lower part of the eyeball.

5. Fat and mucus accumulating in the female sex organs are frequently indicated by a yellow coating on the lower central rim of the eye. Vaginal discharges, ovarian cysts, fibroid tumors, and similar disorders are also possibly shown as white/gray mucus.

Another clue to approaching cancer is a change in skin color. When cancer develops, a greenish shade will often appear in certain areas of the skin. The appearance of this color represents a process of biological degeneration. To better understand this, let us consider the order of colors in the natural world. Among the seven primary colors, red has the longest wavelength and is the warmest, brightest, and most active. Therefore, we classify red as yang. The opposite colors—purple, blue, and green—have shorter wavelengths and are cooler, darker, and more still or passive. We therefore classify them as yin. Red is the color of the more yang animal kingdom and is readily apparent in the color of the blood and general pigmentation of the skin. On the other hand, green is the color of the more yin vegetable realm and is the color of chlorophyll. Eating represents the process whereby we transform green vegetable-quality life into red animal-quality blood. It is based on the ability to change magnesium, which lies at the center of the chlorophyll molecule, into iron, the element that forms the basis of the hemoglobin in our blood.

More yin colors—purple, blue, or gray—appear in the sky and atmosphere, both of which are more expanded or yin components of the environment, as well as often near the time of death. More yang colors—yellow, brown, and orange—appear in the more compact world of minerals. During the transformation of vegetable life into human blood cells, waste products are eliminated through functions such as urination and bowel movements. These represent in-between stages in the transformation of vegetable into human life and therefore are yellow and brown, the colors that lie in between green and red in the color spectrum.

Cancer represents a reverse evolutionary process in which body cells decompose and change back toward more primordial vegetable life. Multiplication of these degenerating cells gives rise to tumors and manifests in a greenish shade appearing on the skin. This shading does not appear on the entire body or near the tumor itself but in certain areas along the respective meridians of electromagnetic energy corresponding with the location of the cancer. These meridians or pathways run the length of the body and form the basis for shiatsu (Oriental massage), acupuncture, the martial arts, and some home remedies. The light green color signifying cancer tends to show up on the hands or feet. Several examples are listed below.

TABLE 20.   VISUAL DIAGNOSIS USING COLOR

Cancer Type	Region Where Greenish Shade Might Appear
Colon	Outside of either hand in the indented area between thumb and forefinger
Small intestine	Outside of the little finger
Lung/breast	Either or both cheeks and on the inside of the wrists
Stomach	Along the outside front of either leg, especially below the knee or in the extended area of the second and third toes
Bladder/uterus, ovaries/prostate	Around either ankle on the outside of the leg
Liver/gallbladder	Around the top of the foot in the outside central area, with its area extending to the fourth toe
Spleen/lymph	Inside the foot from the outer root of the big toe toward the area below the anklebone

Please note that the appearance of a green hue on the body does not necessarily indicate the presence of cancer or a precancerous condition. In some cases, hues and shadings are transitory and quickly come and go, especially following exposure to chemical toxins or other extreme substances. It is vitally important that you do not conclude you have cancer or another serious illness on the basis of a transitory appearance. (You may see green on your skin or face because you are apprehensive, while others may not!) You may then internalize the imagery and make yourself sick. Rather, take visual cues like this as a potential warning to be checked out and confirmed by other approaches, including medical, if necessary, and make dietary, lifestyle, and emotional changes in your life.

SEASONAL APPEARANCE OF SYMPTOMS

The season of the year in which symptoms first appear or the time of day in which discomfort is greatest can also help us determine the nature and location of the sickness. Heart and small intestine ailments arise more frequently in summer and in the late morning or at noontime. Spleen-, stomach-, pancreas-, and lymph-related disorders arise more during the late summer or in the afternoon. Lung and large intestine troubles often surface in the autumn and during the middle to late afternoon. Kidney, bladder, and reproductive difficulties are particularly prevalent in wintertime and during the evening or night. Gallbladder and liver disorders commonly arise in spring and are especially noticeable in early morning. In general, the incidence of cancer increases with cold weather in autumn to early winter, as excess accumulation from the summer is manifested in the formation of tumors. At this time of year breast, skin, and other more yin-type cancers appear because of the high volume of sugar, soft drinks, and dairy food that are consumed in the summertime. Conversely, in winter people tend to eat more meat, poultry, eggs, and other strong yang foods, giving rise to proportionately more yang cancers in the spring, including those of the colon, liver, ovaries, and prostate. Of course, these are general, not absolute tendencies. Cancer may appear in any specific form at any time of the year.

Modern medicine is beginning to study the influence of some of these circadian rhythms on health and sickness. For example, medical researchers have found that heart attacks are almost twice as likely to occur in the hours after waking. As we have seen, the circulatory system is more active in the morning and at midday. Another reason is that modern people tend to eat heavy breakfasts, with an emphasis on bacon, eggs, ham, and other animal food. On top of their yang condition, these excessively yang foods can precipitate a heart attack.

Similarly, researchers report that women with breast cancer face four times the risk of recurrence and death if they have surgery near the time of their menstrual period, compared to women who have operations in mid-cycle. From the macrobiotic view, this is easy to understand. Before the menstrual period a woman becomes more yang and should naturally make balance by taking lighter food, less animal food, and less seasoning. However, if she is eating meat, eggs, chicken, and other strong contractive foods, she becomes very yang (and often tight, irritable, angry, etc.). To offset this, in turn, she is often attracted to extreme yin in the form of sugar, sweets, light dairy food, alcohol, and other relaxing items that make her weak. Overall, extremes of meat and sugar intake make the blood acidic. In this condition, surgery—which is both extremely yangizing (shocking the system) and yinnizing (weakening it through severing the natural energy flow and through the effects of anesthesia)—can lead to increased risk of death or recurrence of the disease (especially through the impaired lymphatic system). As a rule, a woman is attracted to discharge at the full moon, not only in the form of menstruation but also in a tendency toward more frequent shopping, spending money, cleaning the house, and going to the doctor's or dentist's. Unless her intuition is good and she is eating well, she may endanger her health and safety by extreme behavior.

In respect to natural immunity, the number of T cells that counterbalance infections and tumors is at a high in the winter and at a yearly low in June. The reason for this, once again, is that during the winter people are usually eating stronger food, with stronger cooking, more salt, and more animal food. This creates a more yang condition in the blood and lymph system, which produces more lymphocytes. In the spring and early summer, people begin to eat proportionately more raw foods, fruits, sugars and sweets, beverages, and other stronger yin foods. Naturally, their blood and body fluids become weaker. In this way, combining our understanding of diet and environment with the unifying principle of yin and yang, we can begin to understand the cycles and rhythms of health and sickness.

There are many other factors to consider and other traditional diagnostic procedures we may use to help detect cancer before it develops or, if it has already appeared, before it spreads further. These supplementary methods include taking pulses on both wrists and touching the pressure points on the skin along the meridians of electromagnetic energy.

In contrast to modern medicine, traditional diagnosis does not require elaborate or expensive technology, and the methods employed are simple, safe, and accurate. Our own senses are the only tools employed. As our understanding of physiognomy develops, we realize that we are our own machines, and our own intuition and judgment are superior to the most advanced computer. What we see, hear, smell, taste, and touch can tell us the story of an individual's past, present, and probable future. The outer echoes the inner; the inner mirrors the outer. Learning to perceive the development of just one person can lead us to begin to understand the destiny of humanity. The person to begin with is oneself.

12

Combining Macrobiotics with Other Approaches

INTRODUCTION

Many people, including many people in usual good health as well as patients and their families, want to know whether the macrobiotic approach can be combined with other dietary or nutritional systems, supplements, vitamins, exercise and bodywork of various kinds, mental and spiritual exercises, and especially with modern medicine. Are any of these recommended, or will they prevent or hinder improvement?

Just as the macrobiotic way of eating is not a set diet but a body of principles that can be flexibly adapted according to many factors, including personal condition and needs, the macrobiotic way of healing is not a set, rigid approach but a dynamic, ever-changing process that can embrace or complement virtually any other healing technique or modality.

For thousands of generations our ancestors followed a more natural way of life, focusing on daily food preparation and the gathering of wild plants and herbs (supplemented sometimes by animal-quality products) to sustain, nourish, and heal themselves. Principal food—whole cereal grains in most climates and environments—was recognized as the foundation or staff of life. Other foods, drinks, and natural substances could then be used to assist in maintaining usual good health as well as overcome sickness, accident, war, natural catastrophe, and other difficulties.

Hippocrates, the father of modern medicine, was thoroughly macrobiotic in his approach, and for the next two thousand years Western as well as Eastern people and those in other parts of the world essentially observed the principle of "let food be thy medicine and thy medicine be food."

In the last several centuries, the advent of modern science and medicine has introduced many new diagnostic technologies, healing techniques, and nutritional theories and products. Some of these are extremely beneficial; others are often helpful but at the same time may carry health or safety risks, and some are dangerous and are to be avoided except when there is no other alternative.

The traditional macrobiotic way continues to offer a foundation of health and happiness, but the artificial landscape and environment of the modern world often make it difficult to practice. Organic food is increasingly contaminated with genetically modified organisms (GMOs), chemicals, and other toxins, and the nutrients in most common foods have declined about 25 to 50 percent in the last generation.

Meanwhile, the pace of modern life continues to accelerate, global warming threatens to disrupt the four seasons and the world's food supply, and artificial electromagnetic radiation from global networks are disrupting nature, especially honeybees and other beneficial insects, birds, bats, and other pollinators on which our sustenance depends.

In these emergency circumstances, adjustments and modifications to the macrobiotic way of eating and life may need to be observed temporarily. In fact, very few if any people who go to macrobiotics for help in preventing or recovering from illness have not already tried other approaches and currently may be taking special foods, supplements, or medications for their condition. Naturally, they want to know whether these should be continued, discontinued, or modified in some way.

The key to integrating macrobiotics with other approaches is to understand that it is not a single approach among many or opposed to anything else. Rather, macrobiotics—the "large view of life"—incorporates all nutritional and healing approaches, including modern medicine, under one canopy, like a giant tree that shelters all of life. The goal is to develop your intuition and use the philosophy of harmony and balance—namely, the principles of yin and yang, expansion and contraction—to know if and when conventional, alternative, or complementary approaches and techniques are needed and helpful and how to select among them. All approaches to healing, however dangerous (including chemotherapy or experimental cancer techniques), may be used under certain circumstances and be considered part of the macrobiotic way. The difficulty is determining what those circumstances are. Macrobiotics does not reject anything as totally negative, destructive, or evil and sets itself apart from life as a whole.

THE MANDALA OF HEALING

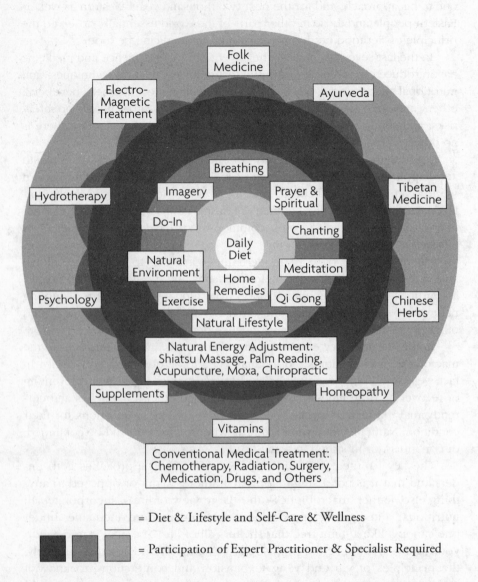

= Diet & Lifestyle and Self-Care & Wellness

= Participation of Expert Practitioner & Specialist Required

For the purpose of embracing the diverse traditions and products of human culture and tradition, including modern medicine and new nutritional and energetic techniques, the Mandala of Healing has been developed. *Mandala* is the traditional Sanskrit or Indian word for "wheel" or "universal model" and is a map illustrating core teachings. At the center of the mandala is dietary practice, namely, the macrobiotic way of eating. This approach itself is constantly evolving to take into account changing environmental and climactic conditions, social and economic factors, and personal needs.

In principal, a balanced daily diet will help prevent sickness and harm. But if imbalance arises, special dishes, special drinks, and home remedies (most of which are based on traditional foods such as the ginger compress, ume-sho-kuzu drink, and kombu plaster) represent the next, or second, circle of healing.

The third circle represents natural lifestyle approaches and includes simple activities and exercises that can be used to strengthen mind and body, stimulate energy flow, and promote better metabolism at various levels. Examples are Do-in, or self-massage, yoga, tai chi and qi gong, walking, painting and drawing, dance, singing, playing or listening to music, prayer, meditation, mind control, and other simple, basic practices that can be performed by the individual easily, safely, and without any special cost.

The fourth circle of healing involves natural energy adjustments. Examples include acupuncture (the use of needles to stimulate energy flow), moxibustion (the use of a dried herb for similar purposes), shiatsu or massage that makes use of clay or oils, aromatherapy, chiropractic, osteopathy, neurolinguistic programming, and others. Again, these external applications may be helpful depending on the case, but they usually require a specialist, specialized diagnosis and evaluation, and moderate cost.

The fifth circle of the mandala includes supplements, vitamins, minerals, herbs, and other largely nutritional products. They include both traditional substances such as Chinese herbs and modern ones such as genistein (soy-based) tablets. For the most part they originate from natural plants or animals, but the way they are processed may be very calm and peaceful (like macrobiotic cooking) or very highly processed (like fast foods). They may also contain other ingredients of low quality (such as gelatin, or animal-based, capsules), and they can be rather expensive and in some cases require an expert to prescribe or administer (for example, Chinese herbs). Compared to the first three circles, circles four and five represents moving beyond self-reliance to dependence on authorities, companies, and health claims that may or may not be true and beneficial.

The sixth circle includes traditional, alternative, and complementary medicine. It also includes electromagnetic treatment and a variety of machines and vibrational devices. Again, these external applications may be helpful depending on the case, but they are often invasive, require experts, and may incur significant cost.

The seventh circle includes conventional medical procedures. The most innocuous are blood tests, EKGs, and other simple lab tests. A variety of pills, drugs, and medications carry low, moderate, and high risks, especially selective serotonin reuptake inhibitors (SSRIs) and other psychiatric drugs. Other risky procedures include surgery (which may range from mild to life-threatening but which can damage meridian flow), radiation of different kinds (MRIs, CT scans, X-rays, mammograms), chemotherapy, and many experimental medications.

Except for accidents, emergencies, and life-and-death situations, many medical procedures are unnecessary; they are aimed at destroying disease rather than identifying the underlying cause of the imbalance. However, in any given case they may be beneficial (especially in small, controlled amounts or frequencies), necessary, or life-saving.

The mandala encourages us to develop our intuition and to keep an open mind or what traditionally was known in Zen as Beginner's Mind—a childlike awareness that marvels at the infinite universe, maintains faith in its order and goodness, and recognizes that all energy ultimately is one.

DIET: THE FOUNDATION

The standard macrobiotic way of eating is the universal foundation for health and happiness and can be modified for climate and environment, cultural and religious traditions, age, sex, level of activity, condition of health, and personal needs and dreams. No food or drink traditionally consumed by humanity is forbidden, and none is a cure-all or panacea for all conditions or all people. Balance, moderation, and common sense are the key. Today, except for a very few remaining traditional cultures and religious communities, we all live in two worlds: the modern world of fast-paced, high-energy technology, communications, and highly processed, largely contaminated foods, and the natural world in which humanity's biological and spiritual development depends primarily on grains, vegetables, and other plant quality foods with a small, modest amount of animal food if desired.

Is it all right to continue to eat foods that are not generally encouraged in the macrobiotic way of eating? Yes—but! Anything may be consumed, and it should be consumed joyfully, without guilt, remorse, or other negative emotions. But all foods have energetic effects, and those foods that are to be avoided or limited are discouraged because they tend to create imbalance and sickness. Disease is not negative, bad, or sinful. It arises over time because of energetic imbalance, especially the way we eat. But if it prompts us to change our view of life, our diet, and our lifestyle, heart disease or cancer may be the best thing that ever happened to us. Hence, all foods and beverages may be eaten, especially for those in usual good health. Taking extreme items, such as meat and sugar, commonly produce extreme effects but often can be tolerated in small doses on infrequent occasions. If extreme foods become habitual, then imbalance will set in, leading eventually to acute or chronic illness. For those who are already sick, especially those with cancer, it is strongly recommended that extreme items be avoided or limited.

Practically, it is not wise to change at once; it is better to make a slow, gradual transition to the new way. It is better to take several weeks or months to implement the macrobiotic approach than try to do it overnight or too quickly. Go at your own pace, continuing to eat at least partly in the old way as long as necessary without fear or regret. The important thing is to make progress. In fact, if you go as slowly as possible, you will find that you have changed completely before you know it. The harder and faster you try, the more difficult it is. The easier and slower you go, the less difficult it becomes. And if you lapse, don't worry about it. Try to figure out why you are attracted to extremes. Usually it is because of some common mistake in cooking or food selection. This is your homework: the study of yin and yang. Two steps forward, one step backward. Don't worry about making mistakes, lacking the will, or jeopardizing your improvement. Just start anew, fresh each day, and do the best you can. Before you know it, you will graduate to a higher level of understanding and practice.

HERBS, VITAMINS, MINERALS, AND OTHER NUTRITIONAL SUPPLEMENTS

Many nutritional supplements are promoted for preventing and relieving illness. These include aloe vera, comfrey, ginkgo biloba, red clover, and dozens of other herbs; vitamin A and beta-carotene, vitamin B complex, vitamin C, vitamin D, vitamin E, and other vitamins; calcium, selenium, zinc, and other minerals; and green tea, pomegranate, kampyo, wild yam, and other food-based supplements.

In principle, the macrobiotic way of eating, based on organically and naturally grown foods, traditionally or minimally processed fare, and cooking with love and conscious intention, includes all the Ki (or life energy) and nutrients to ensure optimal health and well-being. For many years the macrobiotic community discouraged the consumption of supplements of any kind. By the early twenty-first century, however, it became clear that we live in a world that is increasingly chaotic and contaminated so that even good-quality foods are often compromised. To compensate, many macrobiotic friends, families, and teachers who had strictly avoided supplements are resorting to vitamins, herbs, enzymes, or other special substances to compensate for the sharp decline in food quality and Ki energy. In the United States, the food quality has especially deteriorated, while it is still fairly good in Europe, Japan, and other parts of the world.

Since this trend is new, it is not yet possible to recommend any specific supplements. It may take years or even a generation for a consensus to emerge about what works and what doesn't. Instead, the following principles for using supplements can be considered:

1. As the proverb goes, "If it's not broken, don't fix it." If you are growing your own food, if you are buying locally grown food of high quality, and if you are enjoying good health, vitality, and a calm,

peaceful mind with your present way of eating, then there is no need to take or experiment with supplements. Thousands of macrobiotic individuals, families, and households around the world feel no need for supplements and get along perfectly well without them.

2.   Some cases may require supplementation for a limited period of time, such as individuals currently in transition from unhealthful eating habits to a well-balanced macrobiotic diet; individuals who are not eating a well-balanced macrobiotic diet but are only partially doing so; individuals who have developed a serious ailment that may require supplemental, conventional, or alternative approaches until they establish a reasonably healthy condition and begin to practice a macrobiotic way of life; and healthy individuals whose natural or macrobiotic-quality food is compromised by pollution, GMOs, or other toxins and who feel they need a temporary supplement because of low energy, fatigue, stress, or symptoms that don't improve.

3.   Such individuals should seek the highest quality supplements available: (a) supplements prepared at home using natural, whole food ingredients such as macrobiotic home remedies. Examples include ume-sho-kuzu drink, daikon tea, etc.; (b) segments or extracts of natural plants and vegetables and/or their combinations that people can make themselves or purchase if available. These supplements may also include naturally processed food products. "Naturally processed" means juicing, heating, pressing, drying, diluting, crushing, roasting, boiling, freezing, and other similar natural processes that do not involve the application of chemical substances or chemical processing. Examples include vegetable juices, fruit juices, herbal teas, Chinese herbal medicine, spirulina, blue green algae, green magma, and various homeopathic substances; (c) products that contain natural minerals but are not coated, mixed, or treated with chemical substances. Examples include calcium, iron, magnesium, zinc, etc.; (d) products that contain less than 20 percent (of the total weight of the product) meat- or animal-based substances and that contain no chemical additives, chemical processing, or GMO animal feed. Examples include Oriental medicines, folk medicines, and products containing oyster shells, fossils, bones, skin, or eggs; (e) products that contain natural plant, mineral, and animal substances as well as chemical substances or chemical processing (as long as they do not produce harmful effects).

4.   The highest commercial-quality supplements are generally organically grown, minimally or traditionally processed, and all plant or vegan quality. Learn to read labels and become savvy about hidden

sugar, dairy, and animal products that may be disguised with innocuous labels (for example, casein is dairy protein).

5. If you take supplements with animal ingredients, seek those that are derived from organically raised animals and not chemically fed or raised with GM soy, corn, or other compromised animal feed.

6. Generally, plant quality is superior to animal quality. Animal quality is preferable to foods chemically manufactured or artificially produced. For example, traditionally made soy foods such as miso, tofu, and tempeh produce effects completely different from modern, highly processed soy foods such as textured vegetable protein, genistein, and soy ice cream that may be chemically manufactured or treated.

7. Take supplements in small amounts and as infrequently as possible. Manufacturers' suggested recommended doses are often exaggerated and designed to get the customer to take (and hence purchase) more than he needs. As a rule of thumb, start with half the recommended dose and work up if necessary; also take half as often as recommended, such as once a day rather than twice. See if you experience any benefit. If not, increase the dose or frequency, and if no effect or a negative effect comes at the recommended level, discontinue.

8. If you are already taking supplements and want to stop them, it is better to stop gradually rather than all at once. Decrease by a small amount or cut back in frequency and gradually taper off. As a rule (see Modern Medicine, page 164), do not discontinue medically prescribed supplements or drugs without consulting a physician. But for over-the-counter items, especially nutritional supplements, use your own judgment and common sense. Make it an adventure and discover what works and what doesn't. Keep a food/supplement journal or daily diary and begin to correlate your activity level, health, mind, and spirit with what you eat. Study yin and yang and the energetics of food. Sharpen your intuition. Over time you will see clear trends.

9. When you have healed or improved and your intuition tells you that you no longer need to take the vitamins, herbs, or enzymes, start to taper off. It is hoped that a slow exit strategy will enable your body to adjust to any withdrawal symptoms. It may be that you will reach a plateau and need to remain there for a while. Don't worry. There is no absolute right or wrong or something unmacrobiotic about

continuing supplements or medication. Whatever works for you and enables you to maintain your health and realize your goals is what is important.

ALTERNATIVE AND COMPLEMENTARY THERAPIES

Some of the most popular dietary, lifestyle, and other alternative approaches are described here:

1. Antioxidants are healthful compounds found in whole grains, vegetables, fruits, and other largely plant-quality foods. The standard macrobiotic way of eating and a balanced vegan or vegetarian diet generally supplies adequate amounts of antioxidants. A wide variety of antioxidants is available in pill form, including selenium, vitamin E, and beta-carotene. However, the source of this supplementation may be of low quality or contaminated, and recent medical studies suggest that taking antioxidants in pill form is counterproductive. For example, in 2008 a study in the *Mayo Clinic Proceedings* found that beta-carotene supplements increased the risk for lung cancer among smokers and that selenium supplements may benefit men but not women. As a rule, as most nutritionists agree, avoid antioxidant supplementation if possible and get these healthful substances through whole foods.

2. Apricot pits, laetrile, amygdalin, and vitamin B_{17} have been associated with reducing leukemia and other forms of cancer. They contain nitrilosides and a trace of cyanide that are said to kill cancer cells. The sale of laetrile across state lines or international borders is prohibited in the United States by the FDA, which says it is toxic. But laetrile is available from clinics in Mexico and from some physicians. Traditionally, apricots have been part of a healthy diet in many societies such as the Hunza, the long-lived people in the Himalayas. Modern apricot derivatives such as laetrile and vitamin B_{17} may be helpful for leukemia and other types of cancer as part of a balanced whole foods diet.

    Interestingly, the umeboshi plum that is widely used in the macrobiotic community has one of the highest concentrations of laetrile. The umeboshi is actually a member of the apricot family, not the plum. The ume's laetrile is located in the seed. This in turn is situated in the hard inedible pit of the ume. It can be accessed by hitting the pit with a hammer. The seed can be carbonized in a 450-degree oven for eight to ten minutes, after which it turns black.

Grind into a powder and use for a variety of ills, including stomach and intestinal ills, colds, diarrhea, nausea, fevers, coughs, and motion sickness. They are also good for a variety of cancers, including intestinal cancer and leukemia. The shells of the seed may also be made into a tea.

There are no magic foods, pills, or bullets in life, and overreliance on any one product or nutrient is not recommended. Apricot products may be helpful for certain conditions but not others. Other popular anti-cancer fruits include pomegranates, grapes, and schisandra (a traditional berry from China). Similar qualifications apply.

3. Ayurveda is the traditional medicine of India. It is based on a deep understanding of nature and universal law and has traditionally been practiced by millions of people to maintain their health and well-being. Today it still offers guidance. However, Ayurveda and its offshoot—the yogic diet, of which there are many varieties—commonly do not take into consideration very different climates and environments in North America and Europe and the Indian subcontinent. Hence, diet and medicine focusing on curry, spices, herbs, aromatic oils, and other expansive substances that may be beneficial in a tropical or subtropical region could be counterproductive in a temperate area. Similarly, the Tibetan diet high in animal products is appropriate in the high Himalayas to protect from cold and elevated altitudes, but when exported to India, Britain, or America, it often leads to declining health. The principles of Ayurveda, Tibetan medicine, African medicine, and other traditional medicines around the world are sound and reliable. Their implementation is often flawed, however, especially when adhered to in different climates and environments.

4. Cacao and bitter chocolate have been found in some medical studies to reduce the risk of certain cancers and other disorders. From the macrobiotic perspective, this extremely yin substance (especially dark chocolate without cane sugar) may be temporarily helpful for yang conditions such as ovarian or prostate cancer, but for many others, especially breast cancer and those with strong yin factors, it could be disastrous.

5. Chanting and other spiritual practices involving sound and music are generally helpful, but like other forms of energy, chants, songs, and musical genres produce different effects on mind, body, and spirit. Some chants (for example, "Om Namyo Renge Kyo," are extremely yangizing and may be helpful for yin conditions but detrimental for

yang ones. Similarly, yin chants (such as "Alleluia") may be helpful to soothe and relax yang conditions but too expansive for yin conditions. Traditional chants that are more balanced include "Su," "Om" (Aum), "Amen," and "Allah." Gregorian chants, as a rule, are also more balanced and soothing, Zen chants are generally yang, and many (but not all) Sanskrit chants are yin.

6. Chorella is a type of single-cell algae that grows in fresh water. It is also known as green or blue-green algae or sun chorella and comes in the form of pills, powders, and liquid extracts. High in chlorophyll, the substance that gives plants a green color, chorella supplements reportedly help prevent or relieve cancer, guard against infection, promote natural immunity, and confer other benefits. Freshwater algae is extremely yin, or expansive in nature, and as a supplement to a balanced diet may help offset yang conditions, including prostate, colon, and ovarian cancer. However, it could aggravate yin conditions, including breast cancer, most leukemias and lymphomas, and other more expansive conditions. In general, the standard macrobiotic diet emphasizes algae in the form of sea vegetables. Not only are these multicellular foods richer in vitamins and minerals than single-cell algae, but they come from a saline environment—corresponding with human blood and the circulatory system—that contributes more balanced energy than lake and river plants which grow in a salt-free environment.

7. Colonics refers to various techniques used to cleanse or purge the bowels and lower digestive system. The methods commonly make use of enemas (sometimes with coffee or other food or beverage) to purge stagnated and toxic material from the bowels. The procedures are often successful, but they put tremendous strain, pressure, and tension on intestines and other organs. Colitis, fluid and electrolyte imbalances, and in some cases septicemia (blood poisoning) have resulted from its application. In our experience it is far better to use the ginger compress on the abdomen and other less strenuous, more peaceful methods of facilitating discharge and a return to normalcy.

8. Enzymes and probiotics are widely available to promote better digestion, assimilation, and metabolism, especially in the small intestine. As with other supplements, quality, quantity, and frequency of use are important considerations. Some macrobiotic teachers and counselors recommend these substances for some of their clients and have found them to be helpful, while others have not. Since everyone's metabolism is different, it is hard to give any general

guidance. A double-blind study published in the *Lancet* in 2008 studied 296 patients at risk for severe pancreatisis. Those who were given probiotics required substantially more intensive care and surgical intervention, and had higher death rates than those given placebos.

9. The Gerson diet developed by Max Gerson in the mid-twentieth century is a natural foods diet based on restoring proper cell metabolism. The diet is high in potassium and low in sodium, includes plenty of fruits and vegetables, and avoids or limits animal and dairy products, fats, and sugars. The Gerson diet also stresses the use of ground coffee enemas, which may be stressful.

10. Green tea is made from the leaves of the tea bush or plant and has traditionally been used in Asia for relaxation and healing. Because it contains some caffeine and has a slightly expansive effect, it is classified as yin and in small amounts can be helpful for some strong yang conditions such as colon, liver, ovarian, and prostate cancer. It may also be taken occasionally by those in usual good health for sociability and enjoyment. Many current medical studies are showing the benefits of green tea for cancer and other conditions, but be aware that these benefits are experienced largely by a yang, meat-eating population that the yin components of green tea help offset. For people eating more plant-quality foods, it could have an opposite effect. Macrobiotics generally discourages the daily or regular use of green tea for this reason. Kukicha (or bancha tea) that is made from the stems and twigs of the tea bush (and are essentially caffeine-free) is far better for daily health and more soothing than green tea.

11. Herbs have traditionally been used around the world and are an important part of traditional medicine. In the past, people grew up knowing the flora and fauna of their region, including medicinal herbs, roots, and other plants. Unfortunately, that knowledge is no longer common, and today use of herbs requires specialized knowledge and experience. Hence, reliance on specialists, high costs, and other complications may arise. Further, since herbs grow primarily in the wild, they are usually much stronger energetically than ordinary foods. They can be very effective if properly used and administered, but if taken in excess or without professional guidance, they can stress mind and body and be counterproductive. Some people, for example, turn to Chinese herbs for many conditions including cancer. In principle, Chinese herbology is possibly the oldest and most advanced. However, in practice, people who use Chinese

herbs often develop troubles when toxins discharged by the herbs overburden the liver, the main organ of discharge, or the kidneys, intestines, lungs, and other sites where energy is actively exchanged with the environment. Be cautious.

12. Saunas, hot springs, and sweat lodges have also been used success-fully by many cultures for healing. The aim is to work up a sweat and release toxins from the body. There are a variety of types, and each produces slightly different effects. Since heat is a very yang factor, these methods will primarily benefit those with a more yin constitution or condition. Those who are yang may be repelled by the strong heat or experience overactive heart and circulatory sys-tems. Japanese hot springs or baths, for example, combine strong yin and yang—fire and water—and primarily benefit a yang popu-lation that eats a large amount of fish and seafood, salt, pickles, condiments, and other salt-based items. Such springs or baths are often too extreme for macrobiotic individuals or those whose con-dition is more balanced. Again, be mindful and moderate in using fire and water to heal.

13. Juice fasts, raw foods, and vegetarian diets have been used to heal from cancer and other disorders. These approaches are strongly yin and will attract and benefit yang individuals who have consumed substantial amounts of animal food in the past. Juice, fruit, oil, spices, and raw foods all promote rapid discharge, and people on these diets typically feel terrific in the beginning as excess and tox-ins come out. However, if eaten over time, they usually become weaker and weaker as the initial high peaks and their energy level go down. A generation ago, Nathan Pritikin developed a special diet to prevent heart disease. It included substantial fruit, raw foods, and more yin items. The Pritikin diet did help guard against heart attacks but often left the person weaker and vulnerable to yin disorders such as leukemia, which ultimately claimed Pritikin. One of the criticisms of macrobiotics over the years is that it does not include enough fruits, juices, and fresh foods. There is some truth to this observa-tion, and in recent years more macrobiotic individuals and families are eating more of these items and feeling lighter and more relaxed.

14. Lycopene, a substance in tomatoes and other foods, has been found to have strong anti-cancer effects, especially in men with prostate cancer. The standard macrobiotic diet for a temperate climate dis-couraged the consumption of tomatoes and other nightshades (potatoes, peppers, eggplants, and others) for many years. How-ever, it became clear that men with this disease did in fact benefit

from consuming some tomato products. Because tomatoes are extremely yin, we recommended that a small amount of miso be added to tomato sauce to help balance spaghetti or whatever dish it is served with. Because of global warming and other yang climatic and atmospheric conditions, the entire macrobiotic way of eating has lightened up in recent years. In principle, we still urge caution on eating nightshades, especially as primary vegetables or on a daily basis. But practically speaking, a majority of macrobiotic individuals in temperate regions today occasionally eat a small amount of tomatoes, potatoes, and other foods that we strictly avoided in the past. It is another example of the flexibility of the macrobiotic way and its constant adaptation to changing circumstances.

15.   Mushrooms including shiitake, maiitake, and others, are offered for relief from various disorders. We have used and recommended these items for many years, but, once again, they should be used in small quantities and infrequently because they are extremely yin. Mushrooms are easier for yang individuals to eat and help eliminate fat and oil from the body. Yin people may become weaker from taking too many mushrooms. If cancer is present, fresh shiitake should be avoided, dried shiitake are preferable.

16.   Music therapy encompasses many dimensions, from masking pain and improving memory and concentration to stabilizing the emotions and lifting the spirit. Sound and music are important parts of a comprehensive healing approach. Singing a happy song every day has long been a cardinal lifestyle guideline.

17.   Omega-3 and omega-6 oils and the ratio between them is one of the most popular new nutritional approaches to health and well-being. The standard macrobiotic way of eating generally contains an ideal balance of these nutrients. Like other nutritional theories, the omega oil approach focuses on one set of parameters to the exclusion of others and offers a limited framework. We need a balance of nutrients, and reductionist approaches encourage people to seek supplements and take excessive doses, resulting in the opposite of what they intend.

18.   Rain forest herbs are touted for their botanical and medicinal properties. They are wonderful, especially for people who live in the rain forest. They are totally unecological for people living in different climates and environments. Harvesting them usually results in shrinking the rain forests and threatens traditional cultures. It is best to avoid them.

19. Reflexology utilizes pressure on the feet, hands, or other parts of the body to relieve a variety of ailments and balance the flow of energy. There are several types including zone therapy and reflex therapy. Medical studies generally show that they are helpful in controlling pain, promoting relaxation, and stimulating well-being. In macrobiotics we focus primarily on acupressure, a form of massage that can be done individually (in the form of Do-in) or by a family member, friend, or practitioner (shiatsu). Such methods are an important part of a comprehensive approach to health and well-being.

20. Reiki is a contemporary form of healing using the hands or palms. Its roots go back to the laying on of hands (found in the Bible, the Koran, and other traditional texts) and can be extremely beneficial. In our classes we teach palm healing (which harnesses the infinite energy of heaven and earth) to energize, relax, and harmonize the body, mind, and spirit. The direct use of energy like this from the cosmos is one of the highest forms of healing. In extraordinarily difficult cases where diet is not working or the patient is unable to eat, we have used palm healing to get energy moving again. In some cases it has resulted in almost miraculous recoveries. Palm healing, laying on of hands, Reiki, and therapeutic touch (a comparable movement in the nursing community) can be successfully integrated into a comprehensive approach to illness. Medical studies show that it can help reduce pain in some patients with advanced cancer. The key is to learn and master it yourself or find a practitioner who has a deep understanding and is sensitive to your condition and needs.

21. Shamanism, witch doctors, medical men and women, and other forms of spiritual healing are found worldwide and can be an important dimension of healing. The key once again is personal study or finding an experienced practitioner. In most cases, people with illness do not need to avail themselves of such esoteric methods. Traditional prayer, meditation, and self-reflection are generally safer, simpler, and free. If performed with a pure or grateful heart, they are also much more effective.

22. Shark cartilage comes from material extracted from the heads and fins of sharks. The skeletons of these fish are made up almost entirely of cartilage, a type of connective tissue, instead of bones. Glycoproteins, calcium salts, and complex sugars known as mucopolysaccharides are found in shark cartilage, and according to proponents, they im-

pede the growth of new blood vessels, or angiogenesis, a process associated with the growth and spread of tumors. In the macrobiotic view, the shark is a very yang creature, and shark cartilage as a supplement to a balanced diet may be helpful for more yin conditions, including certain cancers. However, shark energy is so extreme— aggressive and predatory—that consuming it may contribute to overly powerful emotions and thoughts. There is also an analogy with cow's milk. Compared to human beings, the skeletal structure of cows is about four times larger, and consuming their milk can lead to bone, spine, and joint problems, including osteoporosis. Similarly, since sharks are mostly cartilage and very little bone, the human skeletal structure may suffer as a result of the ingestion of this substance.

23. Soy foods are widely promoted as anti-cancer agents by both traditional healers and some medical researchers. However, other scientists and physicians strongly warn against the ingestion of soy, especially for breast cancer and other women's ailments, because soy is high in phytoestrogens that can elevate female hormones and increase disease risk. In short, there is a major controversy about the role and value of soy in cancer regimens. Traditional soy foods, especially fermented ones such as miso, shoyu, tempeh, and natto, have been consumed for thousands of years in Asia and have not been associated with an increased cancer risk. On the contrary, almost all studies show they are protective and substantially reduce the risk of cancer. Tofu, which is not fermented, can also be part of a healthy way of eating, but women with breast cancer should use it moderately. The main problem with soy today is that modern, highly processed items such as soy milk, textured soy protein, genistein pills, and other soy products are not traditionally consumed or are manufactured in vast mechanized food factories. These products are generally not suitable for ordinary use, much less for healing, and should be avoided except as party foods. Unfortunately, many medical studies on soy use these artificial soy products and make no distinction between them and traditional ones in drawing conclusions.

24. Sprouts and wheatgrass are promoted by some alternative regimens. Classified as strongly yin, they may help detoxify the body and be beneficial as part of a balanced diet for yang conditions, including yang tumors. However, they may be counterproductive and produce harmful effects for yin conditions and diseases. A small, modest amount of sprouts (including wheatgrass, if desired) falls within the

guidelines of the standard macrobiotic way of eating. But, once again, excessive consumption of any one food, ingredient, or nutrient is not advisable.

25. Pet therapy has become a recognized area of medical research. People who interact with animals often heal more quickly, have less pain, and are happier than those who do not. In respect to cancer, dogs that can sniff out tumors have recently been in the news, and one hospital has a house cat with a gift for knowing when a cancer patient will die. The cat curls up and comforts the dying person for several hours in advance of the time of death. Even in today's modern world, many animals, especially those eating more natural foods, remain extremely intuitive and can give aid and comfort and lift the spirits of both the well and the ill. Everyone is attracted to a different animal, often the one that governs his or her birth sign in Western or Oriental astrology. Birds in particular are psychic and spiritual, and traditionally conveyed messages between heaven and earth. Watching and listening to birds can be done from a sickbed or hospital window and may prove restful and enlightening. In the celebrated words of Dr. Albert Schweitzer's philosophy of reverence for life: "I am life that wills to live in the midst of life that wills to live." Developing the will is important in healing from cancer or any other condition. The other beings with whom we share the planet can teach and assist us in strengthening our resolve and inner development.

   Dogs and cats, especially those who eat chemically processed pet food or modern foods left over from the dinner table, are liable to get cancer. Dr. Norman Ralston, a macrobiotic veterinarian and president of the Holistic Veterinarians Association of America, developed a comprehensive approach that appears in his book *Raising Healthy Pets*.

26. Vitamin therapy is used for many conditions and disorders. The traditional macrobiotic approach is that a balanced daily diet should provide all the vitamins necessary for optimal health, including B_{12}, D, and other vitamins that until recently many medical associations said could be obtained only from animal sources. More recent scientific research has confirmed that these vitamins are available in plant foods, including many regular foods in the standard macrobiotic diet. The medical profession agrees that vitamins taken in the form of pills and supplements are often counterproductive, and it is better to obtain nutrients in whole foods. However, because of global warming and worsening environmental conditions, including

the decline in organic and natural food quality, it may be necessary to take a particular vitamin temporarily as part of a comprehensive approach to healing. In this case the guidelines given above about quality, quantity, and frequency should be observed.

Among vitamins, vitamin D is unique in that it is primarily stimulated by sunlight. It is found in a few foods such as fish and other animal products, as well as sun-dried vegetables and other plants. Medical studies have strongly linked adequate intake of vitamin D with preventing cancer and other diseases. For example, people who live in higher latitudes with less exposure to the sun have more cancers of the colon, pancreas, prostate, ovaries, and breast than those in sunnier climes. This could also result from people in northern regions consuming more yang diets, including animal food, salt, and other heavier fare. The first four malignancies mentioned above are yang in nature, and breast cancer often has strong yang as well as yin factors. Still, the benefits of vitamin D are not just epidemiological. Prevention studies have shown that the risk of colon and breast cancer can be substantially reduced by taking vitamin D supplements of 300 to 2,000 IU daily.

For adequate natural vitamin D from the sun, according to medical authorities, during the spring, summer, and autumn you can expose your arms and legs to the midday sun daily for ten to fifteen minutes before applying sunscreen. If you are not living in a sunny climate or don't get outside much (for example, taking a twenty- to thirty-minute walk every day as macrobiotic lifestyle guidelines recommend), you may consider increasing your fish and seafood intake, taking sun-dried foods, and temporarily trying a vitamin D supplement (of vegan rather than animal quality).

27.   Yoga, tai chi, martial arts, sports, and other activities and exercises are also part of an active, healthy way of life. Aerobic activities that utilize a variety of limbs, muscles, and systems are generally preferable to isometric or static activities that focus on only one arm, leg, or muscular motion (for example, weight lifting). Relative to each other, physical activities can be classified as relatively or strongly yin, yang, or more balanced in the middle. For yang conditions, softer or gentler exercises are recommended, while for yin ones, slightly more active are preferred for balance. The many styles within each type often make classification confusing. For example, there are very dynamic yang styles of yoga such as Iyengar and Kundalini as well as more yin ones like Jnana and Bhakti. Similarly, karate and kung fu tend to be yang, while tai chi is more yin, and aikido is more in between. Among popular sports, football is extremely yang, basketball

combines strong yin and yang, and baseball is more balanced. Jogging is very yangizing, watching TV is very yinnizing, and walking is in between. Heart and cancer patients should generally engage in milder, less exhaustive, gentler activities even though an extremely contractive sport such as speedriding (parachuting off mountain tops with a glider on skis) would appear to balance an extremely expansive condition (if it doesn't kill them first!). In general, a yin individual has poorer judgment in respect to physical activities than a yang one.

MODERN MEDICINE

From the macrobiotic view, about 90 percent of modern medicine is unnecessary, overly complex, and potentially harmful. Its strongest point is treating accidents and emergencies. This view is increasingly echoed by the medical profession itself, which has officially classified medical error as the third leading cause of death in this country. (Other estimates put it at number one, higher than both heart disease and cancer.) Unnecessary surgeries and X-rays, faulty drugs and prescriptions, hospital-caused infections, and other medical errors claim the lives of an estimated 750,000 to 1 million Americans every year. The saddest part is that all of these are preventable.

Over the last generation the rise of complementary and alternative medicine (CAM) has attempted to provide safe, effective diagnosis and treatment, including many of the methods described above. The lack of universal health care in the United States is a national disgrace that has needlessly increased pain and death, shifting the burden of suffering to the poor, the homeless, individuals and families from ethnic backgrounds that are discriminated against, and others who are under- or uninsured.

CAM—or holistic medicine, as it is often called—spans the first five circles of the Mandala of Healing. Conventional or experimental medicine covers the last two levels. In seeking medical treatment, the following may be kept in mind:

1. Should I have medical tests? If you suspect cancer or serious illness because of recurrent or unusual symptoms, it is advisable to seek a medical diagnosis. You don't have to follow the doctor's advice; that is entirely up to you. But it is wise to be informed about your condition and get as much information as possible. It can be helpful to you in selecting alternative approaches. You don't want to expose yourself to further risk with unnecessary or harmful tests, of course, so you have to be selective. As a rule, blood tests, EEGs, EKGs, other heart tests, and other less invasive procedures are relatively safe. More invasive and potentially hazardous tests such as mammograms,

MRIs, CT scans, colonoscopies, and biopsies should be taken as a last step rather than a first one. Do not hesitate to have one of these more complex, expensive, and risky procedures done if necessary. But don't rush into them just because you are told that everyone of a certain age or profile should be screened periodically.

2. What is my real condition? Unfortunately, modern diagnostic methods, including MRIs, CTs, mammograms, X-rays, and biopsies, are frequently inaccurate and have a high degree of error. They may also contribute to the condition they are designed to diagnose or another serious disorder. For cancer it is advisable to get a second opinion or have several different types of tests performed to determine whether you really have cancer. In principle, macrobiotic diagnosis, especially physiognomy or visual diagnosis, can determine whether cancer is present, but in any given case it depends on the skill of the practitioner or counselor. Even the most experienced macrobiotic counselor can make mistakes, so it is best to have independent medical tests performed (imperfect as they may be) and let the counselor base his or her recommendations, at least in part, on the medical information you provide. It is very difficult to know whom to trust, so ultimately it comes down to your own intuition. Seeking guidance with a sincere heart should lead you in a healthy, positive direction. Further guidelines on selecting a practitioner or counselor are below.

3. Should I have the cancer removed surgically? Should I undergo chemotherapy? Is radiation appropriate? What about a new experimental drug or treatment? These are all legitimate concerns, and there are no right or wrong answers. Overall, these are symptomatic approaches that seek to eradicate disease rather than address and correct its origins and causes. To this extent they are unnecessary and ill-advised. But in any given case they may be necessary and lifesaving. Do not rush into them or rule them out. The safest thing is to take a middle way, seeing your physician periodically, getting his or her opinion, getting a second opinion if necessary, and then trying as best you can to heal with diet, lifestyle, and other holistic methods as your primary focus. If you experience improvement, continue in the new way gradually until it becomes clear that medical treatment is unnecessary. If your condition declines or does not improve over time, do not hesitate to avail yourself of medical means.

4. Will medical treatment interfere with macrobiotic healing? In some cases it will make healing more difficult, especially if vital organs are

removed or weakened by drugs, surgery, or radiation. On the other hand, medical treatment is sometimes effective and even essential. We have seen some difficult cancer cases that did not respond in whole or part to dietary or lifestyle change but did heal with chemotherapy, radiation, surgery, or experimental drugs. The most common example is where the macrobiotic way cleanses the body so thoroughly that all tumors go away except one. The healing power of food eliminates the metastases from the body, but some of the old fat and oil and other metabolic discharge energy gathers in the primary site. It may start to grow larger, harden, and not lend itself to usual compresses, special drinks or dishes, or further dietary methods. In this case chemotherapy, radiation, or experimental drugs may be powerful enough to trigger the final discharge and eliminate the last tumor. (Palm healing often is also more powerful than diet or home care in a case like this, so try it if other methods don't succeed.) Don't close your mind to extreme methods, use common sense, and do whatever it takes to get well. But do so as a last resort. Unfortunately, we have also seen some macrobiotic friends get sick over the years and refuse medical attention when needed. In these cases medical treatment was part of their macrobiotic recovery because they had become too one-sided or fanatical in their practice and lost their balance and intuition. Be wise, embrace all forms of healing, and don't become prisoners of ideology or abstract theories. If you are currently undergoing medical treatment or taking medication, the macrobiotic way will still be beneficial. It is not either/or.

5. When is it appropriate to discontinue medication? Ideally, you should discuss this with your doctor. As improvement with the macrobiotic way of eating is experienced, you may then gradually decide to taper off supplements, drugs, and other medications. Go slowly and start with over-the-counter items, vitamins and supplements, and less vital substances. Take your time, for example, reducing the strength by 10, 25, or up to 50 percent over several days, weeks, or months, and then gradually taper off. Essential medications, such as certain heart drugs, insulin, and other substances that maintain vital functions may also eventually be decreased in some cases. However, in others they may need to be maintained indefinitely. This will depend on each individual and his or her condition. Hopefully, reliance on medications overall will decrease, but if you reach a plateau and have to continue with certain items, don't worry. The important thing is to live a joyful, happy life, and if medication supports that goal, don't hesitate to make use of it. That may be part of your overall macrobiotic practice, leading to a long, healthful life.

UNDERSTANDING NUTRITIONAL
AND MEDICAL RESEARCH

Scientific and medical research has become the gold standard for dietary, nutritional, and medical guidelines in modern society. Double-blind tests, clinical trials, laboratory studies, and epidemiological surveys are all designed to minimize statistical errors, social and cultural bias, and personal influences that can distort results. Still, the integrity and validity of medical research continue to be called into question, especially over funding. Numerous scandals have arisen in recent years when it was disclosed that pharmaceutical companies, food manufacturers, or other special interests funded the studies; that the principal researchers were paid consultants with potential conflicts of interest; or that the medical journals in which the research appeared accepted substantial advertising revenue from drug or other firms that benefited from favorable articles and reviews. Further, most research is conducted by universities, laboratories, or government agencies that are dependent on the industries whose research they evaluate for grants, subsidies, and funding. Without the support of special interests, in many cases, they could not exist. Hence, most research today is tainted to begin with and not truly impartial.

Still, much can be learned from scientific and medical studies even if their underlying premise and sponsorship is open to doubt. For the ordinary person, including the cancer patient and his or her family, the biggest concern is how to make sense of conflicting results. For example, tamoxifen appears to be helpful in treating breast cancer, but it can cause or increase the risk of ovarian tumors. Or take another example: Alcohol is a major risk factor for many types of cancer, diabetes, and other disorders, but studies consistently show that individuals who drink a glass of wine regularly have fewer heart attacks (the principal cause of death in modern society). And, finally, as we have mentioned, there is the soy controversy. Some studies suggest that it is protective against cancer, and others that it is a promoter.

How to make sense of confusing and conflicting studies like these? From the macrobiotic view, the key is to use yin and yang, the philosophy of harmony and balance, to interpret the results. Tamoxifen is very yang—strong, contractive—so it may help shrink breast tumors that are classified as very yin (externally located and in the upper body). The ovaries, on the other hand, are very yang (internally located and in the lower body). A yang application such as tamoxifen aggravates and worsens tight, contractive ovaries, increasing the risk for malignancy. In the case of alcohol, wine is very yin, and as part of the modern way of eating it can enhance the risk of breast cancer (which, as we have seen, is also predominantly yin). Coronary heart disease, on the other hand, is very yang, so wine will help dissolve fat, oil, and cholesterol in the blood that contributes to blocking of the arteries. In the case of soy foods, as noted above, the effects of traditional soy products such as miso, shoyu, tempeh, and natto are the opposite of modern highly processed soy foods. In these and many other instances, we have to be discriminating and understand that the same food can produce different effects in different people depending on their constitution, condition, environment, climate, age, sex, level of activity, personal needs, and other factors. We have to have a flexible, dynamic view of energy rather than a rigid, fixed one.

Finally, the same principles apply to medical testing. Commonly, individuals will be told by their physician after routine blood tests that they are seriously deficient in certain vitamins, minerals, or other nutrients. Their doctor then warns them that they need, say, B_{12} injections or supplements (made with extreme animal products), more calcium (often in supplement form from dairy), or other nutrients to bring their levels up to "normal." The problem here is that "normal" is based on mean or average values for a modern meat- and sugar-eating population. It is not normal in the sense of what a free human being needs to survive and thrive in the natural world. Despite substantially better nutritional guidelines in recent years and the shift from the meat-based Four Food Groups to the plant-based Food Guide Pyramid, modern nutritional and medical norms are skewed to a small, affluent (and two-thirds overweight and obese!) fraction of the planet. To educate yourself on what is normal, check out the nutritional guidelines of the World Health Organization, the international medical arm of the United Nations. Its recommendations for daily intake of protein, fat, carbohydrates, and other nutrients are substantially lower than those of the U.S. government and medical associations in this country. They are based on the way 85 percent of the world normally eats, predominantly grains and vegetables.

If you are eating in a more vegetarian, vegan, or macrobiotic direction, you must know that your blood values will be in the low normal range or below normal. Do not needlessly be alarmed and think there is something wrong. Yes, grain- and plant-eating people can develop deficiencies and need to be mindful. But the kinds of deficiencies often observed by physicians are usually not deficiencies at all but normal, healthy levels that modern society does not currently recognize or accept. You can save yourself a lot of anxiety, money, and exposure to potentially harmful supplements by educating yourself on the limits of modern nutrition and medical science and discovering what is appropriate for you.

SEEKING A PHYSICIAN, COUNSELOR, OR HOLISTIC PROFESSIONAL

What should you look for in choosing a doctor, nutritionist, macrobiotic counselor, or other health care professional? The following guidelines may be helpful:

1. The approach is not as important as the practitioner. A skillful physician or teacher will be able to help you proceed in a healthier direction regardless of the discipline, specialty, or school of thought practiced. Whether it's Reiki, osteopathy, internal medicine, psychoanalysis, or macrobiotics, the consciousness and character of the healer is more important than the methodology.

2. Seek help from someone you don't know personally. As Jesus says in the Gospel of Thomas, "A prophet is without honor in his own country, and a physician cannot heal those who know him." You are too emotionally attached to friends, family, or other persons you know to benefit from their guidance and vice versa.

3. Look for someone who is knowledgeable and experienced. Age, sex, and other peripheral characteristics, including universities attended, degrees and honors awarded, and training received, are not as important as practical experience dealing with people from many walks of life and treating a wide variety of conditions. As a rule, avoid specialists because their understanding may be too narrow and limited for a comprehensive approach.

4. Look for someone who embraces all healing modalities, from complementary and alternative medicine to macrobiotics and modern medicine. There are fanatics and true believers in all fields who believe their way alone is valid. Avoid such practitioners.

5. Look for someone who is compassionate, caring, and has good communication skills. Most physicians are warmhearted, as are most family counselors, psychiatrists, and others with a background in psychology. The same is true of many priests, rabbis, ministers, and imans. They commonly have the sensitivity and the capacity to deal with feelings and emotions, not just abstract theory, blood work, and meridian flow, and they are concerned about your mental and spiritual health as well as your physical well-being.

6. Look for someone who has healed themselves of a serious illness (though not necessarily the same as yours). Suffering fundamentally changes a person and creates a sympathy, understanding, and bond with the client and his or her family that is often missing in those who have not personally experienced illness or tragedy in their lives.

7. Stay with the counselor or professional you have selected as long as possible and give that person time to help you achieve slow, steady improvement. Do not seek instant results or the impossible. Do not

go shopping from doctor to doctor and counselor to counselor or ask them to comment or criticize one another's advice or approach. Healing takes time, especially a serious condition such as heart disease or cancer. It may take four to six months for appreciable results to appear, and another year or longer for complete recovery. Don't be impatient; go step by step and persevere inwardly if you experience a setback.

8. Don't stick with someone whose approach or advice you profoundly disagree with or whom your intuition tells you to leave. Don't stay with someone for emotional or economic reasons (such as family ties or medical coverage) or because you don't want to hurt his or her feelings. Remember, it's your life at stake, and that person is there to help you. Voice your concerns, ask questions, and don't take anything on blind faith.

9. Rely on yourself as much as possible. Study, read, write, observe, and reflect constantly. Become a student of life. Don't hesitate to ask for help. Be grateful for what you receive and share your understanding, insights, and experience with others.

10. Create a supportive environment for yourself. This includes keeping your living and working space as clean, orderly, and environmentally friendly as possible. It includes relating harmoniously to other household members, keeping in regular touch with friends, family, and others, and finding a proper balance between activity and rest, including periodic breaks or vacations. Taking advantage of and participating in community activities will also help sustain you; these activities may include religious, cultural, artistic, and social events. There are many public and private health and human resources available. Reach out, if necessary, and don't become isolated. People are fundamentally good, and the more trust you show, the more you will be trusted and be able to help and guide others.

13

Cancer and
Planetary Health

We all need to realize that cancer is not solely the concern of cancer patients, their families, or the medical profession. Cancer is merely one dramatic symptom out of many of the deep misconceptions and ultimately self-destructive tendencies upon which we have built modern civilization. In a very real sense we all have cancer and will be affected by the disease until a new, peaceful way of life is established in place of the old.

As we have seen, cancer is not a disease of certain cells or certain organs but the means of self-protection for an entire diseased organism. If the cancer is artificially removed without changing the underlying ways of eating and the habits that give rise to the disease, this balance is disrupted and the whole may collapse. In modern society there are many parallels between the way we approach cancer and the way we approach relations between men and women, the breakup of the family, crime and social disorder, international conflict, the energy crisis, and destruction of the natural environment.

"Medicine is a social science, and politics is medicine writ large," Rudolf Virchow, the German pathologist, observed more than a century ago. In medicine now we are governed by modern concepts of cellular sovereignty—the notion that what happens in the cell or its nucleus is totally independent of the organism as a whole or its environment. Over the years modern science has convinced us that disease is the result of external invasion or an aberration in an isolated gene, hormone, or other cellular component over which we have no voluntary control or moral responsibility.

Scientists assure us that if the specific factor that is causing the epidemic or abnormal cell growth can be pinpointed, a biochemical solution can be found to block its harmful effects.

Military metaphors are now used routinely to describe bodily processes and to prescribe treating. In "Closing in on Cancer," an article in the *New York Times,* we are informed that "these scientists want to understand how the enemy, the cancer cell, masquerades as a normal cell, slipping past the sentinels of the immune system undetected. . . . Antibodies that circulate through the bloodstream are on constant patrol. . . . The body is alerted and dispatches special killer cells and a barrage of chemical artillery to dispose of the threat. . . . It is hoped that these 'poison-tagged' antibodies will act as miniature smart bombs, delivering their lethal payload to the diseased tissue—and nowhere else."

Science News voiced a similar image: "What do you do with a semipowerful guided missile? Monoclonal antibodies, the proteins produced by immune system/cancer cell hybrids, have become important seek-and-bind weapons in diagnosing cancer and other illnesses. But the missiles are not as good at search-and-destroy missions—researchers have had only limited success in using monoclonal antibodies alone against cancer. Now, others are arming the antibodies with radioactivity, drugs, or toxins."

The *Boston Globe* science columnist, in an article entitled "The Human Body's 'Cell Wars' Defense," compared the body's strategic defenses to the space-based Star Wars missile defense system: "We live in a sea of alien viruses and microorganisms. Many are harmful. Some are deadly. The body is protected by a stupendous array of traps, triggers, walls, moats, and chemical alarms. Some of the body's cells act as patrols, sentries, infantry, and artillery to defend the integrity of the larger society. The 'cell wars' defense system never rests."

Increasingly, modern medicine is becoming nuclearized. At the present time there are 6,000 CT scanners employed in hospitals in the United States, producing a total of 60 million imaging studies each year. In the industrialized world, 25 percent of all patients undergo nuclear medical procedures during diagnosis or treatment. While CT and other scans are often helpful in diagnosis, they are inherently risky. A typical scan can expose a patient to up to three times as much radiation as people within one mile of ground zero at Hiroshima and Nagasaki in the world's first atomic bombings.

The purely mechanical approach to science tends to trivialize traditional values and ways of life. Medically speaking, we choose to control illnesses using drugs and electronic means. Without truly understanding the causes of disease, we remove parts of the body, mechanically stimulate our organs, and gradually artificialize our bodies. On the psychological level we understand only mechanical behavior: If we give this chemical treatment or that nuclear procedure, the patient will react this or that way. But what are the effects of such treatment? How is the treatment affecting the energy of the entire person? This we do not know.

It almost never occurs to us that we have brought disease, pain, and suffering on ourselves because of a longtime imbalance in our way of eating, thinking, or living. In the war on cancer, heart disease, and other afflictions, as we have seen, treatments involve a variety of successively more violent means to protect healthy cells and conquer unhealthy ones. These methods are similar in design and execution to those implemented on a larger scale by the military and political leaders to protect citizens from attack in the name of national sovereignty.

Our social ills follow a development similar to our personal ills. The pattern of progressive degeneration from less to more serious conflict can be seen in disputes between families, communities, states, and nations. These conflicts generally proceed from arguments and threats to violent outbursts and aggressive behavior, from confrontation and polarization to terrorism and war. Disharmony is never the fault of only one side, yet we act as if it were and adopt an adversarial rather than a cooperative attitude. Instead of seeking a peaceful solution that reconciles and takes into account the welfare and needs of all concerned, including the environment and the next generation, we take refuge in our own short-range goals.

Terrorism, revolt, and riots occur only in proportion to society's reliance on excessive military strength and neglect of underlying social factors that create disorder in the first place. The futility of suppressing revolution with force has been demonstrated in the Middle East, Afghanistan, and many other areas of recent conflict.

At the global level, this antagonistic approach has led to the doctrine of national sovereignty. In order to halt terrorism and the spread of chemical, biological, and nuclear weapons, we must transcend our allegiance to individual nation-states and begin to see ourselves as citizens of a common planet. As long as countries see themselves as separate entities, they will retain the right to build and use nuclear weapons to protect their own national security. If all states banded together and formed a world federation, limiting their sovereignty, there would no longer be competing paramount national interests to defend. Until recently the United Nations lacked authority to intervene in the internal affairs of member states. With the end of the cold war, however, the United Nations has begun to take a more active role in the Middle East, East Africa, the Balkans, and other areas of conflict. Of course, unless the health and judgment of United Nations leaders and personnel are sound, another system of oppression may arise on a world scale. Thus, it is important that basic human rights, as well as diverse political, economic, social, and cultural systems, be respected.

How many times have we seen some social problem, from crime to terrorism, from drugs to the breakdown of family values, described as a spreading cancer in the community? Like cancer in an individual, our major social problems are characterized by uncontrolled growth—excessive consumption and development—and our treatments are violent and self-destructive. In all fields of life the use or threat of excessive force proves counterproductive. The violent means with which we produce our foods, treat our bodies, and deal with conflicts must be replaced with peaceful and harmonious methods.

OVERCOMING DUALISM

We are now at a turning point in history. One segment of modern science and medicine is moving in the direction of biotechnology, the artificial manipulation of the environment, including the creation of new life-forms in the laboratory. During the last generation, the number of radiation-induced mutant varieties of seeds available for use in modern agriculture skyrocketed from fifteen to thirteen thousand. Sixty percent of the durum wheat in Italy, for example, is a gamma-induced mutant variety. The U.S. government approved the genetic modification of seeds and foods without comprehensive long-term testing of their possible effects on health and without consumer labeling. The object is to provide foods that are tastier and more varied, but the effects on human health and the environment may be catastrophic. Foods will no longer have strong chi, or natural electromagnetic energy. By blurring the boundary between species, genes from cattle, sheep, fish, and other animals may be blended into common grains, beans, vegetables, and fruits, creating even more chaotic energy and vibration. The effects on the environment—the delicate ecosystem in which everything is interrelated—cannot be gauged in the laboratory. The loss of biodiversity—the sum total of the earth's genetic variety—is inevitable as traditional strains are replaced. Disaster—from predators, disease, altered weather patterns and climate cycles, and mutations—is inexorable.

Meanwhile, dozens of countries have approved the use of food irradiation—an extremely dangerous and destructive technology that exposes food to highly ionized nuclear radiation—in order to prolong shelf life of spices, grains, ·chicken, meat, fruits, vegetables, and other food. The potential health hazards of irradiation include reduced nutritional value of foods, creation of unique radiolytic products not found previously in foods, stimulation of carcinogenic aflatoxin-producing molds, initiation of tumors, kidney damage, and genetic abnormalities as shown in laboratory testing, production of harmful bacteria, and creation of radiation-resistant strains of mutated microorganisms.

We may decide to go further on the road to the mechanization and artificialization of the human species, or we may decide to start turning toward more natural ways of living and caring for ourselves. This is the point of decision. The further degeneration of the soil; the continuing spread of cancer, heart disease, and immune-deficiency diseases; and the outbreak of nuclear war are not inevitable. To stop or prevent such catastrophes we must develop a new orientation toward life. Specifically, we must begin to seek the most basic causes and to implement the most basic solutions rather than continue the present course of treating each problem separately in terms of its symptoms alone. Issues of war and peace, and sickness and health, affect us all in one way or another and in all domains of modern life. The responsibility for finding and implementing solutions should not be left to those with the government, the military, or the medical and scientific communities alone. Global health and security will emerge only through a cooperative effort involving people at all levels of society.

Modern civilization, by orienting itself against rather than with nature, has deprived itself of the capacity to evolve with the environment. Cancer, immune-deficiency diseases, global terrorism, and environmental destruction are only the most extreme manifestations of this adversarial orientation. Instead of considering the larger ecological, social, and biological causes of the breakdown of modern life, we have focused our attention until now in the opposite direction, viewing conflict mainly as an isolated disorder affecting certain cells within the body, criminal elements within society, and terrorist networks and dissident factions within nation-states. The remedies we employ, in our hospitals, legislatures, and world forums, involve containment of or relentless hostility toward the disruptive forces, all the while ignoring the overall conditions that caused the disorder to develop.

The modern way of thinking that has culminated in this dead end can be described as dualistic. Dualistic thinking divides good from bad, friend from enemy, and health from sickness, seeing the one as desirable and the other as undesirable. This divisive mode of thought actually underlies all of modern society, including education and religion, politics and economics, science and industry, communication and the arts. As long as our basic point of view is one-sided, it is impossible to cure fundamentally any sickness or put an end to family disputes, criminal activity, social unrest, or conflict between nations.

From a larger perspective—such as that of the earth as a whole—we can see that no enemies really exist. On the contrary, all factors, however antagonistic to our own limited personal or national objectives, are complementary. All phenomena contain the seed of their polar opposite and are mutually influencing and changing into one another. By balancing extremes—reducing excesses, filling up empty spaces—nature makes for greater diversity and harmony as the spiral of life unfolds.

Sickness is a natural adjustment, the result of the wisdom of the body trying to keep us in natural balance. Degenerative disease is only the final stage in the sequence of events through which individuals in the modern world tend to pass because we fail to appreciate the beneficial nature of disease symptoms. In reality, disease is defending and protecting us by either localizing or eliminating undesirable factors from our body. It is a wonderful defense and adjustment mechanism that enables us to live one, two, five, or ten more years without changing our unnatural diet and artificial way of life. On the other hand, if we are willing to self-reflect, take responsibility for our sickness, and change our orientation, disease will cooperate with us and generally go away if it has not reached an irreversible stage.

As modern medicine is now just beginning to discover, cancer and other serious illnesses can be prevented, and in many cases relieved naturally, without violent treatments by adopting a balanced diet centered around whole cereal grains and vegetables, together with other traditional basic supplemental foods, the administration of safe, simple home care, positive thinking, and other lifestyle changes. Thousands of people with cancer and heart disease, including many given up as terminal, have recovered their health and vitality by adopting natural, holistic approaches, including those presented in this book. Hundreds of thousands have prevented the onset of degenerative disease by changing their way of eating and living. Along with the change in diet, many persons with illness have taken the initiative to apply traditional home remedies to reduce symptoms and discharge toxic material through the skin or urine. These applications are safe, simple, and self-administered, and work by helping to activate circulation and by enabling the body's own electromagnetic healing energy to flow smoothly to the affected region.

The natural macrobiotic approach to cooking and relief of illness is peaceful and gentle. All factors are considered complementary, and the emphasis is on restoring balance and equilibrium. For thousands of years humanity viewed life not as a battle in which enemies had to be violently subdued or destroyed, but as a game of limitless adventure and discovery in which opposites are gently harmonized. Health and peace will naturally follow from adopting this view.

HEALING THE EARTH

By shifting from the modern diet high in meat and sugar and processed foods to a diet centered around whole grains and vegetables, we are benefiting not only our personal health but also the health of the planet as a whole. "The quantity of nutritious vegetable matter, consumed in fattening the carcase of an ox," Shelley, the English poet, observed, "would afford ten times the sustenance, undepraving indeed, and incapable of generating disease, if gathered immediately from the bosom of the earth."

In the nearly two centuries since, particularly in the last generation and the last decade, the effects of the modern way of eating—centered around beef eating and cattle production—on world health, world hunger, and the environment have become better understood.

The underlying cause of poverty and hunger in much of the world today is the modern agricultural system that utilizes the majority of arable land for livestock production and cash crops such as tomatoes, sugar, coffee, and bananas. In emerging economies, tens of millions of families growing grains and vegetables have been uprooted from their ancestral lands by large cattle ranches, sugar plantations, and other agricultural developments. Seeking food and jobs, they have crowded into cities and metropolitan areas, creating huge slums, contributing to unemployment, and becoming part of a downward spiral of hunger, disease, crime, and destitution.

About 30 percent of the world grain harvest goes to cattle and other livestock rather than to direct human consumption. There is more than enough food to feed everyone on the planet. The problem is that most of it goes to feeding cows to produce meat and dairy food. As society returns to a more plant-centered diet, world poverty and hunger will automatically decrease.

Diet and Global Warming

Cutting back on animal food may do more to preserve the planet than buying a hybrid automobile, according to a new United Nations study on the impact of meat eating on the environment. Billions of cattle that are bred for hamburgers, steaks, and milk emit more greenhouse gases that contribute to global warming than all "the cars, planes, and other forms of transport put together."

"The livestock sector emerges as one of the top two or three most significant contributors to the most serious environmental problems, at every scale from local to global," *Livestock's Long Shadow,* the new Food and Agricultural Organization (FAO) study, explained in early 2007. "The findings of this report suggest that it should be a major policy focus when dealing with problems of land degradation, climate change and air pollution, water shortage and water pollution, and loss of biodiversity.

"Livestock's contribution to environmental problems is on a massive scale and its potential contribution to their solution is equally large. The impact is so significant that it needs to be addressed with urgency. Major reductions in impact could be achieved at reasonable cost." Among the findings in the four-hundred-page investigation are these:

- Global meat production will double from 229 million tons in 1999/2001 to 465 million tons in 2050, and milk will jump from 580 to 1.043 million tons. The environmental impact per unit of livestock production must be cut by half just to avoid increasing the level of damage beyond its current level.
- As the largest user of land, the livestock sector accounts for 26 percent of the ice-free surface of the planet, and food grown to feed cattle and

other livestock takes one-third of the planet's total cultivatable land. In all, livestock production accounts for 70 percent of all farmland and 30 percent of the earth's land surface.

- The livestock sector is responsible for 18 percent of greenhouse gas emissions measured in CO_2 equivalent. "This is more than the transport sector." This includes 9 percent of CO_2 emissions, especially from deforestation to clear pastureland; 37 percent of methane (which has 23 times the global warming potential of CO_2), especially from cattle flatulence; and 65 percent of nitrous oxide (296 times the global warming potential of CO_2), especially from animal manure. Livestock are also responsible for nearly two-thirds of ammonia emissions, a main cause of acid rain.

- The livestock sector accounts for 8 percent of human water use, primarily for the irrigation of feed crops, and appears to be "the largest source of water pollution, 'dead' zones in coastal areas, degradation of coral reefs, human health problems, emergence of antibiotic resistance, and many others. The main sources of pollution are from animal wastes, antibiotics and hormones, chemicals from tanneries, fertilizers and pesticides used for feed crops, and sediments from eroded pastures." In the United States, livestock are responsible for 55 percent of soil erosion and sediment, 37 percent of pesticide use, 50 percent of antibiotic use, and one-third of nitrogen and phosphorus contamination of freshwater resources.

- Livestock account for about 20 percent of the earth's animal biomass, and the 30 percent of the surface of the planet they occupy preempt what was once habitat for wildlife. "Indeed, the livestock sector may well be the leading player in the reduction of biodiversity, since it is the major driver of deforestation, as well as one of the leading drivers of land degradation, pollution, climate change, overfishing, sedimentation of coastal areas, and facilitation of invasions by alien species." Some 306 of 825 imperiled ecosystems identified by the World Wildlife Fund reported livestock as a current threat. Of the 35 global hotspots for biodiversity singled out by Conservation International, 23 involve livestock production. The World Conservation Union's Red List of Threatened Species reports that most of the world's threatened species are experiencing habitat loss as a result of livestock production.

Beyond improving the efficiency of livestock production to reduce environmental impacts, the UN report said that it was essential to correctly factor in the real social and environmental costs associated with animal food production. It noted that government subsidies often perversely encourage environmentally damaging activities. "A top priority is to achieve prices and fees that reflect the full economic and environmental costs, including all externalities. One requirement for prices to influence behavior is that there should be secure and if possible tradable rights to water, land, use of common land and waste sinks."

The report called for the selective taxing and/or fees for resource use, inputs, and wastes, as well as incentives for rewarding sustainable practices. "An important general lesson is that the livestock sector has such deep and wide-ranging environmental impacts that it should rank as one of the leading focuses for environmental policy: efforts here can produce large and multiple payoffs. Indeed, as societies develop, it is likely that environmental considerations, along with human health issues, will become the dominant policy considerations for the sector." (The complete report is available online at virtualcentre.org.)

In human beings, cancer is a disease of chronic excess. On the planet, the environmental crisis is the result of modern civilization's chronically excessive consumption of the world's natural resources. In fact, the magnitude of the current crisis has led many people to conclude that the Earth itself is terminally ill. Metaphors comparing some of these problems to cancer, heart disease, and AIDS are becoming more frequent. The buildup of toxic deposits in the land is like tumors developing in vital organs. The pollution of streams and rivers is like leukemia and lymphoma. The thinning of the ozone layer is like loss of the planet's natural immunity. In human beings, cancer thrives in oxygen-depleted cells or in an environment in which carbon dioxide, carcinogens, radioactive particles, and other toxic wastes accumulate. We need oxygen to metabolize our food properly and produce strong blood. We cannot make efficient use of caloric energy without enough oxygen. The medical profession has recently been recommending consumption of whole grains and fresh vegetables high in vitamins A, C, and E—the antioxidants—because they help regulate the availability of oxygen to the body. On a planetary scale, the buildup of carbon dioxide and other toxins indicates that the Earth as a whole is developing a malignant condition.

A diet based on animal foods is dangerous to the environment. Researchers at Caltech reported that cooking meat contributes to air pollution by releasing hydrocarbons, furans, steroids, and pesticide residues. In Los Angeles, long noted for its smog, the greatest source of atmospheric pollution was barbecued beef, exceeding pollution from fireplaces, gasoline- and diesel-powered vehicles, dust from roadwork, forest fires, chemical processing, metallurgy, jet aircraft, and cigarettes.

Clearly the planet is in urgent need of healing. For many years our macrobiotic community has been saying that the outer environment reflects the inner environment and that awareness of ecology begins at the dinner table. Personal health cannot be separated from planetary health, and wholesome natural foods are the bridge between the two. If we are healthy, the environment is naturally healthy and clean. If we are sick, the environment around us begins to suffer. In turn, the quality of the outside environment determines the quality of our life. If our environment is clean and wholesome, we can maintain our health and happiness. If the environment is polluted, we easily become sick and unhappy.

THE ROAD AHEAD

Despite continuing biological degeneration of humanity and the worsening global environmental condition, there are signs of hope and change. Modern science and medicine are clearly moving in a healthier direction as the benefits of a grain- and vegetable-centered diet become more widely known. Over the next twenty-five years we can expect these trends:

- The incidence of heart attack, stroke, and other cardiovascular diseases will continue to drop sharply in the United States. In other countries, where it is currently on the rise, heart disease will also begin to fall as a result of increased nutritional awareness. However, with rising affluence it will move into emerging economies. Recently, heart disease surpassed infectious disease as the most prevalent disorder in developing regions.
- Cancer rates will begin to decline for breast cancer, lung cancer, and colon cancer, as fat consumption drops and fiber intake rises. The overall death toll from the War on Cancer will begin to fall for the first time in the United States and other affluent countries. But as with heart disease, cancer rates will skyrocket in China, India, and other modernizing economies.
- Diet and nutrition will emerge as the key factors in the prevention and treatment of AIDS and other immune-deficiency diseases.
- Populations exposed to nuclear radiation, pollution, and other environmental toxins, in addition to artificial electromagnetic fields, will incorporate miso soup, sea vegetables, and other foods that protect against contaminants in their daily diets.
- Healthier foods will be introduced into schools, hospitals, clinics, prisons, businesses, and other institutions, leading to less aggressive and antisocial behavior, increased efficiency and cooperation, and better human relations.
- Organic and natural agriculture will gradually displace chemical agriculture and become recognized as inseparable from preserving the environment and maintaining planetary health.

As T. Colin Campbell and Chen Junshi, the directors of the China Health Study, observed, "The occurrence of most human diseases is usually the result of exposure to many factors occurring over a long period of time." Modern medicine's analytic approach—isolating one nutrient or component and seeking a specific cause-and-effect mechanism—must be balanced by the synthetic approach in which the balance of the diet as a whole, as well as its relation to lifestyle and environmental factors, is considered.

In the future, dietary and nutritional research methods will also need to pay more attention to food quality. For example, are the foods whole or refined? Traditionally processed or artificially processed? Organically or chemically grown? Consumed seasonally or year-round? Besides scientific and medical studies, there are other avenues to knowledge and understanding, including cultural tradition, spiritual development, literary and artistic creation, and intuition and self-reflection. The medicine of the future will integrate ancient and modern, Eastern and Western, Northern and Southern, synthetic and analytic, and other complementary strands that make up the tapestry of our daily lives. As Campbell and Junshi remind us, we need always to keep in mind "the big picture"—or what has traditionally been called the macrobiotic view.

Essentially, the health revolution is over. All the basic theoretical and practical information is now available to end the epidemic of degenerative disease sweeping the world and to preserve the natural environment. In medical research during the next generation, we can expect the focus of epidemiological and case-control studies to shift to monitoring and comparing people eating the usual modern diet, the macrobiotic diet, and other more plant-centered diets. At the theoretical level, scientists will continue to develop concepts of cocarcinogenicity, synergy, oncogenes, and initiation/promotion, which are now in the formative stages, to explain conflicting results and describe complementary and antagonistic relationships. Science as a whole will move toward adopting a modern form of the traditional yin/yang principle, and a new prevention-oriented medicine centered on diet and nutrition will develop (see Table 21).

As the health and environmental revolution transforms modern society, the macrobiotic community will begin to shift its focus in coming decades to developing principles of a new science and developing a healthy, practical source of energy. Quantum conversion—the controlled, peaceful change of elements into one another (also traditionally known as alchemy or transmutation)—promises in the future to be a healthy, natural alternative to nuclear power, genetic engineering, chemicalization, irradiation, and other artificial sources of energy, products, and processes. The almost limitless natural energies streaming into our planet from the sun, moon, solar system, galaxy, and infinite universe, as well as the turning of the Earth on its axis itself, will be harnessed to provide a simple, safe method of generating energy.

Televisions, computers, automobiles, airplanes, and other modern conveniences will be powered by healthy, natural forms of electromagnetic energy rather than by the potentially harmful artificial methods at present. The competition for limited resources—gas, oil, gold, and other precious metals—will become a thing of the past, further reducing a source of conflict and war.

TABLE 21.   THE YIN AND YANG NATURE OF THE HUMAN BODY

Yang	Yin
Blood system	Lymph system
Nervous system	Digestive system
Bones and muscles	Organs, glands, tissues
Deep inner organs and structures	Peripheral organs and structures
Testosterone and male hormones	Estrogen and female hormones
DNA	RNA
Red blood cells	White blood cells
Growth-suppressing genes	Growth-enhancing genes
Inhibiting neurotransmitters	Activating transmitters
Collagen	Elastin
Sodium ions	Potassium ions
Catabolic agents such as sodium compounds	Anabolic agents such as sterols, alcohols, and amines
Interleukin, interferon, and monoclonal antibodies	Cortisone and other yin drugs
Echinacea and other yang herbs	Goldenseal and other yin herbs

In the twenty-first century the seeds of a new golden age may develop that will last for another ten thousand years—if we can safely pass through this time. By solving the riddle of cancer, heart disease, AIDS, and other degenerative disorders, we can heal the planet and bring health, happiness, and peace to endless generations.

PART 2

A Guide to Different Cancers

INTRODUCTION

This section is intended to serve as a guide to helping people recover from the more common types of cancer in modern society. The chapters may be read as a complementary unit to the first part of the book, which emphasizes cancer prevention. Chapters may also be read individually for information on how to approach cancer in a particular site. Since many similar foods and types of home care are recommended, the actual recipes and instructions have been gathered together in Part III.

The guidelines suggested here are general in nature and will differ slightly for each person. After reading this book, it is recommended that individuals with cancer or their families who wish to pursue this approach see a qualified macrobiotic teacher or a medical doctor who has been trained in this way of life. Information on personal guidance sessions is available in the Resources section on page 569.

In the chapters in this section of the book, each type of cancer will be described under the following headings:

Frequency notes the extent of the disease, standard forms of medical treatment, and the current survival rates for persons undergoing treatment. Statistics are from the latest reports of the American Cancer Society, National Cancer Institute, and U.S. Vital Statistics.

Structure examines in brief the physiology of the organ or body system.

Cause of Cancer discusses the progressive development of disease and the types of foods, beverages, and other substances that commonly give rise to the malignancy. Usually no one food can be said to cause cancer; rather, it is the overall way of eating that has persisted over a long period of time that needs to be changed. Yin and yang are used as tools of balance to help explain this process. A full explanation of these terms is presented in Chapter 6.

The main categories of food are summarized as follows:

STRONG YANG FOODS AND SUBSTANCES

Refined salt

Eggs

Meat

Cheese

Poultry

Fish

Seafood

Some medications (steroids, blood thickeners, etc.)

BALANCED FOODS

Whole cereal grains

Beans and bean products

Sea vegetables

Root, round, and leafy vegetables

Temperate climate fruit

Seeds and nuts

Spring or well water

Nonaromatic, nonstimulant teas

Natural sea salt

STRONG YIN FOODS AND SUBSTANCES

White rice, white flour

Tropical fruits and vegetables

Milk, cream, yogurt

Oils

Herbs and spices (pepper, curry, nutmeg, etc.)

Aromatic and stimulant beverages (coffee, black tea, mint tea, etc.)

Honey, sugar, and refined sweeteners

Alcohol

Foods containing chemicals, preservatives, dyes, pesticides

Drugs (marijuana, cocaine, etc.)

Some medications (tranquilizers, antidepressants, etc.)

Medical Evidence presents data from medical studies and scientific reports linking cancer with dietary, environmental, and lifestyle factors. Sources after each item give the author or principal researcher's name, the book or professional medical journal in which the material appeared, date of publication if not included in the general discussion, and volume and page numbers.

Diagnosis contrasts modern hospital techniques with simple visual methods of detection. The diagnostic methods described here are part of our observations based on the living tradition of the Far East and are explained more fully in Chapter 8 of Part I and in *How to See Your Health: The Book of Oriental Diagnosis* by Michio Kushi (New York and Tokyo: Japan Publications, 1980).

Dietary Recommendations explains how to help relieve a particular cancer by changing the daily way of eating. Of course, the specific guidelines for each person will differ on account of his or her condition, constitution, environment, and personal needs. Ideally, the person with cancer who wishes to begin this approach will see a qualified macrobiotic teacher (see page 569 for Resources). The guidelines in this book are offered for people living in temperate climates such as most of the United States, Europe, Russia, China, and Japan. Those living in other areas should see Appendix II with guidelines for tropical and semitropical areas and for polar and semipolar areas, which include slight adjustments that need to be made with the environment. A variety of less common cancers are not discussed in this book. If it cannot be clearly determined whether the condition is more yin or yang in origin, a centrally balanced diet may safely be followed, such as the one described in the chapter on lung cancer. Macrobiotic cooking instruction is essential for orientation to the new diet.

In the event that a person with cancer has received or is currently undergoing medical treatment, as well as certain nutritional therapies or procedures, the dietary guidelines may need to be further modified for his or her unique situation and needs. These modifications may include proportionately increasing the volume of food consumed, especially protein, complex carbohydrate, minerals, vitamins, or saturated fat of vegetable or animal quality. For instance, chemotherapy affects protein and fat absorption. A carefully balanced macrobiotic diet would include more sources of protein and fat, such as fish and oils. More sweets, such as barley malt, may be employed in such a case, because chemotherapy also causes a craving for sweets. Cooked fruits could then supplement the usual grains, soup, legumes, and vegetables. Radiation treatment calls for increased consumption of miso soup and seaweed, which are taken along with whole grains and vegetables. Some persons with low energy or weight loss may initially need to increase the amount of fish consumed or use more unrefined vegetable oil in cooking. It is advisable for such a person to consult his or her medical doctor, nutritional consultant, or other appropriate professional. Together with proper food preparation and cooking, it may be necessary to continue periodic medical checkups to monitor the person's changing condition as these adjustments are implemented. The most important consideration is the cooperation and support of the person's family and physician. The physician must understand that the macrobiotic approach is not harmful and that it can complement whatever medical procedure is being used.

Special Drinks and Dishes presents additional beverages or side dishes that may be beneficial in some cases. The use of these special preparations, including the amount, frequency, and duration of use, will depend on each person's condition. It is advisable to see a qualified macrobiotic teacher about their use.

The time frames given are averages, and the starting point begins after beginning the new way of eating. Recipes on how to prepare special drinks and dishes are given in Part III.

Home Care lists various compresses and other applications that can be prepared in the home to reduce pain and help discharge toxic excess through the skin or urine. These remedies are inexpensive, easy to prepare, and, if used properly, safe. However, if unnecessarily applied, overused, or incorrectly administered, they may be slightly counterproductive. Their application will differ a little with the individual, and seeing an experienced macrobiotic teacher is recommended. Instructions on how to prepare home cares are given in Part III.

Emotional Considerations looks at the positive and negative emotions associated with disease in the organ or site, foods that contribute or suppress these emotions, relationship advice, and planetary correspondences.

Other Considerations offers some way-of-life suggestions and other types of activity that may be used in conjunction with the dietary approach. Please read or reread the chapter on exercise, lifestyle, and the power of the mind in Part I. For further information on supplementary breathing, fitness, or meditative exercises, see *The Do-in Way* by Michio Kushi (New York: Square One, 2007).

Personal Experience looks at actual accounts of men and women who have recovered from cancer using the approach presented in this book. Many of these friends have sought guidance from us or our associates, and after restoring their health they have gone on to become wonderful macrobiotic teachers, helping many people. Their stories are drawn largely from case histories collected and published by the East West Foundation, One Peaceful World, Planetary Health/Amberwaves, and other macrobiotic organizations and institutes past and present. While these accounts are largely anecdotal, with varying degrees of medical documentation, we hope that they will provide a stimulus for researchers to conduct further studies of the relation between diet and cancer, including the macrobiotic approach.

Bone Cancer

FREQUENCY

This year an estimated 12,120 Americans will die of bone and joint cancer and connective tissue tumors, and 22,270 new cases will surface. Bone cancer appears in a variety of forms. The most lethal is multiple myeloma, accounting for more than 90 percent of bone cancer deaths. It is one of the fastest-rising cancers in the United States and around the world. Over the last thirty years, death rates from multiple myeloma in this country have increased more than 100 percent.

Multiple myeloma affects both bone tissue and the plasma cells of the blood and usually develops in adults over fifty. This condition is characterized by the spontaneous fracture of the bones, including the vertebrae, ribs, pelvis, and skull, as cancer cells replace normal cells. Other bone cancers include osteogenic sarcoma, a tumor affecting children and young adults that begins in the bone and cartilage and often spreads to the bone marrow, muscles, liver, and lungs; Ewing's sarcoma, another cancer of childhood, appears in the marrow of the longer bones and spreads to other bones and organs; chondrosarcoma, a slow-growing tumor that originates in the cartilage of the large bones and affects primarily middle-aged people; chordoma, a rare tumor found at the base of the skull or end of the spine; and rhabdomyosarcoma, a soft-tissue tumor in the fat and muscles that spreads rapidly and usually affects children mostly between the ages of two and six. Primary bone cancer is comparatively rare. However, the bones are frequently the site of cancer spreading from other sites.

Amputation is prescribed for many bone cancers, though most myelomas are too advanced for surgery. Radiation therapy and chemotherapy are often used as supplemental treatments. The five-year survival rate for multiple myeloma is about 33 percent. For other bone cancers, it varies with the type and reaches up to 50 percent.

STRUCTURE

The skeletal and muscular system supports the body framework and governs mobility and physical interaction with the environment. The bones also serve to protect vital inner organs and store calcium, phosphorous, and other minerals that are needed for metabolism. Bone is considered both a tissue and an organ, and is composed of specialized cells called osteocytes, which are imbedded in a matrix. The matrix includes small fibers and an adhering substance made up of mineral salts. The skeletal structure is also composed of cartilage, which is more flexible than bone; joints, which are junctions between two or more bones; muscles, which control tension and body movement, and make up half the body weight; and tendons, which connect muscles and bones.

Bone tissue is made up of thin layers called lamellae. In fully developed bone, these lamellae are classified as either spongy or compact. The skull and ribs, for instance, are more porous or spongelike in structure, while the long bones of the legs and arms consist of a central canal surrounded by concentrically arranged plates of bone tissue. Blood vessels and nerves run through the canals, transporting nutrients and wastes to and from the osteocytes. The bone marrow consists of the soft tissues in the medullary canals of the compact bones and in the interstices of spongy bones.

Bone tissue is constantly changing in order to adapt to stress and varying environmental factors. The bones of infants and children are softer than adults and more subject to malformation or fracture. In the course of aging, the proportion of inorganic mineral salts in the bones increases, slowing their growth. In elderly people this can cause bones to become brittle and break more easily.

CAUSE OF CANCER

The dense, compact bones are classified as yang in structure, and tumors in this part of the body arise primarily from excess accumulation of refined salt and minerals in combination with excessive animal-quality protein and saturated fat. Foods that can produce this overly contracted condition include meat, eggs, poultry, fish and seafood, and hard salty cheese.

In addition to these yang influences, strong yin factors are also sometimes involved in bone cancer formation, especially in the case of multiple myeloma. In this disease the cells of the bone marrow revert to red blood cells, enhancing the susceptibility of the skeletal system to fracture. This condition reflects stagnated intestinal activity caused by excessive consumption of extreme foods in both the yang and yin categories. The latter includes dairy food, refined flour products, sugar and other sweets, coffee and stimulants, soft drinks, tropical fruits and vegetables, drugs and medications, and all kinds of chemicalized or artificially processed foods. The bones and deep inner organs are particularly susceptible to radioactive substances, such as strontium 90, that displace calcium and other minerals in the tissue. Radioactive elements accumulate in the food chain and are consumed principally in animal foods such as milk and beef. (For a complete description of the relationship between cancer and radiation, see the chapter on leukemia.)

MEDICAL EVIDENCE

In 1970, Japanese scientists at the National Cancer Center Research Institute reported that shiitake mushrooms had a strong anti-tumor effect. In experiments with mice, polysaccharide preparations from various natural sources, including the shiitake mushroom commonly available in Tokyo markets, markedly inhibited the growth of induced sarcomas, resulting in "almost complete regression of tumors . . . with no sign of toxicity."[1]

In 1974, Japanese scientists reported that several varieties of kombu and mojaban, common sea vegetables eaten in Asia and traditionally used as a decoction for cancer in Chinese herbal medicine, were effective in laboratory experiments in the treatment of tumors. In three of four samples tested, inhibition rates in mice with implanted sarcomas ranged from 89 to 95 percent. The researchers reported that "the tumor underwent complete regression in more than half of the mice of each treated group." Similar experiments on mice with leukemia showed promising results.[2]

DIAGNOSIS

Modern medicine commonly tests for bone cancer by a variety of methods, including chest and skeletal surveys, acid and alkaline phosphatase tests, serum calcium tests, and a bone biopsy. For multiple myeloma, detection usually includes a myelogram. In this procedure a dye is injected into the spinal fluid and X-rayed for possible malignancies.

Traditional Asian diagnosis forgoes technological methods of detection that can be harmful to health in favor of simple visual observations, acupressure techniques involving touching certain spots on the body, and other safe but accurate procedures. In this way development of serious illness, including cancer, can be diagnosed long before it reaches a critical stage and corrective dietary adjustments taken.

In general, the quality of a person's native constitution can be seen in the bone structure, while the quality of the individual's year-to-year, month-to-month, or day-to-day condition appears more in the muscles, skin, and other peripheral areas of the body. The constitution can be judged by feeling the bones, especially in the area of the shoulders, arms, and legs. Stronger and bolder bones indicate a stronger, more yang constitution, while thinner and weaker bones indicate a more yin, weak, and fragile condition. The former type of person has a tendency to be more active in physical and social life, while the latter tends to be more active in mental and artistic life.

Softer muscles show a more yin constitution, nourished by fluid, vegetables, and fruits, while tighter muscles show a more yang constitution, nourished by grains, beans, and animal food, with more minerals. The condition of the skin is also an indication. However, in comparison with the bones, the condition of the muscles and skin is more changeable through diet and exercise since they are composed of more protein and fat, while the bones are composed of more minerals. Accordingly, while the muscles and skin show the constitution developed during the periods of pregnancy and growth, they also show the present physical and mental conditions. Softer muscles and fine skin indicate a more adaptable and mentally oriented nature, while tighter and harder muscles and skin show a nature that is more physically oriented and active.

These are general tendencies and differ depending on the individual. In visual diagnosis, both constitution and condition are taken into account in determining relative health or sickness and are examined in assessing the digestive, circulatory, nervous, and excretory systems as well as the skeletal and musculature system.

Bone cancer is a yang disorder and especially affects those who are sturdy in build or lean with very strong constitutions. The development of this form of malignancy can be determined by a variety of observations. Facial color is either red-brown or milky white, and in both cases facial and body skin appears oily.

In bone cancer cases, a green coloration often appears along the spleen meridian, especially from the inside of the big toe up the outside of the leg. Also, in some cases, fatty spots with a green shade appear on the outside of the foot below the ankle. The inside of the wrist may also show a dark green or dark blue color. The outer edge of the palm may become red-white, while the edge of the back of the hand may be green.

In many cases of bone cancer the toenails may become white or cracked, and calluses often appear on the tips of the toes or between them. Hard mucus accumulation and calcification also arise on the forehead and are a possible indication of this condition. A yellow-white color, also showing mucus buildup, often appears on the lower white of the eye. The fingertips, especially the second section, often become white, and the second and third set of knuckles tend to be hard. From these and other signs, developing bone cancer can be detected and protected against naturally.

DIETARY RECOMMENDATIONS

Bone cancer can be caused primarily by longtime overconsumption of animal food, especially beef, pork, poultry, eggs, cheese and other dairy food, fish and seafood, and salted and baked foods. Consumption of these and other foods high in fat, protein, and salt should be discontinued. At the same time contributing to bone cancer is the overconsumption of all fatty and oily foods, both of animal and vegetable quality, including sugar, honey, chocolate, carob, and other sweeteners, spices, stimulants, and aromatic foods and drinks, as well as foods that form fat and mucus, such as flour products. These should be limited or avoided completely. Soft drinks, chemical additives, alcohol, and all artificially processed food and beverages are to be avoided because they are considered possible contributing factors. The following are general dietary guidelines for the relief and prevention of bone cancer:

- Whole Grains: Fifty to 60 percent of daily consumption, by volume, should be whole cereal grains. The first day, prepare plain short- or medium-grain brown rice pressure-cooked or cooked in a heavy cast-iron or ceramic pot with a heavy lid. The following days, prepare brown rice cooked with 20 to 30 percent millet, then rice with 20 to 30 percent barley, then rice with 20 to 30 percent aduki beans or lentils, and then plain rice again. A delicious morning porridge can be made by taking leftover rice, adding a little more water to soften it, and seasoning it with a little miso at the end and simmering two to three minutes more. In daily cooking the ratio of grain to water should be about 1:2. For seasoning, cook with a postage-stamp-sized piece of kombu instead of salt. Other grains can be used occasionally, including whole wheat berries, rye, corn, and whole oats, though oats should be avoided for the first month. However, buckwheat should be avoided for about six months because it is very contractive and may harden the tumor. Seitan is also very yang and should be minimized. Flour products, even unrefined whole wheat bread, chapatis, pancakes, and cookies should be totally avoided or limited in volume for a few months. Whole grain pasta and noodles may be eaten a couple of times a week. Fried rice or noodles may be consumed once or twice a week.

- Soup: Five to 10 percent of daily consumption should be soup, consisting of one or two cups or bowls cooked with wakame sea vegetable and various vegetables seasoned lightly with miso or shoyu. To help relieve this condition, pieces of fresh daikon, turnip, or radish can be added almost daily. Occasionally a small amount of shiitake mushrooms may be added to the soup. The miso may be barley miso, brown rice miso, or soybean (hatcho) miso and should be naturally aged two to three years. The taste of the soup should be milder than usual. Grain soups, bean soups, and other soups may be taken from time to time.

- Vegetables: Twenty to 30 percent of daily consumption should be vegetables, cooked in a variety of forms, mainly steamed and boiled. While oil is not usually recommended for most cancer patients, for bone cancer one dish of sautéed vegetables cooked with unrefined sesame oil should be eaten daily or every other day. Sweet vegetables such as cabbage, onions, pumpkin, and winter squash can be used most often, although root and leafy vegetables are also to be used regularly. Vegetables may be seasoned during cooking with sea salt, miso, or shoyu, and the taste should be milder than usual. As a rule of thumb, the following dishes may be prepared, although the frequency may differ from person to person: nishime-style vegetables, three times a week; a squash-aduki-kombu dish, three times a week; dried daikon, one cup three times a week; carrots and carrot tops or daikon and daikon tops, three times a week; blanched vegetables, five to seven times a week; pressed salads, several times a week; raw salad, avoid; steamed greens, five to seven times a week; sautéed vegetables, prepared with water the first month, and then with sesame oil lightly brushed on the pan once or twice a week after that; kinpira, two-thirds of a cup, two times a week; dried tofu, tofu, tempeh, or seitan with vegetables, two times a week.

- Beans: Five percent of daily consumption should be small beans, such as aduki beans, lentils, chickpeas, or black soybeans, cooked together with sea vegetables such as kombu or with onions and carrots. Black soybeans are highly recommended for regular use for this form of cancer. Beans can be cooked with 10 to 20 percent kombu or other sea vegetable, 30 to 50 percent fall-season squash, or 10 to 30 percent onions and carrots. Season lightly with sea salt, miso, or shoyu. Other beans may be used altogether two to three times a month. For seasoning, a small volume of unrefined sea salt or shoyu or miso can be used. Bean products such as tempeh, natto, and dried or cooked tofu may be used occasionally but in moderate amounts.

- Sea Vegetables: Five percent or less of daily consumption should be sea vegetable dishes, including wakame and kombu, when cooking grain, in soup, etc. A sheet of toasted nori may also be taken daily. A small dish of hijiki or arame should be prepared two times a week. All other sea vegetables are optional.
- Condiments: Condiments that should be available on the table are go-mashio (sesame salt), on the average made with one part salt to eighteen to twenty parts sesame seeds, kelp or wakame powder, umeboshi plum, and tekka, although all other regular macrobiotic condiments may be used if desired. These condiments may be used daily on grains and vegetables, but the amount should be moderate to suit individual appetite and taste.
- Pickles: Pickles, made at home in a variety of ways, are to be eaten daily, one tablespoon in all, although salty pickles are to be minimized. Rice bran (nuka) pickles are the most suitable.
- Animal Food: Fish and other animal food is to be avoided. However, in the event that animal food is craved, a small volume of white-meat fish may be eaten once every ten days to two weeks. The fish should be prepared steamed, boiled, or poached, and garnished with grated daikon or ginger. Strictly avoid blue-meat and red-meat fish and all shellfish.
- Fruit: The less the better until the condition improves. If cravings develop, a small volume of cooked fruit with a pinch of sea salt or dried fruit (also preferably cooked) may be eaten. Avoid all fruit juices and cider temporarily, as well as raisins, currants, and other highly concentrated fruits.
- Sweets and Snacks: Overuse of sweets is connected with bone disorders, so it is very important to avoid all sweets and desserts, including good-quality macrobiotic desserts, until the condition improves. To satisfy a sweet tooth, use sweet vegetables every day in cooking, drink sweet vegetable drinks, or prepare sweet vegetable jam. If cravings arise, a small amount of amasake, barley malt, or rice syrup may be eaten. If cravings persist, a little cider, apple juice, or chestnut may be prepared. Mochi, rice balls, vegetable sushi, and other grain-based snacks may be eaten frequently. Limit rice cakes, popcorn, and other dry or baked snacks, because they may harden the tumor.
- Nuts and Seeds: Nuts and nut butters are to be avoided due to their high fat and protein content, except for chestnuts. Unsalted blanched seeds such as sunflower seeds and pumpkin seeds may be consumed as a snack, up to one cup total per week.
- Seasonings: Unrefined sea salt, shoyu, and miso are to be used moderately in order to avoid unnecessary thirst. Avoid mirin and garlic. If you become particularly thirsty after a meal or between meals, you

should cut back on these seasonings until the normal level of thirst returns.

- Beverages: Drinks and other dietary practices can follow the general recommendations in Part I, with bancha twig tea as the principal drink at meals. One cup of carrot juice twice a week is very good for this condition. Strictly avoid the beverages on the "infrequent" and "avoid" list, and don't drink grain coffee for the first two to three months after starting this new way of eating.

The most important thing in connection with dietary practice is chewing very well until the food becomes liquid in the mouth and well mixed with saliva. Chew very, very well, at least fifty times and preferably one hundred times per mouthful. It is also important to avoid overeating and eating within three hours of sleeping.

As noted in the introduction to Part II, individuals who have received or who are currently undergoing medical treatment may have to make further dietary modifications.

SPECIAL DRINKS AND DISHES

One or more special drinks or side dishes may be needed, depending on the individual case, to help reduce excess protein and fat, which are the cause of the cancer; to reduce cholesterol levels; and to assist recovery. Please see a qualified macrobiotic teacher for guidance. Amounts and frequencies listed are averages for each drink or dish; these will differ from person to person. Further directions are in Chapter 36.

- Sweet Vegetable Drink: Take one to two cups every day.
- Zosui with Sweet Vegetables and Nori: Season with a small amount of miso, shoyu, or sea salt. Seasoning is not necessary for ten days in the event you have no appetite for salt.
- Brown Rice Milk with Sweetener: For loss of appetite, take this drink as often as possible, one bowl to a couple of bowls a day.
- Miso Soup with Okara and Vegetables: Make a mild soup and have it three to four times a week for two to three weeks.
- Shiso Powder: One-half to one teaspoon of shiso powder can be sprinkled daily on grain and vegetable dishes. This is made from roasting and grinding the dried leaves that accompany umeboshi plums.
- Kuzu Drink with Grated Daikon: A cup of this drink is also beneficial for this condition and may be consumed frequently.
- Ume-Sho-Bancha Tea: Up to one cup can be consumed with half a sheet of crushed toasted nori sea vegetable a few times a week.

- Carp and Burdock Soup: For strength, bone cancer patients may occasionally prepare this soup (koi koku). Mochi or tempeh may also be added to miso soup frequently to restore vitality and generate energy.

HOME CARE

- Compress Guidelines: For a small number of bone tumors, a compress may be needed to help gradually draw out excess mucus and fat. Please see a qualified macrobiotic teacher for guidance on the proper use and frequency of a compress or plaster. Several types are used depending on the person's condition. Soak a towel in hot water, squeeze it out, and place it on the affected area for three to five minutes to stimulate circulation, and then apply the compress or plaster.
- Hato Mugi with Cabbage Plaster: For bone pain, spread this plaster over cotton linen about one inch thick. Apply it directly to the painful part for three to four hours twice a day; or sleep with it until the next morning.
- Sesame Oil–Ginger Rub: After having radiation therapy, the muscles sometimes get stiff, and pain is experienced when moving. In this case, use this rub. After ten minutes, clean the skin with a warm towel. Do it twice a day.
- Body Scrub: A body scrub with a hot, wet towel, especially on the abdominal and spinal regions, will help activate circulation and energy flow.

EMOTIONAL CONSIDERATIONS

The bones and skeletal structure are associated with form, structure, and stability. Bone problems are often accompanied by lack of order in one's personal life, brittleness, and instability.

High-quality foods that nourish the bones and help develop positive emotions include whole grains, particularly buckwheat, teff, wild rice, and other darker grains; beans and bean products, especially black beans and other darker beans; leafy green vegetables; sea vegetables; seeds and nuts; white-meat fish; and good-quality sea salt.

Foods that harm the bones and contribute to negative emotions include dairy food, especially milk; meat, poultry, eggs, and strong fish and seafood; white flour; sugar and other highly refined sweets; chemicalized and artificial foods; and other extremely contractive or expansive foods and beverages.

While spontaneity and playfulness play an important role in relationships, it is important to maintain basic order and structure. Unstable relationships at work or in the home, feelings of insecurity, and stress and tension can lead to bone, joint, and skeletal problems.

On a planetary scale, the bones correlate with the Earth's mineral deposits. Bone cancer corresponds with mineral depletion.

OTHER CONSIDERATIONS

Daily physical exercise that does not produce exhaustion is recommended. Ten to fifteen minutes of daily breathing exercises, especially emphasizing long exhalation, is also beneficial. These physical and breathing exercises contribute to relaxing tensions in the body and mind as well as harmonizing physical metabolism.

Keeping air quality clean and fresh is important for maintenance of general health. For that purpose, green leafy plants can be placed in the house, and the windows can be periodically opened to allow circulation of fresh air. Don't smoke, because this will tighten the bones.

Avoid wearing wool and synthetic fibers. At the minimum, wear cotton underwear and use cotton sheets and pillowcases.

Avoid watching television for long stretches. Radiation is especially weakening to the bones. Similarly, avoid other artificial sources of electromagnetic energy such as video terminals, smoke detectors, and handheld electrical appliances, which can weaken the bones and skeletal system.

Bone cancer patients should particularly avoid damp and humid environments.

PERSONAL EXPERIENCE

BONE CANCER (METASTASIZED FROM THE BREAST)

In November 1980, Bonnie Kramer, a twenty-seven-year-old mother from Torrington, Connecticut, felt discomfort under her arm. She discovered a pea-sized ball that "seemed to float" when touched, but she was not overly concerned about it. She underwent a mammogram the following February, and the results were negative.

During the winter, the lump went through periods of increasing and decreasing in size, and Bonnie started to experience constant pain in her left breast along with fatigue and a milky white discharge from the nipple. Her breasts were enlarged and tender. She also had an unusual number of colds and flu.

A biopsy in February 1982 revealed cancer, and soon afterward Bonnie entered Winsted Memorial Hospital for the removal of her left breast and several lymph nodes under her arm. She also began chemotherapy and was scheduled to undergo six weeks of radiation. The side effects were not severe, although she was irritable at times, lost some hair, and became nauseated after each treatment. Bonnie completed her treatments in March 1983 and was considered by her doctors to be free of cancer. However, periodic bone and liver scans were advised as a precaution. Feeling better, she took a job as a director of social services at a skilled nursing facility and helped raise funds for the American Cancer Society.

Three years later, in April 1986, while playing ball with her son, Bonnie felt a pull in her lower back. The pain continued off and on, and by early 1987 had become unbearable. "The pain returned with a vengeance," she recalls. "It just would not go away, and the nurses at work became very concerned. The pain radiated to my face. With each menstrual cycle I was bloated, suffering with intense cramps." She underwent a bone scan that revealed tumors on her pelvis and upper back. Her doctors advised radiation and aggressive chemotherapy. Bonnie was "numbed to speechlessness" at the news and "couldn't stop crying." As she recalls, "I had to deal with this; that's all I knew. I prayed for strength and guidance in the midst of all the drama. Then, suddenly, out of nowhere, it hit me! Honestly, just like that the answer came. I knew from my readings that more and more was being learned about nutrition and cancer. I remembered my sister telling me about an article she had read several years before, concerning a doctor whose cancer went into remission through a change in diet. It didn't seem relevant to me then, but, suddenly, now it did. 'Oh my God!' I thought. 'That's what I need to do—find out more about this diet—but how?'"

Bonnie's friend went to a local health food store and bought one of my books to read. She found it completely logical but overwhelming. She went to the health food store and bought staple foods and stopped eating meat, sugar, and dairy foods. She also underwent radiation therapy and a hysterectomy. After recovering from surgery, Bonnie decided to attend a seminar presented by the Kushi Institute.

Bonnie supplemented her practice of macrobiotics by taking weekly cooking classes with Sara Lapenta, a Kushi Institute cooking teacher who lived nearby. By May 1987 a blood test revealed that Bonnie's enzyme levels had returned to normal. A bone scan in September showed that the tumors had greatly decreased in size. A friend who worked in the radiation unit at the hospital told Bonnie that she had never seen a report like that before. In September 1988 another bone scan revealed the presence of scar tissue but no tumors. Bonnie's doctor told her that her remission might have been due to the surgery and radiation, but that macrobiotics may also have helped her. By August 1988 a bone scan produced a totally normal result, with no tumors or scar tissue. Her doctor was now very impressed and fully supportive of her macrobiotic lifestyle.

Bonnie described her experience: "I noticed immediate changes in myself and in my son, Ben, who joined in my meals for the first summer. Our allergies seemed to disappear, and Ben no longer got strep throat. We felt stronger, more energetic, more organized, and very well. I had good spirits and stable moods. As my confidence increased, so did the sense of inner peace. I loved feeling at one with nature, at one with God."

Bonnie went on to become a leading macrobiotic cook and teacher. Believing that "happiness is real only if it can be shared with others," she helped people in her area through classes, food, and guidance. She has dedicated herself to realizing one peaceful world and is grateful to have found a way to "help make this concept a reality."[3] She has been cancer-free for more than twenty years.

Brain Cancer

FREQUENCY

Brain tumors and cancer of the central nervous system will kill an estimated 12,740 Americans this year, and 20,500 new cases will develop. Men between ages fifty and sixty are most at risk, but the incidence in women has greatly increased in recent years. Brain cancer is the ninth leading cause of death from malignancy. Brain tumors are the second leading cause of cancer death for children and young adults under twenty and among men twenty to twenty-nine. Brain cancer has also increased among the elderly, with the incidence of brain tumors more than doubling from 1968 to 1985, but since then has stabilized. In the United States, incidence has peaked and is beginning to decline. Major risk factors are being male, Caucasian, elderly, or living in an urban area.

A majority of brain tumors affect the brain tissue itself and are called gliomas. These are subdivided into four main types: (1) glioblastoma multiforme, a malignant tumor that affects both children and adults, and one that may spread quickly through the cerebrum, cerebellum, brain stem, and spinal cord; (2) astrocytoma, a tumor found mostly in children, affects the cerebellum and brain stem; (3) ependymoma, another childhood tumor, which grows in the ventricles of the brain; (4) oligodendroglioma, a slow-growing tumor that affects the white matter in the frontal lobe and is found in both children and adults.

Other brain tumors include medulloblastoma, a childhood cancer that spreads from the cerebellum to other regions of the brain and central nervous system; meningioma, a tumor that affects the membrane covering the brain and spinal cord; pituitary adenoma, a tumor that affects the hypothalamus and optic nerve; gaulioneuroblastoma, a malignancy that spreads quickly through the nerve cells; neurofibrosarcoma, a cancer affecting the peripheral nervous system; and neuroblastoma, a tumor that affects children three years old or younger and spreads through the nervous network in various regions including the chest, neck, abdomen, lower back, eye, and adrenal glands. About 15 percent of brain tumors have metastasized from other organs, especially the lungs, kidney, breast, or the lymph nodes in the case of Hodgkin's disease.

Because of their location within one of the most sensitive parts of the body, many brain tumors are considered untreatable by modern science. However, depending on the type and staging, surgery and radiation therapy are often employed. The operation is called a craniotomy and involves removing part of the skull, excising the malignant tissue, and putting back the excised bone. The risk of damaging the brain during such a procedure is high.

When surgery is ruled out, radiation is commonly used, especially for medulloblastomas and ependymomas. However, X-ray treatments may cause permanent damage to the spinal cord, especially in children. Hormone therapy is sometimes used in conjunction with surgery to decrease the swelling or control metastases. Steroids are given and are followed up by drugs such as prednisone, which may be administered intravenously or intramuscularly for the rest of the patient's life. Other methods of treating brain tumors include hypothermia (lowering the temperature of the brain or body), cryosurgery (freezing), and implanting radio sensitizers to enhance radiation therapy. Death rates from brain cancer have declined about 10 percent in both sexes over the last twenty years. The present survival rate for all forms of brain tumors is about 34 percent.

STRUCTURE

The human nervous system has two anatomical divisions: the central nervous system, which includes the brain and spinal cord, and the peripheral nervous system, which includes all the nervous structures outside of the skull and vertebral canal, such as the craniospinal nerves and the orthosympathetic branch of the autonomic nervous system. The central nervous system acts as a switchboard for incoming impulses from receptors and outgoing impulses to effectors; it regulates all body activities except for chemically controlled ones and is the seat for the higher consciousness processes.

The autonomic nervous system is not considered an anatomical division but a functional unit that handles the involuntary, unconscious body activities, such as the beating of the heart, breathing, digestive peristalsis, and so on. The autonomic system in turn is composed of two antagonistic branches: the parasympathetic (yang) and the orthosympathetic (yin). The parasympathetic nerves have a more central position of origin in the body, beginning in the brain stem and sacral region of the spinal cord and passing outward through four pairs of cranial nerves and three pairs of sacral nerves. The orthosympathetic nerves have a more peripheral position, beginning in the central section of the spine and passing outward through the corresponding spinal nerves. In almost all organs, tissues, and smooth muscles there are pairs of autonomic nerves, one orthosympathetic and one parasympathetic, which act in opposite ways. When the parasympathetic nerves act on expanded (yin) organs, such as the bronchi of the lungs or the wall of the digestive tract, there is naturally a resultant contraction. Their action on compact organs (yang), such as the iris of the eye or cardiac muscles, brings about expansion or dilation. The orthosympathetic nerves have a complementary opposite effect. They inhibit hollow organs, such as the bladder, and stimulate compact ones, such as the uterus, during pregnancy.

The two major divisions of the brain are the large forebrain, including the cerebrum, and the more compact hindbrain, including the cerebellum. Since the forebrain is more open and expanded, it is classified as yin, while the smaller, more compact hindbrain is yang. The brain can also be divided into its more central region, known as the midbrain, and more peripheral region, called the cortex. In order for communication to proceed smoothly, incoming and outgoing impulses need to be balanced. Within the brain, the more compact or central regions tend to be areas where images and impulses are received, while outgoing communication originates in the more peripheral or expanded areas. Thus nervous impulses from the eyes, ears, nose, skin, and other sense organs gather in the midbrain, while images, dreams, and thoughts are dispatched outward from the more peripheral cortex regions. Also, in terms of receiving and dispatching, the hindbrain receives incoming vibrations and stores them as memory, while outgoing vibrations, including our images of the future, arise in the forebrain.

CAUSE OF CANCER

In the last several years there has been considerable research concerning the relationship between the right and left hemispheres of the brain. Studies show that the left hemisphere in most people is the origin of more simple or mechanical action and consciousness, while the right hemisphere produces more complex and creative thinking. In terms of language, more simple or basic expressions originate in the left hemisphere, while the right hemisphere creates more refined and original expression. Imagination, which is based mostly on futuristic thinking, develops more in the right hemisphere, while analytical thinking, based more on actual past experiences, arises in the left hemisphere.

Our modern technological civilization has arisen due to the active development of left-hemisphere thinking. This more focused, yang type of thinking and activity has resulted from a way of eating centered around meat, dairy food, and other animal products. Imbalance in one direction produces a corresponding pull in the other. To balance the increasing amounts of food, modern society has witnessed a proliferation of extreme substances in the yin category, including alcohol, spices, coffee and other stimulants, refined sugar, imported tropical fruits and vegetables, chemical additives, and a variety of drugs, including tranquilizers, birth control pills, and hallucinogens.

In many modern countries, especially during the last forty years, young people have been exposed to these types of food from birth, and many have experimented and become regular users of marijuana, hashish, cocaine, or LSD. These extremely yin substances have produced a rapid shift in thinking from the left side of the brain, which is predominant in modern society, toward the right side, and also from the back of the brain more toward the front. As a result, many young people started looking more toward the future while neglecting or forgetting previous traditions, including the relationship with their parents, elders, and ancestors. Similarly, they lost interest in school, business or professional careers, and the political and economic condition of society. Instead, they turned to music, the arts, spiritual teachers from the East, and other nonlinear pursuits.

In many cases the continuous intake of yin-type foods and drugs has led to very unbalanced conditions and expression. By moving to the other extreme, vegetarians, who eat primarily fruits, juices, and raw foods, and members of the counterculture risk a variety of illnesses. These include mental disease, herpes, multiple sclerosis, leukemia, and brain cancer.

Tumors that affect the outer regions of the brain or the nerve cells of the peripheral nervous system are caused primarily by foods, drinks, and medications or drugs in the yin category. These forms of brain malfunction or nervous disorders are more commonly found in children or young adults who have grown up on sugar-coated breakfast cereals, honey, chocolate, and other sweeteners, orange juice, soda pop, ice cream, and oily and greasy foods, as well as many chemical additives, in conjunction with a constant intake of milk, butter, and other dairy foods.

Tumors in the inner region of the brain or spinal cord are more yang in structure and location. They arise primarily from consumption of excess animal food, including meat, poultry, eggs, and cheese, and refined salt, and thus tend to affect older persons. As a whole, the brain and central nervous system are extremely compact (yang) and therefore a magnet that attracts drugs, medications, synthetic vitamins, food and mineral supplements, and other extremely expansive (yin) substances. By avoiding these things and centering the diet, the brain and nervous system can maintain their normal functions.

MEDICAL EVIDENCE

In a case-control study of adults residing in Nebraska with glioma, a brain tumor, scientists at the Human Nutrition Research Center on Aging at Tufts University in Boston reported that consumption of fiber-rich beans, dark yellow vegetables, and dietary fiber substantially reduced the risk of adult glioma.[1]

In 1993 scientists reported that diets rich in soy foods, especially miso soup, produced genistein, a natural substance that blocked the growth of new blood vessels that feed a tumor. Researchers from Children's University Hospital in Heidelberg, Germany, reported that genistein also deterred cancer cells from multiplying and could have significant implications for the prevention and treatment of solid malignancies, including those of the brain, breast, and prostate.[2]

Inflammation of the brain is associated with an increase in brain cancer. Dietary fats are a major source of inflammation because they produce eicosanoids, or chemical messengers, that influence inflammation. The type of fats that are especially inflammatory include saturated fats, hydrogenated fats, and transfats. Inflammation also promotes angiogenesis, or the development of new blood vessels that nourish tumor growth. High copper foods, including shellfish, organ meats, and chocolate sauces, syrups, and candies prepared in copper cookware, are major sources of excess copper in the human body.[3]

DIAGNOSIS

Brain tumors are commonly detected by X-rays or CT scans to the skull, spinal cord, and chest. Other medical techniques may include an electroencephalogram, cerebral angiogram, brain scan, spinal puncture, and myelogram.

Oriental medicine uses a variety of simple observations to ascertain the condition of the nervous system. A purplish red color around the eyes shows an overworked nervous system caused mainly by the consumption of drugs, chemicals, medications, refined simple sugars, and other extreme foods and drinks from the yin category. The parasympathetic system is especially affected by these substances. However, the orthosympathetic system will also be weakened, making all body reflexes and functions less sharp. The immediate effect can often be seen in the eyes, where the pupils contract, and in the vascular system, where the blood vessels dilate. After continued drug use, however, the parasympathetic nerves become worn out, expanding more and more. The pupils then dilate and the vessels contract.

The middle region of the forehead also shows the condition of the nervous system. A red color here shows nervousness, oversensitivity, excitability, and instability due to the overconsumption of yin-type foods, drinks, stimulants, and drugs. A white color is caused by an excessive intake of dairy products, especially milk, cream, and yogurt, together with excessive liquid. Nervous functions are generally slow and dull, and mental activities are cloudy and unclear. A yellow color indicates alertness but a tendency toward narrow-mindedness and inflexibility. The major cause is an excessive intake of eggs, poultry, and dairy food. Dark spots or patches on the forehead indicate the elimination of excessive sugars, fruits, honey, milk sugar, and other sweets as well as chemicals and drugs. Red pimples or spots on the middle the forehead show the elimination of sugar and fruits combined with refined white flour products or dairy products.

The middle layer or ridge of the ear reflects the condition of the entire nervous system. A red color here indicates nervous disorders. The earlobe corresponds to the brain, and pimples, discolorations, or other abnormalities in this region may show developing cysts or tumors.

A loose mouth shows a variety of disorders, including nervous-system malfunctions. This condition also usually reflects trouble in the small intestine, the brain's complementary opposite organ.

The color on the back of the hand may also indicate nervous problems. If marijuana, hashish, or other hallucinogenic substances, as well as medications, are used repeatedly for some time, the body will begin to discharge these toxins, and the color of the hands and fingers will change to red or purple.

Rough skin also shows nervous disorders caused by extreme yin-type foods or drugs. This condition may be accompanied by an irregular pulse, excessive perspiration, frequent urination, diarrhea, vertigo, excessive sensitivity, and emotional instability.

The sensitively trained hand can also locate the approximate region of brain tumors and cancer by detecting vibrations produced and discharged from each part of the brain. In some cases, brain tumors may cause paralysis, seizure, loss of sight, and loss of physical and mental coordination. By examining the paralyzed parts and functions of the body, indirect detection of the area of the brain affected can be done.

Generally, brain tumors are comparatively easier than other cancers to relieve through proper eating. This is because they tend to grow slowly in this very compact region, and the abundance of blood supply to the brain means that a change in blood quality from an altered diet will quickly affect the condition of the brain and nervous system.

DIETARY RECOMMENDATIONS

There are two basic types of brain tumors. The harder carcinoma type, usually occurring deep inside the brain, is caused by the gathering of excess protein and fat, especially of animal quality. Animal products, including eggs, meat, poultry, dairy food, and oily, fatty fish, and other strong yang foods should be strictly avoided. Sugar and other strong yin foods may enhance this type of tumor. The second type of brain tumor, sarcoma, is softer and usually occurs more on the surface of the brain. It is caused primarily by the consumption of extreme yin foods and beverages, especially milk, butter, cream, yogurt, sugar and sweets, and excessive fruit and juice. The growth of brain tumors is promoted by chemicals in artificially processed food as well as exposure to industrial pollutants, although these are usually not the primary cause. It is therefore advisable to avoid the continued use of all synthetic food products and for people with this condition to restore their health in a relatively fresh and clean atmospheric environment. Although they are not direct causes of brain tumors, spices, stimulants, alcohol, and aromatic beverages and substances are to be avoided because they tend to accelerate tumor growth. Because of their potential for contributing to cancer creation and growth, flour products, especially refined flour treated with oil, fat, and sweets, as well as an overconsumption of liquid, are also to be avoided. Nutritional advice for infants and young children, including those with brain tumors, is given in the chapter on children's cancer.

Following are general dietary guidelines for older children and adults.

- Whole Grains: Forty to 50 percent of daily consumption, by volume, should be whole cereal grains. The first day prepare plain short- or medium-grain brown rice, pressure-cooked or cooked in a heavy cast-iron or ceramic pot with a heavy lid. On the following days prepare rice with 20 to 30 percent millet, then rice with 20 to 30 percent barley, then rice with 20 to 30 percent aduki beans or lentils, and then plain rice again. A delicious morning porridge can be made by taking leftover rice, adding a little more water to soften, seasoning with a little miso, and simmering for two to three minutes more. In ordinary cooking the ratio of grain to water should be about 1:2. For seasoning, cook with a postage-stamp-sized piece of kombu or a pinch of sea salt, depending on the person's condition. After the first month, these grains can be prepared once or twice a week in the form of fried grains with vegetables. Other grains can be used occasionally, including whole wheat berries, rye, corn, and whole oats, although oats should be avoided for the first month. For more yang tumors deep inside the brain or in the back of the head, avoid buckwheat and seitan for several months. For tumors on the periphery or surface of the head and toward the front, buckwheat and seitan may be taken occasionally. Good-quality sourdough bread may be enjoyed two to three times a week, and noodles (udon for more yang cancers, and both udon and soba for more yin cancers) may also be eaten two to three times a week. Avoid all hard-baked products until the condition improves, including cookies, cake, pie, crackers, muffins, and the like.

- Soup: Five to 10 percent of daily consumption, consisting of one or two cups or bowls per day cooked with wakame sea vegetable and various land vegetables such as onions and carrots seasoned with miso or shoyu. Occasionally a small amount of shiitake mushrooms may be added to the soup. Lotus root should be used often in soup. The miso may be barley miso, brown rice miso, or soybean (hatcho) miso and should be naturally aged for two to three years. To satisfy a sweet tooth, millet soup with sweet vegetables such as squash, cabbage, onions, and carrots may be prepared often. These vegetables can be sautéed with a little sesame oil before cooking in the soup. Among vegetables, more round vegetables are preferred, such as onions, pumpkin, and winter squash, although other root and green leafy vegetables may also occasionally be used in soup. Grain, bean, and other soups may be eaten from time to time. Less frequently, a small portion of white-meat fish or small dried fish can also be cooked in the soup with vegetables, sea vegetables, and/or grains. After the first month, when no oil should be consumed, two to three times a week vegetables may be lightly sautéed in a small amount of sesame or corn oil before cooking them in the soup.

- Vegetables: Twenty to 30 percent of daily consumption can be cooked in a variety of forms. Dishes can be prepared using round vegetables together with root vegetables, such as carrots, burdock, daikon, and turnip. Avoid oil for the first one to two months, after which some dishes may be sautéed with a moderate amount of sesame or corn oil. As a general rule, the following dishes may be prepared, although the frequency may differ from person to person: nishime-style vegetables, three times a week for those with more yang tumors and four times for those with more yin tumors; a squash-aduki-kombu dish, three times a week; dried daikon, one cup, three times a week; carrots and carrot tops or daikon and daikon tops, three times a week; blanched vegetables, five to seven times a week; pressed salads, several times a week; raw salad and salad dressing, avoid; steamed greens, five to seven times a week; sautéed vegetables, twice a week, using water the first month and then sesame oil; kinpira, two-thirds of a cup, two times a week, using water the first month and then sautéing in oil (this dish is particularly beneficial for brain tumors); tofu, dried tofu, tempeh, or seitan with vegetables, two times a week.

- Beans: Five percent of daily consumption; ones such as aduki beans, lentils, chickpeas, or black soybeans may be used, cooked together with sea vegetables such as kombu or with onions and carrots. Other beans may be used two to three times a month. For seasoning, a small amount of unrefined sea salt or shoyu or miso can be used. Bean products such as tempeh, natto, and dried or cooked tofu may be used occasionally but in moderate amounts.

- Sea Vegetables: Five percent or less of daily consumption of sea vegetable dishes, including wakame and kombu when cooking grain, in soup, etc. A sheet of toasted nori may also be eaten daily. A small dish of hijiki or arame should be prepared two times a week. All other sea vegetables are optional. Sea vegetables can be cooked with other vegetables or sautéed with a small amount of sesame oil after softening them by soaking and boiling lightly in water.

- Condiments: Condiments that may be available on the table are gomashio (sesame salt), usually made with one part salt to eighteen parts sesame seeds (reduced to 1:16 after two months); kelp or wakame powder; umeboshi plum; and tekka, although all other regular macrobiotic condiments may be used if desired. These condiments may be used daily on grains and vegetables, but the amounts should be moderate to suit individual appetite and taste. One to two teaspoons a day of sliced lotus root cooked together with kombu and a bit of grated ginger, seasoned with shoyu, is especially good for this condition. Several small pieces of kombu cooked with shoyu can also be helpful if consumed daily with any meal. This is called shio kombu or salty kombu.

- Pickles: Pickles, made at home in a variety of ways, are to be eaten daily, one tablespoon in all, although the consumption of salty pickles should to be minimal.

- Animal Food: Meat, poultry, eggs, and other strong animal food is to be avoided. A small volume of white-meat fish may be eaten once every two weeks by those with more yang cancers and once a week by those with more yin tumors. The fish should be steamed, boiled, or poached, and garnished with grated daikon or ginger. After two months, fish may be eaten twice a week if desired. Strictly avoid blue-meat and red-meat fish and all shellfish.

- Fruit: None is best, and the less the better, including both tropical and temperate-climate fruit, until the condition improves. If cravings develop, a small amount of cooked fruit with a pinch of sea salt or dried fruit (also preferably cooked) may be eaten. Avoid all fruit juices and cider temporarily, as well as raisins, currants, and other highly concentrated fruits.

- Sweets and Snacks: Avoid all sweets and desserts, including good-quality macrobiotic desserts, until the condition improves. To satisfy a sweet tooth, use sweet vegetables every day in cooking, drink sweet vegetable drinks (see special drinks below), and use sweet vegetable jam and a small amount of amasake. Mochi, rice balls, vegetable sushi, and other grain-based snacks may be eaten frequently. Limit rice cakes, popcorn, and other dry or baked snacks because they may harden the tumor. In the event of cravings, a small amount of barley malt or rice syrup may be consumed.

- Nuts and Seeds: Nuts and nut butters are to be avoided due to their high fat and protein content, except for chestnuts. Unsalted blanched seeds such as squash seeds and pumpkin seeds may be consumed as a snack, up to one cup total per week. Avoid sunflower seeds.

- Seasonings: Unrefined sea salt, shoyu, and miso are to be used moderately in order to avoid unnecessary thirst. Avoid mirin and garlic. If you become particularly thirsty after a meal or between meals, you should cut back on these seasonings until the normal level of thirst returns.

- Beverages: Drinks and other dietary practices can follow the general recommendations in Part I, including bancha twig tea as the main beverage. Strictly avoid the beverages on the "infrequent" and "avoid" list and don't drink grain coffee for the first two to three months after starting this new way of eating.

The most important thing in connection with dietary practice is chewing very well, until all food becomes liquid in the mouth and well mixed with saliva. Chew very, very well, at least fifty times but preferably a hundred times per mouthful. It is also important to avoid overeating and eating within three hours of sleeping.

As noted in the introduction to Part II, individuals who have received or who are currently undergoing medical treatment may need to make further dietary modifications.

SPECIAL DRINKS AND DISHES

One or more special drinks or side dishes may need to be consumed, depending on the individual case, to help reduce excess protein and fat, which cause cancer; to reduce cholesterol levels; and to assist recovery. Please see a qualified macrobiotic teacher for guidance. Amounts and frequencies given here are averages for each drink or dish; these will differ from person to person. Further directions are in Chapter 36.

- Dried Daikon, Shiitake, Cabbage, Burdock, and Roasted Rice Tea: Drink one small cup every morning and every evening for three weeks. After that, reduce it to once a day and continue for another three weeks.

- Shio-Kombu: Eat two to three pieces every day at mealtime.
- Ume-Sho-Kuzu: Drink one small cup every other day or once every three days for one month. After that, reduce it to one cup every four to five days and continue for another month.

HOME CARE

- Cabbage Leaf Compress: Apply on the diseased part of the head and keep changing it to cool it down. (In this case, ice cubes should not be used.)
- Massage: All five toes on each foot should be massaged. Pull the big toes strongly for ten to fifteen minutes. Do this two to three times every day.
- If the person has a seizure, as in epilepsy, or loses consciousness, immediately cool the whole head, including the forehead, with a cold towel compress. Massage all the toes well (especially the big toes). If conscious, give ume-sho-bancha using a spoon. Bancha tea with gomashio may be given instead. Seek medical attention if necessary.
- Grated Daikon with Carrot and Shoyu: If some liquid has accumulated around the tumor, eat one small cup every day for five days. After that, continue it once every other day for ten days, followed by two to three times a week for another three to four weeks. In this case, using a cabbage leaf compress as instructed above may also be helpful in relieving this condition.

EMOTIONAL CONSIDERATIONS

Healthy brain functioning is associated with tranquility, cheerfulness, spirituality, and other positive emotions. Impaired brain functioning may lead to hyperactivity, mania, pessimism, and other negative emotions.

High-quality foods that nourish the brain and help develop positive emotions include whole grains, particularly maize; beans and bean products; leafy green vegetables; sea vegetables; fruit, seeds, and nuts; and good-quality oil, sea salt, and other seasonings.

Foods that harm the brain and contribute to negative emotions include meat, poultry, eggs, dairy food, and strong fish and seafood; white flour; sugar, chocolate, and other highly refined sweets; chemicalized and artificial foods; too many raw foods; too many stimulants and other beverages; alcohol; and other extremely contractive or expansive items.

In relationships it is important to communicate calmly and clearly and not become agitated, controlling, or withdrawn. For those who are not able to make themselves understood, mental and emotional disturbances may follow, including the suppression of thoughts and emotions. A thoughtful, optimistic, and amusing or lightly humorous approach often works best.

On a planetary scale, the brain and central nervous system correlate with the Earth's natural electromagnetic field. Brain disorders correlate globally with artificial electromagnetic radiation from cellular networks, fiber optics, satellites, power lines, and other communications and energy systems.

OTHER CONSIDERATIONS

Good exercise is always helpful, but do not exercise to the point of exhaustion. Deep-breathing exercises, massage, and tai chi–type movements are generally preferable to strenuous activities. Walking is excellent.

Maintaining clean, fresh air inside the home is important, and for this purpose green plants can be placed in each room. Indoor air circulation can also be maintained by frequently opening the windows.

Avoid frequent exposure to artificial radiation, including medical and dental X-rays, smoke detectors, television, and video terminals, which often emit radiation toward the face or head.

Brain tumors and cancer can be accelerated if the intestinal functions are stagnated, for example, from constipation or menstrual difficulties. Accordingly, keeping the bowels smooth and the menstrual function regular are very helpful and can also help relieve pressure and pain in the head regions. An enema for inducing elimination may be needed as well as a massage or ginger compress applied on the abdomen. Douching to eliminate stagnated fat and mucus in the uterine region may also be necessary.

Avoid wearing shoes or socks while indoors. Walk barefoot or on the grass or soil outside when possible to stimulate the flow of electromagnetic energy from the earth to the nervous system.

Avoid clothing that is synthetic, especially underwear, stockings, socks, hats, and scarves. Wigs and hairpieces should also be avoided. Synthetic rugs, curtains, furniture, blankets, and other home furnishings should gradually be replaced with more natural materials.

Long hot baths or showers should be avoided in order to prevent depletion of minerals from the body. Limit bathing to a few times a week.

Brain and nervous disorders are often accompanied by excitability, hypersensitivity, despondency, or lowered will to live. Short but regular periods of meditation—including visualization, prayer, chanting, yoga, or other exercises—can help calm the mind and center the thoughts.

Mental nourishment is as important to self-development as physical sustenance. Avoid loud and frenzied music, chaotic art, brutal and violent films, and depressing magazines and literature. Within moderation, select strong, meaningful mental outlets. Reading, music, and arts that help create a positive attitude should be selected.

PERSONAL EXPERIENCE

BRAIN TUMOR

In August 1986, Mona Sanders had just turned thirty-seven and was enjoying life. However, after a grand mal seizure that sent her sprawling onto a tennis court, hospital tests and two surgeries showed that she had an anaplastic astrocytoma, grade 3. The brain tumor, the size of a small grapefruit, was fast growing and, according to physicians, inoperable.

The diagnosis devastated Mona, and she began to experience nausea, vomiting, and numbness in her right leg. "I had always enjoyed life, living by my own decisions—until now," she recalled. "The doctors' prognosis rang through my mind: It was bad. It would never go away. Chemo might be able to slow its growth. It was close to a motor area, and I would eventually lose control. A wheelchair was in the future. Six to eighteen months to live."

An aunt from New Orleans recommended macrobiotics, and Mona began reading *Recovery* by Elaine Nussbaum (see her personal account in Chapter 19). Mona reasoned that if Elaine, also a housewife, could heal herself, she could, too, even though she lived in a small town in northeast Mississippi where no one had ever heard of macrobiotics.

Checking with the American Cancer Society hotline to see if there was anything else she could do, Mona was told, "Nothing. Good luck." The line went dead. "We'll see about that!" Mona said to herself.

Several days later, in January 1987, Mona went to Boston to begin macrobiotics. Although she was on many pills and her thinking was cloudy, she videotaped the seminar and reviewed the tapes when she returned home. In February, Mona returned to Boston and came to see me for personal guidance and instruction.

With the help of several macrobiotic cooks, Mona began to experience the benefits of the diet. In addition, she used imaging and visualization to help shrink the tumor, imagining it decreasing in size from the size of a grapefruit to a golf ball, to a pinhead, and then to nothing.

Medical tests confirmed the steady remission of her malignancy, and a CT scan in April, just four months after she started macrobiotics, showed no evidence of cancer. Since then, she has remained cancer-free.

"Today, with God's help and the love and support of my husband, children, family, and friends, I am alive with the chance to work, play, and love," Mona reports. "I want to share my experiences with others to spare them the anguish I went through and to offer a practical alternative to degenerative disease."[4]

Breast Cancer

FREQUENCY

Breast cancer is the most common form of cancer in American women, and its incidence is on the rise (see Table 22). Between 1935 and 1965 the rate of new cases of breast cancer increased 18 percent, and between 1965 and 1975 it increased 50 percent. Since 1980, the breast cancer incidence has risen about 3 percent a year, now affecting one in every eight women in the United States. Over the last several years the incidence among postmenopausal women has decreased about 4 percent annually since the medical profession reversed course and discouraged the use of hormone replacement therapy (HRT).

Twenty-six percent of new cancer cases in women involve the breast. After lung cancer, it is the second most deadly malignancy. Breast cancer currently accounts for about 15 percent of female cancer deaths in this country and is the leading cause of cancer death for American women aged forty to forty-five. This year an estimated 178,480 new cases of invasive breast cancer will develop, and 62,030 new cases of in situ breast cancer will occur. An estimated 40,910 people in this country will die from the disease. Around the world, where it is the fifth leading lethal malignancy (after lung, stomach, liver, and colon cancer), the death rate from breast cancer differs widely. In Britain it is about one-third higher than in the United States, while in Japan it is 80 percent lower. A majority of patients with breast cancer develop

TABLE 22. BREAST CANCER INCIDENCE

1940: 1 in 20 American women
1950: 1 in 15
1960: 1 in 14
1970: 1 in 13
1980: 1 in 11
1987: 1 in 10
1991: 1 in 9
2000: 1 in 8

metastases. Malignant tumors may spread to the lungs, bone, brain, or lymph nodes. Breast cancer may also occur in men, but it is rare (only 1 percent the rate of women). Some medical studies have found an elevated risk among men working in police departments, the military, or other professions exposed to radar, microwave radiation, or other artificial electromagnetic fields.

Risk factors for breast cancer include aging, a personal or family history of breast cancer, high breast tissue density, inherited genetic mutations in the BRCA1 and 2 genes (affecting about one in three hundred women), hyperplasia, and high-dose radiation to the chest from medical procedures. Reproductive factors that elevate risk include beginning menstruation at an early age and ending later in life, never having children, recent use of oral contraceptives, and giving birth to a first child after age thirty. Overweight or obesity after menopause, the use of hormone replacement therapy, physical inactivity, and consumption of one or more alcoholic beverages daily are modifiable lifestyle factors that enhance risk of this disease. Environmental risks include exposure to pesticides, PCBs, and other toxins.

A balanced diet, breastfeeding, moderate or vigorous physical activity, and maintaining a healthy body weight are associated with a lower risk of breast cancer. Stress management, a support network, positive self-image, and other lifestyle modifications are also beneficial.

After decades of increasing breast cancer mortality, there has been a slight decrease since the 1990s. This appears to be the result of healthier eating, earlier detection, and better medical treatment.

Surgery is the most common method of treating breast cancer. The operation is called a mastectomy and includes several types of incisions, depending on the development of the tumor and the age and condition of the patient. A lumpectomy excises the cancerous lump and a small amount of surrounding tissue. A subcutaneous mastectomy removes internal breast tissue, leaving the skin intact. A simple mastectomy removes the breast. A modified mastectomy removes the breast and lymph nodes in the armpit. A Halsted radical mastectomy removes the entire breast plus the lymph nodes and the pectoral muscles of the chest wall. In addition to these operations, the adrenal glands, pituitary gland, or ovaries are sometimes removed in order to regulate secretions and try to reduce tumor growth.

Radiation may be employed as an alternative or supplement to surgery. Chemotherapy is sometimes used to control metastases and to stop recurrence of the original tumor. Hormone therapy may be employed as an adjunct or alternative to chemotherapy: estrogens, antiestrogens, progestins, androgens, or adrenocortical steroids are given to control tumor growth and mestastases. For certain types of breast cancer, the drug tamoxifen has reduced recurrence and mortality, but it also increases the risk of endometrial cancer, pulmonary emboli, and deep-vein thrombosis.

Survival rates have increased in recent years. The five-year survival rate for localized breast cancer (which has not spread to lymph nodes or other locations outside the breast) is 98 percent; for regional spread, 83 percent; and for distant spread (metastases) 26 percent.

STRUCTURE

The female breasts or mammary glands consist chiefly of a round, compressed mass of glandular tissue known as the corpus mammae. This tissue is made up of fifteen to twenty separate lobes connected by fat. Each lobe contains a milk duct, which leads to the nipple and is further subdivided into lobules and alveoli. The breast is encased in a layer of fat tissue called the adipose capsule and is attached to the chest wall by connective tissue.

CAUSE OF CANCER

If we continue to eat poorly over a long period of time, we eventually exhaust the body's ability to discharge excess wastes and toxins. This can be serious if an underlying layer of fat has developed under the skin, which prevents discharge toward the surface of the body. Repeated overconsumption of milk, cheese, and other dairy products, eggs, meat, poultry, and other fatty, oily, or greasy foods brings about this stage. When it has been reached, internal deposits of mucus or fat begin to form, initially in areas with some direct access to the outside such as the sinuses, the inner ear, the lungs, the kidneys, the reproductive organs, and the breasts.

The accumulation of excess in the breast often results in a hardening of the breasts and the formation of cysts. Excess usually accumulates here in the form of mucus and deposits of fatty acid, both of which take the form of a sticky or heavy liquid. These deposits develop into cysts in the same way that water solidifies into ice, and the process is accelerated by the intake of ice cream, milk, soft drinks, fruit juice, and other foods that produce a cooling or freezing effect.

Women who have breast-fed are less likely to develop breast cysts or tumors. Women who do not nurse their children miss this opportunity to discharge through the breasts and therefore face a greater possibility of accumulating excess in this region of their bodies.

Many nutritionists and doctors are now aware of the relationship between the intake of saturated fats, cholesterol, and degenerative disease but often overlook the effects of sugar and dairy products, both of which contribute greatly to heart disease, cancer, and other illnesses. (See Chapter 27 on pancreatic cancer for a discussion of sugar metabolism and the role of refined sugars in tumor formation, including breast cancer.)

The consumption of milk and other dairy foods in our society usually begins in infancy or early childhood. One of the major biological changes in modern times has been the progressive decline of breast-feeding. In traditional cultures, mothers usually nurse their babies for one year or more. At the beginning of the twentieth century, about 60 percent of the babies in the United States were breast-fed. By the 1970s that number had fallen sharply. Since then, breast-feeding has experienced a rejuvenation, with 70 percent of new mothers in this country nursing their babies in the hospital, 36 percent for six months, and 17 percent for twelve months. The goal of the U.S. Centers for Disease Control (CDC) is to increase these numbers by 2010 to 75 percent, 50 percent, and 25 percent, respectively.

In composition, cow's milk and human milk are very different. Cow's milk contains about four times as much calcium, three times as much protein, and two-thirds as much carbohydrate as human milk. The different structure and growth rate of calves and human babies account for the varying proportion of these ingredients. For example, at birth the brain and nervous system of the calf is fully developed, and the large amount of calcium and protein is needed to increase its bone structure and muscular development. A baby calf often puts on 75 pounds in the first six weeks. In contrast, the body of the human infant is designed to grow slowly, gaining only 2 to 3 pounds in the first six weeks. The infant's brain, however, is only 23 percent mature at birth, and the nutrients in mother's milk are needed to complete its central nervous system.

In addition, mother's milk contains antibodies that resist the growth of undesirable bacteria and viruses, provide immunity against disease and infection (especially against rickettsia, salmonella, polio, influenza, strep, and staph), promote strong white blood cells, which destroy harmful bacteria, and produce *B. bifidum,* a unique type of healthy bacteria found in the intestines of babies that creates resistance to a large variety of microorganisms.

Another ingredient in milk is lactose, a simple sugar that is digested by lactase, an enzyme produced in the intestine. In most traditional societies, lactase is no longer produced after the baby is weaned from its mother's milk between ages two and four. As a result, ingestion of dairy products after that age produces indigestion, diarrhea, cramps, allergy, or other illnesses. This condition is called lactose intolerance.

In the West, however, dairy products have become a dietary staple over the course of many generations. Biologically, lactase continues to be produced in the intestine after early childhood, allowing dairy foods to be consumed into adulthood and later life. Among Caucasians, lactose intolerance is low. Only 2 percent of Danes, 7 percent of Swiss, and 8 percent of white Americans cannot digest milk and other dairy products. In contrast, about 70 percent of black Americans are lactose intolerant, as well as 90 percent of Bantus, 85 percent of Japanese, 80 percent of Inuit, 78 percent of Arabs, and 58 percent of Israeli Jews.

Despite the body's ability to adapt to long-term dairy consumption, the excessive intake of fat and cholesterol in milk, cheese, butter, ice cream, and similar foods has taken a heavy toll as the consumption of these foods has increased. Overall, however, dairy consumption is down as a result of medical research linking milk, cream, butter, and other dairy products with certain cancers, heart disease, and other chronic disorders. As the new century began, the per capita intake of dairy food in the United States stood at 593 pounds a year, including 22.6 gallons of milk. This is down from 703 pounds per person in the 1950s, including 36 gallons of milk (mostly whole in contrast to today's milk which is primarily lower in fat). In the United States there is now one cow for every three people, down from one for every two a half century ago.

In composition, milk is 28 percent fat, cheese is 50 percent, butter is 95 percent, and yogurt is 15 percent. Fatty acids and cholesterol from these foods can build up around the organs and tissues, contributing to heart disease, cancer, and other degenerative conditions. Mentally and psychologically, dairy foods affect the brain and nervous system, contributing to dullness, passivity, and dependence. Studies show that people from ethnic groups who are lactose intolerant tend to have higher IQs than those who are not. The fat from cow's milk also insulates and impedes the flow of electromagnetic energy through the body, diminishing sexual polarity and attraction between men and women.

The quality of milk and dairy food consumed today has also changed from the past. The milk itself has changed from its natural state through modern heating procedures, homogenization, sterilization, and the addition of other ingredients such as vitamin D. In an effort to make them produce greater quantities of milk, modern dairy cows are fed a variety of hormones, antibodies, and other chemicals that further dilute the quality of the milk. Today, 75 percent of all U.S. dairy cows are artificially inseminated, and through superovulation and embryo transfer a cow can now theoretically give birth to a dozen calves a year instead of only one.

As a result, the dairy products available today are different from those consumed by previous generations. Until modern times, most cultures limited their dairy products to fermented foods such as yogurt, kefir, or other foods containing enzymes and bacteria, allowing them to be broken down in the digestive process in the absence of lactase. Cultured products such as yogurt are superior to other dairy foods. However, they still cannot be recommended for regular consumption because they are now not traditionally and naturally processed and cannot be properly assimilated by people with sedentary lifestyles. A fermented vegetable food such as miso, tempeh, natto, or shoyu is preferable if processed naturally and is an important part of a cancer prevention diet.

In the past, animal milk (especially goat, sheep, or donkey milk) was used for infants whose mothers could not breast-feed, for certain medicinal purposes, or in small quantities with other dairy products for personal enjoyment on special occasions. The abuse of dairy food in the modern diet and its degenerating artificial quality are major factors in the rise of breast cancer, heart disease, and other serious illnesses. The quality of our food determines the quality of our blood. The quality of blood, in turn, determines the quality of mother's milk and the biological strength of the next generation.

Genetically modified (GM) foods also pose a serious health problem, especially milk made with bovine growth hormone (BGH). Today, an estimated 30 percent of the cows in the United States are in herds injected with BGH, a GM growth hormone that increases yields. In medical studies, BGH has been linked with increased mastitis and other diseases in dairy cows and in breast cancer in humans. The European Union, Canada, and much of the rest of the world have banned the use of BGH. However, it is still legal in the United States. Responding to consumer concerns, major dairies across the country, as well as natural foods stores, have started eliminating BGH milk from their shelves or introduced non-BGH product lines.

GM enzymes are also used in cheese production, and Consumers Union reports that 60 percent of all hard cheese products on American shelves are made with an engineered form of rennet. Feed given to dairy cows (and other livestock) also commonly include GM ingredients, so it must be assumed that all non-organic dairy products, even those labeled BGH-free, include GMOs (genetically modified organisms).

Processed foods containing GM dairy ingredients may include whipped cream, cottage cheese, milk shakes, cocoa, candies, cookies, bread, cake mixes, sauces and dressings, canned soups, etc.

GUIDELINES FOR SOY FOODS

With the decline of dairy consumption, many individuals, families, schools, and communities have transitioned or switched to soy foods, especially soy milk, tofu, soy burgers, soy hot dogs, and analogues of other animal food products. Soybeans and soy foods have traditionally been eaten in Asia for thousands of years and contributed to a healthy, happy way of life. Many modern medical studies have found that soy products help protect against breast cancer, other malignancies, and other chronic conditions and disorders.

However, modern soy foods are significantly different in quality from traditionally produced or homemade soy foods. Please review the following guidelines for the use of soy products. These suggestions are for everyone in good health as well as those with a serious condition such as breast cancer.

1. Always buy or use organically grown soybeans or certified 100 percent organic soy products. Today, 75 percent of the soybeans grown in the United States (and to a lesser extent in other countries) are made with genetically modified soybeans. These are potentially harmful and should be strictly avoided. Unfortunately, some organically grown soybeans and soy foods have been contaminated by GM soy growing nearby. This is a major problem in the American natural foods industry, and some companies (such as Eden, a macrobiotic company based in Michigan) have their own in-house GM testing laboratory and go the extra mile to ensure that their products are GM-free.

2. On a regular basis (daily or several times a week), eat primarily traditionally made soy products. These include miso, tofu, shoyu (soy sauce), and tempeh. As much as possible, prepare or purchase the basic, plain varieties. Those that include herbs, spices, oils, and other special ingredients may be used from time to time but not for daily or occasional use.

3. On an occasional or infrequent basis, kinako (toasted soybean flour), tamari (a thick sauce and by-product of the miso-making process), yuba (soybean curd skins often used in Chinese restaurants to simulate animal food), and other traditional soy foods may also be eaten in small amounts.

4. Avoid or limit modern, highly processed soy foods (whether or not organic), including textured vegetable protein made from soy, soy powders (such as genistein), soy ice cream, soy hot dogs, and other similar products. These products are not traditionally made or consumed and may have negative side effects.

5. Soy milk has become increasingly popular as an alternative to dairy milk. Traditionally made soy milk, especially the kind you make at home as part of the tofu-making process, is fine and may be consumed occasionally. However, nearly all the commercial soy milk on the market, including organic soy milk, sugar-free soy milk, and other relatively high-quality soy milks, are generally highly processed. They may be used infrequently for enjoyment (such as putting soy milk on cereal or porridge now and then). But they are unsuitable for

daily use, especially by children. The beans used to produce commercial soy milk are not always cooked thoroughly; excessive kombu (a strong yang sea vegetable) are often added to balance their high-pressure, high-speed processing; and excessive oil or other ingredients may also be added. As a rule, treat soy milk as a party food for pleasure on special occasions but not for regular use. Breast cancer patients are strongly advised to avoid soy milk entirely until their condition improves. The same advice applies to commercialized rice milk, oat milk, and similar beverages, although grain-based drinks appear to have slightly less negative effects than 100 percent soy.

6.   Observe the same approach when considering the use of other modern soy foods such as soy ice creams, soy yogurt, soy puddings, etc. These are party foods, not for regular or even occasional use (two to three times a week). In selecting these items, avoid those with processed sugar or too much oil, salt, or other ingredients. Traditionally in the Far East, soy (which is yin) was not combined with sweets (also yin). Today's soy snacks and desserts (such as tofu cheese cake and tiramisu) are very delicious and satisfying, but their energy as a rule is not balanced. They are extremely yin. They should be used very sparingly for holidays, special occasions, etc.

7.   Soybean oil is a monsaturated plant oil and healthier than saturated oils such as palm and coconut. However, for regular daily cooking, sesame or other polyunsaturated oil is recommended. Chinese restaurants frequently use soybean oil, and that is suitable now and then when eating out. But be mindful and limit its use at home as much as possible.

MEDICAL EVIDENCE

•   In an address before the Belgium Cancer Congress in 1923, Frederick L. Hoffman, cancer statistician for the Prudential Life Insurance Company, reported that cancer was unknown among the Indians of Bolivia and Peru. "I was unable to see a single case of malignant disease. All the physicians whom I interviewed on the subject were emphatically of the opinion that cancer of the breast among Indian women was never met with. Similar investigations of mine among the Navajo and Zuni Indians of Arizona and New Mexico have yielded identical results." Hoffman associated the rise of cancer in industrial society with overnutrition and the introduction of refined and artificial foods.[1]

- In 1942, Albert Tannenbaum, M.D., cancer researcher at Michael Reese Hospital in Chicago, reported that mice on a caloric-restricted diet had substantially fewer induced breast tumors, lung tumors, and sarcoma than mice on an unrestricted diet.[2]
- In regions where total and long-term breast-feeding is practiced, breast cancer is rare. In 1969, Canadian medical researcher Otto Schaefer, M.D., reported that over a fifteen-year period only one case of breast cancer was observed in a group of Inuit whose population grew from nine thousand to thirteen thousand. In populations of Inuit where breast cancer was very low but on the increase, Dr. Schaefer cited a decrease in the duration of breast-feeding or its complete elimination as a contributing factor. A 1964 study of breast cancer patients at Roswell Park Institute in New York found that breast-feeding for seventeen months decreased the risk of breast cancer. Women who had lactated for a total of thirty-six months had a more reduced risk. As for possibly transmitting some cancer-causing substance through mother's milk, two other recent studies showed no difference in the breast cancer incidence in daughters who were breast-fed by mothers who later were found to have cancer.[3]
- In a 1975 case-control study of seventy-seven breast cancer cases and seven controls, five categories of foods were associated with breast cancer: fried foods, fried potatoes, hard fat used for frying, nonmilk dairy products, and white bread. The researcher also reported that Seventh-Day Adventist women age thirty-five to fifty-four have 26 percent less breast cancer than the general population, and women in the church over fifty-five have 30 percent less. The Seventh-Day Adventists, about 50 percent of whom are vegetarian, emphasize whole grains, vegetables, and fruit in their diet, and avoid meat, poultry, fish, coffee, tea, alcohol, spices, and refined foods.[4]
- A 1976 study of the relationship of diet and breast cancer in forty-one countries found that a high intake of refined sugar was associated with increased incidence of the disease.[5]
- Women following a macrobiotic diet are less likely to develop breast cancer, researchers at New England Medical Center in Boston reported in 1981. The scientists found that macrobiotic women process estrogen differently from other women and eliminate it more quickly from their body. The study involved forty-five pre- and postmenopausal women, about half of whom were macrobiotic and half nonvegetarian. The women consumed about the same number of total calories. Although the macrobiotic women took in only one-third as much animal protein and animal fat, they excreted two to three times as much estrogen. High levels of estrogen have been associated with the development of breast cancer. "The difference in estrogen

metabolism may explain the lower incidence of breast cancer in vegetarian [macrobiotic] women," the study concluded.[6]

- A fifty-year study of diet and breast cancer mortality in England and
  Wales between 1928 and 1977 showed that at the onset of World War
  II breast cancer mortality markedly fell as consumption of sugar,
  meat, and fat declined and consumption of grains and vegetables increased. By 1954 consumption of these foodstuffs returned to prewar levels. Breast cancer mortality did not return to prewar levels
  until some fifteen years later, suggesting a lag time between the ingestion and appearance of the disease.[7]

- In a 1984 experiment at Harvard School of Public Health, laboratory
  animals fed a control diet with 5 percent *Laminaria* (kombu), a
  brown sea vegetable, developed induced mammary cancer later
  than animals not fed seaweed. "Seaweed has shown consistent anti-
  tumor activity in several in vivo animal tests," the researcher concluded. "In extrapolating these results to the Japanese population,
  seaweed may be an important factor in explaining the low rates of
  certain cancers in Japan. Breast cancer shows a threefold-lower rate
  among premenopausal Japanese women and a ninefold-lower rate
  among post-menopausal women in Japan than reported for women
  in the United States. Since low levels of exposure to some toxic substances have been shown to be carcinogenic, it may be that low levels of daily intake of food with anti-tumor properties may reduce
  cancer incidence."[8]

- In Japan a 1987 experiment consisting of tests on six groups of female rats showed that adding sea vegetables to the diet had a significant inhibitory effect on induced mammary tumorigenesis.
  "Tumor incidences were 35 percent (7/20), 35 percent (7/20), and 50
  percent (9/18), respectively [for groups fed nori, kombu, and another
  type of kombu], whereas that in the control group was 69 percent
  (20/29)," investigators reported. The onset of tumors was also delayed in the seaweed groups, and the weight of tumors was lower.[9]

- Whole grains, cereals, and other foods high in fiber may help protect
  against breast cancer. In laboratory tests, scientists at the American
  Health Foundation found in 1991 that a high-fiber diet reduced induced cancer in rats by about 50 percent. "We found that by doubling the amount of fiber in a diet that is similar to our Western diet,
  you can significantly reduce the amount of mammary cancer," concluded researcher Leonard Cohen.[10]

- In 1993 scientists reported that diets rich in soy foods, especially
  miso soup, produced genistein, a natural substance that blocked the
  growth of new blood vessels that feed a tumor. Researchers from
  Children's University Hospital in Heidelberg, Germany, reported that

genistein also deterred cancer cells from multiplying and could have significant implications for the prevention and treatment of solid malignancies, including those of the brain, breast, and prostate.[11]

- Women in Japan who frequently eat miso are less likely to develop breast cancer, according to a new ten-year study of twenty-one thousand middle-aged women. Among the 179 women who developed breast cancer, those who reported eating miso soup and other foods high in isoflavones, a compound in soy that appears to protect against tumor development, were less likely to be diagnosed with the disease. Interestingly, the highest rate of breast cancer among women who ate the least miso was still lower than that in similarly aged women in Western countries.[12]

- More than 200 chemicals in common consumer products and the atmosphere cause breast cancer in animal tests, according to an American Cancer Society study. American women are exposed to 97 of the 216 chemicals that cause tumors in animals, including industrial solvents, pesticides, dyes, gasoline and diesel exhaust compounds, cosmetic ingredients, hormones, pharmaceuticals, radiation, and a chemical in chlorinated drinking water. "These compounds are widely detected in human tissues and in environments such as homes where women spend time," the study found. "Almost all of the chemicals were mutagenic, and most caused tumors in multiple organs and species." Only 1,000 of the 80,000 chemicals registered in the U.S. have been subject to animal tests.[13]

DIAGNOSIS

A majority of breast lumps are discovered by palpation by the woman or her partner. Although 80 percent of lumps are classified as benign, doctors like to take a soft-tissue X-ray (called a mammogram) of the entire breast. If a malignancy is suspected, a biopsy will be taken to determine whether the growth is a cyst or a tumor. Hormone tests, X-rays of the chest and skeleton, bone marrow aspiration, and scans of gallium, liver, and bone will generally follow. Until the mid-1970s mammography was widely offered as a preventive measure to detect cancer in the early stages. In 1976, however, Dr. John Bailar III, editor of the *Journal of the National Cancer Institute,* reported that the radiation of breast X-rays could cause as many deaths as could be saved through early detection. Since then, the radiation dosage for mammography has sharply declined in many cases. The American Cancer Society currently recommends monthly breast self-examination by women twenty years or older, a screening mammogram by age forty, an annual or biennial mammogram from forty to forty-nine, and an annual mammogram after fifty.

In addition, a physical examination by a doctor is recommended every three years for women age twenty to forty and annually over forty. The mammography controversy flared up again in 1993 when the National Cancer Institute reported that a comprehensive review of data showed that there was no benefit from the procedure for women under fifty and that mammograms failed to detect up to 40 percent of tumors.

In addition to self-examination of the breasts, Oriental medicine looks for signs of developing mammary disorders in the condition and complexion of the cheeks. As a result of parallel embryonic development, the cheeks reflect underlying changes in the chest region, including the lungs and breasts, and in the reproductive region.

Cheeks with well-developed, firm flesh and a clean, clear skin color show sound respiratory and digestive functions, especially if there are no wrinkles or pimples in the area. Red or pink cheeks, except during vigorous exercise or when out in cold weather, show abnormal expansion of the blood capillaries caused by heart and circulatory disorders due to the overconsumption of yin foods and drinks, including fruits, juices, sugar, and drugs. Milky white cheeks are caused by the overconsumption of dairy products such as milk, cheese, cream, and yogurt. A pinkish shade mixed with the white indicates excessive intake of flour products and fruits. Both these colors indicate accumulation of fat and mucus in various regions of the body, including the breasts, lungs, intestines, and reproductive organs.

Fatty spots that are dark, red, or white in color on the cheeks are a sign of fat accumulation in either the lungs or breast and often accompany the beginning of cyst or tumor formation. Coffee and other stimulants such as aromatic beverages may contribute to the appearance of this color on the cheeks. Pimples on the cheeks show the elimination of excessive fat and mucus caused by the intake of animal food, dairy products, and oils and fats. If these pimples are whitish in color, the main cause is milk and sugar. If yellowish, the cause is cheese, poultry, and eggs. A green shade on the cheeks shows that cancer is developing in the breasts, lungs, or large intestine.

Certain colors and marks appearing on the white of the eye also indicate abnormal conditions in the corresponding areas of the body. In the case of the breasts, a transparent or pale white color in the upper outer region of the eye shows the presence of stagnated fat and mucus, which may be growing into a cyst or tumor. Cataracts also may indicate cyst formation. If these colorings or swellings occur in the right eye, the right breast is affected; if in the left eye, the left breast.

Green vessels appearing along the Heart Governor meridian or Lung meridian from the wrist toward the elbow on the inner, softer side of the arm also show the development of cancerous conditions in the breast or lung region. A similar condition is indicated by the appearance of green and dark colors, together with irregular swelling on the inside of the wrist.

In general, tumors in the left breast are caused by predominantly extreme yin factors such as chocolate, sugar, and other sweets and light dairy food such as milk, yogurt, and ice cream. Too much oil and dressings, fruit, potatoes, french fries, hot spices, and sticky, creamy foods may also give rise to malignancies in this area. Tumors in the right breast may also involve some of these factors but are generally caused by proportionately more extreme yang foods, including meat, chicken, tuna, salmon, or other strong red fish, hard cheese, and too much baked goods, including pastries sweetened with sugar and combinations of other flour products and sweets. Too much baked and grilled food and too much salt and salty food may also be main causes.

Tumors on the lower part of the breast tend to be caused by extreme yang, including eggs, cheese, or a combination of the two such as pizza and omelets. Tumors in the upper region of the breast tend to be more yin in origin. Those on the inside are usually more yang, and those toward the outside are more yin.

DIETARY RECOMMENDATIONS

The primary cause of most cases of breast cancer is the longtime consumption of dairy food, including milk, cheese, cottage cheese, yogurt, butter, and ice cream, along with excessive consumption of chicken, eggs, meat, and other fatty animal foods, as well as sweets, sugar, chocolate, honey, and other sweeteners and sugar-treated foods and beverages. All these foods are to be strictly avoided. Tropical fruits, fruit juices (both tropical and temperate-climate), and vegetables of tropical origin such as potatoes, yams, sweet potatoes, asparagus, tomatoes, and eggplant also should not be consumed. Oily and fatty foods should be discontinued, including french fries, salad dressings, and chips; and white flour in the form of white bread, pastries, and other flour products. Because they are excessively mucus-producing, all hard-baked flour products are to be avoided except for the occasional consumption of nonyeasted unleavened whole wheat or rye bread if craved. Chemicalized and artificially produced and treated foods and beverages are to be completely eliminated. Even unsaturated vegetable oil is to be completely avoided or minimized in cooking for a one- or two-month period. All ice-cold foods and drinks should be avoided. Although they are not the cause of breast cancer, all stimulants, spices, coffee, wine and other alcoholic drinks, and aromatic, fragrant beverages and drugs should be avoided because they enhance tumor development. Commercial soy milk, rice milk, and other dairy substitutes are too highly processed and should also be avoided. Birth-control pills, legal and recreational drugs, medications and chemically grown, processed, and treated foods, especially genetically modified foods, may also be contributing factors. Electric or microwave cooking will also further its spread.

There are two main types of breast cancer: (1) the soft type that results from extreme yin substances and influences as described above, and (2) the hard type that results from strong yin foods in combination with strong yang foods, including meat, eggs, poultry, hard cheese, and too many hard-baked flour products and too much salt. The first group includes inflammatory breast cancer that appears as a red inflammation on the surface of the breast and spreads quickly. This form of breast tumor is caused predominantly by extreme yin foods, including excessive oil (both in cooking and salads), sugar, chocolate, and other sweets, dairy food, fruit, stimulants, etc. The following general dietary guidelines are recommended for breast cancer:

- Whole Grains: Forty to 50 percent of daily consumption, by volume, should be whole cereal grains. The first day prepare plain short- or medium-grain brown rice, pressure-cooked or cooked in a heavy cast-iron or ceramic pot with a heavy lid. Then the next day prepare brown rice with 20 to 30 percent millet, then rice with 20 to 30 percent barley, then rice with 20 to 30 percent aduki beans or lentils, and then plain brown rice again. A delicious morning porridge can be made by taking leftover rice, adding a little more water to soften, seasoning with a little miso, and then simmering for two to three minutes more. Except for morning porridge, which may be soft, the grain should be on the firm side rather than creamy. In pressure cooking, the ratio of grain to water should be about 1:2. For seasoning, cook with a postage-stamp-sized piece of kombu instead of salt, although in some cases sea salt may be used depending on the person's condition. Other grains can be used occasionally, including whole wheat berries, rye, corn, and whole oats, although oats should be avoided for the first month. Buckwheat and seitan should be minimized. Good-quality sourdough bread (preferably steamed) may be enjoyed two to three times a week if craved, and noodles, both udon and soba, may also be eaten two to three times a week. Avoid all hard-baked products until the condition improves, including cookies, cake, pie, crackers, muffins, and the like.
- Soup: Five to 10 percent of daily consumption should be soup, consisting of one or two cups or bowls per day cooked with wakame sea vegetable and various land vegetables such as onions and carrots and seasoned with miso or shoyu. Occasionally a small amount of shiitake mushrooms may be added to the soup. The miso may be barley miso, brown rice miso, or soybean (hatcho) miso, and should be naturally aged for two to three years. For breast cancer, millet soup with sweet vegetables such as squash, cabbage, onions, and carrots may be prepared often. Grain soups, bean soups, and other soups may be eaten from time to time, but avoid pureeing soups with oats. For breast can-

cer the consistency of soups and food in general should be neither too creamy nor too salty. If the soup is too salty, a breast lump can remain tight and not heal. Generally, prepare miso soup just once a day and occasionally twice depending on the condition.

- Vegetables: Twenty to 30 percent of daily consumption should be vegetables, cooked in a variety of forms. Root vegetables such as burdock, carrots, and daikon should be used regularly. Round vegetables such as cabbage, onions, and fall-season squash and pumpkin and hard or leafy vegetables such as watercress, broccoli, and dandelion are also recommended and can be prepared separately or together. As a rule of thumb, the following dishes may be prepared, although the frequency may differ from person to person: nishime-style vegetables, three times a week; a squash-aduki-kombu dish three times a week; dried daikon, one cup, three times a week; carrots and carrot tops or daikon and daikon tops, three times a week; blanched vegetables, five to seven times a week; pressed salads, several times a week; raw salad and salad dressing, avoid temporarily; steamed greens, five to seven times a week; sautéed vegetables, two to three times a week, using water instead of oil the first month, and then occasionally a small amount of sesame oil may be brushed on the skillet; kinpira, sautéed in two-thirds of a cup of water two times a week, and then oil may be used after three weeks; dried tofu, tofu, tempeh, or seitan with vegetables, two times a week.

- Beans: Five percent of daily consumption should be small beans such as aduki beans, lentils, chickpeas, or black soybeans, cooked together with sea vegetables such as kombu or with onions and carrots. Other beans may be used two to three times a month. For seasoning, a small amount of unrefined sea salt or shoyu or miso can be used. Bean products such as tempeh, natto, and dried or cooked tofu may be used occasionally but in a moderate amount. Avoid making the tofu too creamy, and use firm rather than soft or silky tofu.

- Sea Vegetables: Five percent or less of sea vegetable dishes, including wakame and kombu, should be included daily when cooking grain, in soup, etc. A sheet of toasted nori may also be taken daily. A small dish of hijiki or arame should be prepared two times a week. All other sea vegetables are optional.

- Condiments: These should be available on the table: gomashio (sesame salt), on the average made with one part salt to eighteen parts sesame seeds (reduced to 1:16 after two months); kelp or wakame powder; umeboshi plum; and tekka, although all other regular macrobiotic condiments may be used if desired. These condiments may be used daily on grains and vegetables, but the amounts should be moderate to suit individual appetite and taste.

- Pickles: Made at home in a variety of ways, pickles are to be eaten daily, one tablespoon in all, although salty pickles are to be minimized.
- Animal Food: Fish and other animal food are to be avoided. However, in the event that animal food is craved, a small amount of white-meat fish may be eaten once every two weeks. The fish should be steamed, boiled, or poached and garnished with grated daikon or ginger. After two months, fish may be eaten once a week. Strictly avoid blue-meat and red-meat fish (especially tuna) and all shellfish.
- Fruit: Avoid all tropical fruits. The less temperate-climate fruit the better until the condition improves. If cravings develop, a small amount of cooked fruit (such as organic apples) with a pinch of sea salt or dried fruit (also preferably cooked) may be eaten. Avoid all fruit juices and cider temporarily, as well as raisins, currants, and other highly concentrated fruits.
- Sweets and Snacks: Limit sweets and desserts, including good-quality macrobiotic desserts, until the condition improves. To satisfy a sweet tooth use sweet vegetables every day in cooking, drink sweet vegetable drinks (see special drinks on page 231), sweet vegetable jam, and amasake (one or two small cups a week). Mochi, rice balls, vegetable sushi, and other grain-based snacks may be eaten frequently. Limit rice cakes, popcorn, and other dry or baked snacks, because they may harden the tumor. In the event of cravings, a small amount of barley malt or rice syrup may be eaten.
- Nuts and Seeds: Nuts and nut butters are to be avoided due to their high fat and protein, except for chestnuts. Unsalted blanched seeds such as sunflower seeds and pumpkin seeds may be consumed as a snack, up to one cup altogether per week.
- Seasonings: Unrefined sea salt, shoyu, and miso are to be used moderately in order to avoid unnecessary thirst. Avoid mirin and garlic. If you become particularly thirsty after a meal or between meals, you should cut back on these seasonings until the normal level of thirst returns.
- Beverages: Drinks and other dietary practices can follow the general recommendations in Part I, including bancha twig tea as the main drink with the meal. Strictly avoid the beverages on the "infrequent" and "avoid" lists, and don't take grain coffee for the first two to three months after starting this new way of eating.

In the event of hunger pains, which women sometimes get with this condition, one or two balls of brown rice with half a umeboshi plum put inside and wrapped with toasted nori may be eaten. However, less overall eating may be beneficial. In some cases, skipping breakfast for a day or on the weekend is very beneficial for breast cancer and many other conditions.

The most important thing in connection with dietary practice is chewing very well, until all food becomes liquid in the mouth and is well mixed with saliva. Chew very well, at least fifty times and preferably one hundred times, per mouthful. It is also important to avoid overeating and eating within three hours of sleeping.

As noted in the introduction to Part II, persons who have received or who are currently undergoing medical treatment may need to make further dietary modifications.

SPECIAL DRINKS AND DISHES

One or more special drinks or side dishes may need to be taken, depending on the individual case. Please see a qualified macrobiotic teacher for guidance. Too many special drinks or dishes and in very large amounts may be counterproductive. Amounts and frequencies given here are averages for each drink or dish; these will differ from person to person. Further directions are in Chapter 36.

- Sweet Vegetable Drink: Take one small cup every day for the first month, then every other day the second month, and then several times a week after that as desired.
- Dried Daikon, Shiitake and Cabbage Tea: Drink one cup every morning and every evening for three weeks; then reduce it to two to three times a week and continue for another month.
- Ume-Sho-Kuzu: Take every three days for one month or occasionally in the event of constipation, tiredness, or fatigue.
- Kinpira Soup: Take two to three times a week for strength and vitality.
- Grated Carrot and Daikon: Eat this preparation every other day for two weeks to help eliminate old fat and oil; and after that, twice a week for another month. You may also add a small amount of water and simmer for two to three minutes.

HOME CARE

- Body Scrub: Scrubbing the whole body, including the abdominal region and the spinal region, with a towel that has been immersed in hot water and squeezed out is very helpful for better circulation of blood, lymph, and other body fluids, as well as for activating physical and mental energies.
- Compress Guidelines: For a small number of breast tumors, a compress may be needed to gradually help draw the excess mucus and

fat from the inner parts of the mammary tissues toward the surface of the skin. Eventually, the fatty mucus, sticky substances, and unclean blood that make up the tumor will dissolve and discharge through the skin or urine and bowel. Please see a qualified macrobiotic teacher for guidance on the proper use and frequency of a compress or plaster. Several types are used depending on the person's condition. Precede the compress or plaster with the application over the affected area of a towel that has been soaked in hot water and squeezed out for three to five minutes to stimulate circulation. Using too many compresses or the wrong ones can be detrimental, so experienced guidance is necessary.

- Hato Mugi and Cabbage Plaster: In some cases this plaster can be applied externally to help facilitate the discharge of toxic matter. Spread the mixture about 1-inch thick on a cotton cloth. Apply the mixture directly on the breast and tie with a cotton strip or bolt of cheesecloth. Leave the plaster on for four hours or more. Repeat once or twice every day. The plaster may be left on overnight.
- Kombu-Cabbage Plaster: This may be applied after surgery to prevent a lump of fat that sometimes appears from growing on the scar. Leave on for about four hours or overnight.
- Cabbage Leaf Compress and Cabbage and Carrot Juice: If you have the lymph nodes removed from the armpit, the arm sometimes swells. In this case, wrap the arm in the cabbage leaf compress and drink the cabbage and carrot juice. This will clear up many cases, but if the swelling persists, please seek medical attention.
- Buckwheat Plaster: In cases where a breast has already been surgically removed and the surrounding lymph nodes, neck, and in some cases the arm have become swollen, a buckwheat plaster can be applied separately following a two- to three-minute application of a ginger compress.
- Medical Attention: In the event the lymph glands under the armpit and along the arm become swollen due to the cancer spreading from the breast through the lymph system, medical attention is often necessary. Again, a qualified macrobiotic teacher, nutritionist, or medical associate or professional should be consulted. Massage is often helpful in reducing such swelling.

EMOTIONAL CONSIDERATIONS

As a symbol of the Earth, the breast is associated with nurture, comfort, and abundance. Breast problems are often accompanied by sadness, loneliness, and feelings of rejection.

High-quality foods that nourish the breast and help develop positive emotions include naturally sweet things such as whole grains, particularly millet and sweet rice; sweet, round vegetables, including cabbage, squash, and onions; tofu, yuba, and other soft, naturally processed soy foods; natural sweeteners, including amasake, rice syrup, barley malt, and honey (in tiny amounts); and round orange or yellow fruits such as peaches, nectarines, and apricots.

Foods that block the breast and contribute to suppressing positive emotions include too much dairy food, especially cheese; meat, poultry, eggs, strong fish and seafood, and other animal products; white flour; sugar, chocolate, and other highly processed sweets; chemicalized and artificial foods; and other extremely contractive or expansive foods and beverages.

In relationships it is important to communicate freely and honestly and not suppress feelings and emotions. If the woman doesn't feel loved and appreciated, she can develop breast problems or be attracted to comfort foods that create blockages in this region.

Breast cancer patients are subject to depression and should do everything possible to maintain a cheerful and calm attitude. Smile, be optimistic, dance, sing, pray, say affirmations, do spiritual practices, and enjoy each day for itself.

On a planetary scale, the breast correlates with rolling hills and valleys, the proverbial land of milk and honey. In today's modern world, breast cancer often mirrors on a small scale toxic waste and deposits in the earth on a large scale.

OTHER CONSIDERATIONS

- In addition to the daily body scrub, soaking the feet at night in hot water, or occasionally in hot gingerroot water, will help bring down the energy of the body and help eliminate excess through the skin.
- Avoid wearing wool and synthetic fibers. At the minimum, wear cotton underwear and use cotton sheets and pillowcases.
- Avoid wearing metallic jewelry, including rings, bracelets, and necklaces. These pick up excess charges from the atmosphere and transmit them to the internal organs via the meridians running along the fingers and hands. It is fine, though, to wear a wedding ring.
- Avoid watching television for long stretches. Radiation weakens the chest area. Similarly, avoid other artificial sources of electromagnetic energy such as video terminals, smoke detectors, and handheld electrical appliances.
- If possible, avoid birth-control pills and estrogen additive therapy. These are extremely weakening and can accelerate breast cancer. Doctors will sometimes recommend estrogen drugs because in medical tests it has been shown that older women taking estrogen get

less heart disease and more women in old age die from heart disease than breast cancer. From an energetic view, most heart disease results from the intake of overly yang foods such as meat, poultry, and eggs, so estrogen, which is classified as extremely yin, will help reduce the risk of heart attack and stroke. However, it contributes to increased risk of breast cancer, which is caused by too much yin. Women who adopt a macrobiotic way of eating commonly experience a rapid improvement in blood values, including reduced cholesterol levels. There is therefore no need to take estrogen to protect against heart ailments if you are eating predominantly grains and vegetables.

- Breast-feed your baby if you are able. There is no danger of transmitting breast cancer to your child, and breast-feeding will have a protective effect on both mother and baby.
- Men who work with radar, cell phones, fiber-optic networks, microwave energy, telephone lines, and other electronic equipment are at high risk for developing breast cancer. Avoidance of artificial electromagnetic energy of all kinds, especially electric-range and microwaved food, is recommended.

PERSONAL EXPERIENCE

METASTATIC BREAST CANCER

In October 1972, Phyllis W. Crabtree, a fifty-year-old homemaker, nursery school teacher, and grandmother from Philadelphia, had an operation for cancer in which her uterus, ovaries, and fallopian tubes were removed. By January 1973 the tumor metastasized, and she had a modified radical mastectomy of the right breast.

In the hospital her son, Philip, who had studied macrobiotic cooking, brought her miso soup, brown rice, and bancha tea. The first food offered to Phyllis by the hospital had been a bowl of Froot Loops.

Breast surgery was a very frightening experience for her. "One of the most terrifying is the signing of that paper which gives a doctor the right to cut out or off any part that he deems necessary," she observed afterward. "By the time I was admitted for the mastectomy, it was my fourth admission in ten weeks, my fourth signing, and this time I knew what they were going to take. For each operation, there was an initial trip for biopsy, an okay from the frozen section, and then a return trip for surgery when more lab work had been completed. Another very simple hospital procedure that was sheer horror for me was the presurgical shave and shower. Watching the surgical nurse shaving my chest from armpit to armpit and washing my breasts for what might have been the last time was a very emotional procedure. Before the biopsy, as I washed (and the tears flowed almost as fast as the shower), I wondered if I would have none, one, or two the next day." Mrs. Crabtree was so distraught from the experience that she had to see a psychiatrist afterward to help her deal with her loss.

Over the next three years she gradually began to implement macrobiotics with the support of her son, daughter, and husband. She cut out sugar from her diet, increased vegetables, and reduced her intake of red meat, dairy food, and martinis. In the summer of 1976, however, the newspapers and television were filled with stories about a connection between cancer and contraceptives and hormone medication. Mrs. Crabtree, who had taken these drugs, became depressed again and suspected that cancer was spreading to her liver.

Once again her son impressed upon her the need to follow the diet closely and to take full responsibility for her condition and recovery. In March 1977 she attended the EWF cancer and diet conference in Boston and came to see me. "I listened and had an appointment with Michio Kushi," she recalled later. "One phrase from the classroom kept haunting me: 'There are no cancer victims, only cancer producers.' Michio recommended a healing diet and sent me off to eat far more strictly than ever before."

The next summer Mrs. Crabtree returned, and I told her that she was 60 percent healed and to continue eating carefully. By the autumn of 1978, Phyllis had completed the five-year "cure" period for her original illness and outlived 85 percent of women who had had similar operations on the uterus and breast.

"I'm grateful to macrobiotics for more than a cancer 'cure,'" she stated. "For myself, there had been an improvement in my aching back (caused by osteoporosis) and a urinary infection (both ailments of thirty years' duration). The migraine headaches are fewer in number and less in intensity and duration. Even my motion sickness has lessened.

"My husband has benefited from the diet through weight control. Michio's lectures in Los Angeles many years ago were instrumental in returning Phil to us from his 'hippy' world. My daughter adopted a baby girl because she had been unable to conceive. She now has three daughters, two of them 'macrobiotically brewed.'"[14]

BREAST CANCER

In February 1986, Anne Kramer was diagnosed with breast cancer and underwent a modified radical mastectomy of her left breast. Doctors found metastatic carcinoma in four lymph nodes, plus microscopic tumor emboli in small auxiliary blood vessels. "My oncologist recommended chemotherapy for a year, possibly longer," Anne recalls. "A second opinion from another oncologist was the same—a year or more of chemotherapy. He suggested that I probably had several thousand cancer cells floating around in my bloodstream. It wasn't a happy picture." Meanwhile, a routine hospital blood test revealed her cholesterol level to be 243.

While recovering from the mastectomy, Anne started to read about scientific research relating diets high in fat content to breast cancer. One study reported that Japanese women eating traditionally had a much lower incidence of breast cancer and a lower recurrence rate compared to Western women eating standard American high-fat foods. Anne decided she wanted to try a low-fat dietary approach but was too weak from chemotherapy to begin. After three months of treatment, including tamoxifen, she learned about macrobiotics from a friend and began to read *The Cancer Prevention Diet.* "I read the book and immediately started cooking meals recommended for my illness," Anne explains. "I knew this macrobiotic diet was what I was looking for. I believed it would help me heal myself of breast cancer. My feelings of helplessness went away. I became more optimistic about the outcome of my disease."

At first it was not easy to shop and prepare the new foods, especially since Anne had almost no energy and felt sick and nauseated most of the time. She attributed this to the chemotherapy treatments. "At least I didn't have to worry about getting hair in the food," she [says, looking] back. "I didn't have any left on my head! I believed in this new diet and followed the directions strictly. Aveline Kushi's peaceful recipes made me feel calm and in charge of my getting well." Anne also performed visualization exercises three times a day.

After two months on the diet, Anne went in for another mammogram on her right breast. She was anxious because her doctor had warned her of the possibility of new tumors where calcification spots had been found. "The mammograms revealed that the calcification spots were gone! I was elated."

In September 1986, Anne decided to stop chemotherapy despite the opposition of her oncologist. "My mind rebelled at the thought of another six months of that poison," she observes. "On several occasions the doctor couldn't perform chemotherapy treatments on me because my white blood cell count was dangerously low. I promised my body I would not undergo any further chemotherapy treatments."

Later that fall Anne met Bonnie Breidenbach, a macrobiotic teacher in the Detroit area who helped her fine-tune her diet. Bonnie also told her about a doctor who had a therapy group for cancer patients. She attended the group sessions for a while and found sharing her feelings and experiences on the diet very encouraging and supportive.

It is now almost seven years later, and Anne is healthy. Repeated mammograms, bone scans, chest X-rays, and blood tests have shown no trace of cancer. Anne is in her early sixties, her cholesterol reading is 170, and she has enrolled in the Kushi Institute Extension Program in Cleveland to learn more about macrobiotics. "I enjoy the program, and I'm enjoying life. I am grateful that my husband is supportive and went on the diet with me from the start. I am also grateful that my child, grandchildren, and eighty-nine-year-old mother are benefiting from this diet as well. I am also thankful to God for giving me illness and health to help me appreciate life."[15]

BREAST CANCER

In 2000, Faye Baxter was diagnosed with breast cancer. Her physicians told her there would be a six-week wait until surgeons could remove the tumor, and then she would have to go on chemotherapy and radiation. During that time Faye, who lived in Great Britain, sought out a macrobiotic counselor and changed her diet. Daphne Watson, who had healed herself of multiple sclerosis on a macrobiotic diet and went on to become a teacher and counselor, met with Faye and gave her dietary and lifestyle guidance. She was encouraged to eat whole grains, miso soup, vegetables, and sea vegetables, and completely avoid sugar, dairy, alcohol, and convenience foods. Regular exercise was also recommended to boost her immunity to disease and detoxify her body.

Within a few weeks Faye began to feel the positive benefits of a change in her way of life. Her pain subsided, she could sleep better, and her lifelong asthma disappeared. She ultimately decided not to have surgery and has continued to remain in good health for the last two and a half years.[16]

BREAST CANCER

When she was forty, Meg Wolff discovered a lump in her right breast, which was later diagnosed as invasive lobular and ductal carcinoma stage 3B. She had already had bone cancer seven years earlier and lost her left leg as a result. She had a mastectomy and was thinking of having the other breast removed, but a specialist told her that a tumor would probably occur within a year. She tried tamoxifen but discontinued it because of side effects.

A naturopathic doctor recommended macrobiotics and Meg found a cook in Maine, where she lived, and started taking classes over the next year and a half. While studying, she met several women who had recovered from breast cancer with diet and eventually Meg went to see Warren Kramer, a counselor in Boston.

"Many things started to improve in my life, including my health," she recalls. "I began sleeping through the night—a problem I had been having for five years. I had also been taking medication for a heart arrhythmia which I eventually weaned myself off with the okay of my doctor. I lost weight, my skin got very clear, and the sinus problem and headaches I had lived with for years finally cleared up." Her thinking became sharper and her memory improved. The ulcerative colitis she had suffered from for four years cleared up.

Meg went on to become a macrobiotic teacher and counselor herself. She started an online resource center to assist others: macrobreast cancersurvivors.com, wrote up her inspiring story in *Becoming Whole: My Complete Recovery from Breast Cancer,* and now lectures to women's groups, health associations, and military centers across the country.[17]

BREAST CANCER

Gayle Stolove discovered a prominent lump, in the upper and outer portion of her left breast, two years before she actually had it diagnosed. The thirty-nine-year-old Floridian discovered it while taking a shower and knew what it was. "I knew I had been living wrong, yet I wanted so desperately for it to not be cancer that I denied, and edged my way around it, for two years, and did not change my lifestyle at all," she recalls.

Finally, in July 1996, when she just couldn't face herself in a mirror anymore, partly because the skin around the "lump" was beginning to pucker and wrinkle, she went to see a surgeon, hoping that she could just have the "lump" removed, and "go on with my life as it was, unchanged by the event."

The surgeon instantly announced that she had "very advanced breast cancer" and recommended immediate bilateral mastectomy. He did this without even a biopsy, although she did have one eventually to confirm the diagnosis.

Gayle felt that a bilateral mastectomy was rather extreme. Two people had come into her life at varying times years earlier, both of whom had healed themselves from cancer through macrobiotics. On the day of her cancer diagnosis, she made a commitment to herself that she would, from that day forward, become macrobiotic.

Referred to macrobiotic counselor Lino Stanchich, Gayle was "fascinated, confused, overwhelmed, yet hopeful as I began the most wonderful journey, way beyond anything I could imagine."

With her counselor's careful guidance, and during nine months of chemotherapy and six weeks of radiation, she began to embrace not only the macrobiotic diet, but also the macrobiotic way of life. As she changed her diet to whole and natural macrobiotic foods, Gayle's whole life changed. Her mind became clearer, her body began to heal, and everyone said she looked "great."

Given six months to a year to live, Gayle has now remained cancer-free for the last twelve years. She is a registered nurse, licensed massage therapist, natural foods chef, and macrobiotic teacher and counselor. She lives in Fort Lauderdale, Florida, and spends her time helping others follow the macrobiotic way.[18] Her Web site is whollymacrobiotics.com.

17

Children's Cancer

FREQUENCY

Cancer is the second leading cause of death in this country of children between the ages of one and fourteen. (Death by accident is number one.) This year an estimated 10,400 American children will be diagnosed with cancer and another 1,545 will die, about a third of them from leukemia. Childhood leukemia in the United States climbed in the 1970s and 1980s but has leveled off and started to drop slightly since then. Other common sites include the bone, bone marrow, lymph nodes, kidneys, and soft tissues. Boys have higher death rates than girls, adolescents more than children, and whites and blacks more than Asians/Pacific Islanders. Hispanics had higher rates than non-Hispanics. Survival rates have steadily increased for medical treatment in recent years, rising from 58 percent at all sites to 79 percent from 1975 to 2002.

The principal malignancies are: (1) acute lymphocytic leukemia (ALL), the most prevalent cancer among children, characterized by diminished granulocytes, the white blood cells that resist infection; (2) osteogenic sarcoma and Ewing's sarcoma, bone cancers; (3) neuroblastoma, which can appear anywhere but mostly appears in the abdomen, where swelling results; (4) rhabdomyosarcoma, the most common soft-tissue sarcoma, which can occur in the head, neck, genito-urinary tract, trunk, or extremities; (5) brain cancers, characterized in the early stages by headaches, blurred or double vision, dizziness, difficulty in walking or handling objects, and nausea; (6) lymphomas and

Hodgkin's disease, which involves the swelling of lymph nodes in the neck, armpit, or groin, general weakness and fever, and other possible symptoms; (7) retinoblastoma, an eye cancer that affects children under the age of four; and (8) Wilms' tumor, a kidney cancer that appears as a swelling or lump in the abdomen.

Medical treatment usually involves radiation or chemotherapy and has greatly improved over the last thirty years. Overall five-year survival has climbed from less than 50 percent in the 1970s to almost 80 percent today.

CAUSE OF CANCER

During the embryonic period, energy and nutrients that support the formation of the body, the mind, and associated functions are supplied through the placenta and the embryonic cord. During pregnancy, from the time of conception to the time of birth, the human embryo increases in weight approximately 3 billion times. The food we eat as human beings recapitulates the entire course of biological evolution.

In the womb we eat the essence of animal food in mother's blood. Until about one year of age we eat the more diluted essence of animal food in mother's milk. After that, whole grains, which coevolved with human beings in the most recent 25-million-year period, become our principal food, initially in soft, easily digestible form. If we don't eat grains during the entire course of our life, we begin to lose our unique human status. Grains are customarily cooked with a pinch of salt or seaweed and eaten with salt- or mineral-rich soup or broth, representing the primordial ocean in which life began and the slightly saline quality of our blood. Plant foods—the major supplement to grains—include ancient and modern vegetables and beans, representing the continuing course of biological evolution on land. Since grains and beans are already fruits, consumption of tree and ground fruits (which coevolved with and gave rise to monkeys and apes), as well as nuts and seeds, is not essential for our development, but these foods may be eaten in moderation for enjoyment and variety.

Animal foods, which share a similar quality with human beings, should generally be avoided or limited; if consumed, they should be eaten in the forms further away from us on the spiral of evolution. Fish and seafood, representing more primitive forms of animal life, are more suitable than birds and mammals. Daily food is the essence of biological life, and the kind, amount, frequency, and way of preparing the food that we eat largely shape and determine our human destiny on this planet.

If a mother's eating habits are imbalanced and her diet consists largely of acid-producing foods—including excessive consumption of animal protein and fat, dairy foods, simple sugars, fruits and fruit juices, soft drinks, chemicalized food and beverages, and others—a baby developed in her womb may be born with deformities, congenital heart disease, or a tendency toward natural immune deficiency that could lead to cancer, AIDS, or other serious disorders. This orientation may manifest during childhood, especially if improper foods continue to be consumed after birth throughout the growing period.

The modern way of life tends to produce a child that is weaker physically and mentally than children in the past. Children today tend to be larger and heavier than necessary. Physical and mental response tends to be duller. On the average, a smaller, thinner, and shorter child is stronger than a larger, fatter, and taller one. Compared with children from a few generations ago, modern children are weaker in their physical and mental resistance, endurance, and response in general. This means that modern newborns are also weaker in natural immunity than in the past.

Because increasing numbers of newborns are physically larger and heavier and many mothers have weak contracting power during delivery, cesarean surgery has tripled in modern society, accounting for about one in every four births. In addition, the use of forceps, drugs, and other emergency measures to assist in delivery has become more widespread. If the newborn does not experience passing through the natural birth canal with strong repeated contractions, the child tends to be weaker in physical endurance and resistance in general.

At the same time, nursing is often intentionally stopped, and artificially produced formula is substituted for mother's milk. During the first few days after delivery, the mother's breast secretes a yellow fluid called colostrum, which has ample immune factors. Throughout the next period of breast-feeding, as regular mother's milk is produced, the newborn continues to receive essential natural immune factors. These include antibodies that resist the growth of undesirable viruses and bacteria, provide immunity against infectious disease (especially against rickettsia, salmonella, polio, influenza, strep, and staph), promote strong white blood cells, and produce B. bifidum, a unique type of healthy bacteria found in the intestines of babies that creates resistance to a large variety of microorganisms. These immune factors decrease as time passes. It is more difficult for the newborn to develop natural immunity, including a strong blood and lymphatic system, if it has not been breast-fed.

The rise of childhood cancer and other degenerative and immune diseases began in the 1950s. At that time dietary habits began to change dramatically when a high-protein, high-fat diet became standardized in the United States and most of the industrialized world. Chemical agriculture replaced organic farming, and grain and flour products were increasingly refined. Commercially prepared fast foods replaced home cooking, and modern advertising elevated sensory appeal and satisfaction, along with packaging, especially through the new medium of television, which was often directed at children. In the 1960s and early 1970s, fast foods, including hamburgers, french fries, pizza, and fried chicken, became popular, further weakening the younger generation. Then in the 1980s and early 1990s, microwave cooking, food irradiation, and other highly artificial methods of preparing and preserving foods became widespread, and finally in 2000, we have genetically engineered food—all contributing to further decline. This vast fundamental change in the modern way of eating naturally altered the biological, mental, and spiritual status of human beings, contributing to degenerative disease. The lack of whole grains and natural minerals in fresh vegetables and sea vegetables has particularly contributed to the decline.

In addition, the last half-century has seen an abuse of medication and pills, the overuse of antibiotics and medical treatment, the rise of recreational drugs, exposure to X-rays and other potentially harmful medical and dental procedures, exposure to electrical generators, television, computers, cell phones, and other appliances and devices that emit artificial electromagnetic energy, and environmental pollution. Out of a misunderstanding of the nature and function of the human body, millions of children (and adults) have had their tonsils removed. The tonsils are one of several important immune glands that serve to cleanse toxins, excess mucus, and other substances from the lymph system. Chronic swelling and inflammation show that they are doing their job of localizing and neutralizing dietary excess. The way to relieve tonsillitis is not to take out the tonsils, but to stop the intake of improper foods and drinks that are overburdening the lymphatic system. If the tonsils are removed, diseases can spread more rapidly.

Together these factors have resulted in the biological decline of modern children. In extreme cases this can result in childhood cancer, especially leukemia, lymphoma, cancer on the surface or in the front of the brain, bone cancer, and central nervous system cancer, which are all classified as more yin.

From the macrobiotic view, the primary dietary causes of childhood malignancies are: (1) dairy food of all kinds, including whole milk, low-fat or skim milk (high in protein), yogurt, butter, cheese, and ice cream; (2) sugar, sweets, chocolate, honey, carob, and foods and candy containing these simple sugars; (3) soft drinks, cold drinks, and drinks served with ice cubes; (4) white flour, white bread, and other refined flour products, including pizza, crackers, muffins, cookies, cakes, and pies; (4) excessive oily and fatty foods of all kinds, including animal and vegetable, including meat, poultry, eggs, salad dressings, mayonnaise, and others; (5) tropical fruits and vegetables, including bananas, mangoes, pineapple, tomatoes, potatoes, eggplant, and others; (6) too much soymilk and other highly processed soy products; (7) too much chemically grown food and foods containing artificial additives, preservatives, and GMOs; (8) too many canned, frozen, precooked, and other prepared foods; and (9) food that is cooked on an electric range or microwave oven, which gives a chaotic energy and vibration.

MEDICAL EVIDENCE

In an analysis of seventeen pesticides, toxins, and other chemical substances in the breast milk of vegetarian and nonvegetarian mothers, scientists found that except for PCBs (which were about equal), "the highest vegetarian value was lower than the lowest value obtained in the [nonvegetarian] sample. . . . [T]he mean vegetarian levels were only one or two percent as high as the average levels in the United States."[1]

DIAGNOSIS

Civilized life as a whole is making people more yin. They are more passive and sedentary. Their thinking is more yin. They are dropping out from disciplines at all levels—family life, schools, religions, work. Today people don't want to do hard work or help others. Parents don't want to make the effort to bring up children, so they take birth-control pills (yin) and have abortions (which is also weakening and makes the woman very yin).

Children today are weaker, more yin, than children used to be. This is shown not just by declining SAT test scores over the last generation, but by physiological signs. These include smaller ears and ears lacking in detached earlobes, weaker bones and teeth, and bodies that are taller and heavier. Children today are becoming lazier. They can't tolerate cold weather, hardships, or difficulties as their grandparents used to. Many lack self-discipline due to a lack of good-quality yang in their diet: whole grains, vegetables, good-quality salt, and mineral-rich seaweed.

While everyone's condition is unique, those susceptible to cancer in childhood often share some of the following characteristics: (1) general fatigue, physically and mentally, with a tendency to become inactive and seek more comfortable situations and surroundings; (2) development of frequent colds and infections accompanied by light fever; (3) skin rashes, similar to allergic reactions; (4) intestinal disorders including gas, constipation, and frequent diarrhea; (5) feeling of nausea; (6) irregular appetite, fluctuating from insatiable to almost no appetite, and frequent cravings for sweets, fruit, pastries, and similar foods; (7) hypoglycemia, including a tendency to be more depressed, irritable, and sad, particularly in the late afternoon; (8) difficulty sleeping at night; (9) peripheral parts of the body are often colder than normal; (10) susceptibility to bruises and cuts and slower than normal healing; (11) swelling of lymph glands; and (12) inability to focus or concentrate on what they are doing.

DIETARY RECOMMENDATIONS

The major cause of cancer in children, including leukemia, lymphoma, brain tumors, and kidney cancer, is the consumption of foods and beverages in the extreme yin category, including sugar, sugar-treated foods and drinks, ice cream, chocolate, carob, honey, soft drinks and soda, tropical fruits, fruit juices, oily and greasy foods, dairy foods, especially butter, milk, and cream, and many chemicals contained in foods, beverages, and supplements. All of these should be avoided in daily eating. However, the consumption of these items is often accompanied by the intake of foods from the extreme yang category, including meat, poultry, eggs, and cheese, in order to achieve a rough counterbalance. Accordingly, all these animal foods are also to be avoided, with the exception of fish and seafood, which can be consumed in small quantities after one month on a stricter diet. Although they are not the direct cause, the following enhance malignant conditions and should also be discontinued: ice-cold food and drinks; hot, stimulating, and aromatic spices; various herbs and herb drinks that have stimulant effects; and vegetables that historically originated in the tropics, including potatoes, tomatoes, and eggplant.

Compared to adults, children are smaller and more compact—more yang—and therefore require less salt, miso, shoyu, and other salty seasonings, and slightly more oil, fruit, sweets, and desserts. When cooking for a family, it is advisable to season according to the children's needs and for adults to add slightly more condiments at the table.

Here we give, first, the dietary guidelines for babies and infants, and then for children. For older children with cancer (those over fifteen), follow the guidelines under the specific cancers in this section of the book.

Guidelines for Babies and Infants

Our diet should change in accordance with the development of our teeth. The ideal food for the human infant is mother's milk, and all the baby's nourishment should come from that source for the first six months. The quantity of breast milk can gradually be decreased over the next six months while soft foods, containing practically no salt, are introduced and proportionately increased. Mother's milk should usually be stopped around the time the first molars appear (twelve to fourteen months), when the baby's diet consists entirely of soft mashed foods.

Harder foods should be introduced around the time the first molars appear and gradually increase in percentage over the next year. By the age of twenty to twenty-four months, mashed foods should be replaced entirely by harder foods, which will comprise the mainstay of the diet.

At the beginning of the third year a child can receive one-third to one-fourth the amount of salt used by an adult, depending on the child's health. A child's intake of salt should continue to be less than an adult's until about the seventh or eighth year.

At age four the standard diet may be introduced, along with mild sea salt, miso, and other seasonings, including ginger. Until this age, infants ideally should not have any animal food, including fish, except in special cases where the child is weak, slightly anemic, or lacks energy. Then give about one tablespoon of white-meat fish or seafood that has been well boiled with vegetables and mashed. At age four, if desired, a small amount of white-meat fish or seafood may be included from time to time for enjoyment. Different tastes appeal to us at different periods of our development. A natural sweet taste particularly nourishes babies and children.

The following dietary recommendations may be followed for healthy infants as well as those with serious sicknesses, including childhood leukemia, lymphoma, or brain or kidney tumors.

- Whole Grains: These can be introduced after eight months to one year as the baby's main food. The cereal should be in the form of a soft whole-grain porridge consisting of four parts brown rice (short-grain), three parts sweet brown rice, and one part barley. The porridge is preferably cooked with a piece of kombu, although this sea vegetable does not always have to be eaten. Millet and oats can be included in this cereal from time to time. However, buckwheat, wheat, and rye are usually not given.

  The porridge may be prepared by pressure-cooking or boiling. To pressure-cook, soak the cereals for two to three hours and pressure-cook with five times more water for one hour or longer, until soft and creamy in consistency. To boil, soak the cereals for two to three hours and boil with ten times more water until one-half of the original volume of water is left. Use a low flame after the rice comes to a boil. If the rice boils over, turn off the flame and start it again when the rice has stopped boiling over.

  If the cereal is introduced to a baby less than five months old, the porridge is best digested when mashed well, preferably in a suribachi or with a mortar and pestle. If the baby is less than one year old, rice syrup or barley malt may be added to maintain a sweet taste similar to mother's milk.

  The proportion of water to grains depends on the age of the baby and usually ranges from 10 to 1, to 7 to 1, to 3 to 1. Younger babies require a softer cereal and thus more water.

  The porridge can also be given to the baby as a replacement for mother's milk if the mother cannot breast-feed.

  Be careful to avoid giving babies porridge or ready-to-eat creamy grain cereals made from flour products.
- Soup: This can be introduced after five months, especially broth. The contents may include vegetables that have been well mashed until creamy in form. No salt, miso, or shoyu should be added before the baby is ten months old. Thereafter, a slightly salty taste may be used for flavoring. However, in such special cases as a baby with green

stools or a baby experiencing digestive difficulties, a salty taste may have to be used, but only in small amounts and for a short period.

- Vegetables: These can be introduced after five to seven months, usually when the teeth are coming in and grains have been given for one month. When introducing vegetables to children, start by giving sweet vegetables such as carrots, cabbage, squash, onions, daikon, and Chinese cabbage. These may be boiled or steamed and should be well cooked and thoroughly mashed. Because it is usually difficult for children to eat greens, parents should make a special effort to see that they are eaten. Sweet greens such as kale and broccoli are generally preferred over slightly bitter-tasting ones such as watercress and mustard greens. Very mild seasoning may be added to vegetables after ten months to encourage the desire to eat them.

- Beans: These can be introduced after eight months, but only small amounts of aduki beans, lentils, or chickpeas, cooked well with kombu and mashed thoroughly, are recommended. Other beans such as kidney beans, soybeans, and navy beans can also be used occasionally, provided they are well cooked until very soft and mashed thoroughly. Beans may be seasoned with a tiny amount of sea salt or shoyu, or sweetened with squash, barley malt, or rice syrup.

- Sea Vegetables: These can be introduced as a separate side dish after the child is one and one-half to two years old. It is preferable to cook grains with kombu, and vegetables and beans may also be cooked with sea vegetables even if they are not always eaten.

- Fruit: Fruit should be given to babies or infants occasionally. Temperate-climate fruit, in season, can be introduced between one and one-half and two years of age in small amounts, about one tablespoon, in cooked and mashed form. However, in some special cases, cooked apples or apple juice may be used temporarily as an adjustment for some conditions.

- Pickles: Those traditionally made quick and light in aging and seasoning can be introduced after the child is two to three years old.

- Beverages: These may include spring or well water (boiled or cooled), bancha twig tea, cereal grain tea, apple juice (warmed or hot), and amasake (which has been boiled with two times as much water and cooled).

For further information on infant and childhood nutrition or health, please refer to my book *Macrobiotic Pregnancy and Care of the Newborn* (New York and Tokyo: Japan Publications, 1984) or contact a qualified macrobiotic teacher or medical professional.

Guidelines for Younger Children

Whole Grains: Forty to 50 percent of daily consumption, by volume, should be whole cereal grains. The first day, prepare plain short- or medium-grain brown rice, pressure-cooked or cooked in a heavy cast-iron or ceramic pot with a heavy lid. On the following days prepare brown rice cooked with 20 to 30 percent millet, then rice with 20 to 30 percent barley, then rice with 20 to 30 percent aduki beans or lentils, and then plain rice again. A delicious morning porridge can be made by taking leftover rice, adding a little more water to soften it, seasoning it with a little miso, and simmering for two to three minutes more. In ordinary cooking the ratio of grain to water should be about 1:2. For seasoning, cook with a postage-stamp-sized piece of kombu instead of salt, although in some cases sea salt may be used, depending on the child's condition. Other grains can be used occasionally, including whole wheat berries, rye, corn, and whole oats, although oats should be avoided for the first month. Buckwheat and seitan should be minimized, since they are usually too energizing for children. Good-quality sourdough bread may be enjoyed two to three times a week, and noodles, both udon and soba, may also be eaten two to three times a week. Avoid all hard-baked products until the condition improves, including cookies, cake, pie, crackers, muffins, and the like.

- Soup: Five to 10 percent of daily consumption should be soup, consisting of one or two cups or bowls cooked with wakame sea vegetable and various land vegetables, such as onions and carrots, and seasoned with miso or shoyu. Occasionally a small amount of shiitake mushroom may be added to the soup. The miso may be barley miso, brown rice miso, or soybean (hatcho) miso, and should be naturally aged two to three years. To satisfy a sweet tooth, millet soup with sweet vegetables such as squash, cabbage, onions, and carrots may be prepared often. Grain soups, bean soups, and other soups may be eaten from time to time.

- Vegetables: Twenty to 30 percent of daily consumption should be vegetables, cooked in a variety of forms. In general, leafy vegetables, round, hard vegetables grown near the surface of the earth, and root vegetables can be used in about equal amounts, i.e., one-third of each type daily. During cooking they can be seasoned moderately with sea salt, shoyu, or miso. After the first month, unrefined vegetable oil, especially sesame or corn oil, may be used for sautéing vegetables several times a week, although oil should not be overconsumed. As a general rule the following dishes may be prepared, although the frequency may differ from person to person: nishime-style vegetables, four times a week; a squash-aduki-kombu dish, three times a week; dried daikon, one cup, three times a week; carrots and carrot tops or daikon and daikon tops, three times a week; blanched vegetables, five to seven times a week; pressed salads, several times a week; raw salad and salad dressing, avoid; steamed greens, five to seven times a week; sautéed vegetables, two to three times a week, using a small amount of sesame oil; kinpira, two-thirds of a cup, two times a week; dried tofu, tofu, or tempeh with vegetables, two times a week. Limit seitan.

- Beans: Five percent of small beans, such as aduki beans, lentils, chick-peas, or black soybeans, may be used daily, cooked together with sea vegetables such as kombu or with onions and carrots. Other beans may be used two to three times a month. For seasoning, a small amount of unrefined sea salt or shoyu or miso can be used. Bean products, such as tempeh, natto, and dried or cooked tofu, may be used occasionally, but in moderate amounts.

- Sea Vegetables: Five percent or less sea vegetable dishes, including wakame and kombu, may be eaten daily when cooking grain, in soup, etc. A sheet of toasted nori may also be eaten daily. A small dish of hijiki or arame should be prepared two times a week. All other sea vegetables are optional. Sea vegetables can be cooked with other vegetables or sautéed with a small amount of sesame oil after softening them by soaking and boiling lightly in water.

- Condiments: Those that should be available on the table are go-mashio (sesame salt), on the average made with one part salt to eighteen parts sesame seeds (reduced to 1:16 after two months); kelp or wakame powder; umeboshi plum; and tekka, although all other regular macrobiotic condiments may be used if desired. These condiments may be used daily on grains and vegetables, but the amounts should be moderate to suit individual appetites and tastes.

- Pickles: Made at home in a variety of ways, pickles are to be eaten daily, one tablespoon in all, although salty pickles are to be minimized.

- Animal Food: Meat, poultry, eggs, and other strong animal food are to be avoided. A small amount of white-meat fish may be eaten once or twice a week. The fish should be steamed, boiled, or poached and garnished with grated daikon or ginger. After two months, fish may be eaten twice a week if desired. Strictly avoid blue-meat and red-meat fish and all shellfish.

- Fruit: The less the better, including both tropical and temperate-climate fruit, until the condition improves. If cravings develop, a moderate amount of cooked fruit with a pinch of sea salt or dried fruit (also preferably cooked) may be eaten. Juice, such as apple cider, may be used in moderation.

- Sweets and Snacks: Avoid all sweets and desserts made with sugar, chocolate, honey, carob, maple syrup, and other simple sugars. To satisfy a craving for sweets, use sweet vegetables every day in cook-ing, drink sweet vegetable drinks (see special drinks on page 250), or eat sweet vegetable jam. Mochi, rice balls, vegetable sushi, and other grain-based snacks may be eaten frequently. Limit rice cakes, popcorn, and other dry or baked snacks because they may harden the tumor. Macrobiotic desserts made with good-quality grain-based sweeteners such as amasake, barley malt, or rice syrup may be enjoyed in moderation. Avoid soy ice cream, soy yogurt, and all other highly processed modern soy foods, as well as desserts combining tofu with a sweetener such as tofu cheesecake or tiramisu.

- Nuts and Seeds: Nuts and nut butters are to be limited. Unsalted roasted seeds such as sunflower seeds and pumpkin seeds may be consumed as a snack, up to one cup total per week.
- Seasonings: Unrefined sea salt, shoyu, and miso are to be used moderately in order to avoid unnecessary thirst. Avoid mirin and garlic. If your child becomes particularly thirsty after a meal or between meals, you should cut back on these seasonings until the normal level of thirst returns.
- Beverages: Good spring or well water of natural quality may be used as a daily beverage. Bancha tea may also be drunk frequently. Strictly avoid commercial soy milk, rice milk, oat milk, and other highly processed beverages. Avoid grain coffee for two to three months, and limit juice. Amasake and carrot juice are all right in moderation several times a week.

The most important thing in connection with dietary practice is chewing very well, until all food becomes liquid in the mouth and well mixed with saliva. Chew very well, at least fifty times and preferably one hundred times per mouthful. It is also important to avoid overeating and eating within three hours of sleeping.

As noted in the introduction to Part II, children who have received or who are currently undergoing medical treatment may need to make further dietary modifications.

SPECIAL DRINKS AND PREPARATIONS

Children with cancer may also consume some special drinks and dishes, which, taken in small amounts, can strengthen blood and lymph quality. These dishes include the following:

- Sweet Vegetable Drink: Take one small cup every day for the first month, then every third day the second month.
- Ume-Sho-Kuzu Drink: Take one small cup every two days for two weeks, then one cup a week for three to four weeks. This will help energize and restore vitality.

- Grated Daikon: Grate half of a small cup of fresh daikon and add a few drops of shoyu. Taken occasionally, two or three times a week, this will help digestion and discharge old fat and oil from the body.
- Carp and Burdock Soup (Koi Koku): Cook whole carp with shredded roots, seasoned with miso and a little grated ginger. This soup may be used as the soup dish a few times a week for a period of several weeks. It is very energizing and is to be used only medicinally. See the recipe in Part III.
- Brown Rice Cream: In the event of appetite loss, two to three bowls of genuine brown rice cream can be served daily with a condiment of either gomashio (sesame salt), umeboshi plum, or tekka. This rice cream may also be used occasionally as part of the regular whole grain diet. If the child requires a sweet taste, add sweet vegetable jam, amasake, barley malt, rice syrup, or a small amount of cooked fruits to the cereal.

HOME CARE

- Body Scrub: Scrubbing the whole body, including the abdominal region and the spinal region, with a towel that has been immersed in hot water and squeezed out is very helpful for better circulation of blood, lymph, and other body fluids, as well as for activating physical and mental energies.
- Swelling: Swelling of the spleen and abdominal regions sometimes accompanies children's cancers and is caused by overeating in general, especially protein, and excessive intake of beverages, seasonings, and condiments. In such cases, food consumption should be simplified for several days, up to ten days. During this period, daily consumption may consist of pressure-cooked brown rice and barley, one to two cups of miso soup, a small dish of half dried daikon and half daikon leaves pickled for a long period (over two months) with sea salt and rice bran, a dish of vegetables such as onions, carrots, and cabbage sautéed in sesame oil, and several cups of bancha twig tea. However, this simplified diet should not be continued longer than ten days unless it is under the supervision of an experienced macrobiotic teacher, nutritionist, or medical associate or professional.

EMOTIONAL CONSIDERATIONS

Children require proper nourishment at every level from the nutritional to the mental, from the emotional to the spiritual. Lack of love, care, and kindness may inhibit their emotional development.

Children require a balanced diet with whole grains, beans and bean products, vegetables from land and sea, and a balance of other usual foods. They need more naturally sweet foods than adults and less salt and other contractive foods. Too much animal food, hard-baked food, and salt and salty foods can make them aggressive, angry, and unfeeling, and contribute to other negative emotions. Too much milk, ice cream, and other light dairy foods, sugar and other simple sugars, white flour and other polished grains, raw foods, and liquids can lead to apathy, lack of direction, and the inability to concentrate. Together these extremes can lead to hyperactivity, tantrums, and other emotional difficulties.

OTHER CONSIDERATIONS

- General physical exercise and deep-breathing exercises are recommended, especially outside in the fresh air. Shiatsu massage and other treatments to relax and loosen any physical and psychological stagnations and hardenings are also very helpful.
- Maintaining clean fresh air inside the home is important, and for this purpose green plants can be placed in each room. Indoor air circulation can also be maintained by frequently opening the windows.
- Wearing cotton underwear and avoiding synthetic fabrics are helpful for better skin metabolism and facilitate energy flow through the body.
- Avoid exposure to electromagnetic fields. Keep common handheld appliances, especially cell phones, to a minimum, and shield them if possible. If you have a choice, have the child live, play, and go to school in areas away from an artificial electronic environment.

18

Colon and Rectal Cancer

FREQUENCY

Cancer of the large intestine, including the colon and rectum, is the second most deadly cancer in the United States (lung cancer being number one) and the third most common cancer in men and women. It is also known as colorectal cancer, bowel cancer, and cancer of the gut. This year an estimated 52,180 people in the United States will die of this disease, and about 153,760 new cases will develop. Overall, incidence and mortality have slightly declined in the last twenty years. Rectal cancer is slightly more prevalent in men, colon cancer more frequent in women, and each type is on the increase in both sexes. Colorectal cancer primarily affects urban, affluent people and whites more than blacks, Asians, and other groups. Ninety percent of colon and rectal tumors develop from polyps, benign growths in the lining of the large intestine. About 54 percent of tumors appear in the rectum, 23 percent in the sigmoid colon, 13 percent in the ascending or right colon, 8 percent in the transverse colon, 3 percent in the descending colon, and 1 percent in the anus. Bowel cancer is much less common in the Far East. In Japan the rate is about one-fourth the American incidence.

Current medical treatment calls for surgical removal of part or all of the large intestine. After the tumor and some healthy adjacent tissue are taken out, the ends of the remaining part of the colon are sewn together. If this is not possible, a *colostomy* is performed in which an opening is made in the skin and a disposable plastic bag is worn to collect feces. Radiation and chemotherapy may be administered after surgery in an attempt to control metastases, though some medical studies have shown that these follow-up treatments are no more effective than no treatment and in some cases could contribute to death or further disability. The most common site for the spread of this disease is the liver.

Cancer of the large intestine often spreads to the lungs or liver and, in women, the ovaries. Overall, 64 percent of patients with this disease can expect to live five years or more, although only 10 percent of those with distant metastases survive that long.

Risk factors include aging (90 percent of cases are over fifty), a personal or family history of colorectal cancer and/or polyps, and a personal history of chronic inflammatory bowel disease. Other conditions and behaviors that elevate risk are obesity, physical inactivity, smoking, heavy alcohol consumption, and dietary imbalance, especially the consumption of red or processed meat and a low intake of grains, vegetables, and fruits.

STRUCTURE

The large intestine meets the small intestine at the cecum, turns upward (ascending colon), crosses the abdomen (transverse colon), winds down (descending colon), makes an S-shaped turn (sigmoid colon), and extends straight (rectum) to the anus. Altogether, the entire bowel tract is about five feet long. Like other organs, the large intestine can be classified according to its relative degree of expansion and contraction, or yin and yang. In structure, the large intestine is yin—long, soft, expanded, smooth. In contrast, its complementary opposite, the lungs, are more yang—small, firm, compact, textured.

The major functions of the large intestine are (1) to absorb water, vitamins, and minerals through its mucous-lined tissue to be sent to the liver for distribution through the body, and (2) to eliminate waste and excessive nutrients from the body, including iron, magnesium, calcium, and phosphates. The large intestine's functions are complementary to the lungs, which (1) regulate delivery of oxygen to the heart for distribution in the bloodstream, and (2) regulate elimination of carbon dioxide and other gaseous wastes from the body. Interestingly, the total number of cases of cancer of the large intestine and cancer of the lung are almost the same: 120,000 and 122,000, respectively. Without drawing too much from this correlation, this close incidence may suggest an underlying relationship between the origin and development of these two forms of cancer. Oriental medicine has traditionally treated them as a pair of organs that are antagonistic and complementary to each other.

CAUSE OF CANCER

People living in modern society suffer from a multitude of intestinal disorders. These include diarrhea, constipation, gas, enteritis, colitis, hernia, appendicitis, obesity, hemorrhoids, diverticular disease, and spastic or irritable colon. In general these conditions arise from overeating, inadequate chewing of poor-quality food, overworking, and not enough exercise. The colon becomes further abused because of irregular patterns of eating, especially snacking between meals and eating before bedtime, which put an increased burden on the inner organs.

A sedentary lifestyle, including long hours watching television or the habit of riding in cars for short distances instead of walking, is another major factor contributing to intestinal ailments. In traditional societies, where intestinal disorders and cancer of the colon are rare, people are much more orderly and active. They eat only two or three times a day, rarely eat between meals or before going to sleep, and approach their daily activity as creative participants rather than as passive spectators.

The traditional diet, which has largely protected past generations from cancer and other degenerative diseases, is high in what today we call fiber or roughage. Fiber includes the insoluble cellulose found in the cell walls of cereal grains, vegetables, and fruit; the endosperm of seeds; and the lignins or substances that constitute the woody pulp of growing plants. Whole grains, the best source of fiber, contain about four to five times as much as fruit. In the large intestine, fiber works like a sponge to absorb water, bile acids, and other waste products, giving bulk to the feces and propelling them quickly through the system. Fiber also serves to modify cholesterol metabolism, bind trace metals, and neutralize various irritants, residues, and toxins that accumulate in the intestinal lining. In addition, there are several hundred different kinds of bacteria in the colon that synthesize enzymes and vitamins, especially the B complexes. A regular diet of fibrous whole grains and vegetables is necessary for the proper functioning of these bacteria.

The consumption of meat, dairy products, and other animal foods, on the other hand, weakens the digestive tract and can lead to various colonic disorders. Unlike grains and vegetables, which do not usually putrefy before they are eaten, animal protein starts to decompose as soon as the animal is killed. This process is offset by refrigeration or the addition of preservatives in the form of spices or chemicals. But putrefaction resumes as soon as the animal protein is cooked and eaten, and by the time it reaches the colon, decay has set in. The harmful bacteria from this decay tend to accumulate in the large intestine.

In addition to the synthesizing yang group of bacteria in the colon, there is a yin group of bacteria that decomposes the remaining food particles into elementary compounds. These bacteria can break down a small amount of animal fat and protein in the colon, but the volume of these foods ingested by many people today cannot be properly metabolized. As a result, excess ammonia and bile acids begin to accumulate in the bowel tract. Along with the harmful bacteria produced by the putrefaction of animal food, these substances give rise to mutations in the lining of the large intestine, injure and kill cells, and lower the body's natural immunity to infection.

The shape, size, color, texture, and frequency of the bowel movement indicate the specific condition of the large intestine and overall health of the individual. People consuming a traditional or macrobiotic diet high in whole grains usually pass from 13 to 17 ounces of solid waste a day. Those consuming a high-fat, high-protein diet discharge only 3 to 4 ounces a day. On the whole grain diet, food takes about thirty hours to travel from the mouth through the gastrointestinal tract. On the modern diet, transit time averages two to three days and in elderly people can take up to two weeks. Nearly 100 percent of the foods in humanity's traditional diet contain fiber, and this way of eating produces a bowel movement that is large and long, light in color, soft in consistency, and floats in water. Only 11 percent of the calories from the modern diet come from foods with fiber, and the bowel movement tends to be small, compact, dark in color, hard in consistency, and sinks in water. Lack of fiber in the diet slows down the movement of feces and allows the buildup of harmful bacteria. Furthermore, the muscles of the large intestine must work harder to propel small, compact wastes. As pressure builds, small sacs appear in the lining of the colon called diverticula. These pockets, in turn, can become inflamed as harmful bacteria and waste material become trapped.

Cancer of the large intestine is generally preceded by spastic colon, colitis, or diverticulosis and the growth of polyps. Although usually classified as benign nodules by modern medicine, polyps should be viewed as a precancerous condition. Polyps, or abnormal growths in the mucosa of the colon, represent a defensive measure on the part of the large intestine to limit the passage of harmful material. When the colon can no longer protect itself with benign resistance, full-fledged obstructions in the form of cancerous tumors result. Of course, these blockages may be removed by surgery. But unless daily diet, the source of the disease, is changed, cancer will spread to other organs, and eventually the patient will die.

Nearly 75 percent of intestinal cancer in the United States occurs in the rectum and sigmoid or lower colon—the compact yang end of the gut. This suggests overconsumption of meat, eggs, salty cheeses, poultry, and other extreme yang foods as major causative factors. However, the intestines can also become loose and sluggish from an excessive intake of sugar, alcohol, refined flour, and other extreme yin substances, resulting in cancer of the ascending colon. Tumors in the transverse or descending colon result from a combination of extreme yin and yang foods and beverages.

Over the last decade there has been increased scientific interest in the relationship between diet and colon cancer. Among the major forms of cancer, colon and breast cancer are now generally associated with a high-fat, high-protein diet by epidemiologists and clinical researchers. Still, the progressive development of intestinal sickness is not widely understood. Modern medicine continues to employ a variety of laxatives, enemas, and colonics to speed up elimination, relieve constipation, and reduce pain. In the long run these medications only further expand and weaken an already overactive bowel tract. Additional complications then develop that require a still stronger application of temporary chemical antidotes. We must begin to look at the other end of the digestive system for a permanent solution to intestinal disease. A balanced diet centered around whole grains offers lasting relief from colonic ills and the promise of improved health and vitality in the future.

MEDICAL EVIDENCE

- After serving as a surgeon for the British in Africa from 1941 to 1964, Denis P. Burkitt, M.D., concluded that cancer and other degenerative diseases were rare and in some cases virtually unknown among traditional societies. Over the course of thirteen years the internationally renowned cancer specialist (after whom Burkitt's lymphoma is named) reported that in one South African hospital with two thousand beds, only six patients were observed with polyps, a condition of the colon that sometimes precedes cancer. He attributed the "replacement of carbohydrate foods such as bread and other cereals by fat (and animal fat in particular)" with the rise of cancer and other degenerative diseases during the last century. Burkitt also cited studies showing that forty to fifty years ago the incidence of colon cancer among African Americans was less than among whites but higher than among rural Africans today. In recent years, as American blacks began to eat less grains, especially cornmeal, and more fat and protein, their rate of intestinal cancer rose to that of whites.[1]

- In a 1981 study of twenty-one macrobiotic individuals, Harvard medical researchers reported that the addition of 250 grams of beef per day for four weeks to their regular diet of whole grains and vegetables raised serum cholesterol levels 19 percent. Systolic blood pressure also rose significantly. After the macrobiotic individuals returned to a low-fat diet, cholesterol and blood pressure rates returned to previous levels.[2]

- In a population-based case-control study of over four thousand people in California, Utah, and Minnesota, cancer researchers reported that high whole grain intake was associated with up to 60 percent less risk for colon cancer, while intake of refined grains increased the risk one and a half to two times. Foods high in fiber, vitamin B_6, thiamine, and niacin were also protective.[3]

- In laboratory studies, researchers at Hiroshima Prefectural Women's University reported that 180-day fermented miso significantly reduced the size and incidence of induced colon cancer in rats. Miso could "act as a chemopreventive agent for colon carcinogenesis," the researchers concluded.[4]

- In a review of prospective cohort studies and a meta-analysis, researchers at the University of Hannover in Germany reported that consumption of fruit, vegetables, and whole grains was associated with reduced risk for colon cancer, while intake of refined white flour products, sweets, milk and dairy products, eggs, and red meat enhanced the likelihood of the disease. "As primary prevention, a diet rich in vegetables, fruits, whole grain products, and legumes added by low-fat dairy products, fish, and poultry can be recommended," they concluded. "In contrast the consumption of sweets, refined white flour products, and meat products should be reduced."[5]

DIAGNOSIS

In a doctor's office or hospital, cancer of the large intestine is usually diagnosed through a rectal examination; blood, urine, and stool tests; X-rays; a proctosigmoidoscopy, in which a rigid tube is inserted through the rectum to provide a view of the lower colon; or a colonoscopy, in which the tube is inserted and air is forced in to expand the complete colon for viewing.

Traditional Oriental medicine analyzes the condition of the bowel tract with simple external means rather than complex internal ones. In facial diagnosis, the lower lip corresponds to the large intestine, and by observing its condition we can take preventive or remedial dietary action to counter intestinal disorders, including bowel cancer. A swollen lower lip signifies a swollen yin condition of the large intestine. In modern society, up to 75 percent of the population have swollen lower lips, indicating irregular bowel movements and enteritis or inflammation of the intestinal tract. Usually a swollen lower lip indicates constipation from a combination of excessive yin and yang foods. However, if the lip is wet, diarrhea is indicated. An extremely contracted yang lower lip shows overconsumption of meat and other protein. The virtual absence or receding of the lower lip shows a tendency toward cancer of the sigmoid colon or rectum.

The different colorations of the lower lip further show specific disorders. White indicates fatty mucous deposits in the colon; pale shows weak metabolism of nutrients and anemia; bright red indicates expansion and hyperactivity of the blood capillaries and tissue; yellow around the edges of the lips shows hardening of fatty deposits in the large intestine and blockages in the liver and gallbladder; blue or purple shows stagnation of feces and blood in the colon; and a green shade around the mouth probably indicates colon cancer.

These discolorations may also occur around areas along the meridian of the large intestine, especially on the area around the base of the thumb on the inside of the hand. A blue or green color in this region may indicate developing intestinal cancer. Also, the fleshy part of the outside of the hand between the thumb and index finger often takes on a green or bluish hue in the case of colon cancer. If this coloring appears on the left hand, the descending colon is affected. If it is on the right hand, the ascending colon is diseased.

The condition of the colon is also revealed on the forehead. The right part of the forehead shows the ascending colon, the upper forehead the transverse colon, and the left part the descending colon. Swellings, colorations, patches, pimples, or spots indicate where fat deposits, ulcers, or cancerous growths are developing in the colon.

General skin color also offers clues to intestinal disorders. A purplish shading indicates the consumption of extremely yin foods and beverages; a brown shade indicates excessive yang animal food and yin tropical vegetables and fruits; and yellow, white, or hard fatty skin indicates the consumption of excessive eggs, poultry, cheese, and other dairy foods. These are early warning signs of overactive intestines and general digestive troubles.

DIETARY RECOMMENDATIONS

For cancers of the large intestine—the ascending, transverse, and descending colon and the rectum—it is advisable to eliminate all animal food, including beef, pork, and other kinds of meat, chicken and eggs, and cheese and other dairy food, which are the primary cause of this type of cancer. Even fish and seafood, which may be high in fat and cholesterol, should be avoided for an initial period. Furthermore, any greasy, oily, or fatty foods and beverages are to be stopped. Sugar, sugar-treated food and beverages, refined flour, soft drinks, tropical fruits and vegetables, various nuts and nut butters, spices, stimulants, and aromatic food and drinks are also to be discontinued. Flour products, although not a main cause of this malignancy, may contribute to stagnation and blockages and make recovery more difficult and therefore should be strictly avoided—even good-quality sourdough bread—for an initial period. Dietary guidelines for daily consumption by volume are generally as follows.

- Whole Grains: Forty to 50 percent of daily consumption, by volume, should be whole cereal grains. The first day prepare plain short- or medium-grain brown rice, pressure-cooked or cooked in a heavy cast-iron or ceramic pot with a heavy lid. On subsequent days, alternate brown rice cooked with 20 to 30 percent millet, then rice with 20 to 30 percent barley, then rice with 20 to 30 percent aduki beans or lentils, and then plain rice again. A delicious morning porridge can be made by taking leftover rice, adding a little more water to soften, seasoning with a little miso, and then simmering for two to three minutes more. In ordinary cooking, the ratio of grain to water should be about 1:2. For seasoning, cook with a postage-stamp-sized piece of kombu instead of salt, although in some cases sea salt may be used depending on the person's condition. Other grains can be used occasionally, including whole wheat berries, rye, corn, and whole oats, although oats should be avoided for the first month. However, for a contracted condition such as colorectal cancer, buckwheat and seitan should be limited in use because they are very contracted relative to other grains and grain products. Flour products, even unrefined whole wheat bread, chapatis, pancakes, and cookies, should be totally avoided or limited for a few months. Whole grain pasta and noodles also should not be used more than a couple of times a week in small amounts.

- Soup: Five to 10 percent of daily consumption should be soup, consisting of one or two cups or bowls per day cooked with wakame sea vegetable and various hard green leafy vegetables such as kale or collards, seasoned lightly with miso or shoyu. Occasionally a small amount of shiitake mushrooms may be added to the soup. The miso may be barley miso, brown rice miso, or soybean (hatcho) miso, and should be naturally aged two to three years. Grain soups, bean soups, and other soups may be eaten from time to time.

- Vegetables: Twenty to 30 percent of daily consumption should be vegetables, cooked in a variety of forms, mainly steamed, boiled, and, after one month, occasionally sautéed without oil. For cancer of the ascending colon, lighter and quicker cooking, which preserves freshness and crispness, is preferred over longer cooking with a strong salty taste. Leafy vegetables are preferable to root vegetables for this cancer, although root vegetables should also be used occasionally. For cancer of the transverse colon, leafy vegetables and round vegetables such as cabbage, onions, pumpkin, and squash may be used almost equally. The cooking style should be medium, neither too short nor too long. For cancer of the descending colon and rectum, round and root vegetables should receive more emphasis than leafy vegetables, although the latter are also necessary. For any of these conditions, seasoning with unrefined sea salt, shoyu, and miso or condiments is to be moderate. After one month with limited oil, sautéed vegetables made with unrefined sesame or corn oil can also be consumed frequently.

  As a rule of thumb, the following dishes may be prepared, although the frequency may differ from person to person: nishime-style vegetables, three times a week; a squash-aduki-kombu dish, three times a week; dried daikon, one cup, three times a week; carrots and carrot tops or daikon and daikon tops, three times a week; blanched vegetables, five to seven times a week; pressed salad, several times a week; raw salad, avoid the first month, then once in ten to fourteen days; steamed greens, five to seven times a week; sautéed vegetables, once a week, and then after the first month more often; kinpira, two-thirds of a cup, two times a week; dried tofu, tofu, tempeh, or seitan with vegetables, two times a week.

- Beans: Five percent of daily consumption should be small beans, such as aduki beans, lentils, chickpeas, or black soybeans, cooked together with sea vegetables such as kombu or with onions and carrots. Other beans may be used two to three times a month. For seasoning, a small amount of unrefined sea salt or shoyu or miso can be used. Bean products such as tempeh, natto, and dried or cooked tofu may be used occasionally, but in a moderate amount.

- Sea Vegetables: Five percent or less of sea vegetable dishes, including wakame and kombu, should be included daily when cooking grain, in soup, etc. A sheet of toasted nori may also be taken daily. A small dish of hijiki or arame should be prepared two times a week. All other sea vegetables are optional.

- Condiments: Those that should be available on the table are gomashio (sesame salt), on the average made with one part salt to eighteen parts sesame seeds; kelp or wakame powder; umeboshi plum, and tekka, although all other regular macrobiotic condiments may be used if desired. These condiments may be used daily on grains and vegetables, but the amount should be moderate to suit individual appetites and tastes. As a condiment, a small amount of miso sautéed in sesame oil with the same amount of chopped scallions can be used daily on grains. One teaspoon of sautéed whole dandelions is also helpful for cancer of the large intestine.

- Pickles: Made at home in a variety of ways, pickles are to be eaten daily, one tablespoon in all, although salty pickles are to be minimized. Rice bran (nuka) pickles are the most suitable.

- Animal Food: Fish and other animal food are to be avoided. However, in the event that animal food is craved, a small amount of white-meat fish may be eaten once every ten days for the first three months, then once a week. The fish should be steamed, boiled, or poached and garnished with grated daikon or ginger. Strictly avoid blue-meat and red-meat fish and all shellfish.

- Fruit: The less the better until the condition improves. If cravings develop, a small amount of cooked fruit with a pinch of sea salt or dried fruit (also preferably cooked) may be eaten. Avoid all fruit juices and cider temporarily, as well as raisins, currants, and other highly concentrated fruits.

- Sweets and Snacks: Avoid all sweets and desserts, including good-quality macrobiotic desserts, until the condition improves. To satisfy a sweet tooth, use sweet vegetables every day in cooking, drink sweet vegetable drinks (see special drinks below), and use sweet vegetable jam and amasake. Mochi, rice balls, vegetable sushi, and other grain-based snacks may be eaten frequently. Limit rice cakes, popcorn, and other dry or baked snacks because they may harden the tumor. In the event of cravings, a small amount of barley malt or rice syrup may be eaten.
- Nuts and Seeds: Nuts and nut butters are to be avoided due to their high fat and protein, except for chestnuts. Unsalted blanched seeds such as sunflower seeds and pumpkin seeds may be consumed as a snack, up to one cup altogether per week.
- Seasonings: Unrefined sea salt, shoyu, and miso are to be used moderately in order to avoid unnecessary thirst. Avoid mirin and garlic. If you become particularly thirsty after a meal or between meals, you should cut back on these seasonings until the normal level of thirst returns.
- Beverages: Drinks and other dietary practices can follow the general recommendations in Part I, including bancha twig tea as the main drink. Strictly avoid the beverages on the "infrequent" and "avoid" lists, and don't take grain coffee for the first two to three months after starting this new way of eating.

The most important thing in connection with dietary practice is chewing very well until all food becomes liquid in the mouth and well mixed with saliva. Chew very well, at least fifty times and preferably a hundred times per mouthful. It is also important to avoid overeating and eating within three hours of sleeping.

As noted in the introduction to Part II, people who have received or who are currently undergoing medical treatment may need to make further dietary modifications.

SPECIAL DRINKS AND DISHES

One or more special drinks or side dishes may need to be taken, depending on the individual case. Please see a qualified macrobiotic teacher for guidance. Amounts and frequencies given here are averages for each drink or dish; these will differ from person to person. Further directions are in Chapter 36.

- Sweet Vegetable Drink: Take 1 small cup every day for the first month, then every other day the second month. This will reduce cravings for stronger sweets.

- Brown Rice Porridge with Grated Daikon and Umeboshi: Eat one to two bowls of this porridge every day for one week to ten days; after that, eat it two to four times a week for another three to four weeks.
- Dried Daikon, Daikon Leaves, Roasted Brown Rice and Shiitake Tea: Drink one to two cups every day for two to three weeks; after that, reduce it to three to four times a week and continue for another month.
- Pressed Salad with Daikon and Daikon Leaves and Sea Salt: This salad is beneficial for this condition. Wash the salad with water to remove excess salt before serving. Eat a small amount of this preparation with meals.
- Ume-Kuzu Drink: This drink is helpful to relieve bleeding. Drink one to two small cups every day for three days.
- Water-Sautéed Daikon and Daikon Leaves: These are also recommended. Season with a little miso or shoyu. Eat one small dish of this preparation every day.
- Grated Daikon and Potato Juice: Drink one-third of a small cup of this preparation every day. You may add a little sea salt. But be careful not to drink too much, or it can make you weak.
- Daikon, Daikon Leaves, and Quick Pickles: Wash the salad with water to remove the excess salt before serving. Eat a small amount of this preparation with your meals.

HOME CARE

- Body Scrub: Scrubbing the whole body, including the abdominal region and the spinal region, with a towel that has been immersed in hot water and squeezed out is very helpful for better circulation of blood, lymph, and other body fluids, as well as for activating physical and mental energies.
- Compress Guidelines: For a small number of colon tumors, a compress may be needed to help gradually draw out the excess mucus and fat. Please see a qualified macrobiotic teacher for guidance on the proper use and frequency of a compress or plaster. Several types are used depending on the person's condition. Precede the compress or plaster with the application of a towel that has been soaked in hot water and squeezed out over the affected area for three to five minutes to stimulate circulation.
- Potato Plaster: For intestinal and rectal tumors a potato plaster may be applied for three to four hours following administration of a ginger compress for three to five minutes. This plaster may be repeated daily for several days and then occasionally.
- Buckwheat Plaster: In the event of swelling in the abdominal region, the repeated application of a buckwheat plaster can help absorb

excessive liquid. The buckwheat plaster should be kept warm while being applied.

- Green Vegetable Plaster: In the event of pain, a ginger compress applied for three to five minutes and a plaster of mashed green leafy vegetables mixed with 20 to 30 percent white flour in order to make a paste is helpful. The ginger compress should precede the vegetable plaster. Gentle massage and acupuncture treatment may also help relieve pain and bowel tract stagnation.
- Gas Formation: To eliminate intestinal gas, all food should be chewed very well. It is also helpful to eat less, even skipping breakfast for a period of a few weeks.
- Intestinal Warmth: Avoid exposing the abdominal region to cold air or consuming cold beverages, which have a paralyzing effect on the intestines. Keeping the abdominal region warm is essential for restoring smooth digestive functions. For that purpose a small amount of scallions or garlic cooked in miso soup or in bancha tea, consumed daily or several times a week, is helpful.
- Weight Loss: People with cancer and their physicians are concerned that weight loss is not beneficial, and thus a tendency arises to overconsume, especially food rich in protein and fat. Actually, this practice serves to enhance the cancerous condition, especially in the case of the large intestine. Having an energetic and tireless condition is more of a barometer to health than maintaining previous weight.
- Rice Fasting: For a short period—seven to fourteen days—persons with large-intestine cancer may eat only brown rice served with either umeboshi plum or gomashio (sesame salt) and with toasted nori. The rice and condiments should be chewed very well. In making gomashio, the proportion of roasted sea salt to crushed sesame seeds should be from one to sixteen, to one to eighteen. Along with the brown rice, one to two cups of miso soup and one or two dishes of cooked vegetables may be consumed every day. This limited rice diet is very beneficial to cleansing and revitalizing the intestinal tract. However, it should not be continued longer than two weeks without the proper supervision of a qualified macrobiotic teacher, nutritionist, or medical associate or professional.

EMOTIONAL CONSIDERATIONS

In traditional Eastern medicine and philosophy, a healthy large intestine is associated with feelings of wholeness, happiness, and fulfillment. An unhealthy colon is associated with being scattered or rigid, being sad or melancholy, and lacking the ability to achieve or complete things. In many ways these reflect the eliminatory process. There is a direct correspondence between the bowels and our thoughts and feelings. Physical diarrhea finds a mental and psychological counterpart in verbal diarrhea, fragmented thinking, and emotional instability. Physical constipation is mirrored in a stubborn, narrow, frustrated point of view. Tumors in the colon, especially the descending colon and rectum, are very yang, so this latter tendency is pronounced.

High-quality foods that nourish the large intestine and help develop positive emotions include brown rice and other whole grains; root vegetables such as carrots, parsnips, and radishes; broccoli, cauliflower, and other more compact, condensed vegetables; and pungent foods such as ginger. Foods that block the colon and contribute to suppressing positive emotions include too much cheese and other salty or heavy dairy food; meat, poultry, eggs, strong fish and seafood, and other animal products; bread, hard-baked goods, chips, and other baked foods; grilled and roasted foods; dried and puffed foods; and other more contractive items, including too much salt and other salt-based seasonings. Foods that weaken the colon and stimulate the negative emotions associated with this organ include milk and other lighter dairy food, sugar, alcohol, too much oil, excessive spices and herbs, and other extremely expansive fare.

Overall, colonic energy is contractive, condensed, and moving downward. Hence, to help overcome an overly yang condition, activities and practices that cultivate more light, upward energy are helpful. These include singing, dancing, painting, writing poetry, listening to music, and other creative, artistic pursuits. In respect to relationships, it is important to minimize tension and conflict, to do things that are mutually enjoyable, and to get out—for example, going on a long walk, having a picnic, traveling, or taking a nice holiday. Colonic energy easily gets stuck and needs to be stimulated in order to flow freely.

On a planetary scale the large intestine correlates with the deep oceans. Ocean pollution, sludge and oil spills, dead zones, and toxic chemical dumping are all manifestations of cancer-like destruction on a global scale. Those with colon problems need to be particularly careful to avoid these influences and, if necessary, seek out healthier surroundings.

OTHER CONSIDERATIONS

- Those who suffer with intestinal cancer tend to be depressed, sad, and melancholy. It is important to keep a positive, optimistic, happy mood. Good breathing exercises are very helpful not only for lung metabolism but also for the smooth functioning of the large intestine.
- Avoid wearing wool and synthetic fibers. At the minimum, wear cotton underwear and use cotton sheets and pillowcases.

- Avoid watching television for long stretches. Radiation weakens the intestinal area. Similarly, avoid other artificial sources of electromagnetic energy such as video terminals, smoke detectors, and handheld electrical appliances.

PERSONAL EXPERIENCE

COLON CANCER

Osbon Woodford was born in Macon, Georgia, in the mid-1940s, and nearly all the food that he ate during his first twenty years growing up was homemade. However, it was laced with lard, cooked in lard, and seasoned with grease left over from bacon or fatback. Sugar, in various forms, was also plentiful. Over the next twenty years he lived primarily on fast food and highly processed foods from the supermarkets.

In April 1987, Osbon was diagnosed with colon cancer and several days later underwent surgery at Riverside Methodist Hospital in Columbus, Ohio. Doctors found metastases to eleven lymph nodes, and their prognosis was poor. His wife was told there was nothing that could be done, and he would probably live six months to a year.

Seeking alternatives, Osbon began macrobiotics, eating whole grains, vegetables, legumes, and sea vegetables daily. Along with the change in his way of eating, he reduced his stress level through meditation and self-reflection.

In February 1990, Osbon's oncologist pronounced him cured after his CEA tests repeatedly registered normal-low level and no signs of recurrence or metastasis appeared.[6] Today, more than twenty years later, Osbon remain cancer-free and is teaching macrobiotics in Cleveland, Ohio.

COLON CANCER

In 1982, Cecil Dudley experienced pain in his abdomen, and his doctor prescribed a tranquilizer for "gas." About this same time, Cecil took a course at Ohio State University titled Avoid Dying of Cancer—Now or Later. While the course was attended primarily by medical and nursing students, it was offered without charge to senior citizens. During the course Cecil, who was then seventy-five years old, learned that everyone over fifty should be tested for blood in the feces with a simple test called the hemoccult II slide method.

Cecil conducted the test at home. It proved positive, and a barium enema later revealed that he had a tumor in the colon. Following surgery, Cecil learned about macrobiotics and attended a seminar on diet and degenerative disease at the Kushi Institute, where he learned about cooking, home care, and macrobiotic principles. With the support of his wife, Margaret, he has experienced constant improvement. "I increased my amount of exercise. As a result, I experienced weight control from a lowered fat intake. My cholesterol went from 219 to 137, and I feel physically and mentally more alert and good enough to take several trips a year. My CEA levels are well within the normal range, and there is no sign of a recurrence of the cancer."[7]

COLON CANCER

See also Appendix II, "Illness in the Kushi Family."

Female Reproductive Cancers: Ovary, Uterus, Cervix, and Vagina

FREQUENCY

Cancer of the reproductive organs is the third most common form of cancer in American women (after lung and breast). This year an estimated 28,020 women will die of cancers of the ovary, uterus (endometrium), cervix, vagina, and other reproductive organs, and 78,290 new cases will develop.

Ovarian cancer, which will claim 15,280 lives this year, is rarely detected early and kills most patients in less than a year. There are many varieties of ovarian tumors, both benign and malignant, and precancerous conditions, including dermoid cysts. Standard treatment for ovarian cancer is a hysterectomy (surgical removal of the uterus) and a salpingo-oophorectomy (removal of the ovary and fallopian tubes). This operation may be done through the vagina or the abdomen, and the woman will no longer have menstrual periods or be able to conceive children. An omentectomy is also often performed as a preventive measure, and this operation involves removing a fold of abdominal membrane, which is often the site of metastases. Internal or external radiation treatment may follow surgery, and chemotherapy may be used for maintenance. The five-year survival rate for ovarian cancer is 39 percent.

Cancer of the uterus, especially the endometrium, will account for 50,230 new cases this year and 11,070 deaths. In some parts of the country its incidence jumped 25 to 30 percent. This dramatic rise, almost unparalleled in the history of cancer, has been associated with the use of the birth-control pill by women of child-bearing age and estrogen additive therapy in menopausal women over fifty. The use of tamoxifen has also caused uterine cancer rates to soar, and although legal in the United States, the World Health Organization has designated the drug (used primarily to treat breast cancer) as a carcinogen. Usual treatment for uterine cancer is a total abdominal hysterectomy. The ovaries, fallopian tubes, and pelvic lymph nodes may also be removed depending on the individual case. Radiation treatment and chemotherapy commonly follow, along with hormone therapy, especially large doses of progesterone. The remission rate is about 10 to 15 percent.

Cancer of the cervix appears primarily in women over forty. However, it is on the increase in younger women, and cervical dysplasia and sometimes herpes type 2 virus are considered precancerous conditions. Cervical cancer can spread to other reproductive sites as well as the rectum, bladder, liver, lymph, and bones. It is treated with a hysterectomy, radium implants, or experimental chemotherapy. Cervical dysplasia is often treated with cryosurgery, a procedure in which nitrous oxide or other gas is used to freeze and kill affected cells. This year about 3,670 American women will die of cervical cancer, and 11,150 new cases will develop. The five-year survival rate has improved and is now over 90 percent. In 2006 a cervical cancer vaccine was approved to protect against human papillomavirus (HPV), a virus associated with increased incidence of this malignancy. The vaccine stirred controversy because it was primarily aimed at eleven- and twelve-year-old girls (who are not sexually active) and because numerous side effects and several deaths have been reported (see Cause of Cancer on page 270).

Cancers of the vagina and vulva are rarer, accounting for about 1,670 deaths this year and 5,630 new cases. They affect women mostly over fifty but are increasingly found in younger women as well. Vaginal tumors tend to spread quickly to the pelvic lymph nodes, and vulvar tumors may spread to the vagina, lungs, liver, or bones. Depending on the stage and type, the patient may receive a hysterectomy, a vaginectomy (removal of the vagina), or a vulvectomy (removal of the vulva). Internal radiation implants and external pelvic irradiation may be used to supplement surgery. Survival rates range from 8 to 75 percent.

STRUCTURE

The ovaries are the primary organs of the female reproductive system. Each of these tiny paired organs is about the size of an almond, and the production of eggs (ova) takes place in the follicles. A follicle consists of an ovum surrounded by one or several layers of follicle cells. At birth the ovaries contain about 800,000 follicles. This number decreases until, at menopause, few if any follicles remain. When a follicle has reached maturity, it will either rupture and release its ovum or collapse and decompose. The former process is known as ovulation. The latter process is called atresia and involves the natural degeneration and discharge of follicles from the body during menstruation.

Following ovulation, the egg enters a fingerlike end of the fallopian tube and begins its movement into the uterus. If intercourse has taken place, the egg has the possibility of being fertilized. The union of egg and sperm occurs in the fimbriated end of the uterine tube. If an ovum is fertilized, it begins to develop as it passes through the uterine tube and into the uterus. Implantation of the fertilized ovum in the uterus takes place after about seven to ten days. The uterus or womb averages two and a half inches in length and weighs approximately 1.8 ounces (50 grams). It has a capacity of 0.07 to 0.17 ounces (2 to 5 cubic centimeters) and is tightly constructed. During pregnancy it increases substantially and at full term reaches a length of about 20 inches. The uterus returns to its original condition following delivery.

The lining of the uterus, which is shed during menstruation and is regenerated after about two days, is called the endometrium. The neck of the uterus, connecting the womb with the vagina, is called the cervix. The chief organs of intercourse are the vagina and the vulva, consisting of the major and minor lips, and the clitoris.

CAUSE OF CANCER

Female sexual disorders have risen sharply in recent years. Each year approximately 600,000 American women have hysterectomies. The variety of sexual disorders ranges from menstrual cramps and irregularities to vaginal discharge, blocked fallopian tubes, ovarian cysts, fibroid tumors, and cancer. To understand the origin and development of these illnesses, we must examine the menstrual cycle.

The cycle of menstruation correlates with the process of ovulation. During the first half of the menstrual cycle, between the woman's period and ovulation, the hormone estrogen reaches its peak. During the second half of the menstrual cycle, between ovulation and the onset of the period, the hormone progesterone predominates. The length of time for each stage in the cycle is largely dependent on the types of food that a woman eats. If a woman eats primarily whole grains and cooked vegetables, menstruation usually takes only three days. However, among women who eat a diet high in meat, sugar, and dairy products, five or six days is the norm. The next phase, in which the endometrium regenerates itself, usually takes two days. With proper eating, however, this can be accomplished in only one day. The following stage, in which the follicle matures, lasts about eight days, and ovulation should occur in the part of the cycle that is exactly opposite to the onset of menstruation or, ideally, fourteen days. In healthy women conception usually arises at this time or four to five days after ovulation. During this phase the yellow endocrine body (corpus luteum) found in the ovary in the site of the ruptured follicle matures and secretes progesterone. This hormone influences the changes that take place in the uterine wall during the second half of the menstrual cycle. If not fertilized, the follicle and corpus luteum eventually decompose during this phase and are discharged during menstruation.

If a woman is eating properly, her menstrual cycle should correlate with the monthly lunar cycle, about twenty-eight days. During the full moon, the atmosphere becomes brighter and charged with energy. A woman who regularly eats grains, cooked vegetables, and other yang foods and is physically active will usually menstruate at this time. The condition of the atmosphere will cause her to become more energized, necessitating the discharge during her period. During the new moon, the atmosphere is darker or more yin. Women who menstruate at this time are usually consuming a more expansive diet. After eating properly for some time, a woman begins to menstruate at either the full or new moon, indicating that her condition is in harmony with the natural atmospheric and lunar cycle.

During the first half of the menstrual cycle, women quickly regain balance and can readily follow a more centered diet of whole grains, cooked vegetables, and seasonal fresh fruit. Immediately prior to ovulation, fertility is expressed with general feelings of joy, contentment, and bliss. The woman feels wonderful and exudes cheerfulness and confidence, and her eating remains centered during the few days of ovulation.

During the second half of the cycle, as menstruation approaches, some women experience dissatisfaction, irritability, and constant hunger. Overcooked foods, animal food, and other heavier substances may become unappealing and, if taken in too great a quantity, frequently lead to excessive intake of sweets, fruits, salad, and liquid. In such cases, just prior to menstruation, some women may experience swelling of the breasts and a general bloated feeling. They may continue to crave strong foods in the yin category and to feel impatient and melancholy.

In order to have a smooth menstrual cycle, it is important for the woman to adjust her diet during the two halves of her month. During the first two weeks, between menstruation and ovulation, she should eat plenty of dark, leafy green vegetables along with whole grains and other more substantial foods to which she will be naturally attracted. During the last two weeks, between ovulation and menstruation, she will feel more comfortable if she reduces her intake of overcooked foods and avoids animal food altogether. Otherwise they will produce an increased craving for sweets, fruit, juices, salads, and lighter foods. To prevent this compulsion from arising, the woman can eat more lightly cooked vegetables at this time along with lighter seasonings and less salt. Special dishes, such as mochi, turnip or radish tops, or amasake, are very helpful and will reduce cravings for more extreme foods.

An irregular menstrual cycle results if the diet is imbalanced too much in one direction or the other. For example, if it totals less than twenty-eight days, this usually indicates an overly yang condition from eating excessive animal and overly energizing foods. A cycle longer than average, up to thirty-two or thirty-five days, shows that a woman may well be consuming too many foods in the yin category such as sweets, fruits, and dairy food. Both conditions can be corrected by eating a more central diet of grains and vegetables.

Menstrual cramps are usually caused by an excessive intake of animal products, especially meat, fish, eggs, and dairy food, in combination with too many expansive foods such as sugar, soft drinks, refined flour, and chemically processed foods. Cramps can be eliminated in two to three months on a balanced standard macrobiotic diet.

Excessive menstrual flow can result from overconsuming foods from either the yin or yang category. In the case of too many contractive foods, including animal foods rich in protein and fat, the blood thickens and the flow lasts longer. This is often accompanied by an unpleasant odor. When too many expansive foods are consumed, including foods that slow down the body metabolism, the blood becomes thinner than normal and menstruation is prolonged. When a woman eats a more balanced diet, menstruation will be of shorter duration and the flow will be lighter.

Biologically, women need not eat any animal food except occasional consumption, if desired, of very light white fish or shellfish. An imbalanced diet can give rise to headaches, depression, and emotional outbursts prior to menstruation. This condition has recently been recognized by medical science under the name premenstrual syndrome (PMS). It can be corrected by centering the diet, especially avoiding extremes of meat and sugar and chemicalized food.

Deposits of fat and mucus, coming largely from animal foods, dairy foods, sugar, and refined flour products, often accumulate in the inner organs if an imbalanced way of eating continues over several years. In women this buildup tends to concentrate in the breasts, the uterus, the ovaries, the fallopian tubes, and the vagina. The solidification of mucus or fat around these organs can result in the development of cysts. Those that occur in the comparatively tight ovaries are saturated in quality, or yang, whereas those in the more expanded vagina or vulva contain more grease and mucus— their quality is yin. Most cysts are soft when they begin to form, but with the continuation of an improper diet they harden and often calcify. This type of cyst is something like a stone and is very difficult to dissolve. Some varieties of cysts contain fat and protein and can become extremely hard, in which case they are called dermoid cysts. Tumors represent the final stage in this process as the body attempts to localize the continuing influx of unhealthy nutrients by creating blockages and obstructions in various organs and sites of the body. The accumulation of fat and mucus can also block the fallopian tubes, preventing the passage of egg and sperm and resulting in the inability to conceive.

Foods that when overconsumed create cysts and tumors in the reproductive organs include varied combinations of milk, cheese, ice cream, and other dairy products; sugar, soft drinks, chocolate, and other sweeteners; fruit and fruit juices; nut butters; greasy and oily foods; refined flour and pastries such as croissants, doughnuts, and sweet rolls; and hamburgers and other animal foods. Once again serious reproductive illnesses may be relieved by eliminating extreme foods and centering the diet on whole grains, beans, vegetables, sea vegetables, and small amounts of fruit and seeds.

Recently some cancer specialists have linked the spread of human papillomavirus (HPV) with cancer of the cervix. This type of sexually transmitted disease may be considered a precancerous condition. But like other STDs, HPV infection is largely the effect of poor eating, especially foods high in fat and sugar. A multitude of viruses and other microorganisms live in symbiosis with the human organism and usually will not give rise to disease unless the blood quality is weakened. If the blood quality is strong, the body's immune system will neutralize and destroy any harmful bacteria or other organisms.

One in four teenage girls in the United States now has an STD. The current epidemic of STDs is the result of degenerating blood quality. Widespread consumption of synthetic and artificial foods, on top of meat and sugar, has created a weakened condition in which harmful viruses can thrive. People who eat a balanced diet and over time have strengthened their blood and immune system should remain free of HPV and other infections. The cervical cancer vaccine has raised major ethical and spiritual questions because it is aimed at adolescent girls, and many parents fear it will encourage them to have sexual relations. The vaccine itself has also been associated with a variety of harmful effects, including three reported deaths and 1,600 adverse reactions between June 2006 when it was introduced and April 2007. Dizziness and fainting are commonly reported. The CDC and FDA currently stand by the vaccine, which is administered in three injections over a six-month period and is designed to protect for at least five years. From the macrobiotic perspective, this vaccine is largely unnecessary and potentially dangerous. America's females would be better served by a national campaign focusing on dietary and nutritional education, including proper cooking and home remedies, and on training in personal growth and development and healthy relationships.

MEDICAL EVIDENCE

- In 1674 an English physician named Wiseman associated cancer with the effects of faulty nutrition on the blood and sexual organs.

"This disease might arise from an error in diet, a great acrimony in the meats and drinks meeting with a fault in the first concoction, which, not being afterwards corrected in the intestines, suffered the acrimonious matter to ascend into the blood, where, if it found vent either in the menstrua in women, or by the hemorrhoids or urine in men, the mischief might have been prevented."[1]

- In 1896, Robert Bell, M.D., senior staff member at the Glasgow Hospital for Women, adopted a nutritional approach to tumors of the uterus and breast after twenty years as a cancer surgeon. "I had been taught that this [surgery] was the only method by which malignant disease could be successfully treated, and, at the time, believed this to be true. But failure after failure following each other, without a single break, inclined me to alter my opinion. . . . The disease invariably recurred with renewed virulence, suffering was intensified, and the life of the patient shortened. . . . That cancer is a curable disease, if its local development is recognized in its early stage, and if rational dietetic and therapeutic measures are adopted and rigidly adhered to, there can be no doubt whatever."[2]

- Seventh-Day Adventist women in California ages thirty-five to fifty-four have 84 percent less cervical cancer and 12 percent less ovarian cancer than the national average, according to a 1975 epidemiological study. Female church members over fifty-five have 36 percent less cervical cancer and 47 percent less ovarian cancer. Together both age groups have 40 percent fewer uterine tumors of other kinds. The Seventh-Day Adventists, about half of whom are vegetarian, eat 25 percent less fat and 50 percent more fiber, especially whole grains, vegetables, and fruit, than the general population.[3]

- "Worldwide use of birth control pills, in spite of conclusive evidence of carcinoginicity of estrogens in experimental animals," warned Samuel S. Epstein, M.D., "constitutes the largest uncontrolled experiment in human carcinogenesis ever undertaken." The cancer specialist cited studies estimating that oral contraceptives could cause ten thousand fatalities a year, especially from ovarian cancer.[4]

DIAGNOSIS

Ovarian cancer is generally diagnosed by gynecologists on the basis of a pelvic examination, a Pap smear, and a parancentesis or cul-de-sac aspiration, in which fluid from between the vagina and rectum is drained out by a needle for examination under a microscope. A needle biopsy will be taken if a malignancy is suspected, and metastases will be detected through a mammogram, GI series, or intravenous pyelogram (IVP). Uterine cancer is commonly observed following a pelvic examination and a dilation and curettage (D and C) in which a small amount of tissue is scraped from the inside of the uterus. Metastases will be checked out with X-rays to the chest, IVP, bone and liver scans, and endoscopy of the lower colon and bladder. Cervical, vaginal, and vulver cancers are diagnosed with a pelvic examination, a Pap smear, and a colposcopy, in which a viewing scope transmits a magnified area of the sex organs to a television monitor.

The condition of the reproductive system can be observed directly without technological intervention or potentially harmful X-rays. If the woman has a vaginal discharge, for example, its color can help locate the site and extent of the swelling. If the discharge is yellowish in color, a cyst is developing. A white discharge is less serious but usually leads to development of a soft type of cyst unless the woman changes her way of eating. A green discharge signifies tumorous growth, especially if the color has been occurring for a length of time.

Vaginal discharges, ovarian cysts, and fibroid tumors are frequently indicated by a yellow coating in the lower part of the whites of the eyes. Dark spots in the whites of the eye indicate ovarian cysts or tumors or kidney stones.

The eyelashes also correspond with reproductive functions. Eyelashes that curve outward show degeneration of the sex organs due to consumption of excessive yin foods, especially fruits, juices, and dairy products during early childhood. Eyelashes that curve inward indicate excess intake of strong foods in the yang category, including eggs and meat. In this case there may be menstrual cramps or lack of menstruation due to contraction of the ovaries. Menstrual cramps are also indicated when a woman smiles if a horizontal line or ridge appears between the upper lip and nose.

Split fingernails and abnormal colors on the fingertips, resulting from a chaotic way of eating, indicate malfunctions in the reproductive system as well. If one thumbnail or thumb tip shows these conditions and the other is normal, it indicates that the ovary corresponding to the abnormal side is malfunctioning.

Pimples in the center of the cheeks with a fatty appearance may reflect the formation of cysts in the ovarian region.

Along the bladder meridian, a green shade appearing around either ankle on the outside of the leg indicates developing cancer in the uterus or bladder. Also, a fatty swelling along the ankle region indicates mucus and fat accumulation in the uterine region and may be a sign of a precancerous condition.

DIETARY RECOMMENDATIONS

Cancer in the ovary is largely caused by overconsumption of eggs and other food rich in protein and rich in fat. Uterine cancer is caused more by beef, pork, and chicken. Hard dairy food as well as too much salty, baked, and roasted foods, which make the muscles and tissues tight, also contribute to both ovarian and uterine cancer and should be avoided. Cancer in the cervix or vagina is caused by fat- and cholesterol-rich foods such as those in the case of ovarian and uterine tumors, but also by proportionately more consumption of light dairy food, fruits, and flour products. Cancer in the reproductive region as a whole is accelerated by the intake of synthetic chemicals, including various kinds of drugs and estrogen replacements, as well as artificial birth-control methods and other unnatural regulation of reproductive and menstrual functions. Accordingly, all these things should be avoided. Sugar, sugar-treated foods, and other sweeteners, including artificial ones, should also be avoided. Flour products such as white bread, pancakes, and cookies tend to form mucus and fat and should not be eaten. Food and beverages that possess stimulant, aromatic, and fragrant characteristics, including seasonings such as curry, mustard, and pepper, coffee, alcohol, soft drinks, and herb teas should also be avoided. Oils, even unsaturated vegetable oils, should be minimized. All oily or greasy cooking methods, including deep-frying, are to be avoided until the condition improves. Salad dressings, mayonnaise (dairy or soy), and other oily dressings and spreads are to be avoided. All chemicalized foods and beverages are to be avoided, while those of more organic and natural quality are recommended. Following are general guidelines for daily food consumption:

- Whole Grains: Forty to 50 percent of daily consumption, by volume, should be whole cereal grains. The first day prepare plain short- or medium-grain brown rice, pressure-cooked or cooked in a heavy cast-iron or ceramic pot with a heavy lid. On the following days alternate brown rice cooked with 20 to 30 percent millet, then rice with 20 to 30 percent barley, then rice with 20 to 30 percent aduki beans or lentils, and then plain rice again. A delicious morning porridge can be made by taking leftover rice, adding a little more water to soften it, seasoning with a little miso at the end, and simmering for two to three minutes more. In daily cooking, the ratio of grain to water should be about 1:2. For seasoning, cook with a postage-stamp-sized piece of kombu instead of salt. Other grains can be used occasionally, including whole wheat berries, rye, corn, and whole oats, though oats should be avoided for the first month. However, buckwheat should not be eaten for about six months because it is very contractive and may harden the tumor. Seitan is also very yang and should be minimized. Flour products, even unrefined whole wheat bread, chapatis, pancakes, and cookies, should be totally avoided or limited in volume for a period of a few months, though people with ovarian and other female problems typically like roasted, baked, or crunchy foods. Whole grain pasta and noodles may be eaten a couple times a week.

- Soup: Five to 10 percent of daily consumption should be soup, consisting of one or two cups or bowls per day cooked with wakame sea vegetable and various vegetables, especially daikon and daikon leaves and other green leafy vegetables, seasoned lightly with miso or shoyu. Occasionally a small amount of shiitake mushrooms may be added to the soup. The miso may be barley miso, brown rice miso, or soybean (hatcho) miso, and should be naturally aged two to three years. Grain soups, bean soups, and other soups may be eaten from time to time.

- Vegetables: Twenty to 30 percent of daily consumption should be vegetables, cooked in a variety of forms, mainly steamed, boiled, and, after four to six weeks, occasionally sautéed without oil. Various types of leafy vegetables—green, yellow, and white—can be cooked in different ways, as can various root vegetables such as carrots, turnips, daikon, radishes, lotus root, and burdock roots, although burdock should be used much less frequently than other root vegetables. Round vegetables such as acorn and butternut squash, cabbage, and onions can also be used frequently. Daikon and daikon greens are especially recommended for these conditions.

  As a rule of thumb, the following dishes may be prepared, although the frequency may differ from person to person: nishime-style vegetables, three times a week; a squash-aduki-kombu dish, three times a week; dried daikon, one cup, three times a week; carrots and carrot tops or daikon and daikon tops, three times a week; blanched vegetables, five to seven times a week; pressed salad, several times a week; raw salad, one to two times a week for ovarian cancer and temporarily avoid for the others; steamed greens, five to seven times a week; sautéed vegetables, prepared with water the first month and then with sesame oil lightly brushed on the pan once or twice a week after that; kinpira, two-thirds of a cup, two times a week; dried tofu, tofu, tempeh, or seitan with vegetables, two times a week.

- Beans: Five percent of daily consumption should be small beans, such as aduki beans, lentils, chickpeas, or black soybeans, cooked together with sea vegetables such as kombu or with onions and carrots. Other beans may be used two to three times a month. For seasoning, a small amount of unrefined sea salt or shoyu or miso can be used, and beans can frequently be made with a sweet taste rather than a salty one by adding a little barley malt. Bean products, such as tempeh, natto, and dried or cooked tofu, may be used occasionally but in moderate amounts.

- Sea Vegetables: Five percent or less of sea vegetable dishes, including wakame and kombu, should be included daily when cooking grain, in soup, etc. A sheet of toasted nori may also be taken daily. A small dish of hijiki or arame should be prepared two times a week.

All other sea vegetables are optional. For yang tumors, avoid or limit the use of kombu.

- Condiments: These should be available on the table: gomashio (sesame salt), on the average made with one part salt to eighteen to twenty parts sesame seeds; kelp or wakame powder; umeboshi plum, and tekka, although all other regular macrobiotic condiments may be used if desired. These condiments may be used daily on grains and vegetables, but the amount should be moderate to suit individual appetites and tastes.

- Pickles: Made at home in a variety of ways, pickles are to be eaten daily, one tablespoon in all, although salty pickles are to be minimized. Wash off the salt if too salty.

- Animal Food: Fish and other animal food is to be avoided. However, in the event that animal food is craved, a small amount of white-meat fish may be eaten once every ten days to two weeks. The fish should be steamed, boiled, or poached and garnished with grated daikon or ginger. Strictly avoid blue-meat and red-meat fish and all shellfish.

- Fruit: The less the better until the condition improves except for those with more yang tumors. If cravings develop, a small amount of cooked fruit with a pinch of sea salt or dried fruit (also preferably cooked) may be eaten. Women with ovarian cancer may take a little more fruit than the others, including fresh fruit. Avoid or limit fruit juices and cider as well as raisins, currants, and other very concentrated fruits.

- Sweets and Snacks: Overuse of sweets is associated with these disorders, so it is very important to avoid all sweets and desserts, including good-quality macrobiotic desserts, until the condition improves. To satisfy a sweet tooth, use sweet vegetables every day in cooking, drink sweet vegetable drinks, or prepare sweet vegetable jam. If cravings arise, a small amount of amasake, barley malt, or rice syrup may be eaten. If cravings persist, a little cider, apple juice, or chestnut puree may be prepared. Mochi, rice balls, vegetable sushi, and other grain-based snacks may be eaten frequently. Limit rice cakes, popcorn, and other dry or baked snacks because they may harden the tumor.

- Nuts and Seeds: Nuts and nut butters are to be avoided due to their high fat and protein, except for chestnuts. Unsalted steamed or boiled seeds such as sunflower seeds and pumpkin seeds may be consumed as a snack, up to one cup altogether per week. Minimize roasted seeds.

- Seasonings: Unrefined sea salt, shoyu, and miso are to be used moderately in order to avoid unnecessary thirst. Avoid mirin and garlic. If you become particularly thirsty after a meal or between meals, you should cut back on these seasonings until the normal level of thirst returns.

- Beverages: Drinks and other dietary practices can follow the general recommendations in Part I, including bancha twig tea as the main beverage. Mu tea is highly recommended if consumed for only a few months or occasionally. Mu is a medicinal tea made from either nine or sixteen different herbs that serve to warm the body and strengthen weak female organs. Strictly avoid the beverages on the "infrequent" and "avoid" list and don't take grain coffee for the first two or three months after starting this new way of eating.

The most important thing in connection with dietary practice is chewing very well, until all food becomes liquid in the mouth and well mixed with saliva. Chew very well, at least fifty times and preferably a hundred times per mouthful. It is also important to avoid overeating and eating within three hours of sleeping.

As noted in the introduction to Part II, people who have received or who are currently undergoing medical treatment may need to make further dietary modifications.

SPECIAL DRINKS AND DISHES

One or more special drinks or side dishes may need to be taken, depending on the individual case. Please see a qualified macrobiotic teacher for guidance. Amounts and frequencies given here are averages for each drink or dish; these will differ from person to person. Further directions are in Chapter 36.

- Brown Rice Porridge with Grated Daikon and Lemon: This is helpful for ovarian cancer. Eat one small cup of this gruel every evening for about two weeks. After that, have it every other day or every three days for another three weeks.
- Dried Daikon, Shiitake, and Onion Tea: For ovarian cancer take one small cup of this broth every morning and every evening for about three weeks. After that, take it one to three times a week for another three to four weeks.
- Kumquat Jam: For ovarian cancer finely chop kumquats. (Do not peel them.) Add a small amount of water and a pinch of sea salt, and simmer to make a jam. Eat one tablespoon of this jam every day for three to four weeks. You may also make kumquat tea by dissolving kumquat jam in bancha twig tea or hot water.
- Tangerine Jam and Tangerine Tea: As an alternative to kumquat, tangerine jam or tea may be made following the above recipe.
- Lemon Juice: A small amount of lemon juice may be used from time to time for ovarian tumors to help cleanse the body of dairy. Grate

½ cup of daikon, add water, simmer, and add a little lemon juice. Grated sour green apple cooked with lemon is also good, as is marinated daikon and carrot.

- Beets: Beets may also be used on occasion for ovarian conditions. Take ½ cup of raw beet juice daily for five days and then every other day for ten days, or cook the beets and eat them. Add a little lemon juice if the liver is stagnated.
- Sweet Vegetable Drink: Take one to two small cups to reduce cravings for sweets and, in cases of ovarian cancer, to reduce pain.
- Roasted Brown Rice Porridge with Grated Daikon: For uterine tumors, eat one to two small cups of the porridge every day for about ten days. Then have it every other day for three weeks. After that, reduce it to twice a week and continue for another one month.
- Dried Daikon, Daikon Leaves, and Shiitake Tea: For uterine tumors drink one to three small cups of this broth every day for two to three weeks. After that have it two to three times a week for another month.
- Ume-Shiso Bancha: For uterine tumors drink one small cup of this tea every day for one week. After that, have it every other day or every three days for another two weeks.
- Daikon and Daikon Leaves Sautéed in Water: This combination is especially good for uterine conditions. Eat one small dish of this preparation every day for three to four weeks.
- Grated Daikon and Carrot with Umeboshi, Shiso, Lemon, and Shoyu: For cervical cancer eat one to two small cups of this preparation every day for one week and then every other day for ten more days. After that, have it two to three times a week for another month.
- Dried Daikon, Dried Daikon Leaves, and Mushroom Tea: For cervical cancer drink one to two small cups every day for three to four weeks; thereafter, have it two to three times a week for another month.
- Brown Rice Porridge with Grated Daikon: For cervical cancer lightly season this dish with sea salt or miso. Eat one bowl every day for about ten days. After that, have it two to three times a week for another month.
- Lotus Seed, Seaweed, and Onion Tea: For cervical conditions this tea is helpful to drink often.
- Corn Soup with Lotus Seeds: This dish is also helpful for cervical conditions. Have this soup three to four times a week for four to five weeks.
- Nabe-Style Vegetables: This dish with dipping sauce is also recommended to help relieve cervical tumors and may be eaten often. But do not use udon noodles. Cook shiso leaves, Chinese cabbage, cab-

bage, and other leafy greens together. Tofu or yuba may also be added. Rather than ginger, use nori and chopped scallions for the dipping sauce. If you like, add a squeeze of yuzu (a type of lemon) or lemon juice to the dipping sauce.

HOME CARE

- Body Scrub: Scrubbing the whole body, including the abdominal region and the spinal region, with a towel that has been immersed in hot water and squeezed out is very helpful for better circulation of blood, lymph, and other body fluids, as well as for activating physical and mental energies.

- Compress Guidelines: For a small number of tumors in the female reproductive system, a compress may be needed to help gradually draw out the excess mucus and fat. Please see a qualified macrobiotic teacher for guidance on the proper use and frequency of a compress or plaster. Several types are used depending on the person's condition. Precede the compress or plaster with the application of a towel that has been soaked in hot water and squeezed out over the affected area for three to five minutes to stimulate circulation.

- Daikon Hip Bath: In the event of frequent vaginal discharges, a hip bath will facilitate the elimination of accumulated fat and mucus. Ideally, the water for the hip bath should contain dried leafy greens such as daikon or turnip greens. To prepare this bath, hang several dozen bunches of these leaves to dry, either near a window or outside, but not under direct sunlight. The leaves will first turn yellow and then brown, at which time they are suitable for use. For each evening's bath, boil two or three bunches of dried leaves for ten to twenty minutes in several quarts of water to which you may add a handful of sea salt or kombu sea vegetable. The water will turn brownish in color. Run hot water in the bathtub, add the mixture along with another handful of sea salt, and get into the tub. The water should cover your hips. Wrap a thick cotton towel around your upper body to avoid chills and to absorb perspiration. As the water begins to cool, add more hot water and stay in the tub for ten to fifteen minutes.

  If dried leaves are not available for this bath, use sea vegetables, especially arame. If these cannot be obtained or are too expensive, add two handfuls of sea salt to the bathwater and proceed as above.

  While in the bath, your lower body will become very red as circulation in that area increases and the stagnated fat and mucus inside the sex organs start to loosen. Immediately following the bath, douche with a preparation made with one teaspoon of sea salt, two teaspoons of rice vinegar or lemon juice, and one quart of warm bancha tea. This bath and douche can be done every evening or every other evening for five to ten days and thereafter once every five days or once a week, until mucus and fatty substances are generally eliminated from the uterus and vaginal regions.

- Green Vegetable Plaster: To relieve pain it is also helpful in some cases to apply a paste of mashed green leafy vegetables mixed with flour for one to two hours, after warming the area with a hot towel. This green leafy plaster should be kept warm during the application by placing roasted sea salt wrapped with cotton cloth above the plaster. It is also helpful to apply a very hot compress, such as a ginger compress, repeatedly on the base of the spine.

- Hato Mugi-Potato Plaster: This compress is beneficial for some cases of ovarian cancer. Leave the plaster on for four hours or longer. Repeat twice a day or, if possible, leave the plaster on all night while sleeping. Continue every day for about three weeks.

- Massage: For ovarian cancer, massage the feet and all toes for about fifteen minutes, two to three times every day. If the feet become so cold that you cannot sleep, you may use a hot water bottle, but do not soak your feet in hot water or do a ginger foot bath. For cervical cancer, massage the feet and toes well for fifteen minutes. Repeat two to three times every day.

EMOTIONAL CONSIDERATIONS

Female reproductive problems are associated emotionally with sexuality, intimacy, and regeneration.

High-quality foods that nourish the cervix, ovaries, and other female sexual organs and help develop positive emotions include whole grains, particularly buckwheat, teff, wild rice, and other darker grains; beans and bean products, especially black soybeans and other darker beans; leafy green vegetables; sea vegetables; seeds and nuts; white-meat fish; and good-quality sea salt.

Foods that harm these organs and contribute to negative emotions include dairy food; meat, poultry, eggs; strong fish and seafood; white flour; sugar and other highly refined sweets; chemicalized and artificial foods; and other extremely contractive or expansive foods and beverages.

In respect to relationships it is important to communicate freely and honestly and not suppress feelings and emotions. A woman who feels rejected and unappreciated, is overly aggressive, or engages in secretive relationships may localize her repressed feelings in the ovaries or related organ.

On a planetary scale, the sex organs correlate with the deep oceans, and cancer in this region is akin to ocean pollution.

OTHER CONSIDERATIONS

- Daily physical exercise that does not produce exhaustion is recommended. Ten to fifteen minutes of daily breathing exercises, especially emphasizing long exhalation, is also beneficial. These physical and breathing exercises contribute to relaxing tensions in the body and mind as well as harmonizing physical metabolism.
- Keeping air quality clean and fresh is important for the maintenance of general health. For that purpose, green leafy plants can be placed in the house and the windows periodically opened to allow circulation of fresh air. Don't smoke because this will tighten the ovaries.
- Avoid watching television for long stretches. Radiation weakens the reproductive area. Similarly, avoid other artificial sources of electromagnetic energy such as video terminals, smoke detectors, and handheld electrical appliances, which can weaken the ovaries and the reproductive system.
- Although cancer is naturally accompanied by a decline in energy and vitality, normal sexual practice is not harmful if it does not lead to exhaustion.
- Avoid or limit artificial methods of regulating your period, especially birth-control pills, estrogens, and tubal ligation, which severs the flow of electromagnetic energy through the body. As your eating improves, your menstrual cycle will become more regular and tuned to the lunar cycle, and you can gradually begin natural birth-control methods.
- Avoid or limit abortion and cesarean section if possible. Study natural methods of delivery, and if you are in good health, consider home birth with the assistance of a midwife or other experienced medical person. Breast-feeding will help protect you and your child against future illnesses, including cancer.
- Avoid synthetic underwear and stockings, artificial tampons, chemical douches or toiletries, talcum powder, and other synthetic products that may be irritating or harmful to the reproductive system.
- During the menstrual period, a woman's excess is discharged through the skin as well as through the menstrual flow. It is recommended that a woman not take cold showers or wash her hair with cold water, since both of these tend to draw this excess away from its normal course of discharge. To clean yourself, use a wet towel or sponge.
- Deep relaxation exercises, including Do-in and shiatsu acupressure massage around the lower back prior to menstruation, can help reduce physical and emotional discomfort. Active physical exercises are also important for healthy living.

- In the case of pain, one half hour of palm healing is helpful. This is done simply by putting one hand on a piece of cotton placed over the affected area, synchronizing the breath, keeping a peaceful mind, and allowing the natural energy of the environment to flow through the hand. Palm healing is more effective when a second person performs the healing, but it can be done alone.

PERSONAL EXPERIENCES

UTERINE TUMOR

In 1947 film star Gloria Swanson learned that she had a tumor in her uterus. She went to three gynecologists, and each one recommended an immediate hysterectomy. She finally went to see a specialist who was considered the top woman's doctor in the country. "After examining me," she later recalled in an article for *East West Journal,* "he didn't say exactly what the first three had, but he did say, 'Well, you know this has to come out by Christmas'—which was about five months away."

Instead, Miss Swanson went to California to see Dr. Henry G. Bieler, a physician who treated illness with diet. He said to her, "Now, Gloria, what is the function of a protein?" She said, "It's a cell builder, Dr. Bieler." He asked her, "Are you fully grown?" She said, "Dr. Bieler, don't pull my leg. You know I'm forty-seven." He said, "Well, maybe you're a ditchdigger. Or are you a tennis pro? A football player?" She said, "What are you trying to tell me?"

Dr. Bieler went on to remind Gloria Swanson that she had had a hard time with the birth of her child in 1920. He also reminded her that cancer doesn't develop overnight but can sometimes take twenty years to develop.

"Have you been eating a lot of protein?" he asked her. "Well, I guess I have," she replied. "Well, now, what are you going to do about that, if it's a cell builder?" he inquired. "Do you really think I can starve this to death?" she said. The doctor smiled and said, "You get enough protein, you don't need all that animal protein." Gloria responded, "All right. As of this moment I shall not eat any more animal protein. How long do you think it will take?" The physician replied, "I don't know—a year, two years, maybe three."

For the next two years, despite a heavy travel schedule and demanding routine, Gloria carried around her own food, consisting primarily of whole grains and vegetables and a little bit of fruit. Two and a half years had elapsed by the time she went back to see the famous specialist. "I had a feeling the tumor was gone," she wrote. "He hadn't heard from me since the time he told me what was going to happen around

Christmastime (that would have been a nice Christmas present for somebody—a pathologist, I guess). I hopped up on his table, and he started hunting. Oh, it was fascinating to watch his face. I said, 'It isn't there, is it, Doctor?' 'No,' he said reluctantly. I said, 'Don't you want to know what I did?' 'What do you mean, what you did?' 'Well,' I said, 'I went on a diet.'"

The doctor threw his head back and laughed. "He thought it was very funny," she continued. "A diet: ha-ha-ha. I said, 'It was a non-animal protein diet, Doctor.' He laughed even harder. I said, 'Well, you can laugh; I don't think it's a laughing matter. I'm still a woman, and what's more, I'm very happy about it. But I'm not laughing about it, and I don't think you should laugh either. I'd hoped you might learn something, because I have. And I don't really think you ought to send me a bill.' And I hopped off and went home, and he never did."

In the more than thirty years afterward, until dying of old age, Gloria was extremely active in promoting natural foods and macrobiotics. Several years ago she and her husband, Bill Dufty, author of *Sugar Blues*, joined my wife, Aveline, and me on a visit and speaking tour of Japan. "You're responsible for your own health," Gloria told people who asked her how she maintained her health and beauty for over eighty years. "It's quite true. There's nobody who can chew your food for you. And so if you really want to be well, you have to do it yourself."[5]

UTERINE CANCER WITH METASTASES TO THE BONE AND LUNGS

In April 1980, Elaine Nussbaum had a diagnostic procedure to determine the cause of excessive and prolonged menstrual bleeding. The doctor found a tumor in the connective tissue on the wall of her uterus. She was given twenty radiation treatments, a radium implant, hormone medication, and both oral and intravenous chemotherapy. In August 1980 physicians performed a radical hysterectomy and a bilateral salpingo-oophorectomy, removing her ovaries.

Elaine continued to take chemotherapy. In May 1982 she experienced pain in the lower back that continued to worsen despite medication. She could neither sit nor lie down. In August, after several days standing up for twenty-four hours, sleeping only on her husband's shoulder in a standing position, she went to an orthopedist. He diagnosed a compression fracture and found that her vertebrae were partially collapsed. To prevent complete collapse of her backbone, she was put in a brace that extended from above the chest to the lower pelvic region.

Elaine's pain continued to worsen and spread to her legs. Eventually she could no longer stand. Her husband put her in a recliner and gave her strong painkillers night and day, but the pain continued.

In September she was taken to the hospital for more X-rays and tests. Bone scans showed that the cancer had spread to the lumbar spine and the thoracic spine, and there were malignancies in both lungs.

Elaine received five radiation treatments, followed by chemotherapy, another series of radiation treatments and more chemotherapy. The usual treatment was ten rounds of chemotherapy over intervals of three to four weeks. She felt exhausted, had low vitality, and experienced nausea and pain.

In January 1983, after four cycles of chemo, medical tests showed an increase of activity and progression of the tumor in the spine and no change in Elaine's lungs.

Toward the end of January, Elaine cut her finger opening an envelope in the mail. Infection set in because of her weakness following chemo, and she was unable to ward off the infection. Over the next ten days she received four blood transfusions in the hospital, as well as massive doses of intravenous antibiotics. The doctors decided to put her on less toxic treatment, and it was then that she knew conventional medicine would not work for her.

After researching the alternatives, Elaine decided to start macrobiotics. She weaned herself from meat, dairy food, fruit, sugar, and eventually all thirty-eight pills she had been taking daily.

Beginning the diet in a hospital bed, and still using a wheelchair and a brace, Elaine was able to start using a walker relatively quickly and then a cane. In April a chronic urinary disorder disappeared. In mid-May the brace came off, and on May 22 she walked up and down the street by herself.

In June, Elaine put away her wig. As a result of chemotherapy, all her hair had fallen out, but it now had grown back. Returning the hospital bed to the hospital, she started driving again and resumed her studies. "In six months, I changed from a sick, depressed, pill-popping invalid to a happy, optimistic, and very grateful pain-free person," she recalled.[6]

Elaine went on to complete a master of science degree in nutrition and has taught, lectured, and offered cooking classes around the country. She lectured widely and wrote a bestselling book, *Recovery: From Cancer to Health Through Macrobiotics*. She remained cancer-free for the next twenty-five years and passed away in her sleep in 2006.

OVARIAN AND LYMPHATIC CANCER

The Dobics seemed like a typical happy modern family. Milenka had two wonderful children and a challenging career as a program director for one of the largest radio stations in Belgrade. Her husband, Bosko, was in the import/export field handling agricultural machinery. In 1986, however, tragedy struck. After Milenka experienced migraine headaches, chronic tiredness, and pressure in her head, medical tests showed that she had ovarian cancer, which had already spread to the lymphatic system. Doctors operated and advised chemotherapy and radiation but were not hopeful.

In the hospital a friend, who happened to be a doctor, gave Milenka a copy of *The Cancer Prevention Diet,* and she began to associate her condition with her past way of eating a high amount of animal foods, especially meat, dairy, and oily dishes. Declining further medication, she left the hospital even though her doctors told her she could expect to live only two months.

At home Milenka told her husband and family that she would try to combat her malignancy with diet and wanted to go to the United States to study macrobiotics. With the help of friends and associates at work, funds were raised, and she and Bosko came to America in February 1987. In Boston they attended a seminar on diet and degenerative disease at the Kushi Institute and saw me for a personal guidance session. I explained that the primary cause of her condition was the past intake of cheese and dairy food, but that with proper cooking she could overcome her cancer. "At that moment," Milenka said, looking back, "I felt like my journey was really starting. I had hope now."

Back in Yugoslavia, Milenka started cooking macrobiotically as well as doing self-massage and a daily body scrub, singing songs, and practicing meditation and visualization. Medical tests confirmed that she was improving, and within five months the tumor had disappeared: "To the doctors it seemed like a miracle. They could not understand."

Milenka, Bosko, and their family studied at the Kushi Institute in Becket for several years. They helped organize seminars in their native Yugoslavia and have had a beneficial impact on the health of many people. Today, only twenty years later, Milenka is still cancer-free and one of the leading macrobiotic cooks, teachers, and counselors on the West Coast. Her autobiography, *My Beautiful Life*, has been published in several languages.[7]

OVARIAN CANCER

After being diagnosed with ovarian cancer in 2002, Gerry DeMello had surgery at Dana Farber Cancer Hospital in Boston. Over the next six months she underwent chemotherapy to treat the spreading tumor.

Seeking an alternative approach, she started macrobiotic cooking classes as well as Reiki, visualization, and acupuncture treatments, and responded immediately. Feeling weak and unable to continue medical treatment, she quit chemo but was subsequently hospitalized and told that she would not recover. Her daughter and a friend continued to bring macrobiotic food, and after several days she was released from the

ICU. In early 2003 she was discharged from the hospital after being told that nothing further could be done. Gerry's body was filled with fluid from the waist down, and her right leg was paralyzed. Discontinuing the injections and medications she had been given, she adhered to the diet, and eventually the excess fluid went away and she could walk again.

"Don't wait until you have a life-threatening disease. Start making changes in your life now," she advised others. "Start a macrobiotic diet. Make a commitment to yourself to improve your health and life. You will be amazed at how great you will feel. It is now two years and nine months since the day I found out I had cancer. Everyone is astonished at how my life has turned around."[8]

CERVICAL CANCER

See also Appendix II, "Illness in the Kushi Family."

20

Kidney and Bladder Cancer

FREQUENCY

Cancers of the kidney, bladder, and other parts of the urinary tract will claim an estimated 27,340 American lives this year, and 120,400 new cases will develop. Overall, mortality from bladder cancer has fallen during the last generation, but kidney cancer deaths are on the rise in both sexes. About one-third of all urinary cancers occur in the kidney and two-thirds in the bladder, ureters, and urethra. Kidney cancer occurs about evenly in men and women and is found among both adults and children. Bladder cancer is much more prevalent in men, especially those in the fifty-five to seventy-five age group.

Standard medical treatment calls for surgical removal of the afflicted kidney along with adjacent lymph nodes and adrenal glands in an operation called a radical nephrectomy. In a rarer form of kidney cancer known as renal pelvis carcinoma, the ureter will be removed along with the kidney in a procedure called a neproutererectomy. A person can survive with only one kidney. If both kidneys are removed, a kidney transplant may be performed or kidney dialysis instituted. A kidney dialysis machine performs the functions of the kidneys by filtering fluids through tubes imbedded in the patient's arms. The patient must undergo this treatment two or three times a week for three or four hours' duration each time. Radiation therapy is sometimes used prior to kidney surgery to shrink a tumor. The five-year survival rate for kidney cancer is about 66 percent.

In the case of bladder cancer, superficial tumors are generally removed by burning or cutting with the use of a cystoscope, a flexible tube inserted through the urethra or an abdominal incision. Total removal of the bladder in advanced cases is called a cystectomy. In men the prostate is often malignant and is removed as well. An artificial bladder is then constructed, usually with a section of the small intestine, and connected to a disposable bag on the outside of the body for the elimination of urine. Radiation in the form of external voltage or internally implanted radioactive seeds is also sometimes employed before bladder surgery in order to destroy invasive tumors. Chemotherapy is not used as a primary treatment for urinary cancers but may be used to control pain following surgery. Some 82 percent of bladder cancer patients treated by these methods live five years or more.

STRUCTURE

The two kidneys are bean-shaped organs located in the upper part of the abdominal cavity near the spinal column. The main tasks of the kidneys are to filter impurities from the blood and to discharge excess fluid from the body in the form of urine. About a quart of blood passes through the kidneys every minute, and these organs serve to regulate the amount of salt, water, and other constituents of the bloodstream. Urine is formed in the kidney by filtration of urea and other wastes from the blood vessels and the absorption and excretion of other substances from the filtrate.

In general, urine is amber in color, forms a mildly acidic reaction, and has a slight odor and a salty taste. The quantity of urine discharged varies with the amount of fluids consumed but usually amounts to between 33.8 and 50.7 ounces (1,000 and 1,500 cubic centimeters) a day. The quantity of solids in the urine changes with the diet and is significantly higher following consumption of foods higher in fat and protein. People eating the modern diet excrete about 1.4 to 2.6 ounces (40 to 75 grams) of solid waste daily in their urine, of which 25 percent is urea, 25 percent chlorides, 25 percent sulfate and phosphates, and the rest organic acids, pigments, hormones, and so on. In unhealthy urine, high levels of albumin, sugar, blood, pus, acetone, fat, chyle, cellular material, and bacteria may be present.

The adrenal glands, attached to the upper part of the kidneys, are part of the endocrine system. They secrete hormones, including adrenaline, regulating mental and emotional stress. The ureters are long, narrow tubes that convey the urine from each kidney to the bladder by muscular action. The bladder is a hollow Y-shaped organ situated in the pelvis, which serves as a reservoir for urine. It can hold about one pint. The urethra is the canal through which the urine is discharged from the body. The urethra extends from the neck of the bladder to the genital region. In men, the urethra is divided into the prostatic portion and the penile portion. In women, the urinary system is largely separated from the reproductive system.

CAUSE OF CANCER

Kidney disorders may be divided into two groups: (1) overly contracted, tight, and inflexible (yang) kidney conditions that result in the restriction of blood flow and urination; and (2) loose or swollen (yin) kidney conditions that prevent complete filtration of the blood and can lead to excessive retention or elimination of liquids. Preliminary signs of contracted and hardening kidneys are tossing and turning during sleep, insomnia, nightmares, and rising early in the morning. Tight kidneys are caused by overconsumption of extreme yang foods such as eggs, meat, other animal products, dry baked goods, and commercial salt as well as overactivity and a pressure-filled environment. Initial symptoms of overly expanded kidneys are snoring, groaning, bedwetting, lower back pain, getting up to urinate at night, and getting up late in the morning. This yin condition may be caused by a high intake of beverages (especially milk, fruit juices, and coffee) as well as foods of tropical origin, fruit, sugar, and sweets. A sedentary lifestyle contributes to weak, sluggish kidneys.

Over time, excessive consumption of a combination of extreme yin and yang foodstuffs and beverages can lead to the formation of stones, cysts, or tumors in the urinary tract. These obstructions develop when an excess of solid wastes cannot pass through the fine network of cells in the interior of the kidneys, the ureters, or the bladder. The kidneys are a frequent site of mucus and fatty-acid accumulation. In this condition the kidneys often retain water and become chronically swollen. Since the process of elimination is impaired, excess fluid is often deposited in the legs, producing periodic swelling and weakness. At the same time excessive perspiration will also usually develop. If someone with this swollen condition continues to consume large amounts of expansive foods, the deposited fat and mucus will crystallize into kidney stones. Stones are principally caused by long-term eating of high-fat foods combined with chilled or frozen foods, particularly ice cream, sherbet, yogurt, orange juice, soft drinks, ice water, and other beverages that make the body cold.

Over a long period of time, cysts and stones will culminate in the formation of tumors as the kidney fights back in self-defense to restrict the flow of excess waters and irritating fluids through its system. In the case of bladder cancer, excessive toxins and other irritants in the urine, especially from processed foods and chemicalized water, can ultimately give rise to cancer. Kidney cancer, affecting the more tight, compact part of the urinary system, is a relatively more yang form of cancer. Bladder cancer, affecting the expanded hollow portion of the urinary system, is relatively more yin. To restore balance, a slightly more yin macrobiotic diet is recommended for kidney cancer, and a more yang diet in the case of bladder cancer.

MEDICAL EVIDENCE

- Looking back over four decades of medical work in French Equatorial Africa, Dr. Albert Schweitzer reported that he had never had any cancer cases in his hospital and that its occurrence among the African people was very rare. He attributed the rise of degenerative diseases to the importation of European foods including condensed milk, canned butter, meat and fish preserves, white bread, and especially refined salt. "It is obvious to connect the fact of increase of cancer with the increased use of salt by the natives. In former years there was only available the little salt extracted from the ocean. . . . So it is possible that the formerly very seldom and still infrequent occurrence of cancer in this country is connected with the former very little consumption of salt and the still rare use of it."[1]

- A 1975 epidemiological study reported that Seventh-Day Adventists in California have 72 percent less bladder cancer than the general population. The church members avoid meat, poultry, fish, rich and refined food, coffee, tea, hot condiments, alcohol, and spices, and eat proportionately more whole grains, vegetables, fresh fruit, and nuts.[2]

- Japanese scientists reported that rats fed a diet high in fermented brown rice reduced the incidence of hyperplasia, dysplasia, and carcinoma in the bladders of the experimental group by 92 percent, 49 percent, and 38 percent respectively. The researchers concluded that a brown rice–based diet could be "a promising chemopreventive agent for human urinary bladder cancer."[3]

DIAGNOSIS

When kidney cancer is suspected, modern medicine offers the following diagnostic methods: laboratory tests, including urinalysis; X-rays; an intravenous pyelogram (IVP) to locate tumors; ultrasound examination of the abdomen; a renal angiogram to determine the location and extent of tumor growth; a tomogram of the kidney to distinguish between a cyst and a tumor; and a CT scan of the pelvis and upper abdomen. Sometimes a needle aspiration biopsy is performed, but this procedure has been implicated in spreading cancer along the path of the needle and is increasingly avoided. Many kidneys are nearly completely damaged before being diagnosed as cancerous, and one-third of patients have metastases to other locations. In the case of bladder cancer, diagnostic procedures include lab tests, IVP, cystoscopy, cystogram, bone scan, liver scan, ultrasound, lymphangiogram, and a cystourethrogram in which the bladder and urethra are observed during urination. About 82 percent of bladder cancers are diagnosed in local stages before spreading to regional areas or other organs. In men, bladder surgery can result in impotence.

Traditional visual diagnostic techniques do not rely on potentially harmful X-rays or mechanical invasions of the body. Simple visual methods allow the kidneys to be monitored long before the onset of serious illness and permit corrective dietary adjustments to be made. These nutritional measures will safeguard against the development of kidney troubles in healthy individuals and offset any tendency toward urinary cancer in those who are already sick.

In physiognomy, the area under the eyes corresponds to the kidneys. Darkness or black coloring of the skin in this region signifies kidney stagnation and toxic blood due to kidney malfunction. During adulthood, but increasingly even during youth in modern society, many people develop bags under the lower eyelid. Eyebags may have one of two causes, although the appearance may be similar: (1) a pool of liquid, and (2) pooled mucus. The first type of eyebag appears watery and swollen. Both types of eyebags show disorders of the kidney, bladder, and excretory functions. The first type, due to excess liquid, indicates swelling of the kidney tissues and frequent urination. Excessive intake of any kind of liquid, including all kinds of beverages, fruits, and juices, may cause this condition. The second type of eyebag does not necessarily accompany frequent urination but shows mucus and fat accumulation in the kidney tissue. If small pimples or dark spots appear on these mucous-caused eyebags, accumulated mucus and fat in the kidney tissues may be forming kidney stones. If these eyebags are chronic, mucus accumulation is developing in the ureter, the wall of the bladder, and the reproductive organs (ovaries, fallopian tubes, and the uterus in women and the prostate gland in men), creating bacterial activity, inflammation, itching, vaginal discharge, ovarian cysts, and eventually the growth of tumors and cancers in these areas.

Both types of eyebags also indicate the decline of physical and mental vitality as a natural result of the above conditions. Overloaded body systems, fatigue, laziness, forgetfulness, indecisiveness, and loss of clear judgment are developing. The water-caused eyebag is easily corrected by the restriction of liquid intake, while the mucus-caused eyebag can be corrected by the restriction of all mucus- and fat-forming food, including dairy products, meat, poultry, sugar, refined flour, and all kinds of oil. This type of eyebag takes longer than the watery eyebag to clear up. In visual diagnosis, the right eye and its surrounding area corresponds to the right kidney, the left eye to the left kidney. Relative darkness, swelling, tightness, or other markings indicate which kidney is more affected.

The ears, which are shaped like kidneys, also mirror the internal condition of the urinary tract and should be checked carefully. Redness around the edge of the ear indicates an overly yin condition of the kidneys caused by excessive consumption of sugar, dairy food, fruit, and juices. Overconsumption of oil, fat, and other strong yin items will also overburden the kidneys and show up in ears that are oily to the touch. Moles or warts on the ears show deposits of mucus in the kidneys caused by an accumulation of animal protein. The left ear shows the left kidney, the right ear, the right kidney, and the location of these abnormalities indicates precisely where troubles in the kidneys are occurring. Bumps or pimples on the ears show deposits of fat and developing kidney stones. Deafness is often connected with buildup of fat in the kidney. Excessive wax in the ears indicates fatty deposits in the ureter.

The kidneys can be aggravated by too much fluid consumption, and this generally shows up in wet or damp hands and feet. Kidney disorders, including cancer, are indicated by pain or hardness on the initial point of the kidney meridian at the bottom of the foot. Calluses here represent an effort on the part of the kidneys to discharge excess mucus, protein, and fat through the meridian or energy channel in the foot. Flour products, fats and oils, and sugar and sweets especially give rise to this condition.

Urine itself can be inspected for general clues to the condition of the kidneys and bladder. Urine that is healthy is light gold or yellow in color. Too much salt will turn the urine darker, and too little salt or too yin a diet will result in urine that is much lighter in color. If too much fluid is consumed, urination will become very frequent. Normally, we should urinate about three or four times a day. More than this indicates that too much fluid is being consumed, while less means that not enough is being consumed.

The upper part of the forehead corresponds with the bladder, and lines or ridges in this area indicate trouble in this organ.

Posture is a further clue to kidney condition. Leaning forward while sitting, standing, or walking indicates overly contracted kidneys. This yang condition may also be shown by a stiff back, walking brusquely, or running, or wearing shoes with elevated heels. On the other hand, leaning backward, leaning against things, and slouching, as well as wearing shoes with elevated toes, are all signs of overly expanded (yin) kidneys.

DIETARY RECOMMENDATIONS

Cancer of the kidney is caused mainly by overconsumption of dairy food and animal food rich in saturated fats, together with sugar, chemicals, and artificial beverages. Cheese, eggs, and chicken are a typical combination. Cancer of the bladder is largely caused by overconsumption of dairy foods, sugar products, chemicals, stimulants, fruits, juices, and food that produces fat and mucus. All these foods are to be avoided. The kidneys govern salt metabolism, and use of salt should be minimized in the case of kidney cancer for the first several months. Overconsumption of salt tends to solidify the mass of cancer cells.

Kombu, which is rich in minerals, may be used for seasoning instead. The use of miso and shoyu should also be light. All oily and greasy food as well as all refined flour products, including bread, pancakes, and cookies, are to be avoided. Food and beverages that lower the body temperature, including fruits, icy drinks, and artificial beverages, are to be discontinued. For improvement of urinary cancer, eating baked flour products is not advisable. All spices, including mustard, peppers, and curry, and any fragrant, aromatic condiments and supplements are to be avoided. Following are the general dietary guidelines, by daily volume, for urinary cancer, including cancer of the kidney and bladder.

- Whole Grains: Forty to 50 percent of daily consumption by volume should be whole grain cereals. The first day prepare plain short- or medium-grain brown rice, pressure-cooked or cooked in a heavy cast-iron or ceramic pot with a heavy lid. On the following days alternate brown rice cooked with 20 to 30 percent millet, then rice with 20 to 30 percent barley, then rice with 20 to 30 percent aduki beans or lentils, and then plain rice again. A delicious morning porridge can be made by taking leftover rice, adding a little more water to soften, seasoning with a little miso at the end, and then simmering for two to three minutes more. In daily pressure-cooking, the ratio of grain to water should be about 1:2. For seasoning, cook with a postage-stamp-sized piece of kombu instead of salt. Other grains can be used occasionally, including whole wheat berries, rye, corn, and whole oats, although oats should be avoided for the first month. Avoid buckwheat and limit seitan for either one of these conditions for the first three months. Flour products, even unrefined whole wheat bread, chapatis, pancakes, and cookies, should be totally avoided or limited in amounts for a few months. Whole grain pasta and noodles may be eaten a couple of times a week.
- Soup: Five to 10 percent of daily consumption should be soup, consisting of one or two cups or bowls per day cooked with wakame sea vegetable and various vegetables, especially leafy green and white vegetables, seasoned lightly with miso or shoyu. Occasionally a small amount of shiitake mushrooms may be added to the soup. The miso may be barley miso, brown rice miso, or soybean (hatcho) miso, and should be naturally aged two to three years. Grain soups, bean soups, and other soups may be eaten from time to time.
- Vegetables: Twenty to 30 percent of daily consumption should be vegetables, cooked in a variety of forms, mainly steamed, boiled, and, after one month, occasionally sautéed without oil. Among vegetables, green vegetables are needed to help recover from kidney or

bladder cancer, especially quickly sautéed greens. As a rule of thumb, the following dishes may be prepared, although the frequency may differ from person to person: nishime-style vegetables, three times a week; a squash-aduki-kombu dish, three times a week; dried daikon, one cup, three times a week; carrots and carrot tops or daikon and daikon tops, three times a week; blanched vegetables, five to seven times a week; pressed salad, several times a week; raw salad, avoid the first month, then once in seven to ten days; steamed greens, five to seven times a week; sautéed vegetables, two times a week, prepared with water the first month and then with sesame or corn oil once or twice a week after that; kinpira, two-thirds of a cup, two times a week; dried tofu, tofu, tempeh, or seitan with vegetables, two times a week.

- Beans: Five percent of daily consumption should be small beans, such as aduki beans, lentils, chickpeas, or black soybeans, cooked together with sea vegetables such as kombu or with onions and carrots. Other beans may be used two to three times a month. For seasoning, a small amount of unrefined sea salt or shoyu or miso can be used. Bean products, such as tempeh, natto, and dried or cooked tofu, may be used occasionally, but in a moderate amount. Dried tofu is better for this condition than fresh tofu.

- Sea Vegetables: Five percent or less sea vegetable dishes, including wakame and kombu, should be included daily when cooking grain, in soup, etc. A sheet of toasted nori may also be taken daily. This is especially good for the bladder. A small dish of hijiki or arame should be prepared two times a week. All other sea vegetables are optional.

- Condiments: Those that should be available on the table are gomashio (sesame salt), on the average made with one part salt to eighteen parts sesame seeds; kelp or wakame powder; umeboshi plum; and tekka, although all other regular macrobiotic condiments may be used if desired. These condiments may be used daily on grains and vegetables, but the volume should be moderate to suit individual appetites and tastes. Shiso leaf powder and green nori flakes are especially good for bladder and kidney troubles.

- Pickles: Made at home in a variety of ways, pickles are to be eaten daily, one tablespoon in all, although salty pickles are to be minimized.

- Animal Food: Fish and other animal food are to be avoided. However, in the event that animal food is craved, a small amount of white-meat fish may be eaten once every seven to ten days. The fish should be steamed, boiled, or poached and garnished with grated daikon or ginger. Strictly avoid blue-meat and red-meat fish and all shellfish.

- Fruit: The less the better until the condition improves. If cravings develop, a small volume of cooked fruit with a pinch of sea salt or dried fruit (also preferably cooked) may be eaten. Avoid all fruit juices and cider temporarily, as well as raisins, currants, and other highly concentrated fruits.

- Sweets and Snacks: Avoid all sweets and desserts, including good-quality macrobiotic desserts, until the condition improves. To satisfy a sweet tooth, use sweet vegetables every day in cooking, drink sweet vegetable drinks (see special drinks below), and use sweet vegetable jam and amasake. Mochi, rice balls, vegetable sushi, and other grain-based snacks may be eaten frequently. Limit rice cakes, popcorn, and other dry or baked snacks because they may harden the tumor. In the event of cravings, a small amount of barley malt or rice syrup may be eaten.

- Nuts and Seeds: Nuts and nut butters are to be avoided due to their high fat and protein, except for chestnuts. Unsalted blanched seeds such as sunflower seeds and pumpkin seeds may be consumed as a snack, up to one cup altogether per week.

- Seasonings: Unrefined sea salt, shoyu, and miso are to be used moderately in order to avoid unnecessary thirst. Avoid mirin and garlic. If you become particularly thirsty after a meal or between meals, you should cut back on these seasonings until the normal level of thirst returns.

- Beverages: Drinks and other dietary practices can follow the general recommendations in Part I, including bancha twig tea as the main beverage. Strictly avoid the beverages on the "infrequent" and "avoid" lists, and don't take grain coffee for the first two to three months after starting this new way of eating. All beverages are to be warm or hot. Cold beverages are to be avoided. All liquid intake should be limited to actual thirst. Water quality is especially important with this kind of cancer. Be sure that you are using good-quality spring or well water for cooking and drinking, and avoid tap water, distilled water, and water that is either too high or too low in minerals.

The most important thing in connection with dietary practice is chewing very well, until all food becomes liquid in the mouth and is well mixed with saliva. Chew very well, at least fifty times and preferably a hundred times per mouthful. It is also important to avoid overeating and eating within three hours of sleeping.

As noted in the introduction to Part II, those who have received or who are currently undergoing medical treatment may need to make further dietary modifications.

SPECIAL DRINKS AND DISHES

One or more special drinks or side dishes may need to be taken, depending on the individual case, to help reduce excess protein and fat, which are the cause of the cancer; to reduce cholesterol levels; and to assist recovery. Please see a qualified macrobiotic teacher for guidance. Amounts and frequencies given here are averages for each drink or dish; these will differ from person to person. Further directions are in Chapter 36.

For kidney cancer, one or more of the following may be helpful:

- Sweet Vegetable Drink: Prepare one small cup every day for one month and then every other day the next month.
- Carrot-Daikon Drink: This drink is also beneficial. Take one small cup every day for five days, then every other day for two weeks, and then every three days for the next month.
- Shiitake-Daikon Tea: One small cup of this tea may be drunk once every three days for a month.
- Aduki Juice: The juice of the aduki bean can help restore smooth urination. Drink one or two cups for up to several days.
- Rice Juice: This is the liquid that rises to the surface when cooking brown rice. It may be used daily or regularly as a beverage.
- Beet Juice: This juice may be helpful in some cases. Drink every day for ten days, then every other day for ten days.

For bladder cancer, one or more of the following may be helpful:

- Dried Daikon, Dried Daikon Leaves, Shiitake, Dried Lotus Root, and Roasted Brown Rice Tea: Consume one cup every morning and evening for about three weeks. After that, continue about three times a week for another three to four weeks.
- Hijiki with Dried Daikon and Shiitake: A few drops of sesame oil can be added. Consume ½ to ⅔ cup of this dish every day or every other day.
- Miso-Scallion Condiment: Have 1 teaspoon every day with the main grain at mealtime.
- Ume-Sho-Kuzu or Ume-Sho-Bancha: In case of bleeding, have one to two cups of one of these drinks every day for a few days.
- Cabbage Juice: In case of pain in the abdomen, make raw cabbage juice and then simmer it slightly for about three minutes. Drink one to two cups daily for three to four days.

HOME CARE

- Body Scrub: Scrubbing the whole body, including the abdominal region and the spinal region, with a towel that has been immersed in hot water and squeezed out is very helpful for better circulation of blood, lymph, and other body fluids, as well as for activating physical and mental energies.

- Compress Guidelines: For a small number of tumors in the kidney or bladder, a compress may be needed to help gradually draw out the excess mucus and fat. Please see a qualified macrobiotic teacher for guidance on the proper use and frequency of a compress or plaster. Several types are used depending on the person's condition. Precede the compress or plaster with the application of a towel that has been soaked in hot water and squeezed out over the affected area for three to five minutes to stimulate circulation.
- Potato Plaster or Potato-Cabbage Plaster: For kidney pain, one of these plasters may be applied for three hours preceded by a hot towel for three to five minutes. This may be repeated once or twice a day for several days.
- Lotus-Potato Plaster: This may be helpful for kidney cancer. Apply on the back, in the area of the kidneys, for three to four hours, preceded by the application of a hot towel for three to five minutes. Apply this plaster daily for two to three weeks.
- Palm Healing: This is also helpful to control kidney or bladder region pain and discomfort.
- Ginger Compress: A ginger compress applied for ten to fifteen minutes once a day on the abdomen (but not over the tumor) helps reduce blockage of the urethra. This compress should be repeated for several days.

EMOTIONAL CONSIDERATIONS

Kidney and bladder problems are associated emotionally with sexuality, intimacy, and regeneration.

High-quality foods that nourish the urinary system and help develop positive emotions include whole grains, particularly buckwheat, teff, wild rice, and other darker grains; beans and bean products, especially black soybeans and other darker beans; leafy green vegetables; sea vegetables; seeds and nuts; white-meat fish; and good quality sea salt.

Foods that harm the urinary system and contribute to negative emotions include eggs and dairy food; meat, poultry, and strong fish and seafood, especially tuna and salmon; white flour; sugar, chocolate, and other highly refined sweets; chemicalized and artificial foods; too many beverages, including soft drinks, mineral water, coffee, tea, and other stimulants; alcohol; and other extremely contractive or expansive foods and beverages.

In relationships it is important to communicate freely and honestly and not suppress feelings and emotions. If a person is not able to express himself or herself, repressed feelings may localize in the urinary system. On the other hand, one who knows no limits on self-expression will eventually exhaust his or her Ki and develop problems in this region.

On a planetary scale, the kidneys and bladder correlate with underground rivers and lakes. Imbalance in this region is like the poisoning of the water table.

OTHER CONSIDERATIONS

- Avoid wearing wool and synthetic fibers. Nylon is particularly irritating to the bladder. At the minimum, wear cotton underwear and use cotton sheets and pillowcases especially organic cotton.
- Avoid watching television for long stretches. Radiation weakens the kidneys. Similarly, avoid other artificial sources of electromagnetic energy such as video terminals, smoke detectors, and handheld electrical appliances, which can weaken the kidney and bladder.
- A daily hot bath or shower should be quick and not frequent (that is, not two to three times a day).
- Psychologically, keeping a positive mind and a strong will is important. Also, any comfortably manageable exercise, including walking outdoors, contributes to improvement. Visualization, prayer, meditation, and other spiritual practices performed daily will also be beneficial.
- The kidneys and bladder are particularly susceptible to cold weather and chills. Keep these organs protected and warm at all times, especially during the winter. In the Far East, a cotton band is commonly worn around the abdomen and back to keep these organs warm.

PERSONAL EXPERIENCE

BLADDER CANCER

Sheldon Rice's strong constitution enabled him to escape the illnesses of his peers. Aside from occasional eating imbalances and a chronic bladder problem, he thought he was relatively healthy.

After reading an article describing how Dr. Anthony Sattilaro recovered from terminal prostate cancer with the help of macrobiotics, Sheldon started eating this way and "fell in love with the food, its taste, and the whole concept supporting it." A visit to Murray Snyder, a macrobiotic counselor in Baltimore, encouraged him to make further improvement. In addition to physical changes, his thinking became clearer.

But soon his weight unexpectedly dropped, his skin turned yellow and brown, and his sexual energy disappeared. In eighteen months his weight dropped from 175 to 105 pounds. "I lost so much that my clothes hung off me alarmingly. Friends didn't recognize me on the street. My muscular system was decimated. I could no longer pick up my eight-year-old daughter."

Sheldon continued to ignore his bladder problems despite the pain and difficulty urinating. He became incontinent and had to wear diapers to sleep. Deep tingling developed on his left side, two toes turned black, and urinating became almost impossible.

A medical exam revealed that his bladder was five times its normal size. In the hospital a CT scan showed a deep-seated tumor between the bladder and spine. Instead of a biopsy and probable chemotherapy, Sheldon discharged himself from the hospital and decided to follow a strict macrobiotic diet.

Over the next four years, while enduring numerous physical and emotional changes, he did all his own cooking with little family support and underwent periodic shiatsu treatments with Shizuko Yamamoto in New York.

Over the next year and a half Sheldon discharged sugar through wart-like discolorations on his forearms, became nearly deaf for weeks until accumulated mucus slowly released from his ears, and came down with infections that took months to heal.

A key to healing was proper chewing taught to him by counselor Lino Stanchich. "I chewed every lunch and dinner for a whole hour over a two-year period," he recalls. "Sometimes I would fall asleep with a bite of food in my mouth. I attribute my eventual recovery to this incredible chewing, moderation in food quantity, eating only the food recommended for me, and a relentless will to live."

Eventually, Sheldon separated from his wife, who was not supportive of his new dietary practice, and resettled in Jerusalem. CT scans confirmed that the cancer was gone. "About seven years after I started macrobiotics, I went through a spiritual awakening that lifted me to levels of joy and peace I never knew possible," Sheldon explains. "I was able to put aside all the anger and pain of my unhappy childhood and marriage, and approach higher levels of consciousness in my daily life."

He went on to marry Ginat Corman, a macrobiotic teacher and shiatsu practitioner who had healed herself of breast cancer. They direct a macrobiotic center in Israel and have worked closely on macrobiotic dietary research with cancer researchers at the University of South Carolina.[4]

21

Leukemia

FREQUENCY

Leukemia, a form of cancer affecting the blood, will claim an estimated 21,790 lives in the United States this year, and 44,240 new cases will arise. Leukemia affects males slightly more than females.

Characterized by the uncontrolled production of white blood cells, leukemia is classified into acute and chronic types. The acute variety tends to grow rapidly, affects children more commonly, and spreads to the liver, spleen, and lymph nodes. Patients with acute leukemia are very susceptible to anemia, secondary infections, and hemorrhaging, and may die from these complications. Chronic leukemia develops more slowly and usually affects those in the middle to older age brackets. The four most common forms of leukemia are: (1) acute lymphocytic or lymphoblastic (ALL), the most prevalent cancer among children, characterized by diminished granulocytes, the white blood cells that resist infection; (2) acute myelocytic (AML), the most prevalent leukemia among adults over forty, characterized by a decrease in platelet production; (3) chronic myelocytic or granulocytic (CML), an illness accompanied by an abnormal chromosome and affecting young and middle-aged adults; and (4) chronic lymphocytic (CLL), a disease that affects primarily the elderly and usually involves malfunction of the spleen.

Modern medicine treats leukemias of all types principally with chemotherapy. Surgery or irradiation by X-rays or radioactive phosphorus may also be used if the lymph system is affected or other organs are enlarged. Fresh blood transfusions or bone marrow transplants are sometimes given in order to provide a fresh source of red blood cells, which scientists believe are produced in the bone marrow. In hospitals, leukemia patients will often be isolated in such devices as the Life Island, a bed enclosed with a plastic canopy designed to provide an environment free of microorganisms. For all forms of leukemia, 35 percent of patients live five years or longer following medical treatment.

STRUCTURE

Our slightly salty bloodstream is a replica of the ancient sea in which biological life developed during most of its evolutionary history. The blood consists of liquid in the form of plasma and formed elements consisting of red blood cells, white blood cells, and platelets. The tighter and more compact red blood cells are yang in structure, while the larger, more expanded white blood cells are yin. The platelets, an important factor in blood clotting, are smaller than red blood cells, and because of their contractive ability and size, they are classified as extremely yang. The plasma comprises about 55 percent of the blood by volume, while the various formed elements, which are suspended in the plasma, constitute the remaining 45 percent.

Our bodies contain about 35 trillion red blood cells. Each of these tiny disk-shaped cells is about 7.7 microns in diameter and about 1.9 microns thick. Men have about 5 million per cubic millimeter, and women about 4.5 million per cubic millimeter. The number of red blood cells is dependent on a variety of circumstances, including age, altitude, temperature, and level of activity or rest. For example, as we grow older, the number decreases to what we had at birth.

Hemoglobin comprises between 60 and 80 percent of the red blood cell and consists of hematin, a more condensed form of protein containing iron, and a simpler, larger protein. Hematin attracts oxygen in the lungs and transports it to the cells of the body. Then, as the oxygen-depleted blood returns through the veins, it attracts and transports carbon dioxide back to the lungs, where it is exhaled. This process is essential for life, and the efficiency with which it is accomplished directly influences our health. In a normal adult, about 20 million red blood cells are destroyed every minute, and new red blood cells are continuously formed to replace them. The total volume of hemoglobin in the body is about one kilogram, twenty grams of which are destroyed and rebuilt every day.

The human body contains far fewer white blood cells than red blood cells—about 6,000 per cubic millimeter. They are usually larger than red blood cells, possess a nucleus, and have a power of movement similar to that of an amoeba. White blood cells are attracted to bacteria entering the body, which they envelop and devour. They also gather around inflamed external injuries.

CAUSE OF CANCER

Normal blood is slightly alkaline, with a pH between 7.3 and 7.45, thus giving rise to its mildly salty taste. A pH of less than 7 is acid, while more than 7 is alkaline. If the pH of the blood dips below its normally weak alkaline level and becomes acidic, acidosis arises. Acidity is classified as a yin condition. When the pH factor of the blood moves into the high pH range, the more yang condition of alkalosis occurs. Daily diet is the principal determinant of the blood's relative alkalinity or acidity. More expansive, yin foods and beverages such as sugar, coffee, fruits, juices, milk, and alcohol thin the blood and make it more acidic. Contractive foods, including salt, are overly alkaline and constrict the circulatory system. The body compensates for poor-quality blood by several mechanisms. For example, when we exhale, excess acids are discharged along with carbon dioxide, and the kidneys continuously filter excess acids from the food and discharge them through urination. Also, our blood contains a variety of buffers, such as sodium bicarbonate, which serve to neutralize acids. In this way the blood can maintain a weak alkaline condition despite regular consumption of extreme foods and beverages.

Under certain circumstances, however, blood equilibrium cannot be maintained, and serious disorders, such as leukemia, result. In blood cancer the number of red blood cells decreases, while the number of white blood cells increases dramatically. In some cases leukemia patients may have as many as 1 million white blood cells per cubic millimeter instead of the normal 5,000 to 6,000.

In a normal healthy subject, food reaches the small intestine in the form of chyme, a homogenous liquid that is ready to be absorbed into the bloodstream. The small intestine is akin to a jungle. The villi resemble a forest of hair with millions of bacteria and viruses furthering transmutation by digesting food, changing its quality with their enzymes, and discharging it. Animal foods, strong acids such as sugar and fruits, medications, drugs, and chemicalized food kill these bacteria and cause indigestion, reduce blood production, and create the foundation for serious illness. In properly functioning intestines, molecules of jellified food attach themselves to the ends of the hairs, or villi, become intestinal tissues, and contribute to the production of blood. White blood cells are larger and more flexible than red blood cells, and can be classified as yin. They tend to be produced by the consumption of expansive foods such as sugar, while red blood cells are created by more yang substances. Leukemia, a condition characterized by too many white blood cells, is primarily caused by overconsumption of yin foods, while scurvy, an excess of red blood cells, is a sign of an overly yang diet. (See page 306 a small number of leukemias that are caused by yang factors.)

Scurvy is no longer a problem, of course, because eighteenth-century British sailors learned how to balance their extremely yang diet of salt pork with very yin citrus food. However, leukemia is a modern scourge, and modern medicine has been unable to discover its origin or cure. The rise of leukemia among children and young people has accompanied the explosion of yin foods and beverages manufactured and commonly eaten since World War II. These include snack, party, and dessert foods made with sugar, honey, chocolate, and other sweets; candy and chewing gum; soft drinks, diet colas, and artificial beverages; white bread, rolls, pretzels, and other refined flour products; oranges, bananas, pineapples, and other tropical fruits; french-fried potatoes and potato chips; and milk, cottage cheese, ice cream, milk shakes, and yogurt. Many children today eat a diet with a largely sweet taste that is soft in texture, large in size, and refined or processed in quality. Such a diet will produce an extremely thin quality of blood. Leukemia is also on the rise among Western vegetarians, especially those who eat large amounts of dairy products, fruit, raw foods, curried foods, aromatic herbs, and vitamin pills. Many of these substances are native and natural to tropical or subtropical environments. However, when they become a major part of the diet in temperate climates, serious illnesses will occur.

The increased incidence of leukemia since World War II has often been attributed to nuclear radiation. Estimates of total U.S. cancer deaths from atomic fallout and nuclear power plant emissions over the next generation range from several thousand to a million or more. Epidemiological studies show that residents living near nuclear sites and workers handling nuclear materials have higher cancer rates than other people. While nuclear radiation is dangerous and should be avoided whenever possible, the underlying way of eating governs the degree of susceptibility to cancer in any given instance.

In 1945, for example, a small number of people following a macrobiotic diet lived in Hiroshima and Nagasaki at the time of the first atomic explosions. Among those who survived the initial blast, the individuals who ate macrobiotically were able to function normally and help many other survivors overcome radiation sickness, a form of leukemia, by eating brown rice, well-cooked vegetables, miso soup, sea vegetables, pickled plums, and natural sea salt. From the symptoms of atomic disease they realized that radiation was extremely expansive, or yin, and that the blood could be strengthened or yangized with counterbalancing opposite factors such as a salt-rich grain and a cooked vegetable diet.

In traditional Oriental medicine, the hair on the head corresponds with the hairlike villi of the small intestine. When people's hair began to fall out after the bombings, it indicated trouble in the intestine and severely curtailed blood production. In the decades since the first atomic bombings, scientists have confirmed that miso and sea vegetables contain substances in addition to salt that can help protect the body from radiation by binding and discharging radioactive elements.

At the social level, various government agencies have proposed that nuclear waste materials be stored in salt mines or deposits in order to neutralize their deadly emissions. This is an example of how yin and yang are used in the modern world, although scientists do not understand the underlying principle of balance—namely, macrobiotic philosophy—involved.

There are many other sources of artificial radiation in modern society in addition to nuclear energy. Color television, computers, and cell phones, photocopier machines, air conditioners, smoke detectors, garage-door openers, supermarket checkout scanners, and numerous other appliances and devices contribute to our rapidly growing electronic environment. Some of this radiation is low-level, such as that emitted by an electric hair dryer. Some radiation is stronger, such as that from microwave ovens. Day by day all artificial electromagnetic stimuli have a cumulative effect on health and vitality.

A healthy human body has a marvelous capacity to adjust to its environment, even a radioactive or transistorized one. People following the standard macrobiotic way of eating need have no fear of leukemia or other serious illnesses. Of course, in an emergency situation, such as the accident at Three Mile Island or Chernobyl, a more limited diet should be followed. However, at current world radiation levels, people still eating the modern refined diet have a much lower tolerance for radioactivity and are at risk of developing leukemia and other cancers. Reversing the biological degeneration of modern society is the key to curing atomic sickness and other forms of cancer. Return to a more natural way of farming, eating, and daily life will make nuclear energy unnecessary and contribute to lasting health and enduring peace.

In a small number of cases, leukemia is caused by strong yang factors, especially the overuse of salt, too much baked flour, baked or roasted foods, and other contractive items and cooking methods. In this type of leukemia, which comprises only about 10 to 20 percent of all cases, animal food is usually not a primary factor. Excess animal protein tends to create solid tumors, for example, in the colon and pancreas. In the blood, too much salt and baked carbohydrates hinder red blood cell production. Strong yang environmental factors may also contribute to leukemia. For example, at the beach, the strong, hot sun makes white blood cell counts go up and red blood cell counts go down as yin is attracted to the surface and yang is brought to the center.

MEDICAL EVIDENCE

- In 1944 mice on a 60 percent caloric-restricted diet registered substantially less induced and spontaneous leukemias than mice fed at pleasure. The incidence of blood cancer in a high leukemia strain of mice fell from 65 to 10 percent, and length of life was considerably prolonged.[1]

- In 1972 a Japanese scientist reported that leukemia in chickens could be reversed by feeding them a mixture of whole grains and salt. The experiment was conducted by Keiichi Morishita, M.D., technical chief for the Tokyo Red Cross Blood Center and vice president of the New Blood Association.[2]
- Seventh-Day Adventist women in California have 44 percent less leukemia than the general population, and men have 30 percent less, according to a 1975 study. The members of this religious group tend to consume whole grains, vegetables, fruit, and nuts, and they avoid meat, poultry, rich and refined foods, coffee, tea, hot condiments, spices, and alcohol.[3]
- Genistein, a nutrient found in miso, tempeh, tofu, and other soybean products, may help prevent leukemia. Researchers at the University of Minnesota reported that in laboratory experiments, genistein killed all the detectable cells of B-cell precursor or BCP leukemia, the most common childhood cancer and the second most common adult acute leukemia.[4]
- The growth of human leukemic cells was significantly inhibited by exposing them to a medium with extracts of Japonica brown rice and milled rice. The in vitro study led Taiwanese scientists to conclude that rice could be an important dietary factor in creating immunity against leukemia.[5]

DIAGNOSIS

Blood tests and bone marrow samples are used by doctors to diagnose leukemia. A bone marrow aspiration and biopsy will also be taken if a malignancy is suspected. Chest X-rays, lymphangiogram, liver, spleen, and bone scans, CT scan of the head, and a lumbar puncture may also be administered.

Far Eastern medicine diagnoses the quality of the blood by a variety of simple, safe visual techniques. A white color on the lips indicates a deficiency of hemoglobin, abnormal constriction of the blood capillaries, or stagnation and slowness of blood circulation in general. Anemia, leukemia, and similar blood conditions can produce this lip color.

A whitish color in the pink area inside the lower eyelid also indicates a weakened condition caused by excessive intake of either extreme yin or yang foods. This color also often accompanies leukemia.

Whitish fingernails further indicate underactive blood circulation, low hemoglobin, general anemia, and a tendency toward leukemia or other forms of cancer. Normally healthy people do not have this whitish color in the nails except when the fingers are stretched.

DIETARY RECOMMENDATIONS

The major cause of leukemia is the longtime, continuous consumption of foods and beverages in the extreme yin category, including sugar, sugar-treated foods and drinks, ice cream, chocolate, carob, honey, soft drinks and soda, tropical fruits, fruit juices, oily and greasy foods, dairy foods, especially butter, milk, and cream, and many chemicals contained in foods, beverages, and supplements. All of these should be avoided in daily eating. However, the consumption of these items is often accompanied by the intake of foods from the extreme yang category, including meat, poultry, eggs, and cheese, in order to achieve a rough counterbalance. Accordingly, all these animal foods are also to be avoided with the exception of fish and seafood, which can be consumed occasionally in moderate amounts. Although they are not the direct cause, the following enhance leukemic conditions and should also be discontinued: ice-cold food and drinks; hot, stimulating, and aromatic spices; various herbs and herb drinks that have stimulant effects; and vegetables that historically originated in the tropics, including potatoes, tomatoes, and eggplant.

The nutritional recommendations for young childhood leukemia are included in the chapter on children's cancer. Following are daily dietary guidelines for the prevention and relief of leukemia in older children or adults that is primarily from extreme yin causes.

- Whole Grains: Forty to 50 percent of daily consumption, by volume, should be whole cereal grains. The first day prepare plain short- or medium-grain brown rice, pressure-cooked or cooked in a heavy cast-iron or ceramic pot with a heavy lid. On the following days prepare brown rice cooked with 20 to 30 percent millet, then rice with 20 to 30 percent barley, then rice with 20 to 30 percent aduki beans or lentils, and then plain rice again. A delicious morning porridge can be made by taking leftover rice, adding a little more water to soften it, seasoning with a little miso at the end, and simmering for two to three minutes more. In ordinary cooking, the ratio of grain to water should be about 1:2. For seasoning, cook with a postage-stamp-sized piece of kombu instead of salt, although in some cases sea salt may be used depending on the person's condition. After the first month, fried rice or fried grain with vegetables can be prepared with a little sesame oil once or twice a week. Other grains can be used occasionally, including whole wheat berries, rye, corn, and whole oats, although oats should be avoided for the first month. Buckwheat and seitan should be minimized. Good-quality sourdough bread may be enjoyed two to three times a week, and noodles, both udon and soba, may also be eaten two to three times a week. Avoid all hard-baked products until the condition improves, including cookies, cake, pie, crackers, muffins, and the like.

- Soup: Five to 10 percent of daily consumption should be soup, consisting of one or two cups or bowls per day cooked with wakame sea vegetable and various land vegetables, such as onions and carrots, and seasoned with miso or shoyu. Occasionally a small amount of shiitake mushrooms may be added to the soup. The miso may be barley miso, brown rice miso, or soybean (hatcho) miso, and should be naturally aged two to three years. To satisfy a sweet tooth, millet soup with sweet vegetables such as squash, cabbage, onions, and carrots may be prepared often. Grain soups, bean soups, and other soups may be eaten from time to time. Less frequently, a small portion of white-meat fish or small dried fish can also be cooked into the soup with vegetables, sea vegetables, and/or grains.

- Vegetables: Twenty to 30 percent of daily consumption should be vegetables, cooked in a variety of forms. In general, leafy vegetables, round, hard vegetables grown near the surface of the earth, and root vegetables can be used in about equal amounts, that is, one-third of each type for daily consumption. During cooking they can be seasoned moderately with sea salt, shoyu, or miso. After the first month, unrefined vegetable oil, especially sesame or corn oil, may be used for sautéing vegetables several times a week, although oil should not be overly consumed. As a general rule, the following dishes may be prepared, although the frequency may differ from person to person: nishime-style vegetables, four times a week; a squash-aduki-kombu dish, three times a week; dried daikon, one cup, three times a week; carrots and carrot tops or daikon and daikon tops, three times a week; blanched vegetables, five to seven times a week; pressed salad, several times a week; raw salad and salad dressing, avoid; steamed greens, five to seven times a week; kinpira, two-thirds of a cup, two times a week, and then oil may be used after three weeks; dried tofu, tofu, tempeh, or seitan with vegetables, two times a week.

- Beans: Five percent of daily consumption should be small beans, such as aduki beans, lentils, chickpeas, or black soybeans, cooked together with sea vegetables such as kombu or with onions and carrots. Other beans may be used two to three times a month. For seasoning, a small amount of unrefined sea salt or shoyu or miso can be used. Bean products, such as tempeh, natto, and dried or cooked tofu, may be used occasionally but in moderate amounts.

- Sea Vegetables: Five percent or less of sea vegetable dishes, including wakame and kombu, should be included daily when cooking grain, in soup, etc. A sheet of toasted nori may also be taken daily. A small dish of hijiki or arame should be prepared two times a week. All other sea vegetables are optional. Sea vegetables can be cooked with other vegetables or sautéed with a small amount of sesame oil after softening them by soaking and boiling lightly in water.

- Condiments: Those that should be available on the table are gomashio (sesame salt), on the average made with one part salt to eighteen parts sesame seeds (reduced to 1:16 after two months); kelp or wakame powder; umeboshi plum; and tekka, although all other regular macrobiotic condiments may be used if desired. These condiments may be used daily on grains and vegetables, but the amounts should be moderate to suit individual appetite and taste.

- Pickles: Made at home in a variety of ways, pickles are to be eaten daily, one tablespoon in all, although salty pickles are to be minimized.

- Animal Food: Meat, poultry, eggs, and other strong animal food is to be avoided. A small amount of white-meat fish may be eaten once a week. The fish should be steamed, boiled, or poached and garnished with grated daikon or ginger. After two months, fish may be eaten twice a week if desired. Strictly avoid blue-meat and red-meat fish and all shellfish.

- Fruit: None is the best, and the less the better, including both tropical and temperate-climate fruit, until the condition improves. If cravings develop, a small amount of cooked fruit with a pinch of sea salt or dried fruit (also preferably cooked) may be eaten. Avoid all fruit juices and cider temporarily, as well as raisins, currants, and other highly concentrated fruits.

- Sweets and Snacks: Avoid all sweets and desserts, including good-quality macrobiotic desserts, until the condition improves. To satisfy a sweet tooth, use sweet vegetables every day in cooking, drink sweet vegetable beverages (see special drinks on page 311), and use sweet vegetable jam and a small amount of amasake. Mochi, rice balls, vegetable sushi, and other grain-based snacks may be eaten frequently. Limit rice cakes, popcorn, and other dry or baked snacks because they may harden the tumor. In the event of cravings, a small amount of barley malt or rice syrup may be eaten.

- Nuts and Seeds: Nuts and nut butters are to be avoided due to their high fat and protein, except for chestnuts. Unsalted blanched seeds such as sunflower seeds and pumpkin seeds may be consumed as a snack, up to one cup total per week.

- Seasonings: Unrefined sea salt, shoyu, and miso are to be used moderately in order to avoid unnecessary thirst. Avoid mirin and garlic. If you become particularly thirsty after a meal or between meals, you should cut back on these seasonings until the normal level of thirst returns.

- Beverages: Drinks and other dietary practices can follow the general recommendations in Part I, including bancha twig tea as the main beverage. Strictly avoid the beverages on the "infrequent" and "avoid" lists, and don't take grain coffee for the first two to three months after starting this new way of eating.

The most important thing in connection with dietary practice is chewing very well, until all food becomes liquid in the mouth and is well mixed with saliva. Chew very well, at least fifty times and preferably one hundred times per mouthful. It is also important to avoid overeating and eating within three hours of sleeping.

As noted in the introduction to Part II, people who have received or who are currently undergoing medical treatment may need to make further dietary modifications.

For leukemia arising from more yang cases, use kombu for seasoning grains instead of sea salt until the condition improves. Emphasize sweet vegetables for the more yang type as well as steamed or boiled greens. A specially recommended dish for yang types of leukemia is soybeans cooked with kombu, carrots, and onions with a light miso taste. Black soybeans may also be cooked with a small amount of chopped kombu and cooked for a long time to bring out their natural sweetness. Alternatively, a small amount of amasake, rice malt, or barley malt may be added to beans for those with yang leukemia to give a light, sweet taste. A drop of oil may also be added to beans during cooking.

For yang cases, also avoid animal food with the exception of white-meat fish that may be eaten once a week. After two months, fish may be eaten twice a week if desired, especially by those with the more yin form of leukemia. Those with the more yang type of leukemia should avoid fish and seafood, although a small amount of white-meat fish may be eaten once every ten to fourteen days if craved.

SPECIAL DRINKS AND DISHES

One or more special drinks or side dishes may have to be eaten, depending on the individual case, to help reduce excess protein and fat, which cause the cancer; to reduce cholesterol levels; and to assist recovery. Please see a qualified macrobiotic teacher for guidance. Amounts and frequencies given here are averages for each drink or dish; these will differ from person to person. Further directions are in Chapter 36.

- Miso-Zosui: Prepare frequently with brown rice or brown rice mixed with other grains and eat every day or three to four times a week. You can cook it with burdock, daikon, carrot, cabbage, winter squash or pumpkin, onion, and leafy green vegetables as well as a small amount of wakame, kombu, or nori.
- Brown Rice and Aduki Beans: Prepare with a small piece of kombu. Have this with gomashio or umeboshi, chewing well. Have one to two bowls a day for about ten days.

- Nishime-Style Root Vegetables: Prepare with burdock, carrot, daikon, lotus, jinenjo (mountain potato), and kombu. Have one bowl every day or every other day, chewing well.
- Koi-Koku: For strength and vitality, have one bowl a day for three days. Ten days later, have one bowl of this every day for another three days. Repeat this sequence three times. If fish is not eaten, kinpira soup may be eaten instead.
- Ohagi: This brown rice preparation made with black sesame seed gomashio is helpful.
- Ume-Kuzu or Ume-Sho-Bancha: In case of frequent constipation or diarrhea, have one small cup of either of these drinks every day or every other day for two weeks.

HOME CARE

- Body Scrub: Scrubbing the whole body, including the abdominal region and the spinal region, with a towel that has been immersed in hot water and squeezed out is very helpful for better circulation of blood, lymph, and other body fluids, as well as for activating physical and mental energies.
- Massage or Palm Healing: Massage or palm healing of the abdominal area may help improve digestion.
- Swelling of the spleen and abdominal regions sometimes accompanies leukemia and is caused by overeating in general, especially protein and fat, and an excessive intake of beverages, seasonings, and condiments. In such cases, food consumption should be simplified for a period of several days, up to ten days. During this period, daily consumption may consist of pressure-cooked brown rice and barley, one to two cups of miso soup, a small dish of half-dried daikon and daikon leaves pickled for a long period (over two months) with sea salt and rice bran, a dish of vegetables such as onions, carrots, and cabbage sautéed in sesame oil, and several cups of bancha twig tea. However, this simplified diet should not be continued longer than ten days unless under supervision of an experienced macrobiotic teacher or medical associate.

EMOTIONAL CONSIDERATIONS

Positive emotions associated with the blood are strength, courage, and will. Blood disorders are frequently accompanied by weakness, hesitation, timidity, fear, and a feeling of hopelessness.

High-quality foods that nourish the blood and help develop positive emotions include a balance of all the foods in the standard dietary approach, especially whole grains, beans and bean products, vegetables from land and sea, and other natural foods. In particular, salt quality is very important because the blood corresponds to the deep ocean in which life began. The proper quality, amount, and frequency of salt, miso, shoyu, umeboshi, and other naturally saline foods highly influence the blood quality and the proportion of other foods that are consumed. A major constituent of blood is hemoglobin. Iron-rich foods help strengthen the blood, especially fibrous leafy green vegetables, sea vegetables, and other mineral-rich foods.

Foods that weaken the blood and contribute to negative emotions include too much meat, cheese, poultry, eggs, strong fish and seafood, and other heavy animal products; white flour; excessive fruit, juice, raw foods, and beverages; sugar, chocolate, and other highly processed sweets; chemicalized and artificial foods; alcohol; and other extremely contractive or expansive foods and beverages.

In relationships it is important to have a strong will to persevere and endure the natural ups and downs of life.

On a planetary scale, the blood corresponds to overall air and water circulation. Blood disorders in an individual mirror pollution and toxicity in the natural environment, including artificial electromagnetic radiation.

OTHER CONSIDERATIONS

- General physical exercise and deep-breathing exercises are recommended, especially outside in the fresh air. Shiatsu massage and other treatments to relax and loosen any physical and psychological stagnations and hardenings are also very helpful.
- Maintaining clean fresh air inside the home is important, and for this purpose green plants can be placed in each room. Indoor air circulation can also be maintained by frequently opening the windows.
- Wearing cotton underwear and avoiding synthetic fabrics are helpful for better skin metabolism and facilitate energy flow through the body.
- Avoid exposure to artificial electromagnetic radiation. Keep common handheld appliances to a minimum. If you have a choice, work and live in areas away from an electronic environment.

PERSONAL EXPERIENCES

LEUKEMIA

Christina Pirello and her mother were very close. When Christina's mother was diagnosed with colon cancer in 1982, Christina thought nothing worse could happen. But following her mother's death two years later, Christina's life was turned upside down. "I watched as conventional methods of treatment hastened her deterioration," Christina recalls. "Watching her suffer more with each treatment strengthened my conviction to seek out alternate treatments should I ever find myself in a similar situation. Interestingly, one of her doctors mentioned macrobiotics to me, but it was too late for her, and I forgot all about it."

Growing up, Christina seemed relatively healthy, although she suffered Mediterranean anemia as a child. She always had a hard time healing cuts and scratches and bruised easily. In her teenage years her menstrual cycle was irregular, and she began hormone treatments that continued for fifteen years.

At age fourteen Christina became a vegetarian. She stopped eating meat but ate lots of dairy foods, sugar, and refined foods. After her mother's death, her fatigue worsened, and she felt constantly drained. Meanwhile, bruises began to appear everywhere on her body, and she felt "as though my insides were on fire."

Seeking a new environment, she moved from Florida to Philadelphia, but the susceptibility to bruises and infection continued. Finally, a doctor put her through a series of medical tests and diagnosed her condition as CML. The specialists were not helpful. With experimental chemotherapy and a possible bone marrow transplant, they told her she could live six months to a year. Without treatment, they told her, she could expect to survive three months.

Not wanting to repeat her mother's experience, Christina sought an alternative, and a friend introduced her to Robert Pirello, who had been practicing macrobiotics for eight years. Bob helped her clean out her kitchen and gave her a copy of *The Cancer Prevention Diet*, "telling me to read and cook. I read all night."

Within a few weeks Christina's energy had returned, and gradually her blood tests began to improve. Over the next few months she experienced several major discharges as her body began to rid itself of toxins accumulated in past years. "Although the discharge was always unpleasant and almost impossible to bear, I knew I was improving," Christina recounts. "Each blood test revealed an improvement in my white cell count. The doctors were amazed." Thirteen months after she began practicing macrobiotics, her white blood cell count returned to normal, and for the last twenty-five years Christina has been completely free of leukemia.

She and Bob Pirello went on to marry, and today they are leaders of the macrobiotic community in Philadelphia, giving cooking classes, organizing seminars, and pushing a leading macrobiotic journal. She is also host of *Christina Cooks!*, the popular Emmy-award-winning macrobiotic and gourmet natural foods cooking show on PBS-TV.[6] She has also written several bestselling books on diet, health, and beauty.

LEUKEMIA

After a sailing trip off Cape Cod, New England insurance executive Doug
Blampied felt more tired and rundown than usual. Routine medical tests
showed that he had acute myologenous leukemia as well as cancer of the
spinal fluid.

Doug started chemotherapy and experienced a variety of side effects. He would wake up in the morning nauseated. When he ate, he
would usually vomit, sometimes up to five times a day. He forced himself out of bed to bathe and use the toilet, only to collapse sick and exhausted. He lost his hair, became skeletal, and was weak and listless.

Despite being warned by his doctors that he would soon die, Doug
never lost the will to live. "Even though I felt unbelievably horrible, I didn't
succumb to the idea of quitting. I had too much to do and wasn't finished
with living yet. I would look at my wife and children and know I hadn't
done all the things with them I wanted to do. I made up my mind to overcome this, whatever it took."

Over the next eight months the cancer went into remission, and Doug
had a bone marrow harvest. Within months, however, his cancer count began to rise again, and doctors advised against further chemotherapy. Another bone marrow transplant offered little hope, and Doug and his wife,
Nancy, decided to forgo the operation.

Searching for alternatives, they read *Recalled by Life*, the inspiring
story of Dr. Anthony Satillaro, M.D., the president of the Methodist Hospital in Philadelphia who overcame his own terminal cancer with the
help of macrobiotics. The Blampieds attended classes with Michio Kushi
and other teachers, and began to change their diet. "We decided to go
for it," Nancy recalls. "We got rid of the electric stove, replaced it with a
gas one, cleaned out the cupboards of the foods that weren't good for
Doug, and supplied ourselves with a complete macrobiotic kitchen."

Doug's cancer count dropped almost immediately and stayed down.
Now, eight years after being diagnosed with leukemia, Doug believes the
experience changed his life in many positive ways. "I am a stronger, better
person now. I see myself as more sensitive and understanding, and less directed at unimportant things. I spend more time with my children. I hug
them regularly and let them know that I love them and how much they
mean to me."[7]

RADIATION SICKNESS IN NAGASAKI

At the time of the world's first plutonium atomic bombing, on August 9,
1945, Tatsuichiro Akizuki, M.D., was director of the Department of Internal Medicine at St. Francis Hospital in Nagasaki, Japan. In his book
Dr. Akizuki explained how he was able to save numerous survivors of the

blast from radiation sickness and cancer of the blood: "On August 9, 1945, the atomic bomb was dropped on Nagasaki. Lethal atomic radiation spread over the razed city. For many it was an agonizing death. For a few it was a miracle. Not one co-worker in the hospital suffered or died from radiation. The hospital was located only one mile from the center of the blast. My assistant and I helped many victims who suffered the effects of the bomb. In the hospital there was a large stock of miso and shoyu. We also kept plenty of rice and wakame (seaweed used for soup stock or in miso soup). I had fed my co-workers brown rice and miso soup for some time before the bombing. None of them suffered from atomic radiation. I believe this is because they had been eating miso soup....

"On the tenth of August at 8 A.M., the Uragami Hospital was still burning. It was truly a miracle that there was not a single death in the hospital. I took up again the treatments of the maladies at 9 A.M., praying to God as I could not believe what happened. The supply of medicine was low. The hospital attendants prepared as usual a meal consisting of brown rice, miso soup with Hokkaido pumpkin and wakame, two times per day, at 11 A.M. and 5 P.M. They distributed the trays of brown rice to our grim neighbors and to the wounded.

"At this period the scientific Americans declared that the center of the explosion area would be uninhabitable for the next seventy-five years. We disregarded this horrible declaration and continued, in straw sandals, to go around the city of Nagasaki the next day after the explosions to visit the sick in their homes.

"The third day at the clinic the number of injured grew; they were affected with bleeding gums, diarrhea, hemorrhages with no signs of any considerable wounds. The patients usually said: 'It is because I have breathed a toxic gas that I bleed.' One notices these violet bloody spots under the skin and in the membranes. Is it dysentery or purpura? The fact is very curious that the persons affected by these symptoms are not burned. It happened in the shade at the moment of the explosion. Now we know the symptoms were in reality those of the first stage of radioactive contamination....

"I resolved to try my method—using miso soup, unpolished brown rice, and salt. Sugar is poison to the blood. Obstinately I persuaded the people around me, again and again. I myself was more or less eccentric. I had no knowledge of the new biophysics or atom-biology; no books, no treatise, on atomic disease yet.... I had no idea what kind of ray the atomic detonation might produce. I made a diagnosis and reasoned thus far: it may be radium, Roentgen ray, or gamma ray, which probably destroys hematogenic tissue, and marrow tissue of the human body....

"I gave the cooks and staff strict orders that they should make unpolished whole-grain rice balls, adding some salt to them, make salty thick miso soup at each meal, and never use sugar. When they didn't follow my order, I scolded them without mercy: 'Never take sugar, no sweets, sugar will destroy blood.'

"My mineral method made it possible for me to remain alive and go on working vigorously as a doctor. The radioactivity may not have been a fatal dose but ever since, Brother Iwanaga, Reverend Noguchi, Chief Nurse Miss Murai, I, and other staff members and in-patients kept on living on the lethal ashes of the bombed ruins. It was thanks to this salt mineral method that all of us could work away for people day after day, overcoming fatigue or symptoms of atomic disease, and survived the disaster free from severe symptoms of radioactivity."

In addition to the testimony of Dr. Akizuki, there are additional accounts by survivors of Nagasaki and Hiroshima who healed themselves of radiation sickness, keloid tumors, and other serious effects of the bombing.[8]

RADIATION SICKNESS IN HIROSHIMA

In 1945, Sawako Hirago was a ten-year-old schoolgirl in Hiroshima. In the atomic bombing on August 6, she was exposed to severe radiation that burned her face, head, and legs. The burned parts swelled up to nearly three times their normal size. In the hospital, doctors feared for her recovery because one-third of her body was burned. Her mother gave her palm healing therapy over the abdomen every night, and Sawako ate the only food available: two rice balls and two daikon radish pickles each day. Inside the rice balls was umeboshi (pickled salted plums). Although the medical doctors gave up on her, Sawako survived.

"My mother didn't show me a mirror until I was cured. However, I was able to see my hands and leg, which were very dirty and had a bad, rotten smell. On the rotten spots there were always flies. When the skin healed, I broke it because it was itchy; finally it became a keloidal condition. I didn't see my face until it was finally cured. However, sores remained on my nose and pus remained on my chest. My hands and chest had masses of skin which remained until I was twenty."

Because of her disfiguration, Sawako was ridiculed, nicknamed "Hormone Short," and told she could never marry or have children. After completing school, she became a high school physics teacher and met a young chemistry teacher who ate very simply. The couple married and attended lectures by George Ohsawa, the founder of modern macrobiotics in Japan, and he said that only people practicing macrobiotics would survive future nuclear war.

After talking with Mr. Ohsawa, Sawako gave up the modern refined food that she had been eating since her survival and started eating brown rice and other foods. To her surprise, her problems, including anemia, leukemia, low blood pressure, falling hair, and bleeding from the nose, started to clear up within two months. She was elated. "My face became beautiful."

Sawako went on to have seven healthy children and raised all of them on brown rice, miso soup, vegetables, seaweed, and other healthy food.[9]

JAPANESE A-BOMB SURVIVORS' FOLLOW-UP STUDY

In 2006, Hiroko Furo, a professor at Illinois Wesleyan University, interviewed survivors of the atomic bombing in Hiroshima and Nagasaki and found that 90 percent attributed their health and longevity to miso soup and other healing foods. In addition to many case histories, her booklet includes references to over twenty scientific and medical studies showing the effectiveness of miso and other soybean products on preventing or relieving cancer, including prostate cancer, breast cancer, colon cancer, lung cancer, small intestine cancer, liver cancer, and stomach cancer.[10]

DIET AND RADIATION-RELATED CANCERS IN RUSSIA

In 1985, Lidia Yamchuk and Hanif Shaimardanov, medical doctors in Chelyabinsk, organized Longevity, the first macrobiotic association in the Soviet Union. At their hospital they have used dietary methods and acupuncture to treat many patients, especially those suffering from leukemia, lymphoma, and other disorders associated with exposure to nuclear radiation. Since the early 1950s, wastes from Soviet weapons production had been dumped into Karachay Lake in Chelyabinsk, an industrial city about nine hundred miles east of Moscow. In particular they began incorporating miso soup into the diets of patients suffering from radiation symptoms and cancer. "Miso is helping some of our patients with terminal cancer to survive," Yamchuk and Shaimardanov reported. "Their blood [and blood analysis] became better after they began to use miso in their daily food."

Meanwhile, in Leningrad, Yuri Stavitsky, a young pathologist and medical instructor, volunteered as a radiologist in Chernobyl after the nuclear accident on April 26, 1986. Since then, like many disaster workers, he suffered symptoms associated with radiation disease, including tumors of the thyroid. "Since beginning macrobiotics," he reported, "my condition has greatly improved."

In Leningrad, in 1990, a visiting delegation of macrobiotic teachers from the United States, Japan, Germany, and Yugoslavia gave macrobiotic lectures at the Cardiology Center, the Institute of Cytology (the main cancer research center), and the State Institute for the Continuing Education of Doctors. Zoya Tchoueva, a Leningrad psychiatrist and medical researcher, translated *The Cancer Prevention Diet* into Russian.

In Pushkin, the former country estate of the Russian emperors and a children's convalescent center, town officials and the Agricultural Institute of Leningrad invited the macrobiotic association to set up an ecological village and donated one hundred acres of land for organic production of grains and vegetables. Soviet medical and environmental groups such as Union Chernobyl and Peace to the Children of the World hope to begin distributing miso, sea vegetables, and other macrobiotic-quality foods that may help protect against the effects of harmful nuclear radiation.

In 1992, Galina Sanderson, a filmmaker from Belarus, and her husband, Cliff Sanderson, a natural medical practitioner from the United States, announced plans to establish an international rehabilitation center near Lake Baikal in eastern Siberia for children from Chernobyl and other sites affected by radiation sickness. Michio Kushi was asked to be on the board of directors and provide macrobiotic dietary recommendations for children and their parents. About 3 million children in the former Soviet Union are estimated to have been exposed to high levels of nuclear radiation as a result of the Chernobyl explosion.[11]

22

Liver Cancer

FREQUENCY

An estimated 16,780 Americans will die of liver cancer this year, two-thirds of them male. Another 19,160 new cases will develop, almost evenly divided between men and women. In the United States, deaths from liver and bile duct cancer are growing faster than any other type of malignancy. Between 1990 and 2003, mortality increased by 40 percent in men and 24 percent in women. The overall five-year survival rate is 10 percent, one of the lowest.

Accounting for about 2 percent of primary cancers in this country, the liver is a common site of metastases from other parts of the digestive system, the breast, and the lungs. Globally, liver is the world's third most deadly cancer (after lung and stomach) with 662,000 deaths annually. There is a higher incidence of liver cancer in Asia than in North America or Europe. In China, liver cancer is one of the top three cancers, and it is also high in the Philippines, Hong Kong, and Papua New Guinea, where it is associated with aflatoxin poisoning.

Hepatomas, tumors involving the epithelial lining of both lobes of the liver, and cholingiocarcinomas, which began in the bile ducts and spread to the liver itself, account for half of all liver cancers in the United States. Other varieties include hemangiosarcomas or mixed tumors of sarcoma cells and dilated blood vessels; mixed sarcomas, which spread to other parts of the liver and lymph nodes in the vicinity of the lung and brain; hepatoblastomas, rare granular tumors found in children; and adenocarcinomas, glandular tumors that develop in the bile ducts.

Most liver cancer patients die from liver failure within six months of diagnosis. Only 10 percent currently survive five years or more. Standard medical treatment usually calls for a total hepatic lobectomy, a surgical operation in which the tumor and part or all of the healthy tissue in one lobe around it are removed. For inoperable cancers a chemotherapy technique called hepatic artery infusion is offered. This procedure calls for placing a catheter directly into blood vessels going to the liver in order to concentrate drugs in that organ.

Between 50 and 80 percent of hepatatocellular carcinomas are linked to cirrhosis of the liver, as a result of alcohol consumption. They may also result from hepatitis B or C infection, exposure to chemicals and toxins, and other environmental risks. The most common chemical stressors are polycyclic aromatic hydrocarbons (found in cigarette smoke and charcoal broiling); toxins in petrochemicals, fertilizers, pesticides, and solvents; plastics (such as vinyl chloride); and nitrosamines (found in tobacco smoke, cured meats, latex and rubber products, and cosmetics).

STRUCTURE

The liver is situated in the right side of the abdominal cavity above the intestines and adjacent to the stomach, gallbladder, and pancreas. About the same size as the brain, it weighs approximately 3 pounds and governs many of the body's digestive, circulatory, and excretory functions. Its many operations include filtering toxins from the blood; making and transporting bile; controlling blood sugar levels; converting carbohydrates, fat, and protein into one another; and manufacturing hormones and enzymes. In traditional Far Eastern medicine, the liver is known as the body's general because of its commanding functions. Using a contemporary metaphor, we may liken it to the body's Environmental Protection Agency, which monitors the quality of the internal environment and neutralizes any harmful substances. A person cannot live without a liver. However, even if 80 percent of the organ is removed, it will continue to function, and the missing section often grows back.

CAUSE OF CANCER

When leaving the heart, part of the blood passes to the digestive organs where oxygen is supplied to the tissues, and food that has been absorbed is picked up. Rather than circulating directly through the body, this metabolized material from the intestines and stomach goes directly to the liver. There it is cleansed of impurities before being sent into the bloodstream. A healthy liver can filter a relatively large and continuous amount of toxic substances that enter the body. For instance, the liver can neutralize about one-third of an ounce of alcohol per hour. However, after years of imbalanced food and beverage intake, the liver may grow swollen or hard and lose its natural ability to function.

As a compact, active, and central body organ, the liver is yang in structure and thus particularly affected by overconsumption of beef, pork, poultry, eggs, dairy products, salt, and other strong yang foods. Although liver disorders tend to have a yang origin, the symptoms can be accelerated by expansive yin substances such as alcohol, foods high in fat and oils, flour products, sugar, tropical fruits and vegetables, raw food, and stimulants.

A look at fat metabolism is helpful at this point to understand the mechanism of degenerative disease and tumor formation, including liver cancer, at the cellular level. Lipids are the family name for fats, oils, and fatlike substances, including fatty acids, cholesterol, and lipoproteins. Fats are solid at room temperature, while oils are fluid. Solid lipids tend to contain more saturated fatty acids. Fatty acids are long chains of carbon and hydrogen atoms, including an oxygen molecule at one end. Saturated fatty acids are bonded or saturated to hydrogen atoms. Unsaturated fatty acids lack at least one pair of hydrogen atoms. Polyunsaturated fatty acids are those in which more than one pair is missing.

Fatty acids are the building blocks of fats, just as simple sugars are the fundamental units of carbohydrates. In order to help digest fats, which are insoluble in water and form large globules, the liver secretes bile, a yellowish liquid stored in the gallbladder. In the intestine, bile serves to emulsify fats and enables them to be broken down into fatty acids and glycerol by digestive enzymes.

Lipids are essential to digestion but can be harmful to the body, especially saturated acids like stearic acid, found in animal tissues, which coats the red blood cells, blocks the capillaries, and deprives the heart of oxygen. One of the main constituents of lipids is cholesterol, a naturally occurring substance in the body, which contributes to the maintenance of cell walls and serves as a precursor of bile acids and vitamin D and also as a precursor of some hormones.

Cholesterol is not found in plant foods but is contained in all animal products, especially meat, egg yolks, and dairy products. Since cholesterol is insoluble in the blood, it attaches itself to a protein that is soluble in order to be transported through the body. This combination is called a lipoprotein. However, excess cholesterol in the bloodstream tends to be deposited in artery walls and, as plaque, eventually causes constriction of the arteries and reduces the flow of blood. Normally, fat is absorbed by the lymph and enters the bloodstream near the heart. However, if excess lipids accumulate in the body, eventually some will become deposited in the liver. Such stored fat, primarily from meat and dairy products, is usually the chief source of liver disorders culminating in the development of liver cancer.

Because of increased public awareness of the connections between cholesterol and saturated fat and heart disease, many people have switched to unsaturated fats and oils, including vegetable cooking oils, mayonnaise, margarine, salad dressings, and artificial creamers and spreads. However, unsaturated fats serve to redistribute cholesterol from the blood to the tissues and combine with oxygen to form free radicals. These are unstable and highly reactive substances that can interact with proteins and cause the loss of elasticity in tissues and general weakening of cells. Medical studies show that polyunsaturated lipids actually accelerate tumor development more than saturated fats and oils.

Whole grains also contain polyunsaturated fats, but these are naturally balanced by the right proportion of vitamin E and selenium, which are usually lost in the refining process. Similarly, unrefined cooking oil (in which the vitamin E remains) is a balanced product and, if used in moderate amounts, will contribute to proper metabolism.

The liver also regulates the amount of sugar in the blood. It turns any excess sugar into a starch called glycogen, which is stored in the liver. When blood sugar levels are low, the liver converts glycogen back into sugar and sends it into the blood to nourish body cells. If we consume our principal food as complex carbohydrates such as whole grains, these starches will be broken down into sugar molecules slowly and be properly absorbed in the intestines and sent to the liver. But if we take much of our diet in the form of simple carbohydrates such as refined grains, fruit, sucrose, or honey, decomposition occurs primarily in the stomach, resulting in the release of strong acids and the rapid transfer of sugar to the liver in large quantities. If there is too much sugar already stored as glycogen or if the liver is weak from chronic abuse, excess sugar will get into the bloodstream and contribute to the eventual weakening of the organism.

Cancer of the liver is the culmination of chronic liver illness and may be preceded by hepatitis, jaundice, or cirrhosis. As we have seen, although essentially a yang disease, liver cancer is accelerated by extreme yin substances, including alcohol, sugar, refined flour, and foods containing chemical additives, preservatives, or pesticides. It is interesting to observe that the incidence of hepatoma has risen sharply over the last thirty years. From 1907 to 1954 only sixty-seven cases were known in medical literature. During this period the Mayo Clinic had diagnosed only four cases. Hepatoma, a form of liver cancer affecting the epithelial tissue, appears to be linked with the tremendous explosion of yin foodstuffs following World War II. These include ice cream, soda, citrus fruits, ice-cold drinks, processed and artificial foods, white bread, and a wide range of prescription and nonprescription drugs such as aspirin, birth-control pills, and marijuana. Now each year several thousand Americans develop hepatomas.

MEDICAL EVIDENCE

- In the sixteenth century, Renaissance anatomist Gabriel Fallopius, who described the ovary and after whom the fallopian tubes are named, associated malignant tumors with imbalanced diet and improper liver functioning. "The efficient cause of cancer, however, is a flux of atrabiliary humor, for only in the spleen and the liver can this tumor arise from congestion because it is there that this humor is generated. . . . [T]he cause of the flux is a faulty mixture of the humors due to bad food." Among the foods mentioned as possible causes of cancer were beef and salty and bitter foods.[1]
- In 1945, Dr. Albert Tannenbaum reported that spontaneous hepatomas in male mice were affected by both caloric restriction and a high-fat diet. Mice on a low-fat diet registered 9 percent liver tumors in contrast to 35 percent on a high-fat diet.[2]
- In 1972, Japanese researchers reported that wakame, a common sea vegetable eaten in Asia, suppressed the reabsorption of cholesterol in the liver and intestine in laboratory experiments. Other studies showed that hijiki, another sea vegetable, and shiitake mushrooms also lowered serum cholesterol and improved fat metabolism.[3]
- Mormons, who generally eat a well-balanced diet high in whole grains, vegetables, and fruit, moderate in meat, and low in stimulants and tobacco, have about 45 percent less liver cancer than other Americans, according to a 1980 epidemiological study.[4]
- In a review of the health benefits of shoyu, the quality assurance department of Kikkoman, a major producer, cited recent scientific studies showing that soy sauce enhanced gastric juice secretion, possessed antimicrobial activity against staphylococcus and other bacteria, contained an antihypertensive component, and exhibited anticarcinogenic effects. Laboratory experiments have found that the active ingredients in shoyu inhibit stomach and liver tumors.[5]

DIAGNOSIS

Modern medicine employs a variety of technological methods to diagnose liver cancer. These include blood tests, X-rays, tomograms, CT scan, liver scan, angiogram, and radiologic catheter invasion. If a tumor is suspected, a needle biopsy will follow these tests. An exploratory laparotomy, in which the abdominal wall is surgically opened to examine the inner organs, may also be performed to determine whether the tumor is primary or has metastasized from another area. Currently about 74 percent of liver cancers have spread from local to regional areas by the time they are detected.

The condition of the liver can be simply, safely, and accurately diagnosed by traditional Far Eastern medicine. The potential development of liver troubles, including cancer, can be spotted well ahead of time, allowing preventive or corrective dietary action to be taken. To begin with, the liver's relative condition can be noted by trying to place the fingers under the rib cage on the right side. If you feel pain here or are unable to place your fingers deeply under the ribs, your liver is swollen. You should be able to insert four fingers without feeling pain or tense resistance.

For more precise diagnosis, carefully observe the central region of the forehead immediately above the nose and between the eyebrows. This area corresponds to the liver in traditional Oriental physiognomy. Vertical lines or wrinkles appearing here are a sign of mucus and fat accumulating in the liver and the expansion or hardening of the organ. The deeper and longer the wrinkles, the more serious the condition. If only one or two lines show, the liver is harder and more rigid as a result of too much salt, animal food, and other yang substances as well as overconsumption of food. On the other hand, if the skin around the lines has puffed up, the cause is too much yin such as alcohol, sugar, drugs, fatty, oily food, and processed or artificial foods.

Pimples in this region above the nose show hard fat deposits in the liver or stone formation in the gallbladder due to excess intake of animal fat, including dairy products. Dry, flaky skin in this area, extending sometimes to the region over the eyebrows, indicates an overconsumption of fats and oils from either animal or vegetable sources together with flour products and a lack of adequate whole grains and cooked vegetables. If this area has white or yellow patches as well as vertical lines, development of a cyst or tumor in the liver or formation of a stone in the gallbladder is very likely.

The texture and coloring of the skin further show the condition of the inner organs. In the case of liver troubles, an oily skin condition suggests disorders in the liver, gallbladder, and general digestive system due to an overconsumption of oily foods from either animal or vegetable sources. Yellow shadings on the eyes, lips, hands, feet, or other areas of the skin show disorders of the bile function due to excessive yang food intake including meat, eggs, seafood, poultry, and salt. A blue-gray color, especially on the cheeks, indicates chronic liver hardening caused by yang animal foods aggravated by sugar, alcohol, stimulants, or other extreme yin. Tumor formation in general is indicated by green colorations on the skin. In the case of liver cancer, this hue often shows up along some area of the liver meridian, especially in the part that runs from inside the first toe and up along the inside of the leg to the area below the knee. Also, a green color appearing on the fourth toe and its area and extending to the front of the foot below the anklebone suggests developing liver cancer, duodenal ulcer, or gallstones.

DIETARY RECOMMENDATIONS

Liver cancer is mainly caused by overconsumption of animal food, especially that high in protein and fat, such as chicken, eggs, and cheese, as well as by overconsumption of sugar, sugar-treated foods, stimulants, aromatic food and drink, alcohol, and various chemical additives. (Liver cancer caused by excessive egg consumption is more difficult to relieve.) All these foods and beverages are to be avoided. Refined flour and flour products, even though of vegetable quality, are to be eliminated in order to prevent mucus formation. Although most vegetable oils are unsaturated in quality, their use is to be limited except for the occasional use of unrefined sesame oil, corn oil, and other good-quality oil after one month without using any oil. As a whole, overconsumption of food and drink—even though of a healthy, natural, unchemicalized quality—is to be avoided. Any foods that make the body colder, including fruit juice, soft drinks, icy beverages, and ice cream, are also to be avoided. Refrain, too, from overuse of salt and salty food, as well as overcooking vegetables. All vegetables of tropical origin, including potatoes, sweet potatoes, yams, tomatoes, eggplant, and avocado, even though they are now grown in temperate zones, are to be discontinued. Tropical fruits and juices, too, are to be avoided, as well as spices such as mustard, pepper, and curry; all stimulant seasonings and drinks, including mint, peppermint, and other herb teas; all alcoholic beverages; and coffee and black tea. The following are general guidelines by volume for daily consumption:

- Whole Grains: Forty to 50 percent of daily consumption, by volume, should be whole cereal grains. The first day prepare plain short- or medium-grain brown rice, pressure-cooked or cooked in a heavy cast-iron or ceramic pot with a heavy lid. On the following days, alternate brown rice cooked with 20 to 30 percent millet, then rice with 20 to 30 percent barley, then rice with 20 to 30 percent aduki beans or lentils, and then plain rice again. A delicious morning porridge can be made by taking leftover rice, adding a little more water to soften, seasoning with a little miso, and simmering for two to three minutes more. In ordinary pressure-cooking, the ratio of grain to water should be about 1:2. For seasoning, cook with a postage-stamp-sized piece of kombu instead of salt, although in some cases sea salt may be used, depending on the person's condition. Other grains can be used occasionally, including whole wheat berries, rye, corn, and whole oats, although you should avoid oats for the first month. However, buckwheat and seitan should be limited in use because they are very contracted relative to other grains and grain products. Flour products, even unrefined whole wheat bread, chapatis, pancakes, and cookies, should be totally avoided or limited in volume for a period of a few months. Whole grain pasta and noodles may be eaten a couple of times a week.

- Soup: Five to 10 percent of daily consumption should be soup, consisting of one or two cups or bowls per day cooked with wakame sea vegetable and various vegetables, especially leafy green and white vegetables, and seasoned lightly with miso or shoyu. Occasionally a small amount of shiitake mushrooms may be added to the soup. The miso may be barley miso, brown rice miso, or soybean (hatcho) miso, and should be naturally aged two to three years. Grain soups, bean soups, and other soups may be eaten from time to time.

- Vegetables: Twenty to 30 percent of daily consumption should be vegetables, cooked in a variety of forms, mainly steamed, boiled, and, after one month without oil, occasionally sautéed. Among vegetables, broccoli, leafy green tops of carrots, turnips, daikon, and watercress are especially recommended. Root vegetables such as carrots, daikon, and burdock are also very beneficial, and cabbage, onions, pumpkin, acorn, and butternut squash may also be eaten regularly. As a rule of thumb, the following dishes may be prepared, although the frequency may differ from person to person: nishime-style vegetables, three times a week; a squash-aduki-kombu dish, three times a week; dried daikon, one cup, three times a week; carrots and carrot tops or daikon and daikon tops, three times a week; blanched vegetables, five to seven times a week; pressed salad, several times a week; raw salad, avoid the first month and then once in ten to fourteen days; steamed greens, five to seven times a week; sautéed vegetables, two times a week, prepared with water the first month and then with sesame or corn oil once or twice a week after that; kinpira, two-thirds cup, two times a week; dried tofu, tofu, tempeh, or seitan with vegetables, two times a week.

- Beans: Five percent of daily consumption should be small beans, such as aduki beans, lentils, chickpeas, or black soybeans, cooked together with sea vegetables such as kombu or with onions and carrots. Other beans may be used two to three times a month. For seasoning, a small amount of unrefined sea salt or shoyu or miso can be used. Bean products, such as tempeh, natto, and dried or cooked tofu, may be used occasionally but in moderate amounts.

- Sea Vegetables: Five percent or less of sea vegetable dishes, including wakame and kombu, should be included daily when cooking grain, in soup, etc. A sheet of toasted nori may also be taken daily. A small dish of hijiki or arame should be prepared two times a week. All other sea vegetables are optional.

- Condiments: Those that should be available on the table are go-mashio (sesame salt), on the average made with one part salt to eighteen parts sesame seeds; kelp or wakame powder; umeboshi plum;

and tekka, although all other regular macrobiotic condiments may be used if desired. These condiments may be used daily on grains and vegetables, but the amounts should be moderate to suit individual appetite and taste.

- Pickles: Made at home in a variety of ways, pickles are to be eaten daily, one tablespoon in all, although salty pickles are to be minimized. Rice bran (nuka) pickles are the most suitable.
- Animal Food: Fish and other animal food are to be avoided. However, in the event that animal food is craved, a small amount of white-meat fish may be eaten once every ten days to two weeks. The fish should be steamed, boiled, or poached and garnished with grated daikon or ginger. Strictly avoid blue-meat and red-meat fish and all shellfish.
- Fruit: The less the better until the condition improves. If cravings develop, a small amount of cooked fruit with a pinch of sea salt or dried fruit (also preferably cooked) may be eaten. Avoid all fruit juices and cider temporarily, as well as raisins, currants, and other highly concentrated fruits.
- Sweets and Snacks: Avoid all sweets and desserts, including good-quality macrobiotic desserts, until the condition improves. To satisfy a sweet tooth, use sweet vegetables every day in cooking, drink sweet vegetable beverages (see special drinks on page 329), and use sweet vegetable jam and amasake. Mochi, rice balls, vegetable sushi, and other grain-based snacks may be eaten frequently. Limit rice cakes, popcorn, and other dry or baked snacks because they may harden the tumor. In the event of cravings, a small amount of barley malt or rice syrup may be eaten.
- Nuts and Seeds: Nuts and nut butters are to be avoided due to their high fat and protein, except for chestnuts. Unsalted blanched seeds such as sunflower seeds and pumpkin seeds may be consumed as a snack, up to one cup total per week.
- Seasonings: Unrefined sea salt, shoyu, and miso are to be used moderately in order to avoid unnecessary thirst. Avoid mirin and garlic. If you become particularly thirsty after the meal or between meals, you should cut back on these seasonings until the normal level of thirst returns.
- Beverages: Drinks and other dietary practices can follow the general recommendations in Part I, including bancha twig tea as the main beverage. Strictly avoid the beverages on the "infrequent" and "avoid" lists, and don't take grain coffee for the first two to three months after starting this new way of eating.

The most important thing in connection with dietary practice is chewing very well, until all food becomes liquid in the mouth and well mixed with saliva. Chew very well, at least fifty times and preferably a hundred times per mouthful. It is also important to avoid overeating and eating within three hours of sleeping.

As noted in the introduction to Part II, people who have received or who are currently undergoing medical treatment may need to make further dietary modifications.

SPECIAL DRINKS AND DISHES

One or more special drinks or side dishes may need to be consumed, depending on the individual case, to help reduce excess protein and fat, which are the cause of the cancer; to reduce cholesterol levels; and to assist recovery. Please see a qualified macrobiotic teacher for guidance. Amounts and frequencies given here are averages for each drink or dish; these will differ from person to person. Further directions are in Chapter 36.

- Roasted Buckwheat and Scallion Tea: To help relieve liver tumors, prepare and keep in a thermos and drink one cup a day for one month.
- A person with liver cancer frequently craves a sour taste. Sour foods create more upward energy, while liver tumors arise from the accumulation of more downward energy. A small amount of lemon juice may be consumed frequently in tea or water. Apple juice or apple cider may also be consumed in small amounts and will provide a sour taste. If you develop jaundice, make two to three cups of sour green apple sauce. This can be taken until the jaundice disappears. Be sure to use tart apples to make this.
- Brown Rice and Barley Porridge with Grated Daikon: This dish will help nourish the liver and discharge old fat and oil from the body.
- Dried Daikon, Dried Daikon Leaves, Burdock, Shiitake, and Cabbage Tea: Drink one or two small cups every day. Continue about three weeks. Thereafter, drink it three to four times a week and continue for three or four weeks more.
- Eat as little food as possible and chew very well. The liver is particularly stressed by overeating. The more you chew, the better.

HOME CARE

- Body Scrub: Scrubbing the whole body, including the abdominal region and the spinal region, with a towel that has been immersed in hot water and squeezed out is very helpful for better circulation of blood, lymph, and other body fluids, as well as for activating physical and mental energies.

- Compress Guidelines: For a small number of liver tumors, the following compress may be needed to help gradually draw out excess mucus and fat. Please see a qualified macrobiotic teacher for guidance on the proper use and frequency of a compress or plaster. Precede the compress or plaster with the application of a towel that has been soaked in hot water and squeezed out over the affected area for about three to five minutes to stimulate circulation.

- Hato Mugi-Potato-Cabbage Plaster: In some cases this application is recommended. Spread on cotton linen to a thickness of a little over an inch (about 3 centimeters) and apply directly on the liver. Keep on at least four hours. Repeat twice every day. If applied before bedtime, it may be kept on until morning.

EMOTIONAL CONSIDERATIONS

Positive emotions associated with the liver and gallbladder are patience, strength, and courage. Liver problems are associated with impatience, frustration, and anger.

High-quality foods that nourish the liver and gallbladder and help develop positive emotions include whole grains, particularly wheat and barley; leafy green vegetables; miso, tempeh, and other fermented foods; and sauerkraut, lemon, and other sour-tasting foods.

Foods that block the liver and contribute to suppressing positive emotions include meat, cheese, poultry, eggs, strong fish and seafood, and other heavy animal products; excessive bread and baked goods, especially those made with white flour; sugar, chocolate, and other highly processed sweets; excessive oil and oily, greasy foods; chemicalized and artificial foods; and other extremely contractive or expansive foods and beverages.

In relationships it is important to be patient, strong, and proceed gradually. People who are impatient, reckless, and easily upset may localize their excess emotional energy in this region.

On a planetary scale, the liver corresponds with mountains, volcanoes, earthquakes, and tempests. The gallbladder corresponds with valleys. Imbalance in this region correlates with destruction of the natural environment, such as mining, cloud seeding and weather manipulation, and nuclear testing.

OTHER CONSIDERATIONS

- Daily physical exercise that does not produce exhaustion is recommended. Ten to fifteen minutes of daily breathing exercises, especially emphasizing long exhalation, is also beneficial. These physical and breathing exercises contribute to relaxing tensions in the body and mind as well as harmonizing physical metabolism.

- Keeping air quality clean and fresh is important for maintenance of general health. For that purpose, green leafy plants can be placed in the house and the windows opened periodically to allow circulation of fresh air.
- Avoid wearing wool and synthetic fibers. At the minimum wear cotton underwear and use cotton sheets and pillowcases.
- Avoid watching television for long stretches. Similarly, avoid other artificial sources of electromagnetic energy such as video terminals, smoke detectors, and handheld electrical appliances, which can weaken the liver.

PERSONAL EXPERIENCE

LIVER CANCER

In the spring of 1979, sixty-two-year-old Hilda Sorhagen experienced a tenderness in her liver area, nausea, diarrhea, and constipation. Her color turned brownish yellow, and her friends asked if she had been to Florida because she appeared so dark. For several years she had been ailing and suffered from poor digestion, fatigue, and nervousness. Some years before, her husband had died, and she faced mounting pressures from watching over his business and the demands of raising three teenagers. "I had seen so many doctors for one thing or another without improvement or a positive diagnosis," she recalled of this period. "It was always 'Go for X-rays' or 'See a specialist.' When I did go, I knew no more than before. They found nothing and blamed it on tension."

When her children grew up, she turned over the family business to the son and entered a yoga ashram in Pennsylvania. The community followed an Indian-style vegetarian diet high in dairy foods, spices, sweets, and raw fruit.

When preliminary medical tests failed to find anything, Hilda came to see me in April 1979, and I evaluated her condition as cancerous. Subsequent examination by her family physician confirmed a hardening of the lower part of her liver, and CEA blood tests were elevated in the cancerous range. However, because of her previous unsatisfactory experience with medical diagnoses, she refused X-rays and decided to begin the Cancer Prevention Diet. Although her sister had died from liver cancer two years previously, Hilda's doctors and children were not convinced that she had a malignancy and opposed her decision.

Taking a week off from her yoga work, Hilda came to Boston and took some introductory classes in medicinal cooking, visual diagnosis, and shiatsu massage at the EWF. Upon her return, she found that since all the food in the ashram was prepared in a community kitchen, she could no longer fulfill her commitments to the ashram to her satisfaction. Locating an apartment nearby, she resolved to live and cook by herself. Her children were not supportive of her approach, and she did not want to burden others with taking care of her. Although she often was so weak that she could not get out of bed, she "somehow managed to drag myself into the kitchen to put up a pot of brown rice."

Looking back, she noted: "The first sign of improvement was change in energy, which was immediately noticeable. I felt stronger; I wanted to be more active. I remembered feeling that I wanted to walk up the hill to the meditation room, whereas before I could barely get in the car to drive, even though it was only 1,500 yards away. I wanted to walk, and when I had made it to the top, I met one of the ashram members. He was surprised to see me so early in the morning. I felt such a victory and gratitude that I wept with joy. There was a time when I thought I would never be able to walk that path again."

By the summer of 1980 her condition had improved considerably, and Hilda stayed in several macrobiotic study centers in Philadelphia to develop her cooking further. I saw her again during this period and observed that the tumor had disappeared.

Commenting on her previous way of eating, she recalled, "Michio told me to stop eating raw fruit. I argued that fruit was healthy and one meal a day consisted of fruit only. I pleaded, 'Not even an apple?' and he just looked at me. Now I understand why he looked at me the way I now look at my students when they ask the same question."

In addition to yoga, Hilda is now teaching cooking, and her relationship with her children has changed. They have grown very close. "I have more energy now than my children," she reported in the autumn of 1982. "This lifestyle has helped me to speed up my spiritual evolution, and I have become a more loving person. I will continue to live a macrobiotic way of life because I love the food, and it has saved my life."

In the fall of 1981 a group at the ashram decided to experiment with the macrobiotic diet for six weeks. The results were so remarkable that Guru Amrit Desai, the community's spiritual leader, asked the entire 150-member group to adopt the macrobiotic way of eating. He described the approach as *sattvic,* or balanced, pure, and cleansing, according to the traditional dietary ideals set forth in the Bhagavad Gita and other Hindu scriptures.

As grains, beans, sea vegetables, and fermented foods became the focus of meal planning, the ashram cooks replaced cheese, eggs, spices, and honey, which had been used extensively in the past. Jeffrey Magdow,

M.D., a staff physician at the community's Kripalu Center for Holistic Health, reported about six months after the transition: "In addition to my own personal experience of many benefits through the practice of this diet, I have seen stabilized energy patterns, improved elimination, and a heightened awareness of the effects of foods on mental and physical well-being."[6]

23

Lung Cancer

FREQUENCY

Lung cancer causes more deaths in both sexes, and its incidence is rising more sharply than any other type of cancer. This year an estimated 160,390 Americans will die, accounting for about 29 percent of cancer deaths in this country. Another 213,380 new cases will develop, accounting for about 15 percent of all diagnoses. In men, incidence fell for the first time about twenty years ago and has declined from a high of 102 cases per 100,000 in 1984 to 78.5 cases in 2003, reflecting several decades of reduced-fat consumption and smoking. In the late 1980s, lung cancer surpassed breast cancer as the most lethal malignancy among women (as women's rates of smoking and animal food consumption continued to rise). About 54 percent of lung cancer patients are men, usually between the ages of forty and seventy. In other parts of the world, lung cancer is also the most common cancer (1.4 million new cases in 2002) and the most deadly (1.2 million deaths).

Among risk factors, smoking is foremost, as risk increases with smoking at an early age, the number of cigarettes consumed, and the number of years smoking. Worldwide, lung cancer rates have doubled in the last thirty years, and about 80 percent of cancer in men and 50 percent in women are linked to tobacco use. Other environmental risk factors include exposure to second-hand smoke, radon, asbestos, heavy metals (chromium, cadmium, and arsenic), radiation, air pollution, and other toxins.

The five-year survival rate for lung cancer is 16 percent.

Lung cancers commonly spread to or from the liver, brain, or bone. Ninety percent of cases consist of four types: (1) epidermoid carcinomas, which are located centrally and spread by invasion to nearby tissues, (2) adenocarcinomas, which usually affect only one lobe of the lung but spread to other sites, (3) large-cell carcinomas, which are similar to adenocarino-mas, and (4) oat-cell carcinomas, which are fast-growing. Early detection of lung cancer is not common, and 50 percent of tumors are considered inoperable. Surgery followed by radiation treatment is favored by the medical profession for the first three types. This may take the form of a lobectomy, involving removal of a lobe of the lung, or a pneumonectomy, removal of the entire lung. Oat-cell carcinoma is treated with chemotherapy. Drugs may also be given to those with the other forms of tumors to control pain. Overall, 16 percent of men and women with lung cancer currently survive five years or more. Chemotherapy for oat-cell carcinoma may produce regression lasting one to two years.

STRUCTURE

The lungs are twin respiratory organs situated along with the heart in the thoracic cavity. They are conical in shape and divided into five lobes. There are three on the right side and two on the left. The lobes are further subdivided into bronchi and alveoli. The alveoli consist of thousands of tiny air sacs. During breathing, oxygen enters the lungs and is picked up by the blood. The surface of the alveoli contains an array of blood vessels that total about 100 square yards. Oxygenated blood goes to the heart, from which it is pumped through the arteries to the cells. In the body's cells, oxygen combines with metabolized sugar or fat to produce energy, leaving behind carbon dioxide and water as by-products. The carbon dioxide is picked up by the blood and carried to the lungs, where it is breathed out. The lungs are also a major site for receiving electromagnetic energy from the surrounding environment and for stimulating certain digestive processes, especially the eliminatory function of the large intestine.

CAUSE OF CANCER

Modern medicine has focused considerable attention on lung cancer because of its steady increase. Cigarette smoking has been cited as the major cause, and epidemiologists say up to 80 or 90 percent of lung tumors could be prevented by eliminating tobacco. Other researchers have noted an association between lung cancer and increased pollution in the environment or workplace. In Houston, for example, lung cancer deaths increased by 53 percent during the 1970s. This seemed to correspond with an increase of petrochemical plants and refineries in the area. Lung cancer is also higher among asbestos workers, copper miners, and those who work with lead and zinc. In the last several years the role of diet in protecting against lung cancer has received increased attention. Several medical studies show that people who regularly consume carrots and dark green or yellow vegetables containing beta-carotene, a precursor to vitamin A, have lower lung cancer rates than other people.

Each of these hypotheses is related to understanding the spread of lung cancer. However, the underlying cause of the disease is not smoking, pollution, or a temporary vitamin deficiency, but rather a longtime imbalance in the entire daily way of eating. Situated in the middle region of the body, the lungs are relatively balanced in structure, combining both expanded (yin) and contracted (yang) features. Respiratory disorders, including lung tumors, result from excessive intake of extreme foods from both the yin and yang categories, including meat, eggs, poultry, dairy products, refined flour, sugar, fats and oils, fruits and juices, alcohol, stimulants, chemicals, and drugs.

As we have seen in the progressive development of disease, excess intake of acid, mucous-forming, and fatty foods eventually results in accumulations in various parts of the body, including the sinuses, inner ear, breasts, lungs, kidney, and reproductive organs. In the case of the lungs, aside from the obvious symptoms of coughing and chest congestion, mucus often fills the air sacs, and breathing becomes more difficult. Occasionally, a coat of mucus in the bronchi can be loosened and discharged by coughing, but once the sacs are surrounded, it becomes more firmly lodged and can remain there for a long period. Then, if air pollutants or cigarette smoke enter the lungs, their heavy components, especially various carbon compounds, are attracted to and remain in this sticky environment. In severe cases these deposits can give rise to tumors. However, the underlying cause of this condition is the accumulation of sticky fat and mucus in the alveoli and in the blood and capillaries surrounding them.

The subject of tobacco and its role in cancer is best understood in relation to daily diet. For centuries North American Indians have smoked tobacco without developing cancer and have utilized the plant for many medicinal purposes. One of the main differences between the Indians' use of tobacco and our own is that they ate a balanced diet high in corn and other cereal grains, wild grasses, locally grown or foraged vegetables, fresh seasonal fruit, seeds, and a small to moderate amount of fresh game. Current studies suggest that in societies where a traditional way of eating is still followed and where smoking is widespread there is no clear correlation between smoking and lung cancer.

The quality of modern tobacco is also a contributing factor in the increase of respiratory illnesses. The original Indian tobacco was grown naturally without phosphate fertilizers or artificial pesticides and was air-dried. Modern flue-cured tobacco is subjected to heavy amounts of chemicals during cultivation, and the drying process is sped up from about three months to six days. Commercial cigarettes also often contain 5 to 20 percent sugar by weight, as well as humectants to retain moisture and other synthetic additives to enhance flavor and taste. In countries where tobacco is not flue-cured or mixed with sugar, such as Russia, China, and Taiwan, medical studies generally indicate no significant correlation between smoking and lung cancer. Laboratory studies also show that mice on a low-fat diet will not get lung cancer from smoking, but when put on a high-fat diet, they will develop tumors. Thus chemically refined tobacco and a diet high in fat, sugar, oil, and other sticky foods will combine synergistically and increase the risk of lung cancer.

Similarly, a healthy pair of lungs can withstand and neutralize a great deal of air pollution, metallic dust, or chemical irritants in the environment. This is why nonsmokers who eat a balanced diet are usually not bothered physically by cigarette smoke in their vicinity. Their lungs are working properly and naturally filter airborne particulates with no perceived discomfort. However, nonsmokers whose lungs are coated with fat, mucus, and acid from eating a meat and sugar diet or a vegetarian diet high in dairy foods and sweets will often feel irritated as these particles from the smoke enter and are trapped in their lungs. Of course, cigarette pollution should be avoided, and insofar as possible, it is advisable not to work in or live near chemical industries or hazardous waste sites. However, some people are relatively more immune than others to toxic substances owing to their daily diet and physical constitution or inherited characteristics formed primarily by their mother's diet during pregnancy.

In Far Eastern medicine, tobacco is classified as a yang substance due to its contracting and drying effects. Smokers are generally thinner (more yang) than nonsmokers, and most smokers put on weight (become more yin) when they stop. Thus smoking contracts the body and has an alkalizing effect on the blood. As the Indians found, pure tobacco used in moderation can have a soothing effect and can increase immunity to colds, infections, and chronic ailments brought about by an overly acidic condition.

The principles of contraction (yang) and expansion (yin) can also be used to understand why many people in modern society are attracted to smoking and why they abuse tobacco by consuming it in far greater quantities than the Indians. Nicotine, the major ingredient in tobacco, is very yang. Farmers in the South have often sprayed tobacco juice on crops to ward off parasites and prevent blights. In the body, a similar process occurs. Disease-promoting bacteria cannot thrive in an alkaline environment. The human blood is normally slightly alkaline in pH. A daily diet of whole grains, cooked vegetables, and seasonal fruit produces this slightly yang condition. However, the modern diet containing a large percentage of meat and sugar has a net effect of making the blood acid. Acid-forming foods also include

eggs, poultry, dairy products, refined flour and flour products, and stimulants. In order to restore proper pH and balance acidic (yin) blood, the body
is physiologically attracted to nicotine (yang). Biochemically, nicotine raises
sugar levels in the blood. Chain smokers are often hypoglycemic and suffer
from low blood sugar, and their daily diet also lacks complex carbohydrates.
This condition is brought about by the intake of excessive fat, protein, sugar,
or alcohol and can result in pancreatic and liver malfunction, weak adrenals,
and erratic emotional behavior. The weaker the blood, the greater the desire
to smoke. The more one smokes, the more carbon monoxide is produced in
the blood and the harder the heart has to work.

In addition to excessive yang effects, smoking can produce excessive
yin effects. Recent studies reported that smoking can increase a person's risk
of leukemia by 30 percent. New studies have also found that smokers experience greater memory loss and ability to concentrate than nonsmokers.
Both leukemia and memory loss are classified as strong yin characteristics,
evidently arising from the sugar and chemicals added to modern cigarettes.

The Indians smoked at most only a handful of cigarettes a day and often
went for long periods without smoking at all. And, of course, their tobacco
did not contain sugar or chemicals. Throughout history almost all traditional
societies around the world existed happily without tobacco, and there is no
biological necessity to smoke. Perhaps the North American Indians alone
were attracted to this extreme yang pastime because their own staple food,
corn, is the most expanded yin form of grain, and this was the way they had
found to achieve a balance with their natural environment.

The unifying principle of yin and yang helps us understand the physiology of smoking and the synergistic role chemicalized tobacco plays in overworking the circulatory and respiratory systems and promoting lung cancer.
Although aggravated by tobacco, the epidemic of lung cancer in the West is
primarily a disease of overnutrition and corresponds with the rise of chemical agriculture and changing patterns of food consumption, especially following World War II. Return to a daily way of eating centered on whole
grains, vegetables, locally grown fruit, and a minimum of animal products
will make lung cancer as rare an occurrence as it was in the early part of the
century. The vitamin A and beta-carotene contained in certain foods are protective, although they are examples of several nutritional elements beneficial
to the lungs. Establishment of a regionally based natural system of agriculture will result in a substantial reduction of pollution in the environment as
well as improved health. Less chemicals will be needed for crops, less pe-
troleum for transcontinental shipment of produce and livestock, and less
mining of metals for heavy farm equipment.

In exploring the roots of lung cancer, we find that many social problems
are also related to the way we eat, and these problems cannot be resolved
apart from changing our daily way of eating.

MEDICAL EVIDENCE

- In 1773, Bernard Payrilhe, professor of chemistry at Ecole Sante and professor-royal of the College of Surgery in Paris, urged that cancer be treated by drinking carrot juice. His proposal won first prize from the Academy of Lyon on the subject of "What is cancer?" In a treatise on cancer four years later, he wrote that "with respect to medicinal ailments, barley, rice, etc., will be of great use."[1]

- In the early twentieth century, cancer began to appear among North American Indians as they began to adopt the diet of modern society. In the 1920s, J. L. Bulkley, M.D., a physician who lived among native Alaskans for twelve years, reported that he did not see a trace of cancer and attributed their lack of degenerative disease to a balanced diet. "The common cereals, which they raised, were ground and baked in the ashes of their fires, unleavened, and with little if any seasoning other than salt." A U.S. government official who helped compile health statistics among tribes in the continental United States noted: "Originally the Indians lived mostly on wild game and fish, with corn and dried berries, but, of course, as their conditions have changed, their diet has changed with them. . . . Like the white man, they now live very largely from tin cans and paper bags. . . . During the first years of my service, the scarcity of cancer among the Indians was a subject of comment. Now cases frequently come to my notice."[2]

- In 1958, Hugh Sinclair, a researcher at Oxford University in England, reported that rats will not develop lung cancer by smoking alone, controlling for other factors. "Just let someone feed a rat a high-meat diet, rich in peroxide fat, and see how quickly it gets lung cancer when it smokes cigarettes."[3]

- After twenty years of tobacco research, Dr. Richard Passey of London's Chester Beatty Research Institute reported an association between flue-dried tobacco, especially that to which sugar had been added, and lung cancer. However, he found no significant link between traditional sugar-free, air-dried tobacco and cancer. In one experiment he gave twenty flue-cured high-sugar cigarettes a day to a group of twelve rats and twenty air-dried low-sugar cigarettes to another dozen rats. On the sixty-second day, three rats in the flue-cured group had died. The other high-sugar rats were too weak to continue the experiment, and four more died shortly thereafter. The dead rats had lung lesions and cancerous changes. At this point the daily quota of the air-dried low-sugar group was increased to forty cigarettes a day. After 251 days, six healthy survivors remained. Three died of heatstroke, two died of undetermined causes, and one had an abscess near the kidney but not the lungs. Epidemiological studies show that England and Wales, which have the highest male lung cancer rate in the world, also have the highest sugar content in cigarettes, about 17 percent. France, where tobacco is air-dried and contains only 2 percent sugar, has one-third less lung cancer. The United States, where sugar in tobacco averages 10 percent, has one-half the male lung cancer mortality rate of Great Britain. Still, the U.S. tobacco industry reportedly is the nation's second largest consumer of sugar after the canning industry.[4]

- In 1978 epidemiologists reported that cancer of the lung, breast, and colon increased two to three times among Japanese women between 1950 and 1975. During that period, milk consumption increased 15 times; meat, eggs, and poultry consumption climbed 7.5 times; and rice consumption dropped 70 percent. In Okinawa, with the highest proportion of centenarians, longevity was associated with lowered sugar and salt intake and higher intake of protein and green-yellow vegetables.[5]

- In a 1991 study of several thousand Finnish men, researchers reported a 60 percent lower rate of lung cancer among men who ate diets high in grains, vegetables, and fruits containing carotenoids, vitamin C, and vitamin E.[6]

- In a 1991 Italian study, researchers reported that diet may modify the carcinogenic effect of tobacco in lung cancer. An ecological analysis carried out by the American Health Foundation showed a positive association between lung cancer mortality rates and dietary fats in forty-three countries. In southern Italy people tend to consume more vegetable foods, including cereals, pulses, fruit, vegetables, and vegetable oil, while those in northern Italy tend to consume more animal foods, including beef, eggs, butter, milk, and cheese. The lung cancer rate in southern Italy, however, was almost half that of northern Italy, although the proportion of smokers was slightly higher in the south. The researchers concluded: "Our data suggest that the effect of smoking alone on the development of lung cancer might be modified by dietary habits, in particular the total amount of saturated and polyunsaturated fats and fruit and vegetables consumed."[7]

- Dairy increases lung cancer risk. In a case-control study of 308 men with lung cancer and 504 controls, Swedish researchers reported that higher consumption of milk increased risk of the disease in both smokers and nonsmokers. Lower vegetable intake also raised the risk. There was no significant risk for the disease among light to moderate smokers.[8]

- Broccoli reduces cancer risk. In a review of seven cohort studies and 87 case-control studies around the world, researchers in the Netherlands reported that 67 percent of the studies found that the consumption of broccoli, cabbage, and cauliflower lowered the risk of lung cancer, stomach cancer, colon cancer, and rectal cancer.[9]

- Sugar increases the risk of lung cancer. In a case-control study involving 463 lung cancer patients and 465 controls, Latin American researchers found that consumption of sugar-rich foods increased the risk for lung cancer by up to 55 percent. Foods high in sucrose included rice pudding, marmalade, ice cream, custard, desserts, soft drinks, and coffee with sugar. Risk was highest among patients with small and large cell undifferentiated carcinomas. The study controlled for the potential confounding effects of tobacco smoking, total calories, total fat, vitamin C, and beta-carotene intakes.[10]
- Miso protects against lung cancer. In laboratory studies at Hiroshima University, scientists reported that long-term fermented miso significantly reduces the number of induced lung tumors compared with short-term miso. "The present results thus indicate that dietary supplementation with long-term fermented miso could exert chemopreventive effects on lung carcinogenesis," the researchers concluded.[11]
- Azuki beans inhibit lung cancer and melanoma. In laboratory studies, Japanese scientists reported that a hot water extract of azuki beans significantly reduced the number of lung tumor colonies and the invasion of melanoma cells. A previous study showed that azukis inhibited stomach cancer by 36 to 62 percent in tumor weight relative to controls.[12]

DIAGNOSIS

Doctors employ a variety of means to test for lung cancer, including chest X-rays; chest tomograms; bone, liver, and gallium scans; fluoroscopy; bronchoscopy; and sputum examination. If tumors are indicated, their location will be sought by various types of biopsies as well as thoracoscopy, a surgical procedure in which the lung is deflated and examined, or a mediastinoscopy, a small incision in the front of the neck by which lymph nodes are removed for examination.

Oriental medicine diagnoses the condition of the lungs by observing their corresponding region of the face: the cheeks. Weak and underactive lungs, as well as tuberculosis, are indicated by a sallow, pale, or slightly puffy appearance on the cheeks. The person often experiences poor circulation, labored breathing, weak chest muscles accompanied by rounding and tensing of the shoulders, a drooping posture, and an inclination toward anemia or overweight. Over time, this condition of the lungs can lead to pleurisy, emphysema, asthma, and possible lung or breast cancer. This form of lung condition results from excessive consumption of hard fats, particularly eggs and cheese, as well as dry, baked, and salty foods, which lead to excessive fluid consumption, the lack of fresh or lightly cooked crisp green vegetables, excessive smoking, and a lack of exercise.

An excessive and hyperactive functioning of the lungs is reflected by a variety of other signs. These include pimples on the cheeks, showing excessive storage of fatty acid and mucus as a result primarily of dairy food and sugar. White cheeks indicate excessive animal fats from dairy foods. Red cheeks show overactive blood capillaries in the lungs caused by too much fruit and juices, spices, sugar, and coffee or tea. A drawn, overly tight appearance on the cheeks is produced by overconsumption of salt, fish, or poultry as well as dry or baked goods. This drawn appearance sometimes includes vertical lines on the cheeks indicating restricted blood flow, contracted alveoli, and tightened chest muscles and may lead to pneumonia. Brown blotches on the cheeks represent acidosis resulting from sugar consumption, and this is a serious precancerous condition. Green colorations on the cheeks or a light green shadow on the outer vertical edges of the cheeks is a sign of breast or lung cancer. Beauty marks show a past fever in the lungs, and moles on the cheeks indicate excess protein and sugar intake. The various signs of excess mucus and fat storage in the lungs can indicate developing allergies, nasal congestion, bronchitis, whooping cough, tuberculosis, or cancer. Overactive lungs are often accompanied by constipation or other difficulties in the large intestine, the lung's complementary opposite organ.

A skilled practitioner of Oriental diagnosis will also examine the person's lung meridian, which runs along the arms and the seam between the thumb and first finger, for colors and blemishes. One common sign of lung problems is a weakness or tension in the thumb, the ending of the lung meridian. The practitioner of Far Eastern medicine will also take pulses on the wrist and press the abdominal, chest, and back regions to substantiate the visual diagnosis and diagnose the exact type of lung ailment.

DIETARY RECOMMENDATIONS

Lung tumors are one of the deeper forms of cancer, and usually the lungs are filled in part or in whole with mucus and fatty substances. The primary cause of lung cancer is dairy food, especially cheese. To prevent and relieve lung cancer, all extreme foods from the yang category are to be avoided or minimized, including meat, poultry, eggs, dairy products, and seafood, as well as baked flour products. It is also necessary to avoid extreme foods and beverages from the yin category, including sugar and all other sweets, fruits and juices, spices and stimulants, and alcohol and other drugs, as well as all artificial, chemicalized, and refined food. In preparing food, beware of using an excessive amount of oil. However, after the first month of starting the macrobiotic approach, during which no oil should be used, a moderate amount of unrefined vegetable oil may frequently be used in sautéing vegetables. No raw, uncooked foods should be eaten. Dietary recommendations for daily consumption, by volume, should be as follows.

- Whole Grains: Forty to 50 percent of daily consumption, by volume, should be whole cereal grains. The first day prepare plain short- or medium-grain brown rice, pressure-cooked or cooked in a heavy cast-iron or ceramic pot with a heavy lid. On subsequent days brown rice may be made with 20 to 30 percent millet, then rice with 20 to 30 percent barley, then rice with 20 to 30 percent aduki beans or lentils, and then plain rice again. A delicious morning porridge can be made by taking leftover rice, adding a little more water to soften it, seasoning with a little miso, and simmering for two to three minutes more. In ordinary cooking the ratio of grain to water should be about 1:2. For seasoning, cook with a postage-stamp-sized piece of kombu instead of salt for squamus cell or small cell lung cancer, although sea salt may be used in case of adenocarcinoma and large cell lung cancer. Other grains can be used occasionally, including whole wheat berries, rye, corn, and whole oats, although oats should be avoided for the first month. However, buckwheat and seitan should be limited in use because they are very contracted relative to other grains and grain products. Flour products, even unrefined whole wheat bread, chapatis, pancakes, and cookies, should be totally avoided or limited in volume for a period of a few months. Whole grain pasta and noodles may be eaten a couple of times a week.
- Soup: Five to 10 percent of daily consumption should be soup, consisting of one or two cups or bowls per day cooked with wakame sea vegetable and various hard green leafy or root vegetables and seasoned lightly with miso or shoyu. Occasionally a small amount of shiitake mushrooms may be added to the soup. The miso may be barley miso, brown rice miso, or soybean (hatcho) miso, and should be naturally aged two to three years. Grain soups, bean soups, and other soups may be eaten from time to time.
- Vegetables: Twenty to 30 percent of daily consumption should be vegetables, cooked in a variety of forms, mainly steamed, boiled, and after one month without oil, occasionally sautéed. Among vegetables, broccoli, leafy green tops of carrots, turnips, daikon, and watercress are especially recommended. Root vegetables such as carrots, daikon, and burdock are also very beneficial, and cabbages, onions, pumpkin, and acorn and butternut squash may also be eaten regularly. Lotus root is especially good for all sorts of lung disorders and helps to ease breathing. Lotus root can be used frequently as part of other vegetable dishes.

As a rule of thumb, the following dishes may be prepared, although the frequency may differ from person to person: nishime-style vegetables, three times a week; a squash-aduki-kombi dish, three times a week; dried daikon, one cup, three times a week; carrots and carrot tops or daikon and daikon tops, three times a week; blanched vegetables, five to seven times a week; pressed salad, several times a week; raw salad, avoid the first month and then once in ten to fourteen days; steamed greens, five to seven times a week; sautéed vegetables, two times a week, prepared with water the first month and then with sesame or corn oil once or twice a week after that; kinpira, two-thirds cup, two times a week; dried tofu, tofu, tempeh, or seitan with vegetables, two times a week.

- Beans: Five percent of daily consumption should be small beans, such as aduki beans, lentils, chickpeas, or black soybeans, cooked together with sea vegetables such as kombu or with onions and carrots. Other beans may be used two to three times a month. For seasoning, a small amount of unrefined sea salt or shoyu or miso can be used. Bean products, such as tempeh, natto, and dried or cooked tofu, may be used occasionally but in moderate amounts.

- Sea Vegetables: Five percent or less sea vegetable dishes, including wakame and kombu, should be included daily when cooking grain, in soup, etc. A sheet of toasted nori may also be taken daily. A small dish of hijiki or arame should be prepared two times a week. All other sea vegetables are optional.

- Condiments: Those that should be available on the table are gomashio (sesame salt), on the average made with one part salt to eighteen or twenty parts sesame seeds; kelp or wakame powder; umeboshi plum; and tekka, although all other regular macrobiotic condiments may be used if desired. These condiments may be used daily on grains and vegetables, but the amounts should be moderate to suit individual appetite and taste.

- Pickles: Made at home in a variety of ways, pickles are to be eaten daily, one tablespoon in all, although salty pickles are to be minimized. Rice bran (nuka) pickles are the most suitable.

- Animal Foods: Fish and other animal food are to be avoided. However, in the event that animal food is craved, a small amount of white-meat fish may be eaten once every ten days to two weeks. The fish should be steamed, boiled, or poached and garnished with grated daikon or ginger. Strictly avoid blue-meat and red-meat fish and all shellfish.

- Fruit: The less the better until the condition improves. If cravings develop, a small amount of cooked fruit with a pinch of sea salt or dried fruit (also preferably cooked) may be eaten. Avoid all fruit juices, cider, and raisins, currants, and other very concentrated fruits.

- Sweets and Snacks: Avoid or limit all sweets and desserts, including good-quality macrobiotic desserts, until the condition improves. To satisfy a sweet tooth, use sweet vegetables every day in cooking, drink sweet vegetable drinks (see special drinks below), and use sweet vegetable jam. Mochi, rice balls, vegetable sushi, and other grain-based snacks may be eaten frequently. Limit rice cakes, popcorn, and other dry or baked snacks because they harden the tumor. In the event of cravings, a small amount of amasake, barley malt, or rice syrup may be eaten.
- Nuts and Seeds: Nuts and nut butters are to be avoided due to their high fat and protein, except for chestnuts. Unsalted blanched seeds such as sunflower seeds and pumpkin seeds may be consumed as a snack, up to one cup total per week.
- Seasonings: Unrefined sea salt, shoyu, and miso are to be used moderately in order to avoid unnecessary thirst. Avoid mirin, garlic, and herbs and spices. If you become particularly thirsty after a meal or between meals, you should cut back on these seasonings until the normal level of thirst returns.
- Beverages: Drinks and other dietary practices can follow the general recommendations in Part I, including bancha twig tea as the main beverage. Strictly avoid the beverages on the "infrequent" and "avoid" lists, and don't take grain coffee for the first two to three months after starting this new way of eating.

The most important thing in connection with dietary practice is chewing very well, until all food becomes liquid in the mouth and is well mixed with saliva. Chew very well, at least fifty times and preferably one hundred times per mouthful. It is also important to avoid overeating and eating within three hours of sleeping.

As noted in the introduction to Part II, people who have received or who are currently undergoing medical treatment may need to make further dietary modifications.

SPECIAL DRINKS AND DISHES

One or more special drinks or side dishes may need to be consumed, depending on the individual case. Please see a qualified macrobiotic teacher for guidance. Amounts and frequencies given here are averages for each drink or dish; these will differ from person to person. Further directions are in Chapter 36.

- Sweet Vegetable Drink: Take one small cup every day for the first month, then every other day the second month, and then several times a week after that as desired.

- Dried Daikon, Shiitake, Dried Lotus Root, and Carrot Leaf Tea: Drink two to three small cups of this preparation every day for one month. After that, drink it every other day for another month.
- Grated Daikon and Carrot with Scallion and Shoyu (cooked): Eat one small cup of this preparation every day for ten days, and, after that, once every three days for three weeks.
- Lotus Root Juice: This is helpful to relieve coughing. Drink one-half to two-thirds of a small cup of this juice. You may add a small amount of water and simmer it quickly. It is best to drink it in the evening or at night when you cough. It is helpful to drink it every day for five to ten days. If your coughing has not stopped by then, continue to drink the lotus juice.
- Brown Rice Porridge with Grated Lotus Root: Eat one bowl of this preparation with umeboshi (previously washed in water) every day for ten days and, after that, every other day or every three days for one more month. Note that you may add the remaining gratings that you squeezed from the remedy for lotus root juice mentioned above.
- Lotus Seeds: A small side dish with kombu or wakame seasoned with a moderate amount of shoyu or miso will help the lungs and may be eaten daily.
- Grated Daikon: Grate about ½ cup of fresh daikon, add a few drops of shoyu, and eat two to three times a week.

HOME CARE

- Body Scrub: Scrubbing the whole body, including the abdominal region and the spinal region, with a towel that has been immersed in hot water and squeezed out is very helpful for better circulation of blood, lymph, and other body fluids, as well as for activating physical and mental energies.
- Massage the fingers well, especially the thumbs and forefingers, three to four times every day. It is also helpful to rub both hands together until they are warm, three to four times daily.
- Compress Guidelines: For a small number of lung tumors, a compress may be needed to help gradually draw out excess mucus and fat. Please see a qualified macrobiotic teacher for guidance on the proper use and frequency of a compress or plaster. Several types are used depending on the person's condition. Precede the compress or plaster with the application of a towel that has been soaked in hot water and squeezed out over the affected area for about three to five minutes to stimulate circulation.
- Mustard Plaster: A mustard plaster applied to the chest, preferably both front and back, can also help alleviate severe coughing.

- Lotus Plaster: A lotus-root plaster, consisting of grated lotus root, mixed with white flour to hold consistency and well mixed with 5 to 10 percent grated ginger, may be applied to loosen up the congested lung. This plaster may be kept on for a few hours.

EMOTIONAL CONSIDERATIONS

In traditional Eastern medicine and philosophy, healthy lungs are associated with feelings of wholeness, happiness, and fulfillment. Unhealthy lungs are associated with being scattered or rigid, being sad or melancholy, and lacking the ability to achieve or complete things. In many ways these reflect the breathing process. There is a direct correspondence between breathing and our thoughts and feelings. If our breathing is blocked or disturbed, we feel blocked and unable to function properly. Unhappiness, sadness, and depression may follow.

High-quality foods that nourish the lungs and help develop positive emotions include brown rice and other whole grains; root vegetables such as carrots, parsnips, and radishes; broccoli, cauliflower, and other more compact, condensed vegetables (some of which resemble the lungs in shape); and pungent foods such as ginger. Foods that block the lungs and contribute to suppressing positive emotions include too much cheese and other salty or heavy dairy food; meat, poultry, eggs, strong fish and seafood, and other animal products; bread, hard-baked goods, chips, and other baked foods; grilled and roasted foods; dried and puffed foods; and other more contractive items, including too much salt and other salt-based seasonings. Foods that weaken the lungs and stimulate the negative emotions associated with this organ include milk and other lighter dairy foods, sugar, alcohol, too much oil, excessive spices and herbs, and other extremely expansive fare.

Overall, the lungs help maintain a balance between expansive and contractive energies. It is important to strive for balance in all aspects of life, including balancing activity with rest, the idealistic with the practical, the personal and social. In respect to relationships, it is important to communicate freely and honestly and not suppress feelings and emotions. Lung energy easily gets bottled up and needs to be released in order to flow freely.

Try to keep as hopeful and positive as possible. Depression, sadness, and melancholy commonly accompany lung problems, and singing a happy song every day will lift the spirits as well as facilitate breathing, energy flow, and the discharge process.

On a planetary scale, the lungs correlate with the rain forests. The depletion of the tropical rain forests and the buildup of carbon dioxide in many regions are all manifestations of cancer-like destruction on a global scale. Those with lung problems need to be particularly careful to avoid

the influence of global warming and, if necessary, seek out healthier surroundings.

OTHER CONSIDERATIONS

- A daily body scrub is important. Avoid wearing wool and synthetic
  clothes. At the minimum wear cotton underwear and use cotton
  sheets and pillowcases.
- Smoking and environments in which smoke is found should be
  strictly avoided by people with lung disorders, especially cancer. Nicotine, tars, and other carbon compounds in tobacco become lodged in
  the air sacs of the lungs. This causes a further accumulation of fat,
  mucus, and other dietary substances that cause the tumor to form.
- Lung conditions are closely related to the proper functioning of the
  large intestine. Smooth, regular bowel movements daily can help the
  smooth functioning of the lungs and improve breathing. If the intestines are constipated or stagnated, it is especially necessary to chew
  all food very well, up to one hundred times, and not to overeat. This
  will help restore proper elimination.
- Those who suffer with lung cancer tend to be depressed, sad, and
  melancholy. It is important to keep a positive, optimistic, happy
  mood. Good breathing exercises are very helpful.
- Avoid wearing metallic jewelry, including rings, bracelets, and necklaces. These pick up excess charges from the atmosphere and transmit them to the internal organs via the meridians running along the
  fingers and hands. It is fine, though, to wear a wedding ring.
- Avoid watching television for long stretches. Radiation weakens the
  chest area. Similarly, avoid other artificial sources of electromagnetic
  energy such as video terminals, smoke detectors, and handheld electrical appliances that can weaken the lungs and respiratory system.
- Avoid smoggy and dusty air as well as atmospheres contaminated with
  industrial gases or chemical fumes. Visit the countryside or seashore
  or take long walks in the woods. At home, maintain a clean, orderly
  environment. Carbon dioxide in the house may accelerate tumor
  growth, so place green plants in the living room and other spaces to
  secure a fresh supply of oxygen.
- Avoid inhaling asbestos fibers. Many household products contain
  asbestos, including some types of aprons, potholders, and other
  cooking fabrics, and some floor tiles and other building and construction materials. Use natural materials and furnishings whenever
  possible.

PERSONAL EXPERIENCE

CANCER OF THE LUNG, FEMALE ORGANS, AND INTESTINES

Kim Bright, the cook at Mother Nature's Restaurant in Fairfield, Connecticut, took one look at the curly-haired woman behind the counter and knew she was ill. Offering to help, Kim suggested she come back for a macrobiotic consultation the next day. Elizabeth Masters was so sick that she could no longer work or walk. During the last six months she had undergone many X-rays, blood tests, and other medical procedures. She was diagnosed with hypoglycemia, kidney failure, congestive heart failure, and allergies. The doctors gave her drugs, but she did not get better. She found that red meat made her feel sick, so she quit eating it and started going to a local vegetarian restaurant.

Elizabeth had an appointment with her doctor at noon, but she decided to see Kim earlier in the day, at nine o'clock. She had been praying for a miracle. As she later looked back, perhaps it was no coincidence that a macrobiotic chef happened to be cooking that night.

Kim told Elizabeth that she appeared to have a large tumor in her right lung and cancer of the female organs. She outlined a healing diet emphasizing whole grains and vegetables. "I felt relieved to know that I had been properly diagnosed," Elizabeth recalls. "I intuitively knew from my green color that I had cancer. The diet made sense to me, so I was anxious to start."

Later that day, however, at the doctor's office she received another shock. When further tests and probings showed nothing, Elizabeth and her husband got upset and mentioned that they had seen another "doctor" who suspected cancer. "They scurried around, looked at the tests and X-rays again, and discovered their error," Elizabeth recounted. "Their diagnosis was cancer of the female organs, intestines, and a large tumor in the lower lobe of the right lung. They told me I had only two weeks to live."

But rather than staying in New Haven and having radical surgery and medical treatment at Yale University Hospital, Elizabeth decided to return home to Maine. "Over their objections, I decided to give the diet a try. I could see that food had created my illness, so I wanted to give my body a chance to heal itself with the proper way of eating. I went home to live or die."

Over the years Elizabeth had experienced many difficulties. Born in Missouri to parents who were unable to care for her because of alcohol problems and violence, she grew up at her grandmother's. As a child she suffered from swollen adenoids and tonsils, and a local physician removed them by holding a rusty tin can filled with cotton over her nose and giving her ether. When she awoke, she was offered ice cream but chose hot dogs and sauerkraut instead. She had come to like the fresh meats, eggs, and dairy food of the countryside.

After years of neglect and abuse as a child, Elizabeth left home at fifteen and found a friend to live with. Working hard, going to school, and continuing to eat the modern American diet, she continued to have problems with her menstrual cycle, and her abdomen was always distended. In high school an appendix ruptured, and ovarian cysts were removed surgically. Elizabeth married at age twenty and gave birth to her first child at age twenty-one. The marriage lasted five years. Elizabeth didn't really know what was wrong; she just felt she had to get out. She went to work and began fitting in with the coffee and doughnut for breakfast, hamburger for lunch, and ice cream for supper crowd.

At age twenty-five, Elizabeth married again and had her second child. She worked at a very stressful job in the aircraft industry, ran a cattle ranch, and continued to eat a diet high in animal food. This marriage lasted fifteen years, although her health problems continued—losing weight, gaining weight, distended stomach, emotional outbursts, an enlarged pancreas—for which she took various medical drugs, including Librium, Valium, antibodies, and allergy shots. When this marriage failed, she took a job that required a lot of traveling.

Elizabeth noticed changes in herself that she didn't like, such as low self-esteem (which showed itself in poor personal grooming, excessive weight, compulsive overeating, and excessive alcohol consumption). She lived life in the fast lane. She would eat excessively, then miss three days of work—sleeping all the time—to let her body recover. Again, excessive menstruation, along with diarrhea, low energy, and extreme pain, caught up with her. This was when she sought medical help and became more vegetarian.

After two weeks eating macrobiotically, Elizabeth was still alive. Able to get out of bed and walk for the first time in months, she returned to work. But after a few months it became apparent that she was not really getting better, and she came to see me in Brookline, Massachusetts. I asked if she could quit work and cook for herself. She wasn't sure she would have the courage to quit, but when she returned to work, her boss came in and told her the company had lost the contract it was working on and could no longer keep her as an employee. With the decision made for her, she began to take macrobiotic cooking classes and concentrate solely on her recovery.

That was nine years ago. Today Elizabeth is in good health and lives with her husband in Maine. She has graduated from the Kushi Institute in Becket, speaks and teaches at centers in New England, and spreads macrobiotics wherever she goes. She is a living testament to the power of food, faith in the universe, and the body's amazing healing abilities.[13]

LUNG CANCER

Janet E. Vitt, R.N., had just turned forty-five when she was diagnosed with small cell adenocarcinoma of the lung, stage 4. The cancer had metastasized to her liver, pancreas, abdomen, and lymph system. As a registered nurse in the Cleveland area, she knew that her prognosis was very poor. She had surgery on the abdominal mass and had several chemotherapy treatments, but she lost one-third of her weight and further treatments were not recommended. Through her sister she went to see a macrobiotic counselor, François Roland. "Observing my face and the palms of my hands, François asked questions related to diet. I will never forget the words he said to me, 'You could be healed.'" Meanwhile, her parents and family had come to assist in her final hours. Instead, they started cooking whole grains, organic vegetables, beans, sea vegetables, and preparing special home remedies for Janet. Looking back, she identified cheese as the main cause of her illness. "I was obsessed with cheese. Not a day passed when I didn't eat it. I loved cheese omelettes, I enjoyed cheese on hamburgers, and I added cheese to all my vegetables. On Tuesdays and Thursdays, after aerobics class, I would come home and eat cheese and crackers. I was a cheeseaholic."

After ten months on the new way of eating, the tumors were all gone. In addition, the migraine headaches she suffered from for over twenty years went away. Joint pain in her knees and ankles disappeared, and many other conditions cleared up. "My physicians were amazed at my recovery," she recalled. "At the hospital, the Tumor Board met to compare the new scans with my originals and couldn't believe they were taken of the same person."

Janet went on to complete studies at the Kushi Institute and become a macrobiotic cook and teacher. Cancer-free now for the last ten years, she has helped countless other people adopt a natural way of life.[14]

Lymphatic Cancer: Lymphoma and Hodgkin's Disease

FREQUENCY

Cancer of the lymphatic system will kill 19,730 Americans this year, while 71,380 new cases will develop, including 8,190 cases of Hodgkin's lymphoma and 63,190 cases of non-Hodgkin's lymphoma (NHL). The prevalence of NHL has nearly doubled since the 1970s, partly due to AIDS-related cases. Deaths from Hodgkin's disease have fallen by about two-thirds over the last thirty years, while those from other kinds of lymphoma have risen by almost the same amount.

Lymphoma affects men and women about evenly and is usually divided into types. Hodgkin's disease, which particularly affects people aged fifteen to twenty-four and over fifty, usually involves enlarged lymph nodes in the neck, armpit, or groin. It often spreads to the brain and adjacent lymph nodes. Depending on the stage and cell type, Hodgkin's is treated with radiation and chemotherapy. NHL is usually treated with just chemotherapy, monoclonal antibodies, and, for persistent or recurrent cases, stem cell transplantation. Eighty-six percent of those with Hodgkin's disease survive five years or longer. Non-Hodgkin's lymphomas are divided into eight major types depending on the type of cells affected and their state of differentiation. This form of lymphoma may appear throughout the body and in sites other than the lymph nodes, such as the digestive tract. Non-Hodgkin's lymphomas metastasize in erratic manners. Radiation and chemotherapy are major methods of treatment.

Altogether, the remission rate for these eight lymphomas is 63 percent. There are also several rarer forms of lymphoma such as mycosis fungoides and Burkitt's lymphoma.

Medical risk factors for NHL include organ transplants, severe auto-immune conditions, infection with HIV, human T-cell leukemia/lymphoma virus 1 (HTLV-1), and possibly hepatitis C virus. Burkitt and some non-Hodgkin's types have been linked with Epstein-Barr virus (EBV). Environ-mental risks include occupational exposure to herbicides, chlorinated organic compounds, genetically altered crops, and other toxins.

Between 53 to 57 percent of those with Hodgkin's disease survive five years or longer.

STRUCTURE

The lymphatic system consists of lymph capillaries, vessels, ducts, and nodes, as well as such organs as the spleen and tonsils. The lymphatic system is closely related to the blood system. When blood circulates, some of the fluid and other elements in the blood leak out due to the enormous pressure the blood is under. This clear liquid or lymph accumulates between the cells and blood capillaries. The lymph system transports this substance through a net-work of small, clear tubes and rejoins with the bloodstream near the collar-bone. In structure, the bloodstream is generally more yang, since its main function is to transport red blood cells. The lymph stream, consisting prima-rily of white blood cells, is more yin. Both comprise the circulatory system as a whole and circulate in opposite yet complementary directions. Blood circu-lation begins in the heart, radiates outward to the more peripheral regions, and then returns. Conversely, the flow of lymph begins in the peripheral body tissues and then enters the central bloodstream.

Unlike the bloodstream, the lymphatic system has no central organ to pump the lymph fluid. The flow of lymph is maintained by several factors such as the activity and contraction of the lungs and diaphragm during breath-ing and the movements of the villi and the contractions of the small intes-tine. The spleen is the major organ of the lymphatic system. Located opposite the liver on the left side of the body, the spleen filters substances like bacteria and worn-out red blood cells from the lymph and body fluid. The spleen contributes to the formation of white blood cells, especially lym-phocytes; stores blood and minerals, particularly iron; produces antibodies; and contributes to the production of bile. The liver and spleen are comple-mentary. The liver is yang (compact) in comparison and functions in coordi-nation with the bloodstream. The more yin (expanded) spleen serves as the major focus of the lymphatic system.

Also associated with the lymph are the tonsils. The main function of the tonsils is to localize various types of toxic excess for discharging from the body. For example, after consumption of an extreme food, such as an excessive volume of sugar, oil, fats, soft drinks, fruits, juices, refined flour, or chemicals, additional white blood cells are created in the tonsils to neutralize any harmful bacteria that may form in the lymph, while minerals start to gather in this region as a buffer for the discharge of acids. In the meantime, the tonsils may become inflamed and the body temperature may rise. If at this time the person has the tonsils removed, the fever and inflammation may disappear, but the toxic bodily fluids will continue to circulate throughout the system, and the remaining lymphatic organs will have to work much harder to perform the cleaning and discharge function of the tonsils. The net result is a reduction in the ability of the lymphatic system to efficiently rid the body of toxic excess.

The lymphatic system also contains another major organ, which is located above the heart. Known as the thymus, this organ reaches its largest size at the age of two and then gradually declines until it disappears entirely. The thymus produces white blood cells along with certain types of antibodies.

CAUSE OF CANCER

If the bloodstream is filled with fat and mucus, which are strong in acid, an excess will begin to accumulate in the organs. Since the lungs and kidneys are usually affected first, their functions of filtering and cleansing the blood become less efficient. This situation leads to further deterioration of the blood quality and also affects the lymphatic system. General lymphatic troubles can be summarized into two types. The first involves expansion or inflammation of the lymphatic nodes and organs. In extreme cases this overly yin condition leads to a rupture of the lymphatic vessels. These problems result when the lymph fluid contains too much fatty acid. The other, more yang condition is hardening of the lymph nodes, organs, ducts, and capillaries.

As we have seen, operations such as tonsillectomies contribute to the deterioration of the lymphatic system, since they reduce the ability of this system to cleanse itself. Swollen tonsils and lymph glands result from overconsumption of refined and artificial foods, sugar, soft drinks, tropical fruits and vegetables, milk and dairy products, spices, and other extreme foods from the yin category usually higher in acid. These swellings represent a healthy reaction of the body to localize, neutralize, and discharge this excess. Continued consumption of these foods may produce a chronic deterioration of the quality of the blood and lymph. When the red blood cells begin to lose their capacity to change into normal body cells, the body starts to create a degenerate type of cell that is known as cancerous.

In Hodgkin's disease the lymph nodes and spleen become inflamed, while in lymphomas a malignant tumor develops within the lymphoid tis sue, and the lymphatic organs become swollen. Both diseases involve an increase in the number of white blood cells. Excessive intake of yin-type foods and beverages is the primary cause of most lymphatic cancers. At the same time a decrease in the number of red blood cells reflects a lack of minerals and other balanced foods centered around natural complex carbohydrate in the diet. Compared to other forms of cancer, especially tumors in the deep inner organs, lymphatic cancer and leukemia are relatively easy to relieve.

Lymphatic cancers primarily arise from overexpansion or inflammation of the lymph nodes and organs as a result of too much yin foods and beverages. Hodgkin's disease is the most expansive form of this disease, resulting from an excessive intake of sugar, chocolate, and other sweets; milk, ice cream, and dairy; fruit and juice; oily and greasy foods; alcohol; drugs; and chemicals. Non-Hodgkin's disease also usually involves extreme yin factors but in less volume or frequency. There is also a more yang form of non-Hodgkin's lymphoma caused by taking too much salt, baked flour, and other contractive fare.

MEDICAL EVIDENCE

- People who regularly eat cereal grains, pulses, vegetables, seeds, and nuts are less likely to get lymphoma or Hodgkin's disease than persons who do not usually eat these foods, according to a 1976 epidemiological survey. The sixteen-nation study, based on World Health Organization statistics, found a high correlation between consumption of animal protein, particularly from beef and dairy products, and lymphoma mortality. "Ingestion of cow's milk can produce generalized lymphadenopathy, hepatoslenomegaly, and profound adenoid hypertrophy," the researcher commented on the mechanism of carcinogenesis. "It has been conservatively estimated that more than 100 distinct antigens are released by the normal digestion of cow's milk, which may evoke production of all antibody classes." The studies indicated that beef and dairy food increased the risk of lymphosarcoma and Hodgkin's disease by 70 and 61 percent respectively, while cereal grains lowered the risk by 46 and 38 percent.[1]
- The average American eats 9 pounds of chemical additives a year, including preservatives, flavoring agents, stabilizers, and artificial colors. Red Dye No. 40, found in imitation fruit drinks, soda, hot dogs, jellies, candy, ice cream, and some cosmetics, has been linked to lymphomas in laboratory experiments.[2]
- In a case-control study in Italy, researchers found that high milk intake was associated with an 80 to 90 percent higher risk of non-Hodgkin's lymphoma and soft tissue sarcomas. Ham and liver intake were linked

to higher risk of Hodgkin's disease, while butter increased the risk of myelomas almost three times. Whole grains and vegetables were protective for many lymphoid cancers.[3]

- In a randomized crossover study, researchers at the Northern Ireland Centre for Food and Health, University of Ulster, fed 85 grams of raw watercress daily to thirty healthy men and thirty healthy women (with an age range of nineteen to fifty-five) for eight weeks in addition to their normal diet. Watercress supplementation was associated with reductions in DMA damage in lymphocytes and an increase in lutein and beta-carotene. "The results support the theory that consumption of watercress can be linked to a reduced risk of cancer via decreased damage to DNA and possible modulation of antioxidant status by increasing carotenoid concentrations," the scientists concluded.[4]

DIAGNOSIS

Hodgkin's disease is diagnosed medically by laboratory tests and usually involves the surgical removal of a lymph node to be examined under a microscope for malignancy. If the nodes are not involved, a variety of other methods will be used, including a bone marrow biopsy; lymphangiogram; IVP; liver, spleen, and bone scans; and abdominal or chest CT scan. In some cases the abdominal wall may be opened surgically for inspection, and the spleen will be removed in an operation known as a splenectomy. For non-Hodgkin's lymphomas, an upper and lower GI series is taken, and a spinal tap will be performed to check for metastases to the brain.

Oriental diagnosis focuses primarily on visual features, especially colors, to ascertain the condition of the lymphatic system. A pinkish white color on the lips indicates weakening lymphatic functions and other disorders, including a tendency toward Hodgkin's disease. This color is caused by excessive consumption of dairy products, fats, sugar, and fruits. A reddish yellow color inside the lower eyelids shows disorder in the circulatory system, including the spleen function. This color is caused by an excessive intake of foods from the extreme yang category, such as poultry, eggs, and dairy products, as well as excess yin-type foods, including sugar, fruits, and chemicals.

A white tone to the skin generally indicates contraction of blood capillaries and tissues and inner-organ problems, especially spleen and lymph disorders. This color is caused by excessive yang intake, especially animal food rich in fat, all dairy products, or the overconsumption of salts and minerals. A pale color on the face often arises with a light green shade or tone in the case of lymphoma and Hodgkin's disease due to a lack of balanced minerals and an overall anemic condition.

The temples on the head correspond to the functions of the spleen and other inner organs. Green vessels appearing in this region show abnormal lymph circulation due to an overactive spleen or underactive gallbladder and are caused by excessive fluid and sugar, fats and oils, alcohol and stimulants, and other extreme foods and beverages from the yin category.

The outer layer of the ear shows circulatory and excretory systems. If this area has an abnormally red color, except during vigorous exercise or after being outside in cold weather, it indicates lymphatic and spleen disorders. If the whole nose, not only the tip area, is reddish in color from expansion of the blood capillaries, disorders are indicated also in the spleen and lymph system.

By observing a combination of these and other signs, potential lymph diseases, including cancer, can be detected long before they reach the chronic or degenerative stages and appropriate dietary adjustments made.

DIETARY RECOMMENDATIONS

The major cause of lymphoma and Hodgkin's disease is the longtime continuous consumption of foods and beverages in the extreme yin category, including dairy food of all kinds and sweets that include sugar, sugar-treated foods, and drinks. All of these should be avoided in daily eating. However, the consumption of these items is often accompanied by the intake of foods from the extreme yang category, including chicken and eggs, meat, poultry, and cheese, in order to achieve a rough counterbalance. Accordingly, all these animal foods are also to be avoided, with the exception of fish and seafood, which can be consumed occasionally in small amounts. Although they are not the direct cause, the following enhance lymphomic conditions and should also be discontinued: ice-cold food and drinks; hot, stimulating, and aromatic spices; various herbs and herb drinks that have stimulant effects; and vegetables that historically originated in the tropics, including potatoes, tomatoes, and eggplant. These nightshade plants especially enhance Hodgkin's disease. In preparing food, beware of using an excessive volume of oil. However, after the first month, during which no oil should be used, a moderate amount of unrefined vegetable oil may be used frequently in sautéing vegetables. No raw, uncooked foods should be eaten. For lymphatic cancer it is extremely important to avoid overconsumption of food. Eat less and chew very, very well.

The dietary recommendations for younger children with lymphatic cancer are included in the chapter on children's cancer. Following are daily dietary guidelines, by volume, for the prevention and relief of lymphoma in older children or adults:

- Whole Grains: Forty to 50 percent of daily consumption, by volume, should be whole cereal grains. The first day prepare plain short- or medium-grain brown rice, pressure-cooked or cooked in a heavy cast-iron or ceramic pot with a heavy lid. On the following days prepare brown rice cooked with 20 to 30 percent millet, then rice with 20 to 30 percent barley, then rice with 20 to 30 percent aduki beans or lentils, and then plain rice again. A delicious morning porridge can be made by taking leftover rice, adding a little more water to soften it, seasoning with a little miso, and simmering for two to three minutes more. In ordinary cooking the ratio of grain to water should be about 1:2. For seasoning, for more yin lymphomas, either a pinch of sea salt or a small square of kombu the size of a postage stamp may be used to season the grain during cooking. For the more yang form of lymphoma, use kombu for seasoning grains until the condition improves. After the first month, these grains can be prepared once or twice a week in the form of fried grains with vegetables. Other grains can be used occasionally, including whole wheat berries, rye, corn, and whole oats, although oats should be avoided for the first month. Buckwheat and seitan should be minimized. Good-quality sourdough bread may be enjoyed two to three times a week, and noodles, both udon and soba, may also be eaten two to three times a week.

Avoid all hard baked products until the condition improves, including cookies, cake, pie, crackers, muffins, and the like.

- Soup: Five to 10 percent of daily consumption should be soup, consisting of one or two cups or bowls per day cooked with wakame sea vegetable and various land vegetables such as onions and carrots, seasoned with miso or shoyu. Occasionally a small amount of shiitake mushrooms may be added to the soup. Lotus root should be used often in soup. The miso may be barley miso, brown rice miso, or soybean (hatcho) miso, and should be naturally aged two to three years. To satisfy a sweet tooth, millet soup with sweet vegetables such as squash, cabbage, onions, and carrots may be prepared often.
- Vegetables: Twenty to 30 percent of daily consumption should be vegetables, cooked in a variety of forms. Dishes can be prepared in various ways using round vegetables together with root vegetables, such as carrots, burdock, daikon, and turnip. Unlike in diets for some other cancers, some dishes may be sautéed with a moderate volume of sesame or corn oil, although vegetables should also be cooked frequently using other methods. However, for the first month avoid oil altogether. As a general rule, the following dishes may be prepared, although the frequency may differ from person to person: nishime-style vegetables, four times a week; a squash-aduki-kombu dish, three times a week; dried daikon, one cup, three times a week; carrots and carrot tops or daikon and daikon tops, three times a week; blanched vegetables, five to seven times a week; pressed salad, several times a week; raw salad and salad dressing, avoid; steamed greens, five to

seven times a week; kinpira, two-thirds of a cup, two times a week; dried tofu, tofu, tempeh, or seitan with vegetables, two times a week.

- Beans: Five percent of daily consumption should be small beans, such as aduki beans, lentils, chickpeas, or black soybeans, cooked together with sea vegetables such as kombu or with onions and carrots. Other beans may be used two to three times a month. For seasoning, a small amount of unrefined sea salt or shoyu or miso can be used. Bean products, such as tempeh, natto, and dried or cooked tofu, may be used occasionally but in moderate amounts.

  For more yin cases of lymphoma, follow the standard recommendations for beans and bean products, sea vegetables, and pickles. However, for the yang type of lymphoma, a recommended dish is soybeans cooked with kombu, carrots, and onions, with a light miso taste. Black soybeans may also be cooked with a small amount of chopped kombu and cooked for a long time to bring out their natural sweetness. Alternatively, a small amount of amasake, rice malt, or barley malt may be added to beans for those with yang lymphoma to give a light, sweet taste. A drop of oil may also be added to beans during cooking.

- Sea Vegetables: Five percent or less sea vegetable dishes, including wakame and kombu, should be included daily when cooking grain, in soup, etc. A sheet of toasted nori may also be taken daily. A small dish of hijiki or arame should be prepared two times a week. All other sea vegetables are optional. Sea vegetables can be cooked with other vegetables or sautéed with a small amount of sesame oil after softening them by soaking and boiling lightly in water.

- Condiments: Those that should be available on the table are gomashio (sesame salt), on the average made with one part salt to eighteen parts sesame seeds (reduced to 1:16 after two months); kelp or wakame powder; umeboshi plum; and tekka, although all other regular macrobiotic condiments may be used if desired. These condiments may be used daily on grains and vegetables, but the amount should be moderate to suit individual appetite and taste.

- Pickles: Made at home in a variety of ways, pickles are to be eaten daily, one tablespoon in all, although salty pickles are to be minimized.

- Animal Food: Avoid animal food with the exception of white-meat fish that may be eaten once a week. After two months, fish may be eaten twice a week if desired, especially by those with the more yin form of lymphoma. Those with the more yang type should avoid fish and seafood, although a small amount of white-meat fish may be eaten once every ten to fourteen days if craved.

- Fruit: None is best, but the less the better, including both tropical and temperate-climate fruit, until the condition improves. If cravings develop, a small amount of cooked fruit with a pinch of sea salt or dried fruit (also preferably cooked) may be eaten. Avoid all fruit juices and cider temporarily, as well as raisins, currants, and other highly concentrated fruits.

- Sweets and Snacks: Avoid all sweets and desserts, including good-quality macrobiotic desserts, until the condition improves. To satisfy a sweet tooth, use sweet vegetables every day in cooking, drink sweet vegetable drinks (see special drinks below), or make sweet vegetable jam. Mochi, rice balls, vegetable sushi, and other grain-based snacks may be eaten frequently. Limit rice cakes, popcorn, and other dry or baked snacks because they may harden the tumor. In the event of cravings, a small amount of amasake, barley malt, or rice syrup may be eaten.

- Nuts and Seeds: Nuts and nut butters are to be avoided due to their high fat and protein, except for chestnuts. Unsalted blanched seeds such as sunflower seeds and pumpkin seeds may be consumed as a snack, up to one cup total per week.

- Seasonings: Unrefined sea salt, shoyu, and miso are to be used moderately in order to avoid unnecessary thirst. Avoid mirin and garlic. If you become particularly thirsty after a meal or between meals, you should cut back on these seasonings until the normal level of thirst returns.

- Beverages: Drinks and other dietary practices can follow the general recommendations in Part I, including bancha twig tea as the main beverage. Strictly avoid the beverages on the "infrequent" and "avoid" lists, and don't take grain coffee for the first two to three months after starting this new way of eating.

The most important thing in connection with dietary practice is chewing very well, until all food becomes liquid in the mouth and is well mixed with saliva. Chew very well, at least fifty times and preferably one hundred times, per mouthful. It is also important to avoid overeating and eating within three hours of sleeping.

As noted in the introduction to Part II, people who have received or who are currently undergoing medical treatment may need to make further dietary modifications.

SPECIAL DRINKS AND DISHES

One or more special drinks or side dishes may need to be consumed, depending on the individual case, to help reduce excess protein and fat, which are the cause of the cancer; to reduce cholesterol levels; and to assist recovery. Please see a qualified macrobiotic teacher for guidance. Amounts and frequencies given here are averages for each drink or dish; these will differ from person to person. Further directions are in Chapter 36.

- Kinpira-Style Burdock, Carrot, and Kombu: Prepare a small dish of this every day or every other day for about a month. After that, take it occasionally.
- Dried Daikon, Dried Daikon Leaves, and Burdock Tea: Prepare this tea in a pot and have ½ cup one to two times a day. Keep taking this for three weeks. After that, take it two to three times a week for three to four weeks.
- Sweet Vegetable Drink: Take one cup a day for three to four weeks.
- Brown Rice, Millet, Buckwheat, and Vegetable Porridge: Prepare by adding a little kombu and water. Have one bowl a day for one week, and after that, three times a week for one month.
- Ume-Kuzu Drink: In the case of constipation, have one small cup every day for three to four days; and after that, two to three times a week for about one month.
- In case of excess sweating, have one cup of Ume-Kuzu, Cabbage Tea, Cabbage Tea cooled to room temperature, or Dried Daikon Tea.

HOME CARE

- Body Scrub: Scrubbing the whole body, including the abdominal region and the spinal region, with a towel that has been immersed in hot water and squeezed out is very helpful for better circulation of blood, lymph, and other body fluids, as well as for activating physical and mental energies.
- Compress Guidelines: For a small number of lymphatic tumors, a compress may be needed to gradually help draw out excess mucus and fat. Please see a qualified macrobiotic teacher for guidance on the proper use and frequency of a compress or plaster. Several types are used, depending on the person's condition. Precede the compress or plaster with the application of a towel that has been soaked in hot water and squeezed out over the affected area for about three to five minutes to stimulate circulation.
- Kombu-Cabbage Plaster: Apply on swollen areas. Wrap them with cotton and keep the plaster on for about four hours. Do this twice a day; it is possible to keep this on overnight while you are sleeping. Continue this until the swelling disappears.
- Cabbage Plaster: Directly apply it to the swollen spleen area for about four hours. Change it two to three times a day. Or apply it when you sleep and keep it on overnight.
- Fasting: Swelling of the spleen and abdominal regions sometimes

accompanies lymphatic cancer and is caused by overeating in general, especially protein, and an excessive intake of beverages, seasonings, and condiments. In such cases, food consumption should be simplified for a period of several days up to ten days. During this period, daily consumption may consist of pressure-cooked brown rice and barley, one to two cups of miso soup, a small dish of half dried daikon and half daikon leaves pickled for a long period (over two months) with sea salt and rice bran, a dish of vegetables such as onions, carrots, and cabbage sautéed in sesame oil, and several cups of bancha twig tea. However, this simplified diet should not be continued longer than ten days unless under supervision of an experienced macrobiotic teacher or medical associate.

- Tofu–Green Vegetable Plaster: A plaster of mashed tofu mixed with the same amount of mashed green leafy vegetables is recommended for swollen glands and inflammation of the spleen.
- Buckwheat Plaster: A plaster of buckwheat flour kneaded with warm water or green clay may also be applied to inflamed lymph nodes or glands to help reduce the swelling.
- Sweating: If sweating occurs at night, relief can be provided by eating a small amount of sliced burdock roots and carrot roots, sautéed with sesame oil and seasoned with shoyu.
- Bathing: Hot baths and showers should be taken quickly. Soaking the body for a long time in the tub causes the body to lose important minerals.

EMOTIONAL CONSIDERATIONS

Positive emotions associated with the spleen and lymphatic system are balance, trust, serving others, and compassion. Lymphatic problems may arise from excessive control and manipulation, mistrust, and lack of sympathy and consideration.

High-quality foods that nourish the lymph and help develop positive emotions include naturally sweet things such as whole grains, particularly millet and sweet rice; sweet, round vegetables, including cabbage, squash, and onions; tofu, yuba, and other soft, naturally processed soy foods; natural sweeteners, including amasake, rice syrup, and barley malt; round orange or yellow fruits such as peaches, nectarines, and apricots; and carrot juice, sweet vegetable drink, and other naturally sweet foods.

Foods that weaken the lymph system and contribute to negative emotions include too much meat; cheese, poultry, eggs, strong fish and seafood, and other heavy animal products; white flour; excessive fruit, juice, raw foods, and beverages; sugar, chocolate, and other highly processed sweets; chemicalized and artificial foods; alcohol; and other extremely contractive or expansive foods and beverages.

In relationships it is important to trust one's partner, try to understand things from his or her perspective, and harmonize. Those who are mistrustful, suspicious, and unsympathetic may localize their excess emotional energy in the spleen and lymph.

On a planetary scale, the lymph correlates to rivers, streams, and brooks. Imbalance in this region is comparable to water pollution.

OTHER CONSIDERATIONS

- Good exercise is strengthening to the lymph and circulatory systems, but do not exercise to the point of exhaustion. Deep-breathing exercises, massage, and tai chi–type movements are generally preferable to strenuous activities. Walking is excellent.
- Maintaining clean, fresh air inside the home is important, and for this purpose green plants can be placed in each room. Indoor air circulation can also be maintained by frequently opening the windows.
- Wearing cotton underwear and avoiding synthetic fabrics are helpful for better skin metabolism and facilitate energy flow through the body.
- Avoid exposure to artificial electromagnetic radiation. Keep common handheld appliances to a minimum. If you have a choice, work and live in areas away from an electronic environment.
- Avoid frequent exposure to artificial radiation, including medical and dental X-rays, smoke detectors, television, and video terminals, which are weakening to the lymph and blood.
- Try to be happy, positive, and outgoing. Singing, dancing, and playing are particularly beneficial for improving overall health and mentality and harmonizing with the rhythms of nature.

PERSONAL EXPERIENCE

HODGKIN'S DISEASE

In January 1973 nineteen-year-old Maureen Duney of Belle Mead, New Jersey, discovered a lump in the right side of her throat. In April a biopsy of the lymph node gland proved malignant, and doctors at Memorial Hospital in New York diagnosed her condition as Hodgkin's disease, stage 3 B.

In June, Maureen began radiation therapy, and by August the tumors were dispersed. However, in March 1975 she noticed a thickening in the intestinal area to the left of the navel, and tests showed that the cancer had come back. There was also a tumor on the last rib on her left side.

In September 1975, Maureen began experimental chemotherapy, but after one month friends persuaded her to try macrobiotics. At the end of the month Maureen came to see me, and I recommended the Cancer Prevention Diet and an application of a ginger compress to the spleen and rib areas.

"Mr. Kushi projected that I would be cured in four to six months," she recorded. "I took the information back to my parents, family, and doctors. I began cooking and eating macrobiotically immediately. From September following my first treatment of MOPP [chemotherapy], my sediment rate was 42; in November, after eating macrobiotically for two months, it had dropped to a normal count of 14. I felt alive again, was active daily, my strength increased, and my hair stopped falling out."

Prior to this time Maureen had always been a poor eater. She did not eat as much meat but, in her words, "devoured sweets, ice cream, fruits, liquids, hoagies, and pizza." By early 1976 the Hodgkin's disease was gone, and she no longer suffered from itching or night sweating. "I consume none of the foods that caused my illness at the first," she concluded. "I continue to eat macrobiotically gratefully every day."[5]

HODGKIN'S DISEASE

Emily Bellew, a resident of Columbus, Ohio, was twenty-two and had been married for three years. She was expecting her first child but had a very difficult pregnancy and delivery. She gained 80 pounds, ballooning up to 205 pounds, and craved large amounts of ice cream, red meat, and anything else she could find.

Three days after the birth of her son, Bryan, Emily experienced a swollen and stiff neck. She attributed it to holding him in the wrong position. During her postpartum checkup a few weeks later, she mentioned the sore neck to her doctor. Medical tests found that she had Hodgkin's disease, stage 2 B.

For the next several months Emily underwent radiation treatment. But her condition worsened. The cancer spread to the lower portion of the hip bone, and she had to use a wheelchair. Following chemotherapy treatments for the next several months, the cancer in the hip cleared up, but it had spread to the abdomen. This was followed by another round of chemo and the discovery of a lump in the groin. After two and a half years of treatment, Emily came across a book on macrobiotics and decided that she had nothing to lose. Doctors had now told her that she could expect to live several more months, a year at most.

Emily came to see me where I was giving a seminar. "The next three days changed my life," she recalled. "I heard lectures and attended cooking classes. I also began to eat macrobiotic food for the first time. I took new knowledge and new cookbooks back home and began cooking. I started to feel the difference right away, and it was all so really simple. This was the way our bodies were meant to be nourished."

Within a year the tumors went away, and doctors could find no trace of cancer. Within two more years her weight stabilized at 113 pounds. It is now nine years since Emily walked away from the hospital to begin the "great life."[6]

LYMPHOMA

Judy MacKenney, a fashion designer and homemaker, was diagnosed with non-Hodgkin's lymphoma that would develop to stage 4 within a few weeks. The tumor was situated on the right side of her abdomen, the lymph nodes on the left side of her neck were swollen, and cancer cells were found in her bone marrow. Judy agreed to take oral chemotherapy, but the side effects were devastating. Her body swelled up and con- torted, she developed ulcers, and her stomach burned with pain.

Judy had the same kind of lymphoma as Jacqueline Kennedy Onassis, who died of the disease, and feared she would suffer a similar fate. While attending a support group for exceptional cancer patients inspired by Dr. Bernie Siegel, she came across *The Cancer Prevention Diet* and started macrobiotics. The sweet vegetable drink stabilized her blood sugar, and the ulcers went away. The ume-sho-kuzu strengthened her digestion and restored her energy. Ginger compresses dissolved stagnation and stimu- lated blood circulation and energy flow. "After two weeks I felt notice- able improvement. The pain in my joints and feet disappeared. My innards embraced the nourishing whole food, I started to discover energy I had not felt in years, and I was experiencing peaceful sleep at last," she recalled. Judy went on to recover completely.

With her husband, Larry, she set up a macrobiotic bed-and-breakfast on the gulf coast of Florida. Both Judy and Larry graduated from the Kushi Institute teacher training program and have managed the Way to Health program, sharing their knowledge and experience with many other cancer patients and their families. She has been cancer-free for the last fourteen years.[7]

2 5

Male Reproductive Cancers: Prostate and Testes

FREQUENCY

Prostate cancer—the most common cancer among American men—will cause 27,050 deaths in the next twelve months, and 218,890 new cases will develop. Prostate cancer sharply increased in the late 1980s, decreased in the early 1990s, and has started to rise again since then. Cancer of the testes and other male reproductive organs will claim 670 lives, and doctors will detect 9,200 new instances of the disease. African American men have the highest rates in the world, while it is rare in Africa, Asia, and most of the developing world. Eighty percent of cases are diagnosed in men over sixty-five. Many cases of prostate cancer develop slowly, causing no symptoms and remaining inactive for years. However, others are very aggressive and spread to the bladder, rectum, and travel through the lymph to the bones, liver, lungs, and elsewhere. Americans have one of the highest prostate cancer rates in the world, up to ten times higher, for instance, than the Japanese.

A variety of disorders can affect the prostate gland, including both benign and malignant tumors. Depending on the particular case, the illness is treated with surgery, radiation, and hormone therapy. Techniques include a transurethral resection (TUR), in which a resectoscope is inserted through the penis to kill tumor cells with an electric wire loop; a suprapubic prostectomy, in which the bladder is opened and the prostate removed by the surgeon through the urethra; a retropubic prostectomy, in which the prostate and seminal vesicles are removed without going through the bladder; and a perineal prostectomy, in which the surgeon enters between the legs in front of the rectum. Radioactive seeds may be implanted in the prostate to reduce the tumor, or external megavoltage radiation may be administered. Finally, to control hormone levels and retard tumor growth, estrogens in the form of DES or cortisone may be given orally. In some instances the testicles, adrenal glands, and pituitary gland may be removed to limit the spread of malignancy. Hormone therapy can result in impotence, enlarged breasts, and heart problems. Surgery may result in impotence and sterility.

Death rates for prostate cancer in the United States have declined since the 1990s, but those in African American men remain twice that of whites. The five-year survival rate for testicular cancer has greatly increased in recent years and except for distant stages is nearly 100 percent.

Testicular cancer usually affects the right testicle more than the left, seldom both, and tends to spread to the lungs. A radical orchiectomy, involving removal of one or both testicles, is the standard form of treatment. If both testicles are removed, the operation will render the patient sterile but not impotent. If cancer has spread to the lymph nodes, radiation or chemotherapy will also be administered. If the malignancy is spreading through the blood, a lympadenoctomy may be performed in which all the lymph nodes on one or both sides of the abdomen up to the kidneys will be removed. The death rates for testicular cancer have fallen dramatically in the last generation, down about one-third in the United States and up to two-thirds or more in Britain and other European countries.

STRUCTURE

The testes, located in a sac called the scrotum, are the primary organs of the male reproductive system. They produce sperm and male sex hormones. The peripheral layer of the testes contains about 250 lobules or chambers. Each chamber holds from one to three minute seminiferous tubules in which spermatozoa are formed. Sperm are discharged from each tubule and float upward to the first portion of the duct system, called the epididymis, where they are stored for weeks, months, or even years. The seminal fluid, or semen, is a mixture of sperm from the testes and fluid from several accessory reproductive organs. The main accessory organ is the prostate gland. The prostate is situated below the bladder and surrounds the urethra, connecting the bladder and penis. The prostate secretes enzymes, lipids, and other substances, which enter the seminal fluid and are deposited in the female reproductive tract by the penis during intercourse.

CAUSE OF CANCER

In structure, the prostate is classified as yang because of its relative compactness, location deep inside the body, and the alkaline fluid it secretes, which serves to neutralize the extremely yin acids of the vagina. About 30 percent of men over fifty in the United States have enlarged prostates. As this organ presses against the upper portion of the bladder and urethra, urination becomes difficult and painful. Of these cases, about one in five develops into prostate cancer; however, any enlargement of the prostate should be suspected as a precancerous condition.

Prostate enlargement and blockage of the other semen ducts arise in the same way as hardening of the arteries. They are caused principally by the overconsumption of foods rich in fat and protein in the yang category, including eggs, meat, and dairy products, all of which contain saturated fats, as well as by an excessive intake of foods in the extreme yin category such as sugar, fruits, and refined flour products, which produce fat and mucus. Over time, these deposits accumulate and can turn into cysts or tumors. The blockages resulting from a high-fat diet can also contribute to impotence. However, the inability to achieve an erection is often caused by an intake of too much expansive food, which causes the muscles of the reproductive system to become loose and expanded. Infertility is also caused largely from an excessive intake of yin-type foods, which weaken the quality of the blood, lymph, and other bodily fluids and secretions that determine the quality of the sperm. Prostate problems can be relieved by adopting a cancer prevention diet that emphasizes slightly more yin foods and style of cooking and avoids animal foods.

Testicular cancer may also involve heavy animal food, especially fish eggs, heavily salted meats, condensed dairy foods such as cheese, and high-fat, high-cholesterol shellfish or seafood, as well as oily, greasy foods, especially french fries. However, because the testes are more external than the prostate, extreme yin is often a major factor—especially animal fat, oil, and dairy—and some forms of testicular cancer are predominantly yin.

MEDICAL EVIDENCE

- In 1974 an epidemiologist found a high direct correlation between mortality from prostate cancer in forty-one countries and per capita intake of fats, milk, and meats, especially beef. Research also disclosed that people who regularly consumed rice had less incidence of the disease.[1]
- Seventh-Day Adventist men in California have 55 percent less prostate cancer than other males, according to a 1975 study. The church members tend to avoid meat, poultry, fish, refined foods, alcohol, stimu-

lants, and spices, and consume whole grains, vegetables, and fresh fruits.[2]

- Whole grains and plant-quality foods protect against prostate cancer. In a study of prostate cancer mortality rates in seventy-one countries, researchers at the University of Alabama at Birmingham reported that cereal grains and rice, in particular, were associated strongly with decreased mortality from prostate cancer. Plant oils, soybeans, and onions were also protective, as was exposure to sunlight. Nutrients and foods that correlated with an increase in deaths from this disease included total animal calories, total animal fat calories, meat, animal fat, milk, sugar, alcoholic beverages, and stimulants.[3]

- In a population-based case-control study of 269 subjects and 797 controls, German scientists at the University of Halle-Wittenberg reported that with each additional twenty servings of milk per month consumed in adolescence, the risk for testicular cancer was enhanced by 37 percent. "Our results suggest that milk fat and/or galactose may explain the association between milk and dairy product consumption and seminomatous testicular cancer," the scientists concluded.[4]

DIAGNOSIS

Prostate cancer is usually diagnosed by a rectal examination as well as a battery of laboratory tests, enzyme and hormone assays, and a needle biopsy if a malignancy is suspected. Skeletal and chest X-rays, bone scans, and intravenous pyelogram (IVP) will be used to check for metastases. About 60 percent of prostate tumors are currently detected before spreading to other sites. In the case of testicular cancer, many of these same diagnostic methods are used, as well as an angiogram, lymphangiogram, CT scan of chest or abdomen, and ultrasound examination of the abdomen.

Oriental medicine diagnoses potential male reproductive cancers with a variety of simple visual observations. According to physiognomy, the mouth and lower face correspond with the sex organs, and discolorations, swellings, or other abnormalities in this region may indicate improper functioning of the reproductive system. For instance, vertical wrinkles appearing on the lips show a recession of hormonal function, especially of the gonad hormones, indicating a decline in sexual function. These wrinkles may also appear in case of dehydration from lack of liquid or overconsumption of dry foods and salt, so other signs must also be observed. Generally, fatty wrinkles or sagging in the chin and upper neck indicate prostate problems in men or uterine and ovarian problems in women. Pimples that appear in the center of the cheeks and have a fatty appearance also show the formation of cysts in and around the reproductive organs.

Fat or mucus buildup in the prostate is further indicated by a yellow and white coating of mucus on the lower part of the whites of the eyes. Along the bladder meridian, cancer of the prostate shows up as a light green coloration on the fifth toe and its extended area at the outside of the foot, below the anklebone and behind the Achilles tendon, with fatty swelling along the Achilles tendon.

On the hands, split or uneven nails show disorders in the circulatory, nervous, and reproductive systems caused by chaotic eating habits. If one thumbnail shows this condition and the other thumbnail is normal, the testicle (or ovary in women) corresponding to the abnormal side is malfunctioning. Red, purple, and other abnormal colors appearing on the tips of the fingers also indicate disorders in the gonad region, including possible cancer or precancerous conditions.

From a combination of these and other factors, the condition of the reproductive system can be determined and appropriate corrective nutritional action taken.

DIETARY RECOMMENDATIONS

The main cause of prostate cancer is food high in protein and fat, especially chicken, turkey, beef, pork, eggs, cheese, and other dairy foods, along with salted foods, baked foods, and roasted foods, which make the muscles and tissues tight. All these should be avoided, including fish and seafood, until the condition improves. The main cause of testicular cancer is eggs, meat, cheese, and other foods high in saturated fat and cholesterol. Not only animal food but also sugar, honey, chocolate, carob, and all sugar-treated food and beverages are to be discontinued for both conditions. Flour products, such as refined white bread, pancakes, and cookies, which have the potential to create mucus, are also to be avoided. All stimulants, including mustard, pepper, curry, mint, peppermint, and other aromatic herbs and spices, all alcoholic beverages, and coffee are to be avoided because they enhance tumor growth, although they are not the direct cause of the cancer. All chemicals artificially added or treated during food production and processing should also be avoided. Excessive consumption of oil, even of unsaturated vegetable quality, is to be avoided, as is excessive consumption of salts and salty food and beverages. Fruit and fruit juices, if consumed frequently, can increase the swelling of the tumor, although they can neutralize animal protein and fat. Accordingly, they should be limited. All vegetables of historically tropical origin, such as potatoes, tomatoes, and eggplant, and tropical and subtropical fruits should be avoided. General dietary guidelines by volume of food consumption are as follows:

- Whole Grains: Forty to 50 percent of daily consumption, by volume, should be whole cereal grains. The first day prepare plain short- or medium-grain brown rice, pressure-cooked or cooked in a heavy cast-iron or ceramic pot with a heavy lid. On subsequent days, brown rice may be made with 20 to 30 percent millet, then rice with 20 to 30 percent barley, then rice with 20 to 30 percent aduki beans or lentils, and then plain rice again. A delicious morning porridge can be made by taking leftover rice, adding a little more water to soften it, seasoning with a little miso, and simmering for two to three minutes more. In daily cooking the ratio of grain to water should be about 1:2. For seasoning, cook with a postage-stamp-sized piece of kombu instead of salt. Other grains can be used occasionally, including whole wheat berries, rye, corn, and whole oats, although oats should be avoided for the first month. However, buckwheat should be avoided for about six months because it is very contractive and may harden the tumor. Seitan is also very yang and should be minimized. Flour products, even unrefined whole wheat bread, chapatis, pancakes, and cookies, should be totally avoided or limited in volume for a period of a few months, although people with prostate problems typically like roasted, baked, or crunchy foods. Whole grain pasta and noodles may be eaten a couple of times a week.
- Soup: Five to 10 percent of daily consumption should be soup, consisting of one or two cups or bowls cooked with wakame sea vegetable and various vegetables, especially daikon and daikon leaves and other green leafy vegetables, and seasoned lightly with miso or shoyu. Occasionally a small amount of shiitake mushroom may be added to the soup. The miso may be barley miso, brown rice miso, or soybean (hatcho) miso, and should be naturally aged two to three years. Grain soups, bean soups, and other soups may be eaten from time to time.
- Vegetables: Twenty to 30 percent of daily consumption should be vegetables, cooked in a variety of forms, mainly steamed, boiled, and, after four to six weeks without oil, occasionally sautéed. Various types of leafy vegetables—green, yellow, and white—can be cooked in different styles, as can various root vegetables such as carrots, turnips, daikon, radishes, lotus root, and burdock root, although burdock should be used much less frequently than other root vegetables. Round vegetables such as acorn and butternut squash, cabbage, and onions can also be used frequently. Daikon and daikon greens are especially recommended for these conditions. As a rule of thumb, the following dishes may be prepared, although the frequency may differ from person to person: nishime-style vegetables, three times a week;

a squash-aduki-kombu dish, three times a week; dried daikon, one cup, three times a week; carrots and carrot tops or daikon and daikon tops, three times a week; blanched vegetables, five to seven times a week; pressed salad, five to seven times a week; raw salad, one to two times a week; steamed greens, five to seven times a week; sautéed vegetables, prepared with water the first month and then with sesame oil lightly brushed on the pan, once or twice a week after that; kinpira, two-thirds of a cup, two times a week; dried tofu, tofu, or tempeh with vegetables, two times a week.

- Beans: Five percent of daily consumption should be small beans, such as aduki beans, lentils, chickpeas, or black soybeans, cooked together with sea vegetables such as kombu or with onions and carrots. Other beans may be used two to three times a month. For seasoning, a small amount of unrefined sea salt or shoyu or miso can be used. Bean products, such as tempeh, natto, and dried or cooked tofu, may be used occasionally, but in moderate amounts.

- Sea Vegetables: Five percent or less sea vegetable dishes, including wakame and kombu, should be included daily when cooking grain, in soup, etc. A sheet of toasted nori may also be taken daily. A small dish of hijiki or arame should be prepared two times a week. All other sea vegetables are optional.

- Condiments: Those that should be available on the table are gomashio (sesame salt), on the average made with one part salt to eighteen to twenty parts sesame seeds; kelp or wakame powder; umeboshi plum; and tekka, although all other regular macrobiotic condiments may be used if desired. These condiments may be used daily on grains and vegetables, but the amounts should be moderate to suit individual appetite and taste.

- Pickles: Made at home in a variety of ways, pickles are to be eaten daily, one tablespoon in all, although salty pickles are to be minimized. Rice bran (nuka) pickles are the most suitable.

- Animal Foods: Fish and other animal food are to be avoided. However, in the event that animal food is craved, a small amount of white-meat fish may be eaten once every ten days to two weeks. The fish should be steamed, boiled, or poached and garnished with grated daikon or ginger. Strictly avoid blue-meat and red-meat fish and all shellfish.

- Fruit: The less the better until the condition improves. If cravings develop, a small amount of fresh fruit or cooked fruit with a pinch of sea salt or dried fruit (also preferably cooked) may be eaten. Tree fruits such as apples, peaches, and pears are better than ground fruits such as strawberries and watermelons. Avoid all fruit juices and cider temporarily, as well as raisins, currants, and other highly concentrated fruits.

- Sweets and Snacks: Overuse of sweets is connected with prostate disorders, so it is very important to avoid all sweets and desserts, including good-quality macrobiotic desserts, until the condition improves. To satisfy a sweet tooth, use sweet vegetables every day in cooking, drink sweet vegetable drinks, or prepare sweet vegetable jam. If cravings arise, a small amount of amasake, barley malt, or rice syrup may be eaten. If cravings persist, a little cider, apple juice, or chestnut puree may be prepared. Mochi, rice balls, vegetable sushi, and other grain-based snacks may be eaten frequently. Limit rice cakes, popcorn, and other dry or baked snacks because they may harden the tumor.
- Nuts and Seeds: Nuts and nut butters are to be avoided due to their high amount of fat and protein, except for chestnuts. Unsalted steamed or boiled seeds such as sunflower seeds and pumpkin seeds may be consumed as a snack, up to one cup total per week. Minimize the use of roasted seeds.
- Seasonings: Unrefined sea salt, shoyu, and miso are to be used moderately in order to avoid unnecessary thirst. Avoid mirin and garlic. If you become particularly thirsty after a meal or between meals, you should cut back on these seasonings until the normal level of thirst returns.
- Beverages: Drinks and other dietary practices can follow the general recommendations in Part I, including bancha twig tea as the main beverage. Strictly avoid the beverages on the "infrequent" and "avoid" lists, and don't take grain coffee for the first two to three months after starting this new way of eating.

The most important thing in connection with dietary practice is chewing very well, until all food becomes liquid in the mouth and is well mixed with saliva. Chew very well, at least fifty times and preferably one hundred times per mouthful. It is also important to avoid overeating and eating within three hours of sleeping.

As noted in the introduction to Part II, people who have received or who are currently undergoing medical treatment may need to make further dietary modifications.

SPECIAL DRINKS AND DISHES

One or more special drinks or side dishes may need to be consumed, depending on the individual case, to help reduce excess protein and fat, which are the cause of the cancer; to reduce cholesterol levels; and to assist recovery. Please see a qualified macrobiotic teacher for guidance. Amounts and frequencies given here are averages for each drink or dish; these will differ from person to person. Further directions are in Chapter 36.

- Brown Rice Liquid with Daikon, Umeboshi, and Shiso: Take one to two small cups of this thinly prepared gruel every day for about two weeks and after that three to four times a week for another month.
- Dried Daikon, Daikon Leaves, and Shiitake Tea: Drink one cup of this broth every evening for three weeks. After that, drink it occasionally.
- Miso-Zosui: This dish, made with scallions, may be eaten frequently, two to three times a week.
- Tomato-Miso Sauce with Scallions and Chinese Cabbage: For prostate cancer, take 1 tablespoonful of this tomato sauce at dinnertime.
- Daikon Leaves Quick Pickles (pickled briefly in light sea salt): If they are salty, rinse off the excess salt before eating.
- Brown Rice and Corn Porridge: This dish is also very healing for prostate conditions and may be eaten twice a week.

HOME CARE

- Body Scrub: Scrubbing the whole body, including the abdominal region and the spinal region, with a towel that has been immersed in hot water and squeezed out is very helpful for better circulation of blood, lymph, and other body fluids, as well as for activating physical and mental energies.
- Compress Guidelines: For a small number of tumors in the male reproductive system, a compress may be needed to help gradually draw out excess mucus and fat. Please see a qualified macrobiotic teacher for guidance on the proper use and frequency of a compress or plaster. Several types are used depending on the person's condition. Precede the compress or plaster with the application of a towel that has been soaked in hot water and squeezed out over the affected area for about three to five minutes to stimulate circulation.
- Kombu-Cabbage Plaster: If the lymph nodes are swollen, apply this plaster and leave it on for six hours or more. Repeat once or twice every day. It may also be left on overnight while sleeping. Use this plaster every day for two to three weeks.
- Ume-Sho-Bancha: For pain, take one to two small cups. Kuzu may be substituted for bancha and will have a soothing effect.
- Buckwheat Plaster: For swelling of the abdominal region, apply this plaster for one hour. Keep it warm by placing roasted hot sea salt wrapped in cotton towels on top. (For ease in handling, the hot salt may be placed in a pouch made from a cotton towel and then wrapped with another towel.) Repeat daily for several days.
- Potato-Cabbage Plaster: For testicular cancer, prepare this plaster made from two-thirds potato and one-third cabbage. Apply for three

to four hours on the affected area, preceded by a Ginger Compress for three to five minutes. Repeat daily for two to three weeks.

EMOTIONAL CONSIDERATIONS

Prostate, testicular, and other male reproductive problems are associated emotionally with sexuality, intimacy, and regeneration.

High-quality foods that nourish the prostate and other male sexual organs and help develop positive emotions include whole grains, particularly buckwheat, teff, wild rice, and other darker grains; beans and bean products, especially black soybeans and other darker beans; leafy green vegetables; sea vegetables; seeds and nuts; white-meat fish; and good-quality sea salt.

Foods that harm the prostate and related organs and contribute to negative emotions include dairy food; meat, poultry, eggs; strong fish and seafood; white flour; sugar and other highly refined sweets; chemicalized and artificial foods; and other extremely contractive or expansive foods and beverages.

In relationships it is important to communicate freely and honestly and not suppress feelings and emotions. If a man cannot express himself, feels rejected and unappreciated, is overly aggressive, or engages in secretive relationships, he may localize his repressed feelings in the prostate or related organ.

On a planetary scale, the prostate correlates with the deep oceans, and cancer in this region is akin to ocean pollution.

OTHER CONSIDERATIONS

- Daily physical exercise that does not produce exhaustion is recommended. Ten to fifteen minutes of daily breathing exercises, especially emphasizing long exhalation, is also beneficial. These physical and breathing exercises contribute to relaxing tensions in the body and mind as well as harmonizing physical metabolism.
- Keeping air quality clean and fresh is important for maintenance of general health. For that purpose, green leafy plants can be placed in the house and the windows periodically opened to allow circulation of fresh air. Don't smoke because this will tighten the prostate.
- Avoid wearing wool and synthetic fibers. At the minimum wear cotton underwear and use cotton sheets and pillowcases.
- Avoid watching television for long stretches. Radiation weakens the reproductive area. Similarly, avoid other artificial sources of electromagnetic energy such as video terminals, smoke detectors, and handheld electrical appliances.

- Although cancer is naturally accompanied by a decline in energy and vitality, normal sexual practice is not harmful if it does not lead to exhaustion.
- Vasectomy and other artificial birth-control methods, as well as the use of drugs or medications to control sexual performance, are to be avoided in order to prevent stagnation, interruption of energy flow, or other abnormal functions.

PERSONAL EXPERIENCES

PROSTATE CANCER

At age sixty-three Herb Walley was diagnosed with a prostate tumor. Doctors recommended hormone treatment and put him on stilbesterol. "The side effects are pretty awful for a man who wants to remain masculine," Herb recalled. "Some of the more depressing transformations are breast and nipple enlargement with extreme tenderness, fluid retention throughout the body—the legs in particular—with resulting inconvenience of hourly toilet trips, both day and night. Also, loss of fingernail substance results in painful split and torn nails. There are many other less obvious effects which are equally annoying."

Herb finally persuaded his urologist to diminish the dosage by half. However, the effects didn't appreciably diminish. Although under control, Herb's tumor still remained malignant six years later when a friend introduced him to a book on macrobiotics. Herb read it avidly and met with a macrobiotic teacher at the Kushi Institute who provided more specific guidelines for his condition. "After one month I felt more alive and much less depressed," Herb said, looking back. "I stopped taking all medications and vitamins and made monthly visits to my general practitioner for checkups." Altogether he lost sixty-five pounds of old fat from all over his body.

Ten months later, medical tests showed that the cancer was gone. To be certain, Herb checked into the Dana Farber Cancer Center in Boston, one of the nation's top cancer clinics. After many more tests and a complete bone scan, he was told that he was "clean."

With his wife, Virginia, Herb went on to operate a macrobiotic bed-and-breakfast and returned to New Hampshire. "I am still 'clean,' with almost unlimited energy," Herb reports. "I can eat all I want without gaining weight and look forward to another twenty or thirty years of excitement and happiness."[5]

PROSTATE CANCER

On a beautiful September day in 1979, Ed Hanley was raking oak leaves. Feeling full of vim, vigor, and vitality, he had no reason to suspect he was not in excellent health. But his next-door neighbor talked to him about his prostate operation and the symptoms leading up to it. Ed then began to experience similar symptoms vicariously, and a voice within told him, "Go see the doctor and have a checkup." A routine medical exam subsequently turned up prostate cancer, and bone scans showed "hot spots" on his skull and pelvis.

Doctors initially recommended surgery but then advised against it because it could make the malignancy spread faster. Instead they suggested castration or taking female hormone pills. Ed took the hormones, and over the next two years the cancer remained dormant but then spread to his spine, ribs, and left thighbone.

One evening Ed's eldest son, David, came to his room and said, "I'm terribly upset because I harbor the thought you're dying. I don't want to lose you. Not now. I'm just getting to know you." Father and son hugged, tears flowed, and they both cried. Determined to live, Ed prayed daily for the strength and means to overcome his cancer. At Bible class one day, a friend gave him an article from the *Saturday Evening Post* about Dr. Anthony Satillaro, the president of the Methodist Hospital in Philadelphia, who had terminal prostate cancer that had spread to multiple organs. Satillaro healed himself with macrobiotics at the suggestion of two hitchhikers he had picked up. His miraculous recovery was profiled in the *Post, Life* magazine, and eventually a bestselling book, *Recalled by Life*.

Believing that God's hand was on his shoulder, Ed attended classes at the Kushi Institute and with his wife, Jeanne, took cooking classes. Over the next year he adhered strictly to the diet, got plenty of exercise, and prayed daily.

"Jeanne had become my faithful 'watchdog,'" he recalls. "If I so much as looked at a cut of red meat or poultry in a butcher's showcase, a picture of a martini (dry), or looked longingly at that joint with the big arch, she stared me down and gave me a sermon on the spot. We both shared in the cooking and accumulated a library full of cookbooks."

Three years after the cancer was first diagnosed, Ed was given a clean bill of health by doctors at the University of Chicago. A bone scan, prostate biopsy, and blood and urine tests disclosed no signs of cancer cells. "God had performed His miracle," Ed recalled seven years later, during which time he remained cancer-free.[6]

PROSTATE CANCER

After being diagnosed with prostate cancer in 2001, Thomas Mueller, a forty-five-year-old attorney in Los Angeles, went on a macrobiotic diet. After three months his PSA, an antigen marker for prostate cancer, plummeted from 4.0 to 1.5 ng/ml, indicating that his tumor was regressing.

Influenced by cases such as this, Dr. Dean Ornish, founder of the Prostate Cancer Research Institute (PCRI), studied ninety-three men who, like Mueller, had decided not to undertake conventional medical treatment. Half of the men were randomly allocated to Ornish's vegan diet, while the other half followed a conventional modern way of eating. After a year the PSA of the treated group decreased an average of 0.25 ng/ml, or 4 percent, while those in the control group increased an average of 0.38 ng/ml, or 6 percent.

Blood tests further showed that the cancer cells in the control group were growing eight times faster than those undergoing dietary therapy.

Physicians associated with Ornish theorized that Mueller's progress was even more dramatic than their own because the macrobiotic way of eating brought his blood sugar levels down to unusually low normal levels. As a result, his insulin levels were naturally suppressed, and the researchers speculated that high insulin, a potent growth hormone, as well as glucose caused prostate (and other cancers) to spread.[7]

Oral and Upper Digestive Cancers: Mouth, Larynx, Pharynx, and Esophagus

FREQUENCY

Cancers of the upper digestive system, including the mouth, throat, and esophagus, will account for 7,550 estimated deaths in the United States this year and some 34,360 new cases. Men are about twice as likely to contract these forms of cancer as women. Esophageal cancer is one of the fastest growing malignancies in the United States, and the death rate has increased substantially in recent years. Among sufferers of Barrett's esophagus, a precancerous condition characterized by persistent heartburn or stomach regurgitations, the incidence of esophageal cancer has soared 100 percent, and the age of onset is steadily falling. Death from cancer of the larynx has increased among women over the last generation, although it has remained steady for men. During the same time frame, oral cancer mortality fell among men and rose among women. The incidence of upper digestive cancer is also particularly high in East Asia.

Cancers in the head and neck do not usually metastasize but spread by local invasion. Almost 90 percent of these tumors are classified as squamous-cell carcinomas. They grow slowly and tend to recur within several years of treatment. Cancer of the esophagus often spreads to the liver, the lungs, or the membrane surrounding the lungs.

Surgery and radiation are widely used by modern medicine to treat these forms of cancer. In the case of esophageal cancer, partial removal of the diseased section is rectified by taking a portion of the large intestine and surgically linking it with the remaining part of the esophagus and the stomach. This procedure is called an esophagogastric anastomosis. If the whole esophagus is taken out, the spleen and end of the pancreas are usually removed as well. Again, part of the intestinal wall or plastic tubing will be inserted to connect the severed ends of the digestive tract.

For head and neck tumors, surgery is usually employed to remove the tumor and part of the healthy tissue surrounding it. Plastic surgery follows if this results in the disfiguration of the face. The voice is often lost as a consequence of surgery to the throat area. Radiation therapy may also be used as a primary treatment, depending on the type and size of the tumor. Chemotherapy may be used in conjunction with radiation if the tumor is advanced or has spread to the bone. The survival rate for esophageal cancer is about 16 percent. The five-year cure rate is higher for larynx cancer, 64 percent, and oral cavity and pharynx cancer, 59 percent.

STRUCTURE

The upper digestive tract extends from the lips to the stomach and consists of the mouth, larynx, pharynx, and esophagus. The larynx is also known as the voice box, the pharynx as the throat, and the esophagus as the gullet. Food enters the body through the mouth and moves spirally up and down in the process of chewing. Digestion alternates between alkaline (yang) and acidic (yin) secretions at various stages along the alimentary canal. From the mouth, where alkaline substances are released, food travels to the stomach, where acids are secreted. From there it moves to the duodenum, where alkaline enzymes from the small intestine and pancreas are activated. Finally, remaining foodstuffs are absorbed by the acidic substances in the villi of the small intestine.

In the mouth the digestive process begins with the secretion of saliva, a clear, watery fluid that has a pH of 7.2, making it slightly salty or alkaline. The main function of saliva is to begin gradually breaking down carbohydrates for further absorption in the stomach and complete digestion in the small intestine. Ptyalin, an enzyme in saliva, is released during chewing and initiates this process.

The pharynx is a mucous-lined tube situated at the back of the mouth, nasal cavity, and larynx. Its muscles push food to the esophagus, a flat canal about 10 to 12 inches long extending from the lower neck through the chest to the stomach.

CAUSE OF CANCER

Tumors of the upper digestive system, except for the tongue, are a more yin form of cancer. They are caused primarily by long-term consumption of expansive yin substances, including milk and dairy products, oily and greasy foods, sugar and other sweeteners, tropical fruits and vegetables, coffee and black tea, spices, vitamin pills and protein supplements, alcohol, drugs, and medications. In the Far East a diet centered around refined white rice, the use of sugar and refined oil, the increasing use of chemical seasonings and flavors, and the popular practice of chewing betel-nut leaves, a gumlike wad of spices, are the main factors contributing to the high rise of mouth, throat, and esophageal cancers in that part of the world.

As we have seen, digestion begins in the mouth, and the primary function of saliva is to alkalinize (make more yang) entering foodstuffs. A meal consisting primarily of whole grains and other balanced foods will begin to break down in the mouth as the enzyme in saliva slowly metabolizes starch into maltose, a disaccharide. Thorough chewing is essential for this process, and it is especially necessary to balance the acidity of extreme yin foods, drinks, and medications. If chewing is minimal or light, not enough saliva will be secreted to neutralize the excess volume or strong quality of incoming yin. As a result, these expansive substances will be prematurely absorbed into the blood system in the mouth, throat, esophagus, or stomach. This makes for a thinner condition of the blood and other bodily fluids, ultimately giving rise to illness, loss of vitality, and degeneration of the organism.

The progressive development of disease in the upper digestive system, as in other systems of the body, takes the form of localized inflammations, ulcers, cysts, and, finally, tumors. Mouth cancer is often preceded by leukoplakia, a disease characterized by the growth of thick white patches on the inside of the cheeks, gums, or tongue. Cancer of the esophagus is commonly accompanied by difficulty in swallowing as the gullet moves to restrict the passage of harmful and irritating substances by creating a natural obstruction.

Cancer of the tongue, a small, compact organ, is a more yang form of mouth cancer and is caused by the excessive intake of yin accompanied by overly yang food. Cancer of the tongue could result from long-term consumption of sardines and cream cheese, smoked white fish cooked with spices, overconsumption of salt and fatty, greasy, and oily foods, or other extreme combinations.

Cancer of the throat is caused by consumption of both extreme yin and yang foods and beverages, including overconsumption of greasy and oily foods, dairy foods, flour products, sugar, and other sweeteners.

MEDICAL EVIDENCE

- A 1975 study in the Caspian littoral region of Iran, an area of high esophageal cancer, indicated a lower intake of lentils and other pulses, cooked green vegetables, and other whole foods.[1]
- Mormon males in California have 55 percent less esophageal cancer and females 39 percent less than other Californians. A 1980 epidemiological study associated lowered cancer risk with the Mormons' diet, which is high in whole grains, vegetables, and fruit, moderate in meat, and low in stimulants, alcohol, tobacco, and drugs.[2]
- Dietary Risks of Esophageal Cancer. In a study of esophageal squamous cell cancer risk in a high-incidence region of rural China, researchers at Fudan University in Shanghai reported that the disease was associated in both men and women with pork braised in brown sauce and in men who smoked tobacco, consumed alcohol, and had diets high in salt and chili.[3]

DIAGNOSIS

Cancers of the mouth and throat are commonly detected by X-rays of the chest, skull, and jaw, an upper GI series, various endoscopies, and a biopsy. Esophageal tumors will be diagnosed with these methods as well as liver and bone scans to check for metastases and a bronchoscopy to see whether the tumor has spread to the bronchial tubes.

Cancers of the upper digestive organs can be pinpointed, however, without the intervention of high technology, including potentially harmful X-ray radiation. In visual diagnosis the upper lip corresponds with the condition of the upper digestive system. Specifically, the top part of the upper lip reflects the condition of the esophagus, and the lower part of the upper lip reveals the state of the stomach. Swellings, discolorations, or patches in this region indicate corresponding troubles in the respective digestive organs. For example, a pinkish white hue on the lips shows overconsumption of sugar, fruits, fats, and dairy products. White patches show an excessive intake of dairy foods and fat.

The condition of the gums and mouth cavity offers other clues to general health. Swollen gums, often accompanied by pain and inflammation, are caused by overconsumption of liquid, oil, sugar, fruits, and juices. Receding gums are caused by either the overconsumption of yang foods, including animal food, salts, and dried food, or overconsumption of yin foods, including sugar, honey, chocolate, soft drinks, and fruit juices. Abnormally red or purple gums that are not swollen are caused by a combination of yang animal food or salts and yin sugar, fruits, juices, soft drinks, and chemicals. Similar colors accompanied by swelling are caused by the overconsumption of yin foods and drinks. Pale, whitish gums indicate poor circulation as well as a lack of hemoglobin in the bloodstream due to anemia caused by a nutritional imbalance.

Pimples appearing on the inner wall of the mouth cavity are eliminations of excessive protein, fat, oil (from either animal or plant sources), sugar, or sugar products. Bleeding gums, in most cases, are caused by broken blood capillaries that have been weakened by a lack of salt and other minerals in the bloodstream. In rare cases they can also be caused by an overconsumption of animal food, dry flour products, salts, and minerals, and a lack of fresh fruits and vegetables, as in the case of scurvy. Inflammation deep in the throat, with or without swollen tonsils, is caused by the overconsumption of such yin foods as fruits, juices, sugar, soda, ice-cold drinks, and milk.

The back region of the tongue, the root area below the uvula, also corresponds to the esophagus. Discolorations, inflammation, pimples, or patches here indicate disorders in the gullet.

DIETARY RECOMMENDATIONS

For all cancers in the upper digestive tract, including the mouth, gums, lips, tongue, larynx, pharynx, and esophagus, it is of primary importance that fatty and oily foods, including animal foods such as meat, poultry, eggs, and dairy food of any kind, as well as vegetable oil, be avoided. Sugar, chocolate, fruits, juices, soda, and all food and beverages treated by sweeteners, as well as heavily chemicalized and artificialized food and beverages, are to be avoided. All stimulants including alcohol, coffee, black tea, aromatic herb drinks, curry, mustard, and peppers should be discontinued. Avoid refined flour products and limit even unrefined flour products. Dietary guidelines are as follows:

- Whole Grains: Forty to 50 percent of daily consumption, by volume, should be whole cereal grains. The first day prepare plain short- or medium-grain brown rice, pressure-cooked or cooked in a heavy cast-iron or ceramic pot with a heavy lid. On subsequent days, alternate brown rice pressure-cooked with 20 to 30 percent millet, then rice with 20 to 30 percent barley, then rice with 20 to 30 percent aduki beans or lentils, and then plain rice again. A delicious morning porridge can be made by taking leftover rice, adding a little more water to soften it, seasoning with a little miso, and simmering for two to three minutes more. In ordinary cooking the ratio of grain to water should be about 1:2. For seasoning, cook with a postage-stamp-sized piece of kombu or a pinch of sea salt, depending on the person's condition. Other grains can be used occasionally, including whole wheat berries, rye, corn, buckwheat, and whole oats, although oats should be avoided for the first month. Good-quality sourdough bread may be enjoyed two to three times a week, and noodles, both udon and soba, may also be eaten two to three times a week. Avoid all hard-baked products until the condition improves, including cookies, cake, pie, crackers, muffins, and the like.

- Soup: Five to 10 percent of daily consumption should be soup, consisting of one or two cups or bowls cooked with wakame sea vegetable and various land vegetables such as onions and carrots, seasoned with miso or shoyu. Occasionally a small amount of shiitake mushrooms may be added to the soup. Millet soup made with sweet vegetables is especially beneficial for this condition. The miso used in seasoning soups may be barley miso, brown rice miso, or soybean (hatcho) miso, and should be naturally aged for two to three years.

- Vegetables: Twenty to 30 percent of daily consumption should be vegetables, cooked in a variety of forms. Hard, leafy vegetables are to be emphasized, supplemented with root vegetables and round vegetables such as onions, pumpkin, autumn squash, and cabbage. As a general rule, the following dishes may be prepared, although the frequency may differ from person to person: nishime-style vegetables, four times a week; a squash-aduki-kombu dish, three times a week; dried daikon, one cup, three times a week; carrots and carrot tops or daikon and daikon tops, three times a week; blanched vegetables, five to seven times a week; pressed salad, five to seven times a week; raw salad and salad dressing, avoid; steamed greens, five to seven times a week; sautéed vegetables, two to three times a week, using water the first month and then a small amount of sesame oil thereafter; kinpira, two-thirds of a cup, two times a week; tofu, dried tofu, tempeh, or seitan with vegetables, two times a week.

- Beans: Five percent of daily consumption should be small beans, such as aduki beans, lentils, chickpeas, or black soybeans, cooked together with sea vegetables such as kombu or with onions and carrots. Other beans may be used two or three times a month. For seasoning, a small amount of unrefined sea salt or shoyu or miso can be used. Bean products, such as tempeh, natto, and dried or cooked tofu, may be used occasionally but in moderate amounts.

- Sea Vegetables: Five percent or less sea vegetable dishes, including wakame and kombu. should be included daily when cooking grain, in soup, etc. A sheet of toasted nori may also be taken daily. A small dish of hijiki or arame should be prepared two times a week. All other sea vegetables are optional.

- Condiments: Those that should be available on the table are gomashio (sesame salt), on the average made with one part salt to eighteen parts sesame seeds (reduced to 1:16 after two months); kelp or wakame powder; umeboshi plum; and tekka, although all other regular macrobiotic condiments may be used if desired. These condiments may be used daily on grains and vegetables, but the volume should be moderate to suit individual appetite and taste.

- Pickles: Made at home in a variety of ways, pickles are to be eaten daily, one tablespoon in all, although salty pickles are to be minimized.
- Animal Foods: Meat, poultry, eggs, and other strong animal food are to be avoided. A small volume of white-meat fish may be eaten once a week. The fish should be steamed, boiled, or poached and garnished with grated daikon or ginger. After two months, fish may be eaten twice a week if desired. Strictly avoid blue-meat and red-meat fish and all shellfish.
- Fruit: None is best, and the less the better, including both tropical and temperate-climate fruit, until the condition improves. If cravings develop, a small amount of cooked fruit with a pinch of sea salt or dried fruit (also preferably cooked) may be eaten. Avoid all fruit juices and cider temporarily, as well as raisins, currants, and other highly concentrated fruits.
- Sweets and Snacks: Avoid all sweets and desserts, including good-quality macrobiotic desserts, until the condition improves. To satisfy a sweet tooth, use sweet vegetables every day in cooking, drink sweet vegetable drinks (see special drinks on page 386), and eat sweet vegetable jam. Mochi, rice balls, vegetable sushi, and other grain-based snacks may be eaten frequently. Limit rice cakes, popcorn, and other dry or baked snacks because they may harden the tumor. In the event of cravings, a small amount of amasake, barley malt, or rice syrup may be consumed.
- Nuts and Seeds: Nuts and nut butters are to be avoided due to their high fat and protein, except for chestnuts. Unsalted blanched seeds such as squash seeds and pumpkin seeds may be consumed as a snack, up to one cup total per week.
- Seasonings: Unrefined sea salt, shoyu, and miso are to be used moderately in order to avoid unnecessary thirst. Avoid mirin and garlic. If you become particularly thirsty after a meal or between meals, you should cut back on these seasonings until the normal level of thirst returns.
- Beverages: Drinks and other dietary practices can follow the general recommendations in Part I, with bancha twig tea as the main beverage. Strictly avoid the beverages on the "infrequent" and "avoid" lists, and don't have grain coffee for the first two to three months after starting this new way of eating.

Chewing thoroughly is essential for all types of cancer but especially for cancers in the mouth and upper alimentary tract. Chew each mouthful fifty times or preferably a hundred times. Liquefying and mixing food well with saliva contributes to the prevention and improvement of this condition. Also, it is important to avoid overconsumption of liquid, although bancha tea or water should be consumed if thirst arises. It is also important to avoid overeating and eating within three hours of sleeping.

As noted in the introduction to Part II, people who have received or who are currently undergoing medical treatment may need to make further dietary modifications.

SPECIAL DRINKS AND DISHES

One or more special drinks or side dishes may need to be consumed, depending on the individual case, to help reduce excess protein and fat, which are the cause of the cancer; to reduce cholesterol levels; and to assist recovery. Please see a qualified macrobiotic teacher for guidance. Amounts and frequencies given here are averages for each drink or dish; these will differ from person to person. Further directions are in Chapter 36.

- Sweet Vegetable Drink: Take one small cup every day for one month and then two to three times a week the second month.
- Carrot-Daikon Drink: Take one small cup two to three times a week for two to four weeks and then once every three days for one month.
- Scallion-Miso Condiment: Take one teaspoon frequently, but avoid a salty or strong taste.
- Ume-Sho-Kuzu: This may be drunk daily for one to two weeks and occasionally afterward to strengthen the blood and for general vitality.
- Kinpira Soup: This dish may be eaten two to three times a week for strength and vitality.
- Soba Noodles: Buckwheat products are strengthening and may be eaten two to three times a week for more yin malignancies. (The more yang types should avoid buckwheat.)
- Grated Daikon: Take a half cup of fresh daikon with a few drops of shoyu two to three times a week. It is good for melting fat deposits.
- Lotus-Daikon-Cabbage Juice: For throat cancer drink this twice a day for ten days, followed by once a day for another ten days, and then every other day or three to four times a week for another three to four weeks.
- Genuine Brown Rice Cream: In the event the person cannot eat or a tube has been inserted, the diet should be liquefied by cooking with more water and by mashing food in a food mill. Homemade rice cream is also helpful and may be eaten with miso soup and other liquefied or mashed foods, including vegetables, beans, and sea vegetables. Carrot and Lotus Root Drink is helpful in this case, too.

HOME CARE

- Body Scrub: Scrubbing the whole body, including the throat and neck, with a towel that has been immersed in hot water and squeezed out is very helpful for better circulation of blood, lymph, and other body fluids, as well as for activating physical and mental energies.
- Compress Guidelines: For a small number of tumors in the upper digestive system, a compress may be needed to help gradually draw out excess mucus and fat. Please see a qualified macrobiotic teacher for guidance on the proper use and frequency of a compress or plaster. Several types are used depending on the person's condition. Precede the compress or plaster with the application of a towel that has been soaked in hot water and squeezed out over the affected area for about three to five minutes to stimulate circulation.
- Hato Mugi-Potato-Cabbage Plaster: Make this throat cancer application and spread it on cotton linen. Apply it directly to the throat for three to four hours, twice a day, or sleep with it overnight. Do this for two to three weeks. This may also be helpful for thyroid cancer.
- Cabbage Plaster: Apply directly to the throat with the same conditions.
- Massage: Massage the toes up to the knees for ten minutes twice a day for one month.
- Palm Healing: Palm healing on the mouth or throat region is also helpful to control pain and discomfort.
- After Surgery: In the event that the esophagus is blocked by a tumorous obstruction and the person is unable to eat, or if the tumor has been removed and a tube has been inserted via the nose, the diet should be liquefied by cooking with more water and by mashing food substances. Rice cream is also helpful and may be consumed with miso soup as well as other mashed and liquefied vegetables, beans, and sea vegetables. Carrot and lotus-root drink is also helpful in this case.

EMOTIONAL CONSIDERATIONS

Positive emotions associated with the upper digestive system are hope, honesty, and openness. Problems in the oral cavity may arise from despair, lack of emotional nourishment, and blocked expression. Neglect, abuse, guilt, and other factors can also contribute to restricting this area.

High-quality foods that nourish the upper digestive system and help develop positive emotions include whole grains, especially barley and wheat; beans and bean products; leafy green vegetables; sea vegetables; fermented foods; and good-quality sea salt, oil, and other seasonings.

Foods that harm this region and contribute to negative emotions especially include chicken and eggs, as well as meat and dairy food; strong fish and seafood; white flour; sugar, chocolate, and other highly refined sweets; chemicalized and artificial foods; too many raw foods; too many stimulants and other beverages; alcohol; excessive salt and salty foods; and other extremely contractive or expansive items.

In relationships it is important to express oneself freely and honestly. If a person is not able to make herself understood, emotional disturbances may follow, including disorders in the mouth, throat, and esophagus.

On a planetary scale, the upper digestive system correlates with deltas, reservoirs, swamps, and other waterways, including those where fresh and saline water meet. Oral cancers mirror the stagnation and toxic buildup in these natural regions.

OTHER CONSIDERATIONS

- Avoid synthetic clothing, especially around the area of the throat, neck, head, and chest, and use cotton underwear, clothing, and sleepwear if possible.
- Maintaining clean fresh air inside the home is important, and for this purpose green plants can be placed in each room. Indoor air circulation can also be maintained by frequently opening the windows.
- Avoid frequent exposure to artificial radiation, including medical and dental X-rays, smoke detectors, television, video terminals, and handheld appliances, which are weakening to the lymph and blood and to the upper digestive system.
- Try to be happy, positive, and outgoing. Singing, dancing, and playing are particularly beneficial in improving overall health and mentality and harmonizing with the rhythms of nature.
- Light exercise, including breathing fresh air outdoors and ten to fifteen minutes a day practicing long exhalations through the nostrils, will promote harmonious mental and physical metabolism and contribute to overall relaxation.

PERSONAL EXPERIENCE

GRANULAR MYOBLASTOMA ON THE VOCAL CORD

In the spring of 1979, Laura Anne Fitzpatrick discovered that her voice had become raspy when she tried out for cheerleader at her high school in Sherborn, Massachusetts. Doctors told her that she had a benign tumor on the vocal cords known as a granular myoblastoma, and in August she had it surgically removed. By January 1980, however, the tumor had reappeared, and Laura underwent a second operation, this time with advanced laser-beam surgery, at University Hospital in Boston. A month later the swelling returned, and doctors feared yet another recurrence of the obstruction.

During this period, Laura and her family saw a television program on macrobiotics. After attending a seminar on cancer and diet at the East West Foundation, Laura came to see me for a consultation, and I recommended the Cancer Prevention Diet. I warned her to avoid oil in cooking completely and advised her to go to bed with a taro plaster wrapped around her neck. Laura's family, including her parents, two sisters, and three brothers still living at home, was very supportive and started the macrobiotic way of eating as well. "John and I both wanted to support Laura, and we also began to eat in this new way as much as we could," her mother later noted. "We changed our stove from electric to gas, and the adventures continued as we truly tried to understand the principles behind the diet."

Laura experienced many changes in her body as the toxins from many previous years of imbalanced eating were rapidly released. She began to feel more energy, and her voice started improving. In the spring of 1980 she returned for a medical checkup, and her doctor was surprised to find that the operation was unnecessary. Laura continued to improve through the fall. However, in November she began to deviate from the diet and use oil in cooking. On Thanksgiving she had turkey. By Christmas her symptoms started to return, and her voice grew weak. The doctors told her the tumor had returned and would have to be removed.

Laura and her family asked the hospital for a two-month reprieve from surgery and returned to see me. Laura recalled of that visit: "[Michio] scolded me humorously, and I decided I was ready to get back to basics and resume the diet he had recommended. . . . I again began to discharge a lot of mucus and felt a tremendous cleansing coming very rapidly. I resumed the taro potato compresses each night. One humorous sidelight of this was that my father's T-shirts were disappearing, and he would find them with mysterious brown spots from the remains of the taro potato. I found that whenever I missed the ginger and taro potato plaster compress for a few days, the mucus would not discharge as freely. I prepared all the compresses by myself, and the routine became normal."

At the college she was now attending, Laura found it difficult to get the proper food and care she needed, but with the help of her family she succeeded. In March 1981 she returned for a medical checkup, and her doctor told her the condition had improved and stabilized, and there was no need for surgery. "I learned from this experience that the diet makes sense," Laura concluded. "I feel I am well on my way to a full and complete recovery." Today, twelve years later, Laura is happily married and in excellent health.[4]

27

Pancreatic Cancer

FREQUENCY

Nearly 33,370 Americans will die from pancreatic cancer this year, and 37,170 new cases will arise. Overall, pancreatic cancer has declined in both men and women in the last twenty years. But prognosis remains poor (overall five-year survival is only 5 percent), and despite its relatively small overall prevalence, it is the fourth leading cause of cancer death in the country.

Affecting primarily those over sixty, it affects men about twice as often as women, but it is rising more rapidly among women. About 90 percent of pancreatic cancers are adenocarcinomas, affecting exocrine cells that perform digestive functions, and most of these are accompanied by pancreatitis and obstruction of the ducts. The other 10 percent are tumors of the islet cells involved with sugar metabolism. Pancreatic cancer may spread to the liver or small intestine.

Modern medical treatment calls for surgery, but because the disease is difficult to diagnose in early stages, many tumors have already metastasized and are considered inoperable. If operable, a partial or total pancreatectomy is performed. The first procedure calls for the removal of part of the organ, adjacent lymph nodes, the duodenum, part of the stomach, and the common bile duct. A total pancreatomy involves removing the whole pancreas. Radiation and chemotherapy may be given after surgery to control pain, but recovery is not a frequent occurrence. Because there is no early detection of this type of malignancy, many patients die within a few months of diagnosis. Pancreatic tumors may spread to the liver or small intestine.

Risk factors include smoking, obesity, diabetes, a sedentary lifestyle, chronic pancreatitis, diabetes, cirrhosis, and exposure to chemicals and toxins.

STRUCTURE

The pancreas is 6 to 8 inches in length and weighs about 3 ounces. It is situated behind the stomach and is connected to the duodenum through a common bile duct with the liver and gallbladder. The sections of the pancreas are known as the head, body, and tail. The head secretes pancreatic juice into the duodenum, and this juice aids in the digestion of carbohydrates, fats, and protein. The body of the pancreas produces enzymes and hormones, including insulin, which regulate sugar levels in the blood. These hormones are secreted by the islets of Langerhans, a network of cells scattered throughout the pancreas, which vary in number from 200,000 to 1.8 million. They are most numerous in the tail portion of the pancreas, which touches the spleen.

CAUSE OF CANCER

Diabetes and hyperinsulinism are the two major degenerative diseases associated with the pancreas and are related to the rise of tumors in this organ. To understand the progressive development of pancreatic disorders, it is necessary to consider the effects of the three different forms of sugar on the body. Simple sugars, or monosaccharides, are found in fruits and honey and include glucose and fructose. Double sugars, or disaccharides, are found in cane sugar and milk and include sucrose and lactose. Complex sugars, or polysaccharides, are found in grains, beans, and vegetables and include cellulose.

In the normal digestive process, complex sugars are decomposed gradually and at a nearly even rate by various enzymes in the mouth, stomach, pancreas, and intestines. Complex sugars enter the bloodstream slowly after being broken down into smaller saccharide units. During the process, the pH of the blood remains slightly alkaline.

In contrast, simple and double sugars are metabolized quickly, causing the blood to become overly acidic. To compensate for this extreme yin condition, the pancreas secretes a yang hormone, insulin, which allows excess sugar in the blood to be removed and enter the cells of the body. This produces a burst of energy as the glucose (the end product of all sugar metabolism) is oxidized and carbon dioxide and water are given off as wastes. Diabetes is a disease characterized by the failure of the pancreas to produce enough insulin to neutralize excess blood sugar. After years of excessive consumption of refined sugar, fruit, dairy products, chemicals, and other highly yin substances, the islet cells in the pancreas become expanded and lose their ability to secrete insulin. Sugar begins to appear in the urine, the body loses water, and reserve minerals are depleted. To offset these symptoms, modern medicine treats diabetes with artificial injections of insulin.

Much of the sugar that enters the bloodstream was originally stored in the liver in the form of glycogen until needed, when it is again changed into glucose. When the amount of glycogen exceeds the liver's storage capacity of about 50 grams, it is released into the bloodstream in the form of fatty acid. This fatty acid is stored first in the more inactive places of the body, such as the buttocks, thighs, and midsection. Then, if refined sugars continue to be eaten, fatty acid becomes attracted to more yang organs such as the heart and kidney, which gradually become encased in a layer of fat and mucus.

This accumulation can also penetrate the inner tissues, weakening the normal functioning of the organs and causing their eventual stoppage, such as in atherosclerosis. The buildup of fat can also lead to various forms of cancer, including tumors of the breast, colon, and reproductive organs. Still another form of degeneration may occur when the body's internal supply of minerals is mobilized to offset the debilitating effects of simple sugar consumption. For example, calcium from the bones and teeth may be depleted to balance the effects of excessive intake of candy and soft drinks.

As a small, compact organ, the pancreas is yang in structure. Pancreatic cancer results primarily from the longtime consumption of eggs, meat, seafood, poultry, refined salt, and other strong yang animal foods high in protein and saturated fat, in combination with refined sugars and other strong yin foods and beverages, chemicals, and drugs. Tumors in the pancreas may follow the development of pancreatitis (the acute or chronic inflammation of the organ) and hyperinsulinism (an overly contractive condition in which blood sugar levels are abnormally low from secretion of too much insulin). The overproduction of insulin attracts fatty acids and coagulates into tumors in the bile duct or the islets of Langerhans. Diabetes may be treated and relieved by adopting a slightly more yang macrobiotic diet consisting of whole grains and vegetables, prepared with a slightly longer cooking time and heavier taste, while cancer of the pancreas can be reversed by a slightly more yin diet consisting primarily of whole grains and vegetables prepared with a little bit less cooking and a lighter taste.

MEDICAL EVIDENCE

- Mormons, whose diet is high in whole grains, vegetables, and fruits, moderate in meat, and low in stimulants, alcohol, and tobacco, have substantially less pancreatic cancer than the general population, according to a 1980 epidemiological survey. Male Mormons have 36 percent less and females 19 percent less. High church officials, who adhere more faithfully to the group's dietary recommendations, have 53 percent less pancreatic cancer.[1]

- In a study of twenty-four patients with pancreatic cancer who adopted a macrobiotic diet, Tulane University researchers found that their mean length of survival was 17.3 months, compared with 6 months for matched controls from a national tumor registry diagnosed during the same time period (1984–85). The one-year survival rate was 54.2 percent in the macrobiotic patients versus 10 percent in the controls. All comparisons were statistically significant.[2]

- In a study of diet related to increased rates of pancreatic cancer in Japan, researchers found that the intake of meats and animal viscera increased the risk of this disease, while vegetables and traditional foods, including tofu, deep-fried tofu, tempura, and raw fish, reduced the risk. "The traditional Japanese foods, which include many plant foods, are preventive against the occurrence of pancreas cancer," the scientists concluded.[3]

- The high consumption of sweetened food and beverages increases the risk of developing pancreatic cancer, according to researchers at the Karolinska Institute. In a study of almost eighty thousand healthy women and men from 1997 to 2005, those who drank two or more fizzy or syrup-based drinks daily ran a 90 percent higher risk of developing pancreatic cancer compared to those who never drank them. Those who added sugar to food or drinks (such as coffee) at least five times a day had a 70 percent higher risk than those who did not. Those who consumed creamed fruit once a day had a 50 percent higher risk.[4]

- Whole grains and other high-fiber foods may lower the risk of pancreatic cancer by 40 percent. In a study of 532 people with pancreatic cancer and 1,701 without the disease, Dr. June M. Chan of the University of California, San Francisco, and associates report that adults who ate two or more servings of whole grains each day almost halved their risk of this disease compared to those who consumed less than one serving. "The risk reductions associated with some whole grain foods and fiber provide general support for the hypothesis that whole grains are better than more refined and sweetened grains for pancreatic cancer prevention," Chan said.[5]

DIAGNOSIS

In the hospital, pancreatic cancer is diagnosed by a variety of means, including lab tests, a fasting blood sugar test, liver scans, upper and lower GI series, CT scan, ultrasound, and an ERCP (endoscopic retrograde cholan-giopancreatography). The ERCP is a kind of endoscope or tube that is swallowed and woven into the duodenum. It contains a tiny catheter that is inserted into the duct of the pancreas, a dye is injected into the pancreas, and X-rays may then be taken. If a tumor is indicated, cell and tissue samples will be taken in a biopsy or a major surgical procedure called a laparotomy, in which the abdominal wall is opened and the inner organs palpated by the surgeon.

Oriental medicine relies on simpler visual cues to ascertain the condition of the pancreas. In facial diagnosis, two major areas correspond with the pancreas: the upper bridge of the nose and the outside of the temples. Swellings, discolorations, or other abnormal markings in these locations indicate pancreatic and sometimes also spleen disorders. For instance, a dark color shows overburdening of the pancreas and elimination of excessive sugars, including cane sugar, honey, syrups, chocolate, fruit, and milk. Red pimples and patches in these regions are caused by excess sugar, sweets, juice, and fruits. Whitish yellow pimples are caused by fats and oils from both animal and vegetable sources, including dairy foods. Dark patches and pimples are caused by excessive sweets or by salt and flour products. Moles here are caused by excess animal-quality protein and fat, and show an overactive spleen and pancreas. A light green color appearing together with whitish, reddish, or dark fatty, oily skin textures in either of these areas indicates possible pancreatic cancer.

Blisters on the eyes may also reflect tumor development in the pancreas. A reddish yellow color in the pink area inside the lower eyelid is caused by consumption of excess yang animal food together with excess yin. A blue-gray color in the middle regions of the white of the eye further suggests cancer in the pancreas.

Above the bridge of the nose, hair growing between the eyebrows shows that the person's mother ate a high amount of dairy food and fatty animal food during the third and fourth months of pregnancy. A person with this type of eyebrows is particularly susceptible to pancreatic, spleen, and liver disorders and should be careful to avoid meat, poultry, eggs, dairy foods, and oily and fatty foods.

Oily skin in general shows disorders in fat metabolism, including pancreatic troubles. A yellowish color of the skin from excess yang foods also shows bile troubles and probable pancreatic malfunctioning.

Finally, cancer of the pancreas, spleen, or lymph is indicated by the presence of a light green color along the spleen meridian. Observe especially the area of the foot below the anklebone extending to the outside of the big toe.

Oriental diagnosis allows us to quickly scan these and other areas and accurately determine the condition of the pancreas and other internal organs. A propensity to cancer can be identified long before it develops and corrective dietary adjustments made.

DIETARY RECOMMENDATIONS

The primary cause of pancreatic cancer is the longtime overconsumption of animal food, especially chicken, eggs, cheese, and shellfish such as shrimp, crabmeat, and lobster, which gradually gather in the pancreas and create a tumor. All animal food should be avoided, including meat, dairy food, and fish and seafood, all of which are high in fat and cholesterol. Pancreatic cancer is also accelerated by the overconsumption of salty food, hard-baked food, and roasted food, as well as sugar and sugar-treated food, soft drinks, spices, stimulants, tropical fruits and fruit juices, and chemicals used in various ways for food production and processing. All these foods and beverages are to be avoided. Although not the cause of pancreatic cancer, refined flour and flour products easily tend to produce mucus and should therefore also be avoided. Commercial seasonings, sauces, and dressings, in which artificial chemical processing is involved, should also be discontinued. It is especially important to avoid all food and drink that make organs, muscles, and tissues tight, including a high amount of salty food. Dietary guidelines are as follows:

- Whole Grains: Forty to 50 percent of daily consumption, by volume, should be whole cereal grains. The first day prepare plain short- or medium-grain brown rice, pressure-cooked or cooked in a heavy cast-iron or ceramic pot with a heavy lid. On subsequent days, alternate brown rice cooked with 20 to 30 percent millet, then rice with 20 to 30 percent barley, then rice with 20 to 30 percent aduki beans or lentils, and then plain rice again. A delicious morning porridge can be made by taking leftover rice, adding a little more water to soften it, seasoning with a little miso, and simmering for two to three minutes more. In daily cooking the ratio of grain to water should be about 1:2. For seasoning, cook with a postage-stamp-sized piece of kombu instead of salt. Other grains can be used occasionally, including whole wheat berries, rye, corn, and whole oats, although oats should be avoided for the first month. Buckwheat should be avoided for about six months because it is very contractive and may harden the tumor. Seitan is also very yang and should be minimized. Flour products, even unrefined whole wheat bread, chapatis, pancakes, and cookies, should be totally avoided or limited in volume for a period of a few months. Whole grain pasta and noodles may be eaten a couple of times a week.
- Soup: Five to 10 percent of daily consumption should be soup, consisting of one or two cups or bowls cooked with wakame sea vegetable and various vegetables, especially sweet round vegetables such as squash, onions, and cabbage, seasoned lightly with miso or shoyu. Occasionally a small amount of shiitake mushrooms may be

added to the soup. The miso may be barley miso, brown rice miso, or soybean (hatcho) miso, and should be naturally aged two to three years. Grain soups, bean soups, and other soups may be eaten from time to time.

- Vegetables: Twenty to 30 percent of daily consumption should be vegetables, cooked in a variety of forms, mainly steamed, boiled, and, after one month without oil, occasionally sautéed. Among vegetables, round vegetables such as squash, pumpkin, onions, and cabbage may be prepared proportionately more, although leafy green vegetables and root vegetables should also be consumed frequently. Lighter cooking, which leaves some freshness and crispness, is recommended. Prepare at least one dish every day in this way. As a rule of thumb, the following dishes may be prepared, although the frequency may differ from person to person: nishime-style vegetables, three times a week; a squash-aduki-kombu dish, three times a week; dried daikon, one cup, three times a week; carrots and carrot tops or daikon and daikon tops, three times a week; blanched vegetables, five to seven times a week; pressed salad, several times a week; raw salad, avoid; steamed greens, five to seven times a week; sautéed vegetables, prepared with sesame oil lightly brushed on the pan, once or twice a week; kinpira, two-thirds of a cup, two times a week; dried tofu, tofu, tempeh, or seitan with vegetables, two times a week.
- Beans: Five percent of daily consumption should be small beans, such as aduki beans, lentils, chickpeas, or black soybeans, cooked together with sea vegetables such as kombu or with onions and carrots. Other beans may be used two to three times a month. For seasoning, a small amount of unrefined sea salt or shoyu or miso can be used. Bean products, such as tempeh, natto, and dried or cooked tofu, may be used occasionally but in moderate amounts.
- Sea Vegetables: Five percent or less of sea vegetable dishes, including wakame and kombu, should be included daily when cooking grain, in soup, etc. A sheet of toasted nori may also be taken daily. A small dish of hijiki or arame should be prepared two times a week. All other sea vegetables are optional.
- Condiments: Those that should be available on the table are gomashio (sesame salt), on the average made with one part salt to eighteen to twenty parts sesame seeds; kelp or wakame powder; umeboshi plum; and tekka, although all other regular macrobiotic condiments may be used if desired. These condiments may be used daily on grains and vegetables, but the amounts should be moderate to suit individual appetites and tastes.
- Pickles: Made at home in a variety of ways, pickles are to be eaten daily, one tablespoon in all, although salty pickles are to be minimized. Rice bran (nuka) pickles are the most suitable.

- Animal Food: Fish and other animal food is to be avoided. However, in the event that animal food is craved, a small amount of white-meat fish may be eaten once every ten days to two weeks. The fish should be steamed, boiled, or poached and garnished with grated daikon or ginger. Strictly avoid blue-meat and red-meat fish and all shellfish.
- Fruit: The less the better until the condition improves. If cravings develop, a small amount of cooked fruit with a pinch of sea salt or dried fruit (also preferably cooked) may be taken. Avoid all fruit juices and cider temporarily, as well as raisins, currants, and other highly concentrated fruits.
- Sweets and Snacks: Overuse of sweets is connected with pancreatic disorders, so it is very important to avoid all sweets and desserts, including good-quality macrobiotic desserts, until the condition improves. To satisfy a sweet tooth, use sweet vegetables every day in cooking, drink sweet vegetable drinks, or eat sweet vegetable jam. If cravings arise, a small amount of amasake, barley malt, or rice syrup may be eaten. If cravings persist, a little cider, apple juice, or chestnut puree may be prepared. Mochi, rice balls, vegetable sushi, and other grain-based snacks may be eaten frequently. Limit rice cakes, popcorn, and other dry or baked snacks because they may harden the tumor.
- Nuts and Seeds: Nuts and nut butters are to be avoided due to their high fat and protein, except for chestnuts. Unsalted blanched seeds such as sunflower seeds and pumpkin seeds may be consumed as a snack, up to one cup total per week.
- Seasonings: Unrefined sea salt, shoyu, and miso are to be used moderately in order to avoid unnecessary thirst. Avoid mirin and garlic. If you become particularly thirsty after a meal or between meals, you should cut back on these seasonings until the normal level of thirst returns.
- Beverages: Drinks and other dietary practices can follow the general recommendations in Part I including bancha twig tea as the main beverage. Strictly avoid the beverages on the "infrequent" and "avoid" lists, and don't have grain coffee for the first two to three months after starting this new way of eating.

The most important thing in connection with dietary practice is chewing very well, until all food becomes liquid in the mouth and is well mixed with saliva. Chew very well, at least fifty times, preferably a hundred times per mouthful. It is also important to avoid overeating and eating within three hours of sleeping.

As noted in the introduction to Part II, people who have received or who are currently undergoing medical treatment may need to make further dietary modifications.

SPECIAL DRINKS AND DISHES

One or more special drinks or side dishes may need to be consumed, depending on the individual case, to help reduce excess protein and fat, which are the cause of the cancer; to reduce cholesterol levels; and to assist recovery. Please see a qualified macrobiotic teacher for guidance. Amounts and frequencies given here are averages for each drink or dish; these will differ from person to person. Further directions are in Chapter 36.

- Sweet Vegetable Drink: Take one small cup every morning and every evening for three to four weeks. After that, reduce it to once every other day and continue for another three to four weeks.
- Fresh Apple Juice and Sweet Vegetable Drink: If jaundice occurs, combine the same amount of fresh apple juice and sweet vegetable drink and simmer for about 2 minutes. Drink two to three small cups of this preparation every day for three to five days.
- Grated Daikon and Carrot with Shiitake Tea: For abdominal swelling, drink two small cups of this broth every day for three to five days.
- Dried Daikon and Shiitake Tea: Drink two small cups of this broth every day for five days.
- Carrot Juice: Carrot juice, preferably heated, may be had several times a week to relax the pancreas or relieve pan.

HOME CARE

- Body Scrub: Scrubbing the whole body, including the abdominal region and the spinal region, with a towel that has been immersed in hot water and squeezed out is very helpful for better circulation of blood, lymph, and other body fluids, as well as for activating physical and mental energies.
- Compress Guidelines: For a small number of pancreatic tumors, a compress may be needed to help gradually draw out excess mucus and fat. Please see a qualified macrobiotic teacher for guidance on the proper use and frequency of a compress or plaster. Several types are used depending on the person's condition. Precede the compress or plaster with the application of a towel that has been soaked in hot water and squeezed out over the affected area for about three to five minutes to stimulate circulation.
- Hato Mugi-Potato-Cabbage Plaster: If the tumor can be felt on the pancreas, or it has gotten harder, make this application and place directly on the affected part. Tie with a cotton strip. Sleep with the plaster, leaving it on for four hours or overnight. Repeat every day for one week to ten days.

- Massage: Massage the feet and all toes well for ten to fifteen minutes, two to three times every day. It is also helpful to massage the body all over to eliminate stiffness, but be careful not to push near the pancreas.
- Hot Foot Soak: Soak the feet in moderately hot water for three to five minutes to promote better circulation.
- Buckwheat Plaster: In the event of swelling from fluid retention in the pancreatic and abdominal regions or from gas formation, which quite often arises (both during the period of cancer development and/or during the period of recovery), a buckwheat plaster can be applied for one to two hours daily for several days. (A kombu plaster may be used instead of a buckwheat plaster to relieve gas formation.) Full-body shiatsu massage or palm healing to the abdominal region, thirty minutes to one hour daily, can also be helpful.

EMOTIONAL CONSIDERATIONS

Positive emotions associated with the pancreas are balance, trust, serving others, and compassion. Pancreatic problems may arise from excessive control and manipulation, mistrust, and lack of sympathy and consideration.

High-quality foods that nourish the pancreas and help develop positive emotions include naturally sweet things such as whole grains, particularly millet and sweet rice; sweet round vegetables, including cabbage, squash, and onions; tofu, yuba, and other soft, naturally processed soy foods; natural sweeteners, including amasake, rice syrup, and barley malt; round orange or yellow fruits such as peaches, nectarines, and apricots; and carrot juice, sweet vegetable drink, and other naturally sweet foods.

Foods that block the pancreas and contribute to suppressing positive emotions include too much meat; cheese, poultry, eggs, strong fish and seafood, and other heavy animal products; white flour; sugar, chocolate, and other highly processed sweets; chemicalized and artificial foods; and other extremely contractive or expansive foods and beverages.

In relationships it is important to trust one's partner, to try to understand things from his or her perspective, and to harmonize. A person who is mistrustful, suspicious, manipulative, and inconsiderate may localize his or her excess emotional energy in the pancreas.

On a planetary scale, the pancreas correlates with the grasslands and savannahs. Imbalance in this region is comparable to soil erosion.

OTHER CONSIDERATIONS

- Daily physical exercise that does not produce exhaustion is recommended. Ten to fifteen minutes of daily breathing exercises, especially emphasizing long exhalation, are also beneficial. These physical and breathing exercises contribute to relaxing tensions in the body and mind as well as harmonizing physical metabolism. Shiatsu, palm healing, and other gentle activities and exercises are helpful.

- Keeping air quality clean and fresh is important for the maintenance of general health. For that purpose, green leafy plants can be placed in the house and the windows periodically opened to allow the circulation of fresh air.
- Avoid wearing wool and synthetic fibers. At the minimum wear cotton underwear and use cotton sheets and pillowcases.
- Avoid watching television for long stretches. Radiation weakens the chest area. Similarly, avoid other artificial sources of electromagnetic energy such as video terminals, smoke detectors, and handheld electrical appliances.

PERSONAL EXPERIENCE

PANCREATIC CANCER

On August 21, 1973, Jean Kohler, a professor of music at Ball State University in Muncie, Indiana, underwent exploratory surgery at Indiana University Medical Center. The fifty-six-year-old pianist had always been healthy and kept fit by gardening and lifting weights. During the summer he had experienced an itching that spread from his leg; he thought he had contracted poison oak. Initial medical tests turned up nothing. However, chief surgeon John Jesseph discovered a tumor the size of a fist on the head of Kohler's pancreas. Moreover, the cancer had spread to the duodenum. Like most other pancreatic cancer patients, Kohler's condition was discovered too late to operate. Dr. Phillip Christiansen, the other doctor in the case, concluded pessimistically, "I know nothing coming out of research in the next ten years that could possibly help him." Kohler was told he would live anywhere from one month to three years and was advised to take chemotherapy to control the pain.

After five days of drug treatment, Kohler suffered badly swollen hands and arms as well as a cough, chills, and general stress. With the help of his wife, Mary Alice, he decided to search for an alternative treatment. An Indiana nutritionist referred him to me, and the Kohlers arrived in Boston for a consultation on September 25. Visual diagnosis, especially the presence of a small blister on Jean's right eye, confirmed the presence of pancreatic cancer.

Kohler expressed a sincere desire to follow the Cancer Prevention Diet for pancreatic tumors outlined above, and I told him that he would be out of danger within three to six months. Prior to this time Jean had consumed meat twice a day, had eaten much canned and packaged food, and had a well-developed sweet tooth. He especially enjoyed milk, cocoa, soft drinks, milk shakes, and desserts topped with whipped cream. A threat of diabetes several years earlier made him switch to diet sodas and saccharin and sucaryl instead of sugar.

In Boston the Kohlers spent a few days learning to cook according to yin and yang. "One of the most amazing and totally unexpected benefits for us personally was that after only five days of macrobiotic food, Jean's hands were suddenly much more flexible," Mary Alice later recalled. "He could reach farther on the keyboard than ever before! This condition has remained to the present time."

On April 7, 1974, after following the diet faithfully for about six months, Kohler returned to Boston. Visual diagnosis indicated that all signs of cancer activity had disappeared. There was a small tumor, the size of a walnut, but it was no longer malignant. Back home Jean continued the Cancer Prevention Diet for another three months and in July was healthy enough to add a little maple syrup to his diet. He continued to improve steadily over the next two years, and his medical tests, including the CEA, which tests for cancer cells in the bloodstream, returned to normal.

For seven years from initial discovery of the tumor, Kohler led a completely normal, active life. In addition to continuing his academic duties and performing musical concerts, he tirelessly wrote letters to scientists around the country about his medical case, delivered hundreds of speeches, and published a book on his recovery. Many thousands of people were helped by his example. As he often said, "The best thing ever to happen to me was having so-called terminal cancer."

The medical world, however, tended to discount his case even though he had compelling scientific documentation. He was often told that only an autopsy would show whether his surgeon's original diagnosis of cancer was accurate and whether it had truly disappeared. In September 1980, Kohler suddenly became ill and checked into Boston's Beth Israel Hospital. Doctors, looking at his medical records, suspected that the pancreatic cancer had come back and asked permission to perform exploratory surgery. Kohler's friends and relatives strongly opposed it, but Jean consented, saying, "I'm too weak to explain, but I have to do this."

On September 14, Kohler died in the hospital. According to Dr. Michael Sobel, the surgeon who had performed two operations on him and examined the autopsy, Jean's death had "nothing to do with cancer." Microscopic signs of previous cancer were discovered that showed that the diagnosis of his original doctors in Indiana had been correct. However, no current cancer activity was found. "For someone to survive seven years with cancer of the pancreas without being treated is ex-

tremely rare if not unheard of," Dr. Sobel commented. Kohler's death was
attributed to a liver infection and complications resulting from hemorrhaging following surgery.

In death, as in life, Jean Kohler showed that cancer is not incurable
and can be reversed by a balanced diet centered around whole grains
and vegetables, accompanied by faith in nature and a strong will to live.[6]

PANCREATIC CANCER

Norman J. Arnold, fifty-two, a resident of Columbia, South Carolina, was
in the prime of his life. President and chief executive officer of the Ben
Arnold Company, he directed the largest wholesaler of wine and alcoholic beverages in the Southeast and among the ten largest in the nation. Active in community affairs, he headed up local chapters of the
Boys Club, the Zoological Society, and the Heart Fund. Appointed to
several state commissions, he served as the committee chairman for the
Governor's Economic Task Force. With his wife and family he was active
in educational, philanthropic, and synagogue activities.

On July 28, 1982, Norman underwent routine gallbladder surgery at
Providence Hospital in Columbia. During the surgery it was discovered
that he had a primary cancer in the head of the pancreas, which had
metastasized to the liver. In consultations with his surgeon and gastroenterologist he was told that he had from three to nine months to live.
Even though the prospects of surviving pancreatic cancer are about nil,
the doctors advised him to start chemotherapy and/or radiation as a
way of "possibly gaining more time." A doctor at Lombardi Cancer Center at Georgetown University recommended a very potent chemotherapy treatment involving three chemicals for "as long as my body could
take it."

Norman had always been an active, energetic, and above-average
amateur athlete and a very optimistic and positive person. The
chemotherapy treatment made him weak and tired, and gave him a deep
feeling of helplessness and hopelessness. "This debilitated feeling was
more painful to me than the actual pain which I endured," he later recalled. "This miserable existence combined with the fact that I did not
want my growing incapacity to be a physical and psychological burden
to my three sons [twins, thirteen, and an older boy, sixteen] and my wife.
I also did not want their last memory of me to be that of an invalid."

During the eight-week period in which he took five chemotherapy
treatments, Norman learned about macrobiotics, made inquiries through
a medical doctor who had relieved his own cancer on the diet, and
arranged to meet with me. "I had heard there were those who promoted
certain nonconventional cancer treatments in order to financially ex-
ploit cancer victims," Arnold noted later. "I was therefore very skeptical

of Mr. Kushi at the outset, but my concern proved to be totally un-
founded."

Norman started eating a macrobiotic regimen, modified for his particular condition, in August 1982. In October he received his fifth and final chemotherapy treatment. On his own initiative Norman decided to
discontinue the chemical injections because he "preferred a more acceptable quality of life, even if that meant less time alive, rather than a
questionably longer existence as a cripple." On the macrobiotic diet he
gradually began to recover his vigor and energy and positive, cheerful attitude: "In time, I found that I had more energy and vitality than I had
had for twenty years. My wife, who also had adhered strictly to the
macrobiotic diet with me, had positive results both physically and psychologically. My sixteen-year-old son, who plays first-string center on
his high school basketball team, discovered that the macrobiotic diet
greatly increased his strength and especially his endurance. My thirteen-
year-old twin boys demonstrated more concentration, mental agility,
and stamina in their schoolwork when eating macrobiotically, as they do
alternate with the 'standard teenage junk food' diet outside our home."

In the nine months following his last chemotherapy treatment, the
various CT scans and ultrasound tests showed the pancreas tumor and
the "spots" on the liver decreasing in size. In the six months since then,
further CT scans, ultrasound, and blood tests showed no evidence of
disease.

Having already outlived his original prognosis by almost two years,
Norman says he is mentally and physically relaxed and functioning better
than he has for many years. "I play vigorous singles tennis matches almost every day and find that I have much more strength and endurance
than I have had for a very long time. Last month I beat my forty-one-
year-old gastroenterologist in a 6–4, 7–5, 6–8, 8–6 match!" Twenty-six
years later he is still in excellent health and cancer-free.[7]

Skin Cancer and Melanoma

FREQUENCY

More than 1 million new cases of skin cancer are diagnosed each year in the United States, and about 2,740 people die annually of this disease. Because detection is comparatively easy, tumors are slow to spread, and survival is high, skin cancer is not included in many cancer statistics. However, there is a more deadly form of skin cancer, called malignant melanoma, that is one of the fastest-rising malignancies in modern society, rising 3 percent a year. This year it will take 8,110 lives, and an estimated 59,940 new cases will arise. This represents an increase of 55 percent in women and 126 percent in men in the last generation.

Eighty percent of common skin cancers are classified as basal-cell carcinomas and occur primarily on the face or the back of the hands. They do not metastasize but spread by invasion to bone and tissue. Risk factors include sensitivity, sunburning easily, difficulty tanning, lowered natural immunity, and occupational exposure to coal tar, pitch, crosote, arsenic compounds, radium, and other toxins.

Skin cancer is often treated by surgery in a doctor's office under local anesthesia. Methods include electrosurgery with a small electric needle and curette, surgical excision with a scalpel, or chemosurgery with zinc chloride or other chemicals to remove the tumor and a portion of normal tissue around it. Radiation is sometimes used, especially on the face where surgery would result in disfigurement. Chemotherapy and immunotherapy may also be employed.

Melanoma affects Caucasians ten times more than people of color and usually appears initially on an existing mole under the skin and spreads quickly through the lymph or blood to the lungs, brain, liver, eye, intestines, reproductive organs, or other sites. Standard treatment is surgery. Melanoma tends to recur, and patients may have many operations, supplemented with chemotherapy. Up to 90 percent of persons who have malignant melanomas removed in the early stages of the disease will survive five years or more. For melanoma that has spread to distant lymph nodes, the remission rate is 15 percent.

STRUCTURE

The main function of the skin, the body's largest organ, is to control the adjustment between the external environment and the internal body condition. The skin protects the body's surface, helps regulate body temperature, and excretes waste material and water through sweat glands. Sweat glands come in two types. The exocrine glands, which are located over the entire surface of the body, serve to cool the body and guard against infection. They secrete a watery solution consisting of various fats, sugar, salts, proteins, and toxins. The second type of gland is called apocrine and is found only in certain areas, such as under the arms, the nipples, the abdomen, and reproductive areas. The apocrine glands secrete stronger solutions and give rise to body odors.

The color of the skin is regulated by melanin, a pigment that varies from brown to black in color. The less melanin in the skin, the lighter the skin color. Such factors as climate, exposure to sunlight, and daily diet influence the production of melanin.

CAUSE OF CANCER

Normally the body is able to eliminate wastes through such normal functions as urination, bowel movements, respiration, and perspiration. Imbalanced foods or beverages will trigger a variety of abnormal discharge mechanisms in the body such as diarrhea, frequent urination, fever, coughing, or sneezing. Chronic discharges are the next step in this process, and continued poor eating will usually take the form of some kind of skin disease. These are common in cases where the kidneys have lost their ability to properly clean the bloodstream. For example, hard, dry skin arises after the bloodstream fills with fat and oil, eventually causing blockage of the pores, hair follicles, and sweat glands.

Over the last ten years the depletion of the ozone layer has contributed to an increase in skin cancer and melanoma. Ordinarily, the layer of ozone above the Earth screens out harmful ultraviolet rays of the sun. In most traditional societies around the world, where people are eating primarily grains and vegetables, skin cancer and melanoma are nonexistent. People have lived and worked in the hot sun for thousands of years without ever getting cancer.

However, among people in modern industrialized countries eating meat and sugar, refined and highly processed food, these forms of cancer were prevalent and were associated with exposure to sunlight even before the ozone started to thin. The reason for this is that overall the sun is more yang—bright, hot, and intense. Exposure to the yang stimulus of the sun draws excess yin—such as fats and oils—to the body's surface. Thus natural sunlight is not the cause of cancer but the catalyst for the body to begin discharging toxic excess to the surface through the skin. This is what we call skin cancer.

The thinning of the ozone layer has complicated this process. Sunlight naturally polarizes into yin and yang wavelengths. The more yang form is called infrared, the more yin ultraviolet. In between is visible light. Ozone—which is a light form of oxygen—is classified as more yin and serves to repel the incoming yin, ultraviolet light of the sun. With the depletion of the ozone layer, more harmful ultraviolet radiation is reaching the earth than previously. Thus people eating the modern diet may be at even greater risk for developing skin cancer or melanoma when exposed to the sun. It is advisable for such people to avoid direct sunlight and wear a hat or stay in the shade. However, the risk is minimal for those eating in a macrobiotic direction, avoiding dairy food, fatty foods, simple sugars, stimulants, and alcohol, as well as all sorts of oily, greasy foods. Such persons may continue to enjoy natural sunlight without undue worry.

Coincidentally, one of the main causes of ozone depletion is modern agriculture and food processing, especially the processing of animal food. Chlorofluorocarbons (CFCs), the main chemical responsible for ozone depletion, are associated with refrigeration and air-conditioning. The modern diet, high in perishable animal food and tropical vegetables, requires refrigeration, while most foods in the macrobiotic way of eating, including whole grains, beans, seeds, nuts, sea vegetables, and others, do not require refrigeration and can be stored naturally in a pantry. Vegetables can be kept in a root cellar or in the garden until used. Some refrigeration may still be needed, but it could be a small unit in contrast to the large modern units with gigantic freezers for ice cream and frozen foods.

Similarly, overreliance on air-conditioning is related to the modern diet. Animal foods cause the body to heat up, and people eating meat, poultry, chicken, eggs, cheese, and similar foods find hot weather uncomfortable (yang repels yang). The demand for air-conditioning would be substantially reduced if people began to shift toward a more natural way of eating, and the planet's as well as our own health would improve. Melanoma, while classified as a skin cancer, is actually more like a muscular disorder, falling in structure between yin skin-surface tumors, occurring on the periphery of the body, and yang bone tumors, occurring in the deep, compact region of the body. Melanoma usually begins to manifest on existing moles. These tiny dark brown mounds under the skin serve to eliminate excess protein and fat from the body. This protein and fat does not necessarily come from the consumption of protein itself but is produced by a combination of consuming too many extreme yin foods, such as sugar, fruits, and chemicals, and general overconsumption of yang foods, including animal foods and especially poultry, eggs, heavy dairy foods, and other high-protein and high-fat foods. Skin cancer can be relieved by adopting a more yang cancer prevention diet, while a centrally balanced way of daily eating is recommended for malignant melanoma.

MEDICAL EVIDENCE

- In 1966 a medical doctor reported that a special protein-restricted diet helped regress melanoma. Dr. Harry B. Demopoulos put five of his patients with advanced malignant melanoma on a diet high in vegetables and fruits and a supplement that decreased serum levels of several amino acids thought to promote tumor growth. In addition, patients were not allowed to eat high-protein foods such as meat and dairy products, nuts and nut butters, as well as potatoes, bread, and flour products. However, they were allowed to eat oils, stimulants, sugar, and syrups. In three of five patients he reported an "abrupt cessation of tumor growth," and "in all three cases one or more tumors completely regressed." The fourth patient improved while on the diet, but the cancer spread when she discontinued it. The fifth patient showed no change.[1]
- Methyl chloromethyl ether, a corrosive liquid used in refining cane sugar and in gelatin production, causes skin and lung cancer in laboratory animals.[2]
- In 1980 investigators reported that soybeans contain substances called protease inhibitors that retard the growth of tumors. In laboratory experiments with mice, skin tumors were blocked when soybeans, lima beans, or other seeds and beans containing this factor were added to the diet.[3]
- In laboratory studies, Japanese scientists reported that a hot water extract of aduki beans significantly reduced the number of lung tumor colonies and the invasion of melanoma cells. A previous study showed that adukis inhibited stomach cancer by 36 to 62 percent in tumor weight relative to controls.[4]

- Sulforaphane, an active ingredient in cauliflower, broccoli, and other cruciferous vegetables, reduced the development of melanoma and metastatic lung tumors by up to 95 percent in laboratory studies, according to scientists at the Amala Cancer Research Centre in Kerala, India.[5]

DIAGNOSIS

Precancerous skin conditions include a variety of lesions and leukoplakia, the growth of white patches on the mucous membranes. Modern medicine distinguishes skin cancer from these conditions by taking a biopsy. In testing for melanoma, patients are usually administered a lymphangiogram, chest X-rays, brain and liver scans, and sometimes a cardiac catheterization.

Oriental medicine tends to look at all skin ailments on a spectrum and focuses on three major characteristics: condition of the skin, skin color, and skin marks. Normal healthy skin should be clean, smooth, slightly shining, and slightly moist. Wet skin indicates an overconsumption of liquid, sugar, and other sweets, and results in a thin quality of the blood, rapid metabolism, a faster pulse, and excessive perspiration and urination. Wet skin can accompany a variety of disorders ranging from diarrhea, fatigue, hair loss, and aches and pains to epilepsy and various hyperactive psychological disorders.

Normal skin is slightly oily, but excessively oily skin—showing up on peripheral parts of the body such as the forehead, nose, cheeks, hair, or palms—shows overconsumption of oil and fats or disorders in fat metabolism. Dry skin also results from overconsumption of fats and oils and is caused by a formation of fat layers under the skin, preventing the elimination of moisture toward the surface. Depending on other related symptoms, dry or oily skin accompanies a wide variety of chronic and degenerative conditions.

Rough skin reflects an overconsumption of protein and heavy fats or an excess intake of sugar, fruit, and drugs. The second, more yin cause is accompanied by more open sweat glands and a slightly red color. People with hardening of the arteries and accumulations of fat and cholesterol around the organs often have rough skin. Doughy skin, which appears white and flabby and lacking in elasticity, indicates overconsumption of dairy products, sugar, and white flour. A variety of illnesses are connected with this condition, affecting primarily the breasts and reproductive organs.

Aside from natural skin colors, many abnormal colors may appear on the skin. In the case of cancer, a light green color, reddish white color, or pinkish red color from excessive yin or yang food reflects decomposition of tissues and cells and development of cysts and tumors.

Abnormal markings on the skin may also reflect a chronic or degenerative condition. Freckles are the elimination of refined carbohydrates, especially sugar, honey, fruit sugar, and milk sugar. Moles are eliminations of excess protein and fat and appear along the corresponding meridians of the organs affected or muscle areas. Warts signify the elimination of a mixture of protein and fat, and indicate developing skin diseases and possible future tumors of the breast, colon, or sex organs. White patches, the result of excess milk, ice cream, and other dairy products, indicate accumulation of fat and mucus throughout the respiratory and reproductive systems. Eczema—dry, hard, raised areas of skin—shows a massive elimination of excess fats, especially from dairy foods and more particularly from cheese and eggs cooked with butter.

According to traditional iridology, clogged skin is indicated by a dark circle on the periphery of the iris of the eye. The color, intensity, and width of the ring varies in each case.

DIETARY RECOMMENDATIONS

Skin cancer is caused primarily by the consumption of extreme yin foods and beverages. For skin cancer, avoid all extremes in the yin category of foods, including refined sugar and foods and beverages treated with sugar such as soft drinks; artificial and chemicalized food; oily and greasy food; all dairy foods, including cheese, milk, butter, cream, and yogurt; all foods having stimulant and aromatic qualities, including curries, mustard, peppers, and various fragrant beverages and teas; all kinds of alcohol; fruits and fruit juices; nuts; and raw vegetables. It is also necessary to avoid extreme foods in the yang category, especially all kinds of fatty, greasy animal food, including meat, poultry, eggs, and oily fish. All foods are to be cooked, and the use of oil should be either avoided or minimized. Fried foods and oily salad dressings are to be avoided. In addition, it is necessary to avoid all flour products, including breads, pancakes, cookies, and cream of wheat–type cereals, except for the occasional use of whole grain flours baked without yeast. Avoid vegetables that originally came from tropical climates and are too expansive (yin) for regular use. These include potatoes, sweet potatoes, tomatoes, eggplant, beets, green peppers, and avocado.

The primary cause of melanoma is chicken, eggs, cheese, and other dairy food, in combination with sugar and sweets, stimulants, and baked flour products, which accelerate its spread. Avoid all these foods as well as those listed above for skin cancer in general.

For both skin cancer and melanoma, all foods are to be cooked, not eaten raw. The use of sea salt, shoyu, miso, and various condiments should be moderate.

Recommended daily food for these forms of cancer, by volume of daily intake, should consist of the following:

- Whole Grains: Forty to 50 percent of daily consumption, by volume, should be whole cereal grains. The first day prepare plain short- or medium-grain brown rice, pressure-cooked or cooked in a heavy cast-iron or ceramic pot with a heavy lid. On the following days prepare brown rice cooked with 20 to 30 percent millet, then rice with 20 to 30 percent barley, then rice with 20 to 30 percent aduki beans or lentils, and then plain rice again. A delicious morning porridge can be made by taking leftover rice, adding a little more water to soften it, seasoning it with a little miso, and simmering it for two or three minutes more. In ordinary cooking the ratio of grain to water should be about 1:2. For seasoning, cook with a postage-stamp-sized piece of kombu or a pinch of sea salt, depending on the person's condition. Other grains can be used occasionally, including whole wheat berries, rye, corn, buckwheat, and whole oats, although oats should be avoided for the first month. Good-quality sourdough bread may be enjoyed two to three times a week, and noodles, both udon and soba, may also be eaten two to three times a week. Avoid all hard-baked products until the condition improves, including cookies, cake, pie, crackers, muffins, and the like.
- Soup: Five to 10 percent of daily consumption should be soup, consisting of one or two cups or bowls cooked with wakame sea vegetable and various land vegetables such as onions and carrots, seasoned with miso or shoyu. Occasionally a small amount of shiitake mushrooms may be added to the soup. Millet soup made with sweet vegetables is especially beneficial for this condition. The miso used in seasoning soups may be barley miso, brown rice miso, or soybean (hatcho) miso, and should be naturally aged two to three years.
- Vegetables: Twenty to 30 percent of daily consumption should be vegetables, cooked in a variety of forms. Among vegetables, round vegetables such as cabbage, onions, pumpkin, and acorn and butternut squash are especially recommended, as well as root vegetables such as burdock, carrots, and daikon. Many other hard, leafy green vegetables are also to be consumed.

As a general rule, the following dishes may be prepared, although the frequency may differ from person to person: nishime-style vegetables, four times a week; a squash-aduki-kombu dish, three times a week; dried daikon, one cup, three times a week; carrots and carrot tops or daikon and daikon tops, three times a week; blanched vegetables, five to seven times a week; pressed salad, five to seven times a week; raw salad and salad dressing, avoid; steamed greens, five to seven times a week; sautéed vegetables, two to three times a week, using water the first one to two months and then a small amount of sesame oil thereafter; kinpira, two-thirds of a cup, two times a week; tofu, dried tofu, tempeh, or seitan with vegetables, two times a week.

- Beans: Five percent of daily consumption should be small beans, such as aduki beans, lentils, chickpeas, or black soybeans, cooked together with sea vegetables such as kombu or with onions and carrots. Other beans may be used two to three times a month. For seasoning, a small amount of unrefined sea salt or shoyu or miso can be used. Bean products, such as tempeh, natto, and dried or cooked tofu, may be used occasionally but in moderate amounts.

- Sea Vegetables: Five percent or less sea vegetable dishes, including wakame and kombu, should be included daily when cooking grain, in soup, etc. A sheet of toasted nori may also be taken daily. A small dish of hijiki or arame should be prepared two times a week. All other sea vegetables are optional.

- Condiments: Those that should be available on the table are gomashio (sesame salt), on the average made with one part salt to eighteen parts sesame seeds (reduced to 1:16 after two months); kelp or wakame powder; umeboshi plum; and tekka, although all other regular macrobiotic condiments may be used if desired. These condiments may be used daily on grains and vegetables, but the amounts should be moderate to suit individual appetite and taste.

- Pickles: Made at home in a variety of ways, pickles are to be eaten daily, one tablespoon in all, although salty pickles are to be minimized.

- Animal Food: Meat, poultry, eggs, and other strong animal food are to be avoided. For melanoma, fish and seafood are also to be avoided, although a small amount of white-meat fish may be eaten once every ten to fourteen days if craved. The fish should be steamed, boiled, or poached and garnished with grated daikon or ginger. Strictly avoid blue-meat and red-meat fish and all shellfish. For skin cancer, depending on the case, a small amount of white-meat fish may be eaten once a week or more frequently after the first month.

- Fruit: None is the best, the less the better, including both tropical and temperate-climate fruit, until the condition improves. If cravings develop, a small volume of cooked fruit with a pinch of sea salt or dried fruit (also preferably cooked) may be taken. Avoid all fruit juices and cider temporarily, as well as raisins, currants, and other highly concentrated fruits.

- Sweets and Snacks: Avoid all sweets and desserts, including good-quality macrobiotic desserts, until the condition improves. To satisfy a sweet tooth, use sweet vegetables every day in cooking, drink sweet vegetable drinks (see special drinks on page 413), and eat sweet vegetable jam. Mochi, rice balls, vegetable sushi, and other grain-based snacks may be eaten frequently. Limit rice cakes, pop-corn, and other dry or baked snacks because they may harden the tumor. In the event of cravings, a small amount of amasake, barley malt, or rice syrup may be eaten.

- Nuts and Seeds: Nuts and nut butters are to be avoided due to their high fat and protein, except for chestnuts. Unsalted blanched seeds such as squash seeds and pumpkin seeds may be consumed as a snack, up to one cup total per week.

- Seasonings: Unrefined sea salt, shoyu, and miso are to be used moder-ately in order to avoid unnecessary thirst. Avoid mirin and garlic. If you become particularly thirsty after a meal or between meals, you should cut back on these seasonings until the normal level of thirst returns.

- Beverages: Drinks and other dietary practices can follow the general recommendations in Part I, with bancha twig tea as the main bever-age. Strictly avoid the beverages on the "infrequent" and "avoid" lists, and don't take grain coffee for the first two to three months after starting this new way of eating.

The most important thing in connection with dietary practice is chew-ing very well, until all food becomes liquid in the mouth and is well mixed with saliva. Chew very well, at least fifty times and preferably a hundred times per mouthful. It is also important to avoid overeating and eating within three hours of sleeping.

As noted in the introduction to Part II, people who have received or who are currently undergoing medical treatment may need to make further dietary modifications.

SPECIAL DRINKS AND DISHES

One or more special drinks or side dishes may need to be consumed, de-pending on the individual case. Please see a qualified macrobiotic teacher for guidance. Amounts and frequencies given here are averages for each drink or dish; these will differ from person to person. Further directions are in Chapter 36.

- Sweet Vegetable Drink: Take one to two small cups every day for three weeks, then about half that amount for the next three weeks, and then stop.

- Dried Daikon, Shiitake, and Kombu Tea: Prepare and store this tea in a thermos and drink one to two cups a day for three weeks. After that, have it every other day, or about three times a week for three more weeks.

- Brown Rice with Marinated Dried Daikon: Prepare this once a day or every other day for about three weeks. After that, eat it one or two times a week for three to four weeks.
- Kombu-Lotus-Shiitake Drink: Drink one small cup daily for three weeks, then twice a week for one month. This is especially good for melanoma.
- Kinpira Soup: For strength and vitality this dish may be consumed two to three times a week.
- Ume-Sho-Kuzu: This drink may be consumed daily for a one- to two-week period and occasionally afterward to strengthen the blood and for general vitality.
- Miso-Scallion Condiment: One teaspoon may be used as a condiment.
- Grated Daikon: Drink half of a fresh cup with a few drops of shoyu two to three times a week to help melt fat deposits.

HOME CARE

- Body Scrub: Vigorous daily brushing of the skin with a squeezed wet towel will help unblock pores and release excess fat and protein through the skin. When washing, avoid using soap. The skin and scalp normally have a slightly acidic pH, and this is upset by most commercial soaps, which are alkaline. Soaps do not really cleanse the skin and can actually prevent excess cholesterol from coming out of pores. Rice bran wrapped in cheesecloth or natural vegetable-quality soaps should be used instead of chemicalized or animal-quality soaps and shampoos.
- Compress Guidelines: For a small number of skin cancer or melanoma cases, a compress may be needed to help gradually draw out excess mucus and fat. Please see a qualified macrobiotic teacher for guidance on the proper use and frequency of a compress or plaster. Several types are used, depending on the person's condition. Precede the compress or plaster with the application of a towel that has been soaked in hot water and squeezed out over the affected area for about three to five minutes to stimulate circulation.
- Kombu-Ginger Compress: Soak a 3-inch piece of kombu. Combine it with half a teaspoon of grated ginger and place over the melanoma or other affected area. Cover with a cotton bandage and leave for several hours or overnight. If the ginger is too hot or stimulating, use just 20 percent ginger with cooked rice and barley. Use every day for a maximum of two weeks.
- Kombu-Grain Compress: Take a 3-inch piece of soaked kombu, combine it with half a teaspoon of cooked rice or barley, and place

over the melanoma or other affected area. Cover with a cotton bandage and leave for several hours or overnight. Use daily for up to two weeks.

- Daikon Compress: A compress made from dried daikon leaves and grated ginger can help speed up the process of discharge. Boil daikon leaves, grate fresh gingerroot, and wrap them in cheesecloth. Turn down the heat and place this "ginger sack" (which should contain a lump of grated ginger about the size of a golf ball) in the water. Then dip a towel into the water, squeeze, and apply to the affected area.
- Rice Bran Wash: A rice bran (nuka) skin wash is also beneficial. Wrap the nuka in cheesecloth, place in hot water, and stir. The nuka will melt, and the water will begin to turn yellow. Wash the affected area with a towel or cloth that has been dipped in this water.
- Wood Ash: The skin may also be washed with wood ash. Place in hot water the ashes that are left over after burning wood in a fireplace and stir very well. Let sit until the ashes settle to the bottom and then use the water to wash the skin. Pat dry with a towel.
- Fresh Daikon: In cases where a person with a skin disease suffers from itching, rub a piece of cut fresh daikon directly on the affected area. If you don't have any daikon, use a scallion or onion.
- Sesame Oil: This oil can be applied directly to the affected area in cases where the skin becomes ruptured. Afterward, cover the area with cotton cloth to protect it from external contact.
- After Surgery: In the event the skin cancer and melanoma have been removed totally or in part by surgery, genuine brown rice cream can be used. Two to three bowls may be consumed each day for the initial several days with a small amount of condiments such as scallion-miso, gomashio (sesame salt), tekka, or umeboshi plum. All other regular dishes such as soup, vegetables, beans and bean products, and seaweed should be continued as usual during this period. After that, regular brown rice and other cereal grains can be introduced gradually. During both periods it is very important to chew the food thoroughly until it assumes a liquid form; one hundred or more times per mouthful is recommended. The removed portion of the skin cancer and melanoma will often restore itself as time passes. Even if the removed section is not restorable, chewing well can sufficiently serve for digestion.

EMOTIONAL CONSIDERATIONS

Positive emotions associated with the skin are confidence, adaptability, and resilience. Skin problems are associated with insecurity, rigidity, and sensory gratification. The cosmetics and fashion industries, which encourage people to beautify themselves with chemicals, synthetic materials, and other harmful substances, stress appearance over inner reality. This leads to a decline in health and the suppression of emotions on a vast scale.

High-quality foods that nourish the skin and help develop positive emotions include whole grains, particularly hato mugi and barley; leafy green vegetables; sea vegetables; and a proper balance of salt and oil.

Foods that block the skin and contribute to negative emotions include oily and fatty foods; meat, cheese, poultry, eggs, fish and seafood, and other animal products; excessive bread and baked goods, especially those made with white flour; sugar, chocolate, and other highly processed sweets; too much fruit and juice; chemicalized and artificial foods; and other extremely contractive or expansive foods and beverages.

In relationships it is important to love and esteem one's self. If a person lacks confidence and is too outwardly (or sometimes too inwardly) directed, he or she may localize his or her excess emotional energy in the skin.

On a planetary scale, the skin corresponds with deserts. Imbalance in this region correlates with desertification and droughts.

OTHER CONSIDERATIONS

- Wool and synthetic fabrics are particularly irritating to the skin. Wear cotton and sleep on all-cotton fabrics to allow your skin to breathe naturally.
- Avoid cosmetics or antiperspirants made with synthetic or toxic ingredients. Most commercial deodorants contain aluminum salts that temporarily close the openings of the sweat glands and stop "wetness." They also contain chemical antibacterial agents that are harmful to the body. Body odor is largely caused by the consumption of animal food, including all kinds of soft dairy foods, and naturally lessens as the diet becomes more centered on grain and vegetable foods. Even natural deodorants should be minimized, since they may contain ingredients such as beeswax, which can also clog pores. Among natural cosmetics, one of the safest is clay. Pure clay or clay powder sprinkled on the body can have an antiperspirant effect. Clay also naturally draws wastes and toxins from the skin and can be used as a basis for a facial mask or a compress.
- A sauna, steam bath, or Japanese hot tub can help open clogged skin pores. However, cancer patients should steam or bathe only occasionally, a few times a week and for a short period of time, such as ten minutes. Prepare a thermos of shoyu-bancha tea or miso soup to drink when you come out in order to replace lost fluids and to thicken the blood. Unless proper foods have been consumed, this

form of inducing sweat is preferable to running, working out in a gym, or other strenuous activity, which may generate more waste products—chiefly urea and lactic acid—that are lost through sweating.

- Do-in or shiatsu massage is beneficial to restoring proper respiration and elimination through the skin. Yoga, martial arts, and other exercises that are grounded in an understanding of the energy meridians can also be used to complement dietary adjustments.
- Avoid direct exposure to the sun as much as possible. Wear a hat or stay in the shade.
- Avoid commercial sunscreen creams that may have chemicals or other harmful ingredients.

PERSONAL EXPERIENCE

SKIN CANCER

In early 1975, Roger Randolph, a sixty-one-year-old lawyer from Tulsa, Oklahoma, observed three red spots on his chest and one on his back that did not go away over the course of several weeks. A skin specialist diagnosed his condition as skin cancer and prescribed two types of medicine: one to be applied to these spots twice daily for three weeks, followed by the other medicine for another three weeks. The doctor said the spots on his chest would probably clear up but recommended surgery or radiation therapy to excise the malignancy on his back before it spread.

Roger discussed his case with his wife and children, and they recommended that he try the macrobiotic approach. Roger agreed and told his doctor that he would experiment with the Cancer Prevention Diet and report back in three months.

On April 28, Roger came to see me, and I examined him carefully. The spots on his chest had cleared up, but the one on his back was definitely malignant. I recommended the diet described above for three months, with particular emphasis on chewing each mouthful fifty to seventy times. "Mr. Kushi said the cancer would probably continue to grow for a month or two," Roger recorded, "but that soon thereafter it would definitely disappear. On May 11, I commenced the strict diet and followed it faithfully for three months."

On August 18, Roger returned for a medical examination, and his doctor was astonished to find that the tumor on his back had disappeared. "He was flabbergasted and suggested that the cure must have been produced by a delayed reaction to the medicine which I had ceased to apply four and a half months earlier," Roger wrote. "He urged me to return in three weeks to verify the cancer was gone."

On September 9, Roger went back and received a clean bill of health. Two months later, in November, he had a final medical check and received a discharge as cured. "In my opinion the macrobiotic diet was the sole cause of the cure," he concluded, "permitting my body to cure itself by providing it with proper nutrition and insulating it from the dreadful food most of us eat."[6]

MALIGNANT MELANOMA

In August 1978, Virginia Brown, a fifty-six-year-old mother and registered nurse from Tunbridge, Vermont, noticed a black mole on her arm that was getting bigger and blacker. She had lost a lot of weight and felt very dull mentally. Doctors at Vermont Medical Center in Burlington performed a biopsy and discovered that she had an advanced case of malignant melanoma (stage 4). The physicians told her that without surgery she could expect to live only six months. "Even though I had been trained and practiced in the medical profession for years," she later recalled, "I could not go along with surgery. I had professed alternatives for years, but did not really practice them."

At home her son and daughter-in-law encouraged her to try macrobiotics, and shortly thereafter she attended the East West Foundation's annual cancer conference, meeting that year in Amherst, Massachusetts. At the conference she listened to fifteen cancer patients discuss their experiences on the diet and was impressed with their accounts.

Prior to that time she had followed the standard American way of eating, high in refined foods and fat, especially animal fat from dairy foods, beef, poultry, and fish. At the time she started the diet, she was so sick that she could hardly make it upstairs and slept most of the day. After three weeks eating the new food, which her children prepared for her, she experienced a change in her energy level, attitude, and mental clarity. "I was a new person; I could get up and walk around."

In September she came to Boston to see me, and I made more specific dietary recommendations and advised her to study proper cooking. With the support of her family, she adhered faithfully to the diet, supplemented by Korean yoga exercises, prayer and meditation, and a two-mile walk each morning after breakfast.

She noted afterward: "I amazed myself at my perseverance, not one of my better qualities. There have been all kinds of days—angry, crying, pain, weakness, tension, sadness, and hopelessness, but also thankful times. . . . The most difficult thing has been to see other loved ones go the chemotherapy and radiation route and suffer so.

"The most impressive thing was when I first saw Michio. He looked at me and said, "You're doing it. You can get rid of it." He had faith. This was such a contrast to the doctors. The way they look at you is unbelievable."

In October 1979 I met with Virginia again and found that she no longer had any cancer in her body. Medical exams subsequently confirmed this diagnosis. After restoring her health, Virginia went on to study at the Kushi Institute and worked in the macrobiotic health program at the Lemuel Shattuck Hospital in Boston, promoting a more natural way of living among other medical professionals and patients.[7]

MELANOMA

In 1983, Marlene McKenna was diagnosed with malignant melanoma. "As a working mother of four children, radio and TV commentator, and investment broker, I was living a very unbalanced life," she explained in an interview in the *Providence Journal*.

In August 1985, Marlene began to complain of severe stomach pains, and in January 1986 doctors discovered that five tumors had spread throughout her body. Two feet of her intestines were removed, and Marlene was told she had six months to a year to live.

Declining all treatments, Marlene turned to macrobiotics at the suggestion of her brother and visited me in Boston. In addition to changing her diet, she replaced her electric stove with a gas stove and began to meditate and practice yoga. A devout Catholic, she also did a lot of inspirational reading and praying.

"I promised God that if He walked me through this and helped me live, I would give Him life with life," she recalls.

Within a year Marlene was on the way to recovery, and doctors found no evidence of further cancer. Feeling well enough to return to public life, she ran for state treasurer in Rhode Island. During the campaign she discovered that she was pregnant. Because of her previous illness and age (forty-two), doctors encouraged her to have an abortion. Marlene refused. "I realized that [having the baby] was part of my promise to give life with life," she explains. Although she lost the election, she gave birth to a healthy baby boy, keeping her promise to God and proving her physicians wrong.

Since then she has opened Shepherd's, a macrobiotic natural foods restaurant in Providence, and is helping people around the country who have heard of her remarkable recovery.[8]

Stomach Cancer

FREQUENCY

In the United States an estimated 11,210 persons will die from stomach cancer this year, and 21,260 new cases will develop. Overall, deaths from stomach cancer have sharply declined by about two-thirds in the United States during the last several decades. This is attributed largely to the decreased consumption of sausage, luncheon meats, and other meats preserved in large amounts of salt or containing nitrosamines. Men suffer the illness about one and a half times as often as women, and blacks slightly more than whites. It is more prevalent in older than in middle-aged or younger persons. Stomach or gastric cancer, as it is also known, accounts for about 2 percent of all new cancers in the United States. In Japan and Korea, however, it is the leading type of cancer, accounting for up to 20 percent of all malignancies. It is also a leading cause of death in other parts of the Far East, Latin America, and Eastern Europe.

Surgical removal of the stomach is the standard treatment. The operation is called a gastrectomy, and the stomach may be partly or totally removed. In total gastrectomies, regional lymph nodes, the spleen, and part of the small intestine are also removed. Chemotherapy or radiation may follow. In the United States about 24 percent of stomach cancer patients survive five years or more. However, because it is often not diagnosed until later stages, many cases are inoperable. Chemotherapy or radiation may also be used, especially to prevent its spread to the blood or lymph system and other organs.

STRUCTURE

The stomach is a relatively hollow gourd-shaped organ located in the upper left of the abdominal cavity between the esophagus and the small intestine. The layers of the stomach include (1) the mucosa, or interior lining of the stomach, which secretes digestive enzymes, (2) the connective tissue between the submucosa and the muscles of the stomach, (3) the muscular coat, which enables the stomach to contract and expand and move decomposing food toward the intestines, and (4) the serosa, or outer coating.

The mucosa contains millions of tubular glands that secrete hydrochloric acid or pepsin as well as small amounts of mucin, anti-anemia materials, and inorganic salts. The upper, expanded region of the stomach, known as the fundus and the body, secretes hydrochloric acid, the stronger of the two acids. The lower, more compact section of the stomach, called the pylorus, secretes pepsin. These acids decompose protein into its various amino acids. Together with muscular peristalsis, enzymatic actions convert solid food into semiliquid chyme, an acid substance that relaxes the lower pyloric valve, allowing the chyme to pass from the stomach into the duodenal section of the small intestine.

CAUSE OF CANCER

In order for the digestive juices in the stomach to be secreted properly, food must first be alkalized by saliva in the mouth. Hence the necessity for thorough chewing of each mouthful of food. Whole grains, especially those cooked with a pinch of sea salt, pass through the stomach to the small intestine where they are absorbed in the villi and converted into red blood cells and other healthy circulatory fluids. In contrast, morsels of food from refined grains such as white flour and white rice, as well as refined sugar, start to be absorbed directly in the stomach and enter the body fluids prematurely, producing a thinner quality of blood and lymph. Stomach cancer results from long-term consumption of extreme yin foods and beverages such as refined grain, flour, sugar and other sweets, soda and ice-cold drinks, alcohol, aromatic and stimulant beverages, chemicals and drugs. Strong yang foods, which overtax the stomach, can also cause cancer, including foods high in animal protein and salts as well as high-fat, oily, and greasy foods. Repeated oversecretion of stomach acids to neutralize and process an excess of these foods results in irritating the stomach lining, ulcerations, and eventually the formation of tumors. Depending on the location and type, stomach cancer can metastasize to nearby lymph nodes, the pancreas, liver, or ovaries (Krukenberg tumor). It can also spread to the lungs, bones, and occasionally the skin through the lymphatic system.

The yin form of stomach cancer, affecting the upper expanded region of the stomach, is caused by overconsumption of extremely expansive substances, especially refined grains, sugar, foods containing chemical additives or preservatives such as MSG, and food grown with chemical fertilizers or pesticides. Cancer in the more compact pylorus in the lower stomach results from overconsumption of meat, eggs, fish, or other overly yang products. Over the last twenty years the rate of stomach cancer in the United States has fallen about 75 percent. In a *Life* magazine article, "The Endless Quest for a Cure," medical writer Jeff Wheelwright concludes: "The trend towards more vegetables, fruit, and fiber in the American diet . . . may be the main reason for the decline."

MEDICAL EVIDENCE

- From 1904 to 1911, British surgeon Robert McCarrison traveled in the Hunza, a remote Himalayan kingdom in the then Northwest Territory of India. There he was astonished to discover a completely healthy culture in which the infectious and degenerative diseases of modern civilization, including colonial India, were unknown. "I never saw a case of asthenic dyspepsia, of gastric or duodenal ulcer, of appendicitis, of mucous colitis, or of cancer," he informed his medical colleagues. McCarrison hypothesized that the unusual health and longevity of the Hunza people was due primarily to their daily diet consisting of whole wheat chapatis, barley, and maize, supplemented by leafy green vegetables, beans and legumes, apricots, and a small amount of dairy products and goat's milk only on feast days. The Hunzas did not eat refined white rice, sugar, black tea, or spices, as did most of the Indian population. In 1927, Sir Robert McCarrison assumed the post of director of nutritional research in India, and to test his theory he began a series of laboratory experiments. Feeding the Hunza diet and the regular Indian diet to rats over a period of four years, he discovered that animals fed the modern, refined diet of Bengal and Madras contracted cysts, abscesses, heart disease, and cancer of the stomach. Rats fed the Hunza whole grain diet remained healthy and free of all disease.[1]
- In 1971 a Japanese cancer researcher reported a significant negative association between per capita tofu intake and stomach cancer.[2]
- In 1981, Japan's National Cancer Center reported that people who eat miso soup daily are 33 percent less likely to contract stomach cancer than those who never eat miso soup. The thirteen-year study,

involving about 265,000 men and women over forty, also found that miso soup is effective in reducing the risk of "hypertensive diseases, ischemic heart disease and all other causes of death."[3]

- The high rate of stomach cancer in Japan caused some Japanese scientists to speculate that a diet high in soy sauce might be a factor. However, in 1991 researchers at the University of Wisconsin observed just the opposite. In laboratory tests, mice given fermented soy sauce experienced 26 percent less cancer than mice on the regular diet. Also, soy-supplemented mice averaged about one-quarter the number of tumors per mouse as the control group. Soy sauce "exhibited a pronounced anticarcinogenic effect," the researchers concluded.[4]

- A number of studies have shown that a diet rich in cruciferous vegetables such as broccoli, cabbage, cauliflower, and Brussels sprouts can lower the risk for cancer of the stomach, breast, and large intestine. In 1992 researchers at Johns Hopkins University School of Medicine reported that they had identified the ingredient in broccoli that worked as a powerful anticancer compound in laboratory experiments. The chemical in broccoli, sulforaphane, boosts the production of an important enzyme known to neutralize carcinogens before they trigger tumor growth. In addition to broccoli, sulforaphane is found in bok choy, ginger, scallions, and other vegetables.[5]

- Japanese researchers at Hiroshima University reported that long-term fermented miso added to the diet of male rats significantly reduced the size of gastric tumors compared to controls.[6]

DIAGNOSIS

Stomach cancer is difficult to diagnose by modern medical methods. Only 18 percent of current stomach cancers are detected in the local stage before spreading to other organs of the body. Cancer of the stomach is commonly confused with other abdominal disorders, especially gastric ulcers, and the patient may feel no unusual symptoms. The normal hospital procedure, called a gastroscopy, allows direct X-ray viewing of the entire stomach. A biopsy is performed if cancer is suspected, and the lining of the stomach may be brushed and washed to obtain cell samples. Follow-up chest and skeletal X-rays and a liver scan are taken to determine possible metastases.

The condition of the stomach is relatively easy to diagnose by traditional Oriental medicine, and the tendency toward acidosis, ulcerations, or tumors can be monitored long before they actually develop so that preventive dietary action can be taken. To diagnose stomach problems, corresponding areas in the face can be observed: the upper lip and the bridge of the nose. The entire digestive system is reflected in the mouth as a whole, and the upper lip mirrors the upper digestive tract, especially the stomach. More specifically, the left side of the upper lip corresponds with the upper, more yin part of the stomach, while the right side shows the lower, more yang region. Swelling in the upper lip shows an expanded stomach condition caused by consumption of refined grains, sugar and other sweeteners, alcohol, and tropical fruit and juices or overeating. A contracted upper lip reflects a tightening in the stomach due to an excessive intake of meat, eggs, salt, or dry baked goods. Both of these conditions reflect overacidity in the stomach, and the tendency or presence of ulcerations may be indicated by inflammation, a blister, or discoloration on the upper lip.

Brown blotches or freckles on the upper part of the bridge of the nose indicate chronic stomach acidosis, ulcerations, hypoglycemic and diabetic tendencies, or possible stomach cancer. In the case of stomach cancer, a slight green tinge may show up in this area. The skin as a whole also shows the condition of the stomach. A splotchy brown or dirty skin color suggests chronic acidity in the stomach as a result of excess sugar or fruit consumption. Discolorations along the stomach meridian, especially in the area below the knee or on top of the foot in the extended region of the second and third toes, are a good indicator of stomach imbalances. Again, a green shading in either of these locations indicates possible stomach cancer.

The near back of the tongue also may be examined to observe developing stomach problems. A dark red color indicates inflammation, ulcerations, and a potential development of stomach cancer. A white or yellow color or white patches indicate accumulations of fat and mucus in the stomach. Blue or purple signifies overconsumption of sugar, soft drinks, alcohol, drugs, medications, and other extreme yin substances. Small mushroom-like eruptions are signs of acidity, ulcerations, and possible nausea and regurgitation.

DIETARY RECOMMENDATIONS

The main cause of stomach cancer is the longtime consumption or overconsumption of foods and drinks that are producing alkaline or acid conditions in the body. Accordingly, it is necessary to avoid all overly expansive foods, including all refined food such as white rice, white bread, and other refined flour products; sugar, honey, chocolate, carob, and similar sweeteners; sugar-treated food and beverages; artificial soda and soft drinks; coffee, black tea, and alcohol; cold, icy beverages; all stimulants and spices, including curry, mustard, and pepper; all aromatic foods and beverages; butter, milk, and cream; chemicalized food, seasonings, and beverages; oily, greasy food; tropical fruits and juices; and vegetables of tropical origin, including potatoes, sweet potatoes, yams, tomatoes, and eggplant. In addition, all extreme yang foods, such as beef, pork, poultry, and eggs; all types of dairy food, including cheese; very salty food; hard-baked flour products such as hard bread and cookies; all baked animal food; and high-protein and high-fat food are to be avoided. The following dietary guidelines should be observed.

- Whole Grains: Forty to 50 percent of daily consumption, by volume, should be whole cereal grains. The first day prepare plain short- or medium-grain brown rice, pressure-cooked or cooked in a heavy cast-iron or ceramic pot with a heavy lid. On subsequent days, alternate brown rice cooked with 20 to 30 percent millet (which is particularly beneficial to the stomach), then rice with 20 to 30 percent barley, then rice with 20 to 30 percent aduki beans or lentils, and then plain rice again. A delicious morning porridge can be made by taking leftover rice or millet, adding a little more water to soften it, seasoning with a little miso, and simmering for two to three minutes more. In ordinary pressure-cooking, the ratio of grain to water should be about 1:2. For seasoning, cook with a postage-stamp-sized piece of kombu or a pinch of sea salt, depending on the person's condition. Other grains can be used occasionally, including whole wheat berries, rye, corn, and whole oats, although oats should be avoided for the first month. Buckwheat and seitan should be minimized. Good-quality sourdough bread may be enjoyed two to three times a week, and noodles, both udon and soba, may also be eaten two to three times a week. Avoid all hard-baked products, including cookies, cake, pie, crackers, muffins, and the like, until the condition improves.
- Soup: Five to 10 percent of daily consumption should be soup, consisting of one or two cups or bowls cooked with wakame sea vegetable and various land vegetables such as onions and carrots, seasoned with miso or shoyu. Occasionally a small amount of shiitake mushrooms may be added to the soup. Autumn squash, cabbage, onions, and other round, sweet vegetables may be used often. Millet-squash soup is especially beneficial for this condition. The miso used in seasoning soups may be barley miso, brown rice miso, or soybean (hatcho) miso, and should be naturally aged two to three years. To satisfy a sweet tooth, millet soup with sweet vegetables such as squash, cabbage, onions, and carrots may be consumed often.
- Vegetables: Twenty to 30 percent of daily consumption should be vegetables, cooked in a variety of forms. Among vegetables, daikon and its greens are particularly recommended for frequent use, as are autumn squash, cabbage, onions, and other round vegetables. As a general rule, the following dishes may be prepared, although the frequency may differ from person to person: nishime-style vegetables, four times a week; a squash-aduki-kombu dish, three times a week; dried daikon, one cup, three times a week; carrots and carrot tops or daikon and daikon tops, three times a week; blanched vegetables, five to seven times a week; pressed salad, several times a week; raw salad

and salad dressing, avoid; steamed greens, five to seven times a week; sautéed vegetables, two to three times a week, using water the first month and then a small amount of sesame oil thereafter; kinpira, two-thirds of a cup, two times a week; tofu, dried tofu, tempeh, or seitan with vegetables, two times a week.

- Beans: Five percent of daily consumption should be small beans, such as aduki beans, lentils, chickpeas, or black soybeans, cooked together with sea vegetables such as kombu or with onions and carrots. Other beans may be used two to three times a month. For seasoning, a small amount of unrefined sea salt or shoyu or miso can be used. Bean products, such as tempeh, natto, and dried or cooked tofu, may be used occasionally but in moderate amounts.

- Sea Vegetables: Five percent or less of sea vegetable dishes, including wakame and kombu, should be included daily when cooking grain, in soup, etc. A sheet of toasted nori may also be taken daily. A small dish of hijiki or arame should be prepared two times a week. All other sea vegetables are optional. Sea vegetables can be cooked with other vegetables or sautéed with a small amount of sesame oil after softening them by soaking and boiling lightly in water.

- Condiments: Those that should be available on the table are go-mashio (sesame salt), on the average made with one part salt to eighteen parts sesame seeds (reduced to 1:16 after two months); kelp or wakame powder; umeboshi plum; and tekka, although all other regular macrobiotic condiments may be used if desired. These condiments may be used daily on grains and vegetables, but the amounts should be moderate to suit individual appetites and tastes.

- Pickles: Made at home in a variety of ways, pickles are to be eaten daily, one tablespoon in all, although salty pickles are to be minimized.

- Animal Food: Meat, poultry, eggs, and other strong animal food are to be avoided. A small amount of white-meat fish may be eaten once a week. The fish should be steamed, boiled, or poached and garnished with grated daikon or ginger. After two months fish may be eaten twice a week if desired. Strictly avoid blue-meat and red-meat fish and all shellfish.

- Fruit: None is best, and the less the better, including both tropical and temperate-climate fruit, until the condition improves. If cravings develop, a small amount of cooked fruit with a pinch of sea salt or dried fruit (also preferably cooked) may be eaten. Avoid all fruit juices and cider temporarily, as well as raisins, currants, and other highly concentrated fruits.

- Sweets and Snacks: Avoid all sweets and desserts, including good-quality macrobiotic desserts, until the condition improves. To satisfy a sweet tooth, use sweet vegetables every day in cooking, drink sweet vegetable drinks (see special drinks below), and eat sweet vegetable jam. Mochi, rice balls, vegetable sushi, and other grain-based snacks may be eaten frequently. Limit rice cakes, popcorn, and other dry or baked snacks because they may harden the tumor. In the event of cravings, a small amount of amasake, barley malt, or rice syrup may be eaten.

- Nuts and Seeds: Nuts and nut butters are to be avoided due to their high fat and protein, except for chestnuts. Unsalted blanched seeds such as sunflower seeds and pumpkin seeds may be consumed as a snack, up to one cup total per week.
- Seasonings: Unrefined sea salt, shoyu, and miso are to be used moderately in order to avoid unnecessary thirst. Avoid mirin and garlic. If you become particularly thirsty after a meal or between meals, you should cut back on these seasonings until the normal level of thirst returns.
- Beverages: Drinks and other dietary practices can follow the general recommendations in Part I, including bancha twig tea as the main beverage. Strictly avoid the beverages on the "infrequent" and "avoid" lists and don't have grain coffee for the first two to three months after starting this new way of eating.

The most important thing in connection with dietary practice is chewing very well, until all food becomes liquid in the mouth and well mixed with saliva. Chew very well, at least fifty times and preferably a hundred times per mouthful. It is also important to avoid overeating and eating within three hours of sleeping.

As noted in the introduction to Part II, people who have received or who are currently undergoing medical treatment may need to make further dietary modifications.

SPECIAL DRINKS AND DISHES

One or more special drinks or side dishes may need to be consumed, depending on the individual case. Please see a qualified macrobiotic teacher for guidance. Amounts and frequencies given here are averages for each drink or dish; these will differ from person to person. Further directions are in Chapter 36.

- Sweet Vegetable Drink: Take one small cup every day for one month and then two to three times a week the second month.
- Millet and Sweet Vegetable Porridge: This soft morning dish may be eaten daily or often.

- Cooked Grated Daikon with Carrot and Shoyu: Eat one small cup of this preparation every day for five days, and after that, eat it two to three times a week for another month.
- Miso-Zosui Brown Rice and Millet: Eat one bowl every day for ten days; after that, eat it three to four times a week for another month.
- Brown Rice with Water-Sautéed Daikon and Daikon Leaves: This dish may also be helpful for this condition.
- Genuine Brown Rice Cream: This dish is helpful if the stomach has been removed. Eat two to three bowls a day for several days with a small amount of condiments such as scallion-miso, gomashio, tekka, or umeboshi plum. Then begin to introduce regular brown rice or other grains. Chewing will enhance healing. Sometimes the part of the stomach taken out will restore itself. If not, thorough chewing will aid digestion.

HOME CARE

- Body Scrub: Scrubbing the whole body, including the abdominal region and the spinal region, with a towel that has been immersed in hot water and squeezed out is very helpful for better circulation of blood, lymph, and other body fluids, as well as for activating physical and mental energies.
- Compress Guidelines: For a small number of tumors in the stomach, a compress may be needed to gradually help draw out excess mucus and fat. Please see a qualified macrobiotic teacher for guidance on the proper use and frequency of a compress or plaster. Several types are used depending on the person's condition. Precede the compress or plaster with the application of a towel that has been soaked in hot water and squeezed out over the affected area for about three to five minutes to stimulate circulation.
- Potato-Cabbage Plaster: This external application may be beneficial for some cases of stomach cancer. Put a hot towel on the affected area for about three minutes to promote better circulation and then apply the potato and cabbage plaster directly on the skin. Tie it with a cotton strip and sleep with it so the plaster does not move. Leave the plaster on for four hours or for the whole night. Repeat daily for two weeks or more.
- Massage: Massage all the toes very well, especially the second and third toes, for about fifteen minutes, three times every day.
- Palm Healing: Application of warmth on the stomach region as well as palm healing for thirty minutes to one hour also can help ease pain or ache in the stomach region.

EMOTIONAL CONSIDERATIONS

Positive emotions associated with the stomach are faith, sympathy, and kindness. Stomach problems may arise from doubt, anxiety, jealousy, and misunderstanding.

High-quality foods that nourish the stomach and help develop positive emotions include naturally sweet things such as whole grains, particularly millet and sweet rice; sweet round vegetables, including cabbage, squash, and onions; tofu, yuba, and other soft, naturally processed soy foods; natural sweeteners, including amasake, rice syrup, and barley malt; round orange or yellow fruits such as peaches, nectarines, and apricots; and carrot juice, sweet vegetable drink, and other naturally sweet foods.

Foods that block the stomach and contribute to negative emotions include too much animal protein, including meat, cheese, poultry, eggs, strong fish, and seafood; white flour, white rice, and other polished grains; sugar, chocolate, and other highly processed sweets; chemicalized and artificial foods, including MSG; and other extremely contractive or expansive foods and beverages.

In relationships it is important to trust one's partner, to try to understand things from his or her perspective, and to harmonize. A person who is doubtful, suspicious, and jealous may localize his or her excess emotional energy in the stomach, creating further anxiety, stress, and disease.

On a planetary scale, the stomach correlates with forests. Imbalance in this region is comparable to acid rain, clear cutting, and other destructive factors.

OTHER CONSIDERATIONS

- Maintaining clean, fresh air inside the home is important, and for this purpose green plants can be placed in each room. Indoor air circulation can also be maintained by frequently opening the windows.
- Wearing cotton underwear and avoiding synthetic fabrics are helpful for better skin metabolism and to facilitate energy flow through the body.
- Avoid frequent exposure to artificial radiation, including medical and dental X-rays, smoke detectors, television, video terminals, and hand-held appliances, which weaken the stomach and digestive system.
- Try to be happy, positive, and outgoing. Singing, dancing, and playing are particularly beneficial in improving overall health and mentality and harmonizing with the rhythms of nature.
- Light exercise, including breathing fresh air outdoors and ten to fifteen minutes a day of practicing long exhalations through the nostrils, will promote harmonious mental and physical metabolism and contribute to overall relaxation.

PERSONAL EXPERIENCES

STOMACH CANCER

In 1983 doctors in New York told Katsuhide Kitatani that he had stomach cancer. After surgery he was put on chemotherapy, but the cancer spread to the lymph system, and he was told that he had only six to twelve months to live. Mr. Kitatani, a senior administrator at the United Nations for many years, started to wind up his affairs. Then one day at a party he ran into a friend who had been suffering from lymph cancer. Mr. Kitatani noticed that all her hair, which had fallen out during medical treatment, had been restored. He asked her how she did it.

She said, "I'm practicing macrobiotics."

"What kind of economics is that?" he asked.

The friend gave him the name of a book to read, and in the fifth or sixth bookstore he looked he finally found the book. It described how a medical doctor—the president of a large American hospital—whose body was riddled with tumors had healed his own terminal condition with the help of a macrobiotic dietary approach. "The diet looked very easy, very Japanese," Mr. Kitatani, who was born in Japan, reflected afterward. "It included plenty of rice, wakame, and miso soup." After arranging a consultation with me in Boston, he started the diet. "I bought three macrobiotic cookbooks and asked my wife to start cooking. I was a very good supervisor." His wife started the diet immediately, but his twin sons were skeptical. Mr. Kitatani's friends were encouraging but also expected him to die shortly.

As his condition improved, Mr. Kitatani looked back on his previous way of eating and the factors that had led to his illness. "I was fifteen when World War II ended. We were starving and had lost the will to produce. We received sugar from the American GIs. Soon I was crawling around on my hands and knees and developed skin disease, but I didn't associate it with what I was eating at the time." Hot springs helped his skin condition. In a U.S. occupation forces camp where he worked, Mr. Kitatani developed a liking for catsup, ice cream, and many other highly processed foods. Later he started working for the United Nations and over the last few decades has been posted all over the world. "Wherever I went, the first question I would ask is: 'Where's the best restaurant?'"

After nine months on his new diet, Mr. Kitatani's cancer went away completely, and he had the unexpected joy of having to replan the rest of his life. He decided that the best way he could help others would be to start a macrobiotic club at the United Nations. "The pace of life is getting quicker and quicker. All around the world people now have access to modern supermarkets and industrially processed food. At the UN we arrange for fertilizers to be shipped, insecticides to be sprayed, and the symptoms of diseases to be eliminated without addressing their underlying causes. People talk till they're blue in the face but don't seem to take action.

"All around the world people are incapacitated and unproductive. UN debates are really selfish and guided by egocentric thinking. The UN has been successful on limited occasions in avoiding conflagrations. In the future, it seems to be that peace will come from individuals who are free of physical and spiritual diseases. Every one of us is an actual or potential peacemaker."

For the last twenty-five years Mr. Kitatani has been cancer-free. After serving as deputy secretary-general of the United Nations specializing in world population issues, he returned to Japan and founded 2050, a global service organization focusing on economic development and sustainability.[7]

30

Thyroid Cancer

FREQUENCY

Thyroid cancer has increased by 73 percent in the United States between 1973 and 1999, making it one of the most rapidly growing malignancies. This year 1,530 people will die and 33,550 new cases will be diagnosed. Women are affected about three times more than men, and thyroid cancer has risen to the seventh most prevalent malignant tumor in American females.

Men are at risk of thyroid cancer until about age seventy-five, while women remain at risk between thirty and fifty-five and then less thereafter. South Asian women are at particularly high risk, apparently because of lifestyle factors described below.

There are four major types of thyroid cancer: (1) papillary, which makes up about 80 percent of tumors and affects the follicular cells and grows slowly; (2) follicular, which makes up 15 percent and also begins in follicular cells and grows slowly; (3) medullary, which accounts for 3 percent and begins in the C cells of the thyroid and also tends to grow slowly; and (4) anaplastic, which affects 2 percent, begins in the follicular cells, and tends to grow and spread very quickly.

Risk factors for papillary thyroid cancer include goiters with benign thyroid nodules or a family history of polyps in the colon or rectum. Inflammation of the thyroid (thyroiditis) may also be a risk factor. The two most common thyroid conditions (overactive and underactive thyroid) are not risk factors for malignancy.

Incipient thyroid cancer usually does not have symptoms, but as it develops, symptoms may include a lump in the thyroid area in the neck, voice changes or hoarseness, swollen lymph nodes in the neck, problems swallowing or breathing, and chronic pain in the neck or throat.

Modern medicine diagnoses thyroid cancer through palpating the thyroid for lumps and feeling nearby lymph nodes for swelling or growths; blood tests, especially abnormal levels of thyroid-stimulating hormone (TSH); ultrasound imaging; a thyroid scan with a radioactive substance; or biopsy.

Standard treatment includes surgery, thyroid hormone treatment, radioactive iodine therapy, external radiation therapy, or chemotherapy. Patients with papillary or follicular thyroid cancer are commonly given radioactive iodine (RAI) about two months after surgery in an effort to destroy any remaining cancer cells in their bodies. Patients undergoing RAI are asked to adopt a low-iodine diet (LID) for about two weeks before testing to deplete the body of its stores of iodine and to continue the diet through testing and treatment.

STRUCTURE

The thyroid is a small gland in the front of the neck just below the larynx (voice box or Adam's apple) that influences many basic metabolic processes. Normally, the thyroid is slightly larger than the American quarter and cannot be felt through the skin. A thin piece of tissue, known as the isthmus, separates the twin lobes of the gland. The hormones produced by the thyroid include thyroid hormone (thyroxin) composed of thyroid follicular cells. Thyroxin helps regulate heart rate, blood pressure, body temperature, and body weight. Another hormone, known as calcitonin, is produced by C cells in the gland and helps regulate calcium levels in the body. Behind the thyroid on the surface of the organ are four or more very small parathyroid glands. They produce parathyroid hormone that also helps maintain calcium levels, especially in the bones and teeth.

CAUSE OF CANCER

Overall, the thyroid, like other endocrine glands, is small, dense, and compact—or very yang. It is easily damaged by overconsumption of meat, poultry, eggs, cheese, and other animal foods, as well as too much salt, hard-baked flour, and other strong contractive items, including some drugs and medications. The endocrine glands also attract extreme yin in the form of metabolic energy from the consumption of sugar, chocolate, honey, and other refined sweeteners; polished grains; fruits and juices; tropical foods; spices, stimulants, and alcohol; and some more expansive drugs and medications.

Overall, thyroid cancer is classified as arising from extremes of both yin and yang. As a small, tight (yang) organ, it is affected by strong animal food, baked food, and salt, and by virtue of its location in the upper body, it also attracts strong upward yin energy from sugar, sweets, oil, light fat and dressings, dairy, and other expansive items.

From an energetic view, many cases of thyroid result from eating too much poultry or eggs and developing physical and energetic structures corresponding to a chicken. Chickens have thick folds in the neck, and people who eat chicken regularly, especially women, often develop similar conditions in their neck and throat.

Modern medicine has studied intensively the possible link of iodine to thyroid cancer. Most people get iodine in shellfish and iodized salt. Not enough iodine in the diet may increase the risk of follicular thyroid cancer. However, other studies show that too much iodine in the diet may also increase the risk of papillary thyroid cancer. As a rule, avoiding dietary extremes, including all shellfish, is recommended for those with this condition. Sea salt should be used in place of table salt, and other foods high in iodine, especially sea vegetables, may temporarily need to be limited until the condition improves. In those cases, where iodine levels are low, sea vegetables and other mineral-rich foods may need to be slightly increased.

MEDICAL EVIDENCE

- In a study of the relationship between frequencies of consumption of selected indicator foods and the risk of thyroid cancer in northern Italy and Switzerland, Italian researchers found a higher association of the disease with refined pasta, refined rice, refined bread, pastry, potatoes, and several types of meat, and significantly so for chicken and poultry, cooked ham, salami, and sausages. Significant direct associations were observed with cheese, butter, and oils other than olive. Most types of vegetables and fruits were protective, especially carrots, green salad, and citrus fruits.[1]
- In a population-based case-control study conducted in Sweden and Norway on the association between dietary habits and the risk of thyroid cancer, scientists report that the disease was associated with the high consumption of butter and cheese.[2]
- Although consumption of whole grain foods seems to reduce the risk of several types of cancer, the potential influence of a diet rich in starches and refined grains is less clear. In a study of the relation

between the frequency of consumption of refined cereals (bread, pasta, or rice) and the risk of selected cancers, Italian scientists found that refined-cereal intake was associated with a high risk up to 60 percent for cancer of the oral cavity, pharynx, esophagus, or larynx; 50 percent for stomach and colon cancer; 30 percent for cancer of the rectum; and 100 percent for thyroid cancer. "Consumption of refined cereals was associated with an increased risk of cancers of the large bowel, the stomach, and other selected digestive and nondigestive sites," the researchers concluded.[3]

- In a study of the relation of thyroid cancer risk and dietary phytoestrogens, which can have both estrogenic and antiestrogenic properties, researchers at the Northern California Cancer Center found that the consumption of traditional and nontraditional soy-based foods and alfalfa sprouts were associated with reduced risk of thyroid cancer. Consumption of "Western" foods with added soy flour or soy protein did not affect risk. Of the seven specific phytoestrogenic compounds examined, the isoflavones, daidzein, genistein, and lignan, secoisolariciresinol, were most strongly associated with risk reduction. Findings were similar for white and Asian women and for pre- and postmenopausal women. "Our findings suggest that thyroid cancer prevention via dietary modification of soy and/or phytoestrogen intake in other forms may be possible but warrants further research at this time," the scientists concluded.[4]

- In a study of 313 case-control pairs in Kuwait to examine the cause of thyroid cancer, the second most common neoplasm among women in this and several other countries in the Gulf region, medical researchers at Kuwait University reported that the high consumption of processed fish products and chicken were independently associated with thyroid cancer that had significant dose-response relationships. Among the thyroid cancer patients who reported high consumption of fish products, a large majority also reported high consumption of fresh fish (98 percent) and shellfish (68 percent). "These data support the hypothesis that hyperplastic thyroid disease is strongly related to thyroid cancer; and that habitual high consumption of various seafoods may be relevant to the aetiology of thyroid cancer. The association with chicken consumption requires further study."[5]

DIAGNOSIS

There is no particular facial feature that corresponds with the thyroid or endocrine system. Symptoms that may accompany thyroid cancer are problems with swallowing, hoarseness, enlarged lymph nodes in the neck, breathing difficulties, and pain in the throat or neck.

DIETARY RECOMMENDATIONS

The primary cause of thyroid cancers is longtime consumption of excessive yin and yang foods and beverages, along with other extreme influences including exposure to radiation, radiation therapy and other medical technology, artificial electromagnetic fields, and exposure to other factors that lower natural immunity to disease. All meat, eggs, poultry, strong fish, dairy, and other animal foods should be discontinued, as well as sugar, chocolate, honey, sweets, spices, herbs, soft drinks, wine, alcohol, fruits and fruit juices, coffee, chemicalized tea, and other stimulants. Foods of tropical origin and oily, greasy foods of all kinds must be minimized. Because they are excessively mucus-producing, all flour products are to be avoided except for the occasional consumption of nonyeasted, unleavened whole wheat or rye bread if craved. Chemicalized and artificially produced and treated foods and beverages are to be completely eliminated. Even unsaturated vegetable oil is to be completely avoided or minimized in cooking for a one- or two-month period. All ice-cold foods and drinks should be avoided.

As a rule, a balanced macrobiotic way of eating should be adopted for thyroid cancer, avoiding extremes of yin and yang. A touch of sea vegetables (high in iodine) may be used for this condition, but too many iodine-rich foods and minerals can aggravate an overly yang type of tumor. Generally, limit or restrict kombu, hiziki, and other stronger sea vegetables and eat arame, wakame, nori, and other milder types. Similarly, miso, shoyu, umeboshi, and other salt-based seasonings may also have to be used lightly or limited temporarily. A balanced macrobiotic way of eating should also be followed to alleviate parathyroid tumors. Dietary guidelines are as follows:

- Whole Grains: Forty to 50 percent of daily consumption, by volume, should be whole cereal grains. The first day prepare plain short- or medium-grain brown rice, pressure-cooked or cooked in a heavy cast-iron or ceramic pot with a heavy lid. On subsequent days, prepare brown rice cooked with 20 to 30 percent millet, then rice with 20 to 30 percent barley, then rice with 20 to 30 percent aduki beans or lentils, and then plain rice again. A delicious morning porridge can be made by taking leftover rice, adding a little more water to soften it, seasoning with a little miso, and simmering for two to three minutes more. Except for morning porridge, which may be soft, the grain should be cooked in a ratio of two parts grain to one part water. Other grains can be used occasionally, including whole wheat berries, rye, corn, and whole oats, although oats should be avoided for the first month. Buckwheat and seitan should be minimized. Good-quality sourdough bread may be enjoyed two to three times a week, and noodles, especially udon and soba, may also be eaten, though generally soba should be limited. Avoid all hard-baked products until the condition improves, including cookies, cakes, pie, crackers, muffins, and the like.

- Soup: Five to 10 percent of daily consumption should be soup, consisting of one or two cups or bowls cooked with wakame sea vegetable and various land vegetables such as onions and carrots, seasoned with very light to moderate miso or shoyu. Occasionally a small amount of shiitake mushrooms may be added to the soup. The miso may be barley miso, brown rice miso, or soybean (hatcho) miso, and should be naturally aged two to three years. To satisfy a desire for a sweet taste, millet soup with sweet vegetables such as squash, cabbage, onions, and carrots may be prepared often. Grain soups, bean soups, and other soups may be eaten from time to time.
- Vegetables: Twenty to 30 percent of daily consumption should be vegetables, cooked in a variety of forms, with plenty of hard, green leafy vegetables, which are good for the liver and detoxification; round vegetables such as squash, cabbage, and onions, which are good for the spleen and immune system; and root vegetables such as daikon, carrot, and burdock, which are strengthening to the intestines and the blood and lymph as a whole. As a rule of thumb, the following dishes may be prepared, although the frequency may differ from person to person: nishime-style vegetables, three to four times a week; a squash-aduki-kombu dish, three times a week; dried daikon, one cup, three times a week; carrots and carrot tops or daikon and daikon tops, three times a week; boiled salad, five to seven times a week; pressed salads, several times a week; raw salad and salad dressing, avoid; steamed greens, five to seven times a week; sautéed vegetables, two times a week using water the first month instead of oil, and then occasionally a small amount of sesame oil may be brushed on the skillet; kinpira, sautéed in water, two-thirds of a cup, two times a week, and then oil may be used after three weeks; dried tofu, tofu, tempeh, or seitan with vegetables, two times a week.
- Beans: Five percent of daily consumption should be small beans, such as aduki beans, lentils, chickpeas, or black soybeans, cooked together with sea vegetables such as kombu or with onions and carrots. Other beans may be used two to three times a month. For seasoning, a small amount of unrefined sea salt or shoyu or miso can be used. Bean products, such as tempeh, natto, and dried or cooked tofu, may be used occasionally, but in moderate amounts. Avoid making the tofu too creamy and use firm, rather than soft, tofu.
- Sea Vegetables: Two percent or less of sea vegetable dishes, including wakame, should be included regularly when cooking grain, in soup, etc. A sheet of toasted nori may also be taken several times a

week. A small dish of arame may be prepared once or twice a week. Minimize kombu, hiziki, and other strong sea vegetables that may be too high in iodine. All other sea vegetables are optional.

- Condiments: Those that should be available on the table are gomashio (sesame salt), on the average made with one part salt to twenty parts sesame seeds (reduced to 1:18 after two months); kombu, kelp, or wakame powder; umeboshi plum; and tekka, although all other regular macrobiotic condiments may be used if desired. These condiments may be used daily on grains and vegetables, but the amounts should be moderate to suit individual appetites and tastes. Umeboshi (one half to one plum a day) and tekka (one-quarter to one-third teaspoon a day) are good for restoring immune ability.

- Pickles: Made at home in a variety of ways, pickles may be eaten daily, one tablespoon in all, although salty pickles are to be minimized.

- Animal Food: Although animal food is to be avoided, a small amount of white-meat fish may be eaten once every week or two weeks. The fish should be steamed, boiled, or poached and garnished with daikon or ginger. After two months, fish may be eaten once or twice a week and may be prepared with other cooking styles, such as broiling, grilling, and baking. Strictly avoid blue-meat and red-meat fish and all shellfish.

- Fruit: None is best, but the less the better, including temperate-climate fruit as well as tropical, until the condition improves. If cravings develop, a small amount of cooked fruit with a pinch of salt or dried fruit may be eaten. Avoid all fruit juices and cider temporarily, as well as raisins, currants, and other highly concentrated fruits.

- Sweets and Snacks: Limit sweets and desserts until the condition improves. Just a little sugar, chocolate, carob, honey, maple syrup, or soy milk could worsen symptoms. To satisfy a sweet tooth, use sweet vegetables every day in cooking, drink sweet the vegetable drink (see special drinks), and use sweet vegetable jam. Mochi, rice balls, vegetable sushi, and other grain-based snacks may be eaten frequently. Limit rice cakes, popcorn, and other dry or baked snacks because they may increase fat beneath the skin and prevent discharge. In the event of cravings, a small amount of grain-based sweeteners such as barley malt or rice syrup may be eaten, as well as a small amount of amasake or good-quality macrobiotic desserts, especially soft ones such as kanten, puddings, and couscous cake.

- Nuts and Seeds: Nuts and nut butters are to be avoided due to their high fat and protein, except for chestnuts. Unsalted blanched seeds such as squash seeds and pumpkin seeds may be consumed as a snack, up to one cup total per week. Sunflower seeds may be eaten only in the summer.

- Seasonings: Unrefined sea salt, shoyu, and miso are to be used lightly in order to avoid unnecessary thirst. Avoid mirin and garlic. If you become particularly thirsty after a meal or between meals, you should cut back on these seasonings until the normal level of thirst returns.

- Beverages: Drinks and other dietary practices can follow the general recommendations in Part I, including bancha twig tea as the main beverage. Strictly avoid the beverages on the "infrequent" and "avoid" lists, including all aromatic, stimulant beverages, and refrain from grain coffee for the first two to three months after starting this new way of eating.

The most important thing in connection with dietary practice is chewing very well, until all food becomes liquid in the mouth and is well mixed with saliva. Chew very well, at least fifty times and preferably a hundred times, per mouthful. It is also important to avoid overeating and eating within three hours of sleeping.

As noted in the introduction to Part II, people who have received or who are currently undergoing medical treatment may need to make further dietary modifications.

SPECIAL DRINKS AND DISHES

Prepare the special Thyroid Drink described in the Home Remedies section.

HOME CARE

- As an external treatment, a compress made from 50 percent regular potato and 50 percent cabbage (with a little flour and water) can be applied to the affected area. Leave on for several hours and apply daily for several weeks or until the condition improves.
- To help treat thyroid problems, shiatsu massage can be performed on the major points along the lung meridian.

EMOTIONAL CONSIDERATIONS

The thyroid governs several hormones, which in turn are related to the emotions. A healthy thyroid and other endocrine glands lead to emotional stability and a calm, steady, cheerful disposition. The thyroid is associated with the throat chakra that governs speech, singing, and other verbal or vocal expression. Suppression of these can lead to thyroid problems. Neglect, abuse, guilt, and other factors can contribute to restricting this area.

High-quality foods that nourish the endocrine system and help develop positive emotions include whole grains; beans and bean products; leafy green vegetables; sea vegetables; and good-quality sea salt, miso, shoyu, and other seasonings.

Foods that harm the thyroid and contribute to negative emotions include especially chicken and eggs, as well as meat, dairy food, and strong fish and seafood; white flour; sugar, chocolate, and other highly refined sweets; chemicalized and artificial foods; too many raw foods; too many stimulants and other beverages; alcohol; and other extremely contractive or expansive items.

In relationships it is important to freely and honestly express oneself. Emotional disturbances, including thyroid disorders, may follow, if a person is not able to make himself or herself understood.

On a planetary scale, the endocrine system correlates with mineral springs, fragrant pools, desert oases, and other nourishing liquid features of the environment.

OTHER CONSIDERATIONS

- The endocrine glands are highly charged by electromagnetic energy from the environment. Their functioning can be improved by stimulating the meridians through acupressure massage, moxabustion, or acupuncture.
- Avoid synthetic clothing, especially next to the skin, confined environments, and exposure to artificial electromagnetic radiation. These impede the natural exchange of energy between the body and the natural environment. They also produce extremely weakening vibrational effects that can contribute to hormone imbalances.
- Those exposed to high levels of radiation, especially from X-rays, are much more likely than others to develop papillary or follicular thyroid cancer. Until the 1950s, medical science in the twentieth century employed high-dose X-rays to treat children with swollen tonsils, acne, and other problems affecting the head and neck. Later, studies linked thyroid cancer with X-ray exposure in childhood. Excessive or repeated exposure to ordinary medical X-rays, including chest X-rays and dental X-rays, could also be harmful. The risks are much less than with 1950s X-rays but still may be cumulative.
- Nuclear radiation is also a risk factor. This includes fallout from atomic weapons testing (such as the testing in the United States, Soviet Union, and elsewhere in the 1950s and 1960s), nuclear power plant accidents (such as Three Mile Island and Chernobyl) in the 1970s and 1980s, and emissions from atomic weapons production plants (such as the Hanford facility in Washington State in the late 1940s). Nuclear fallout contains radioactive iodine (I-131) and other radioactive elements. Individuals exposed to I-131, especially while

growing up, may have an increased risk of thyroid diseases, including thyroid cancer.

- The birth-control pill also slightly increases the risk of thyroid cancer. Unlike other risk factors associated with the pill, the risk for thyroid cancer continues even after use of the pill has stopped.

PERSONAL EXPERIENCE

On the macrobiotic diet, many people with thyroid disorders, including thyroid cancer, have improved, reduced their dependency on thyroid medication, or eliminated it altogether. For example, Rosemary Traill, a longtime macrobiotic counselor from Pittsburgh, told the following to Cancer Research UK, a major medical charity: "I'm working with a young lady right now whose cancer is not only in remission, but also whose allergies and asthma have cleared up and who is also off her thyroid medication. Her children's allergies have cleared up, her husband has lost twenty-five pounds, and her mother has lost twenty pounds."[6]

SPECIAL CONSIDERATION FOR HORMONE THERAPY

Many patients with thyroid conditions besides cancer are treated with hormone therapy and are expected to continue it for the duration of their lives. The thyroid substitutes are generally produced either from pig hormones or synthetic hormones. The question often arises: "Which is preferable?" From the macrobiotic perspective, neither is ideal. Taking hormones from animal sources, in this case swine, contributes animal-quality energy that may lead to aggressive, squeamish, or other pig-like tendencies. Artificial hormones may also result in negative physical or psychological effects and contribute to other disorders. Generally, thyroid patients who are on hormone therapy and then adopt macrobiotics report that they eventually feel more comfortable with the animal product, which is still natural, than with the synthetic or artificial one. Hopefully, over time, the amount and frequency of the dose may gradually be reduced and in some cases be discontinued altogether. Such decisions are best discussed with one's medical doctor or other health care professional and/or family.

PART 3

Practical Approaches

31

Guidelines for People with Cancer

When properly applied, the Cancer Prevention Diet can help restore an excessively yin or yang condition to one of more natural balance. However, slight modifications are needed in every case. Below is a summary of the common types of cancer and the general dietary adjustments for the category in which they fall. Specific nutritional advice for each cancer is given in the individual chapters in Part II under the section "Dietary Recommendations." Cancer patients should consult an experienced macrobiotic counselor or medical associate to make sure the evaluation of their condition is accurate and to help formulate a diet suited to their unique case and personal needs.

Kind of Food	More Yin Cancer	Combination of Both	More Yang Cancer
	Brain (outer regions)	Bladder/Kidney	Bone
		Liver	Brain (inner regions)
	Breast	Lung	
	Esophagus	Melanoma	Colon
	Hodgkin's disease	Leukemia (some cases)	Ovary
			Pancreas
	Leukemia (most cases)	Lymphoma (some cases)	Prostate
			Rectum

(continued)

(continued)

Kind of Food	More Yin Cancer	Combination of Both	More Yang Cancer
	Lymphoma (most cases) Mouth (except tongue) Skin Stomach (upper) Testicular	Spleen Stomach (lower) Tongue Uterus Thyroid	
Grains		Minimize buckwheat	Minimize buckwheat
Soup	Slightly stronger (more miso or shoyu)	Moderate flavor	Milder flavor (less miso or shoyu)
Vegetables	Slightly greater emphasis on root varieties (burdock, carrot, turnip, etc.)	Greater emphasis on ground varieties (cauliflower, acorn and butternut squash, pumpkin)	Greater emphasis on leafy green varieties (daikon, carrot, or turnip greens, kale, watercress, etc.)
Beans	A little more strongly seasoned, use less often	Moderately seasoned and moderate volume	More lightly seasoned, may use regularly
Sea Vegetables	Longer cooking, slightly thicker taste	Moderate cooking, medium taste	Quicker cooking, lighter taste
Pickles	More long-time pickles	More medium-time pickles	More short-time pickles
Condiments	Stronger use	Moderate use	Lighter use
Animal Food	Occasional small amount of white fish or dried fish, only if craved	Avoid completely or minimize	Avoid completely

Kind of Food	More Yin Cancer	Combination of Both	More Yang Cancer
Salad	Avoid raw salad; occasional boiled salad	Limit raw salad; frequent boiled or pressed salad	Occasional raw; frequent boiled or pressed salad
Fruit Dessert	Avoid completely	Small amount of dried or cooked fruit (locally grown and seasonal), if craved	Small amount of dried or cooked fruit (locally grown and seasonal), if craved; occasional fresh fruit in small amounts
Seeds and Nuts	Occasional roasted seeds; avoid nuts	Occasional roasted seeds; limit nuts	Occasional roasted seeds; avoid nuts
Oil	Sesame only, as little as possible. Apply with brush to prevent burning. No raw oil.	Sesame or corn only, as little as possible. Apply with brush to prevent burning. No raw oil.	Sesame or corn for cooking; small amount occasionally for sautéing. No raw oil.
Beverage	Longer-cooked, thicker-tasting tea	Medium-cooked, medium-tasting tea	Shorter-cooked, lighter-tasting tea

32

Making a Smooth
Transition

The transition to a more natural diet and way of life should present no serious conflict. However, sometimes we approach the process too ambitiously and go to great lengths to avoid the foods to which we were previously accustomed. If we rush things and try to change overnight or too quickly, we are bound to make mistakes and within a short period will revert to our former lifestyle or go on to something else. This desire for instant satisfaction is part of the modern consumer mentality, and we can make the mistake of approaching the Cancer Prevention Diet in this way as well as anything else.

In selecting natural foods, we begin to appreciate crops that have matured in the fields and weathered the elements in contrast to those that have been produced in a factory and artificially aged. Similarly, we must respect our own biological rhythms and personal rates of growth. In many cases it has taken ten, twenty, or thirty years or more of poor eating for the cancerous condition to develop. Depending on our own unique situation, it will take several months and, in some cases, a few years to recover our normal digestive, respiratory, circulatory, excretory, and nervous functions. The healing process should not be artificially hurried.

When starting the new way of eating, it is best to begin with just a few basic preparations, such as brown rice, miso soup, a few vegetable dishes, one sea vegetable, and bancha tea. Then, day by day, week by week, we can gradually widen our selection of natural foods and introduce new cooking styles. In the meantime we can still be eating some of the same types of foods we have been eating in the past, including salads and fruit, flour products, and seafood. Rather than eliminating certain categories of food from our diet, it is better initially to reduce their intake and then switch to a better quality of intermediary food until a taste and appreciation for the new foods are developed.

The important thing is to begin to change in the right direction. Ideally the rate of change should be more like walking long distances, where we gradually build up our endurance, rather than like sprinting or marathon running, where we get off to a fast start but inevitably get worn out. If we throw away all of our old food the first day and memorize the yin and yang tables like a catechism, we will soon either leave the diet as abruptly as we adopted it or become missionaries, preaching to the nutritionally unconverted. Such behavior is childish and violates the macrobiotic way of life, which respects all lifestyles and understands opposites as complementary aspects of the whole.

On the other hand there is a danger of taxiing so slowly down the dietary runway that our plane never takes off. Sometimes we can remain in a holding pattern for years, never realizing that we are still on the ground. We are conscious of the importance of proper food and eat whole grains, tofu, and miso soup, but we never really experience looking at things from a healthy perspective. If we adopt a middle way between proceeding too quickly and too slowly, we will soon find ourselves pleasantly aloft.

Of course, these reflections on making a smooth transition apply to people already in relatively healthy condition. Those with cancer or other serious conditions may need to adopt a strict form of the diet without the luxury of integrating it into their previous way of eating. However, in practice the reduction in pain and discomfort quickly convinces the person of the value of the new approach.

As far as obtaining natural foods, growing our own grains and vegetables is best, of course, if the situation allows. We should all try to cultivate a garden even if it is a very small one in an urban environment. Next best is to obtain food at an organic farmers' market or a natural foods co-op so that we can actually experience some of the living energy of the food before it reaches the market shelf or dinner table. In most North American and European cities, there are now natural foods and health food stores that supply most of the staple items in the Cancer Prevention Diet as well as a regular supply of fresh seasonal produce. It is important to shop around and learn what each store offers in terms of quality, availability, service, and price. Buying in bulk saves on packaging and is more ecological and less expensive. Ethnic markets, such as Oriental, Latin American, African American, and Middle Eastern, are also potential sources of basic items, such as grains and beans, and often have a wider selection of vegetables than elsewhere. Increasingly, supermarkets are now offering organic produce as well as whole grains, tofu, and other staples.

As far as possible we should try to make our own bread, tofu, pickles, and traditionally processed foods. Homemade dishes have a much fresher quality, are more delicious, and contribute to the peaceful energy of the home. Each week, each month, or each season of the year we can try our new food preparation or style of cooking and slowly build up a reservoir of experience that can become translated into well-balanced recipes and menus.

During the transition period there will be times when we crave the taste, texture, odor, and other characteristics of previous foods and drinks, especially those we had in childhood. Often, when eating such foods, we suffer from feelings of guilt. These feelings should be put aside and a more relaxed attitude developed. Instead of feeling as if we have committed a sin, we should reflect and try to understand why such cravings arose. Usually during the first weeks or months of the new diet, these cravings reflect a natural discharge process. As our condition improves, the toxins and mucus that have accumulated in our bloodstream and internal organs are eliminated from the body through the bowels, urination, perspiration, and other excretory functions. As they leave the body, the discharged food particles often impress themselves in our consciousness, and we experience them as cravings. At other times, after our condition has stabilized, these occasional cravings signify that our diet is imbalanced in the opposite yin or yang direction from the food to which we are attracted. Thus, if we are attracted to fruit juice or ice cream, our diet is probably too salty, overcooked, and generally yang. If we are attracted to fish, eggs, or other animal products, we are consuming too many sweets, liquids, and other strong yin foods. These promptings are one of the body's ways of alerting us to a disequilibrium in our way of eating.

Rather than suppress these natural urges, it is better to acknowledge and appreciate them and take a tiny amount of the previous type of food from time to time until such cravings lessen and finally go away, as they ultimately will. During the transition period the following table may serve as a guide in substituting better-quality foods for the previous items that we miss.

Cravings	Replacement	Goal
Meat	Fish, seafood	Grains, beans, seitan, tempeh, tofu
Sugar, molasses, chocolate, carob, and other highly refined sweeteners	Honey, maple syrup	Rice syrup, barley malt, and ultimately natural sweeteners from whole grains and vegetables
Dairy food, cheese, milk, cream, butter	Organic dairy food, in small amounts; nuts and nut butters; soy milk	Traditional soy products such as miso and tofu; tahini and other seed butters

Cravings	Replacement	Goal
Tropical and semitropical fruits and juices such as orange, grapefruit, and pineapple; artificial juices and beverages	Organic fruits and fruit juices	Organic temperate-climate fruit (fresh, dried, and cooked) and juices in small amounts and in season
Coffee, black tea, soft drinks, diet drinks	Herb teas, green tea, mineral water	Bancha twig tea, grain coffee, and other traditional nonaromatic teas

During the transition period, instead of coffee or decaffeinated coffee, use grain coffee. To keep awake, take bancha tea with a little barley malt. In the beginning, some people find it difficult to eat brown rice. In this case, take other whole grains and gradually introduce brown rice, or take white rice cooked together with barley or with millet and barley and gradually over the next few weeks add a small amount of brown rice. During this time, as the body begins to rebalance, brown rice will become more appetizing and can be used regularly. Ordinarily we don't use white rice on a daily basis, but in this case it may be used temporarily until the intestines and other organs are able to digest whole grains.

In addition to cravings, the discharge process is often accompanied by some abnormal physical manifestations that may last from three to ten days or, in some cases, up to four months or more, until the quality of the blood fully changes. If our native constitution is strong and well structured, such reactions are usually negligible. However, if our embryonic and childhood development suffered from chaotic dietary habits, if we have ingested many chemicals, drugs, or medications, or if we have had surgery, radiation, or other medical procedure, these discharge reactions may be more pronounced.

Whatever the case may be, we should not worry if these reactions occur. They are part of the natural healing process and signify that our systems are regenerating themselves, dislodging and throwing off the excess that has accumulated over many years. These reactions may be generally classified as follows:

General Fatigue

A feeling of general fatigue may arise among people who have been eating an excessive amount of animal protein and fat. The energetic activity that they have previously experienced was the result of the vigorous caloric discharge of these excessive foods rather than a more healthy, balanced, and

peaceful way of activity. Often these people initially experience physical tiredness and slight mental depression until the new diet starts to serve as an energy supply for activity. Such a period of fatigue usually ends within a month.

Pains and Aches

Pains and aches may sometimes be experienced, especially by people
who have been taking excessive liquid, sugar, fruits, or any other extremely
yin-quality food and beverages. These pains and aches—such as headaches
and pains in the area of the intestines, kidneys, and chest—occur because of
the gradual contraction of abnormally expanded tissues and nerve cells. These
aches and pains disappear—either gradually or suddenly—as soon as these
abnormally expanded areas return to a normal condition. This usually takes
between three and fourteen days, depending on the previous condition.

Fever, Chills, Coughing

As the new diet starts to form a more sound quality of blood, previous
excessive substances—liquid, fat, and many other things—begin to be discharged. If at this time the functions of the kidneys, urinary system, and respiratory system have not yet returned to normal, this discharge sometimes
takes the form of fever, chills, or coughing. These are temporary and disappear in several days without any special treatment.

Abnormal Sweating and Frequent Urination

As in the symptoms described above, unusual sweating may be experienced by some people from time to time for a period of several months, and
other people may experience unusually frequent urination. In their previous
diets, these people have been taking excessive liquid in the form of water,
various beverages, alcohol, fruits, fruit juices, or milk or other dairy food. By
reducing these excessive liquids and fats accumulated in the form of liquid,
the body returns to a normal, balanced, healthy condition. When metabolic
balance has been gradually restored, these discharges will cease.

Skin Discharge and Unusual Body Odors

Among the forms of elimination is the discharge of unusual odors from
the entire body surface through breathing, urination, or bowel movements
and often, in the case of women, through vaginal discharges. This usually
occurs among people who were previously taking excessive volumes of animal fat, dairy food, and sugar. In addition, some people experience—for
only a short period—skin rashes, reddish swelling at the tips of the fingers
and toes, and boils. These types of elimination arise especially among people

who have taken animal fat, dairy food, sugar, spices, chemicals, and drugs, and among those who have had chronic malfunctions of the intestines, kidneys, and liver. However, these eliminations naturally heal and usually disappear within a few months without any special attention.

Diarrhea or Constipation

People who had chronically disturbed intestinal conditions, caused by previous improper dietary habits, may temporarily experience either diarrhea (usually for several days) or constipation (for a period lasting up to twenty days). In this case, diarrhea is a form of discharge of accumulated stagnated matter in the intestines, including unabsorbed food, fat, mucus, and liquid. Constipation is the result of a process of contraction of the intestinal tube, which was abnormally expanded due to the previous diet. As this contraction restores normal elasticity to the intestinal tube, the normal elimination of the bowels resumes.

Decrease of Sexual Desire and Vitality

Some people may feel a weakening of sexual vitality or appetite, not necessarily accompanied by a feeling of fatigue. The reason for such a decline is that the body functions are working to eliminate imbalanced factors from all parts of the body, and excessive vitality is not available to be used for sexual activity. Also, in some cases, the sexual organs are being actively healed by the new quality of blood and are not yet prepared to resume normal activity. These conditions last only for a short period, however, usually a few weeks and, at most, a few months. As soon as this recovery period is over, healthy vitality and desire for sexual activity return.

Temporary Cessation of Menstruation

In a few women there may be a temporary cessation of menstruation. The reason for this cessation is that in the healing of the entire body, once again the vital organs need to receive energy first. Less vital functions, including reproductive activities, are healed later. The period of cessation of menstruation varies with the individual. However, when menstruation begins anew, it is healthy and natural. It begins to adjust to the normal twenty-eight-day lunar cycle and presents no discomfort, as was previously often the case. Mental clarity and emotional clarity are strengthened as well as physical flexibility.

Mental Irritability

Some people who have been taking stimulants, drugs, and medications for long periods experience emotional irritability after changing their dietary practices. This irritability reflects adjustments taking place in the blood and various body functions, following the change to the different quality of food, and generally passes within one week to several weeks, depending on how deeply affected the body systems were by the previous habitual use of drugs and medications. The consumption of sugar, coffee, and alcohol for long periods, as well as longtime smoking, also produces temporary emotional irritability when the new diet is initially practiced.

Other Possible Transitory Experiences

In addition to the above conditions, some people may experience other manifestations of adjustment, such as bad dreams or a feeling of coldness. These, too, will pass.

In many instances, the discharge process is so gradual that none of these more visible temporary conditions arises. However, when they do appear, the symptoms vary from person to person, depending on their inherited constitution and physical condition. They usually require no special treatment, naturally ceasing as the whole body readjusts to normal functioning. In the possible event that the symptoms are severe or uncomfortable, the discharge process can be slowed down by modifying the new diet to include continuous consumption of some previous food in small amounts—about 10 to 30 percent of the meal—until balance is restored. The important thing is to understand that the discharge mechanism is part of the normal healing process, and these symptoms are not to be suppressed by taking drugs or medications, resorting to vitamin or mineral supplements, or going off the diet altogether in the mistaken belief that it is deficient. If there is any uncertainty or question about proper practice that arises during this transition period, a qualified macrobiotic counselor or medical professional should be contacted.

As mentioned earlier, introductory macrobiotic cooking classes are essential for proper orientation to the new way of eating. In addition, it is important to have a community of support consisting of other individuals or families who are eating in this way or in the general direction of more natural foods. Dishes and recipes can then be exchanged and experiences shared in the spirit of adventure and discovery.

Variables in cooking such as salt, oil, pressure, time, and liquid are always changing with the seasons and our own development, and they take time to master. Another factor connected with unsatisfactory cooking is often the use of electricity or microwave. Some families either have recently installed expensive ranges or ovens or live in an apartment where they come furnished with the kitchen. We have found that when people, especially cancer patients, switch to gas heat, they usually get improved results, and a peaceful energy replaces the weakened vibration of the previously prepared food. Although it may appear uneconomical in the short run to invest in another stove, the change in food quality and improved health will be well worth it in the long run. Even a small portable camping stove with one or two propane burners can be set up conveniently in a corner of the kitchen for this purpose. If you have an extreme yang condition, electric cooking may temporarily help you to relax and unwind. In the event that you can only cook with electric, don't worry or become frustrated lest this energy go into your food. Instead, think positively, use affirmations or other mental and spiritual practices to balance the energy, and do the best you can.

All these factors will contribute to a smoother transition and more delicious and satisfying meals.

33

Recipes

This chapter includes many of the basic recipes for the dietary recommendations in this book. People with cancer should be careful to follow the guidelines in the individual chapters in Part II and may need to restrict their use of oil, animal food, fruit, salad, dessert, and other items. Those in good health may wish to consult a macrobiotic cookbook with a wider selection of recipes, such as *Aveline Kushi's Complete Guide to Macrobiotic Cooking* (New York: Warner Books, 1985), Alex and Gale Jack's *Amber Waves of Grain: American Macrobiotic Cooking* (Amberwaves, 2000), or Wendy Esko's *Macrobiotic Cooking for Everyone* (New York: Square One, 2005).

FOOD SELECTION

For variety, these aspects of day-to-day cooking can be changed:

1. The selection and combination of foods within the following categories: grains, soups, vegetables, beans, sea vegetables, condiments, pickles, and beverages
2. The methods of cooking and length of cooking times: boiling, steaming, sautéing, frying, pressure-cooking, etc. (do not overcook or pressure-cook vegetables)

3. The ways of cutting vegetables
4. The amount of water used
5. The amount and kind of seasoning and condiments used
6. The use of a higher or lower flame in cooking foods
7. The seasonal cooking adjustments

PREPARATION

Macrobiotic cooking is unique. The ingredients are simple, and cooking is the key to producing meals that are nutritious, tasty, and attractive. The cook has the ability to change the quality of the food. More cooking—the use of pressure, salt, heat, and time—makes the energy of food more concentrated, while quick cooking and little salt preserve the lighter quality of the food. A good cook controls the health of those for whom he or she cooks by varying the cooking styles.

Methods of Cooking and Food Preparation

REGULAR USE	OCCASIONAL USE
Boiling	Baking
Oil-sautéing	Broiling
Pickling	Deep-frying
Pressing	Raw
Pressure-cooking	Stir-frying
Soup preparation	Tempura
Steaming	
Water-sautéing	
Waterless	

GRAINS

BOILED RICE

1 cup brown rice   *pinch of sea salt*
2 cups spring water

Wash rice and place in heavy cast-iron, ceramic, or stainless steel pot or saucepan. Add water and salt. Cover with a lid. Bring to a boil, lower flame, and simmer about 50 minutes or until all water has been absorbed. Remove and serve.

PRESSURE-COOKED BROWN RICE

1 cup organic brown rice   *pinch of sea salt per cup of rice*
1¼ to 1½ cups spring water per cup of rice

Gently wash and quickly place rice (short- or medium-grain) in a pressure cooker and smooth out surface of rice so it is level. Slowly add spring water down side of pressure cooker so surface of rice remains calm and even. Add sea salt. Place cover on pressure cooker and bring up to pressure slowly. When pressure is up, place a flame deflector underneath and turn flame to low. Cook for 50 minutes. When rice is done, remove pressure cooker from burner and allow to stand for 5 minutes before reducing pressure and opening. With a bamboo rice paddle, lift rice from pot one spoonful at a time and smooth into wooden bowl. Distribute more cooked rice at bottom and less cooked rice at top evenly in bowl. The rice will have a delicious nutty taste and impart a very peaceful feeling.

Note: Each cup of uncooked rice makes about 3 cups of cooked rice. Allow about 1 cup per person. As a rule, make rice fresh every day. But if you make too much or are pressed for time, leftover rice will keep for several days. After rice cools off, place in a closed container in the refrigerator. Warm up by putting rice in a cheesecloth or a piece of unbleached muslin, placing it in a ceramic saucepan or on top of a steamer that fits into a pot or saucepan, adding ¼ to ½ inch of water, and bringing to a boil. After rice has heated for a few minutes, remove from cloth and serve.

VARIATION: One-third of an umeboshi plum may be added instead of salt for each cup of uncooked rice. Long-grain rice may occasionally be used in summer.

BROWN RICE WITH MILLET

2 cups brown rice   *2-inch piece of kombu or pinch of*
½ cup millet   *sea salt*
4½ cups spring water

Wash the grains and place in a heavy pot with water and kombu, or place over fire and add a pinch of sea salt. When contents come to a boil, reduce to a simmer and cook about 50 minutes.

BROWN RICE WITH BARLEY

2 cups brown rice
½ cup barley
4 cups spring water

2-inch piece of kombu or pinch of
sea salt

Wash rice and place in a heavy pot with water and kombu, or add a pinch of sea salt. When ingredients come to a boil, reduce to a simmer and cook about 50 minutes.

SOFT BROWN RICE (Rice Kayu)

1 cup brown rice
5 cups spring water

pinch of sea salt

Wash rice and boil or pressure-cook in water with salt as in previous recipes. However, not all of the water will be absorbed. Rice should be creamy, and some of the grains should be visible after cooking. In case water boils over while pressure-cooking, turn off flame and allow to cool off. Then turn on flame again and continue to cook until done.

Note: Makes a nourishing and appetizing breakfast cereal. Especially recommended for cancer patients and others who have difficulty swallowing or holding food down.

VARIATION: Vegetables such as daikon or Chinese cabbage or an umeboshi plum may be added while cooking. Also, a 1-inch square of dried kombu is highly recommended.

GENUINE BROWN RICE CREAM

1 cup brown rice
10 cups spring water

½ umeboshi plum or a pinch of sea
salt per cup of rice

Dry-roast rice in a cast-iron or stainless steel skillet until golden brown. Place in pot, add water and plum or salt, and bring to a boil. Cover, lower heat, and place a flame deflector beneath pot. Cook until water is one-half of original volume. Let the rice cool and place in cheesecloth or unbleached muslin, tie, and squeeze a creamy liquid out of the pulp through the cloth. Heat the cream again, then serve. Add salt if needed. The remaining pulp is also very good to eat and can be made into a small ball and steamed with grated lotus root or carrot.

Note: Makes a delicious breakfast cereal and is also good for those who have difficulty eating. The lives of many people who otherwise could not eat have been saved with rice cream. The love, care, and energy of the cook can be imparted to the food with his or her hands.

VARIATION: Garnish with scallions, chopped parsley, nori, gomashio, or roasted sunflower seeds.

FRIED RICE

1 tablespoon dark or light sesame oil   *4 cups cooked brown rice*
1 medium onion, sliced diagonally or diced   *1 to 2 tablespoons shoyu*

Brush skillet with sesame oil. Let heat for a minute or less, but do not let oil start to smoke. Add onion and place rice on top. If rice is dry, moisten with a few drops of water. Cover skillet and cook on low flame for 10 to 15 minutes. Add shoyu and cook for another 5 minutes. There is no need to stir. Just mix before serving.

Note: Those in good health may have fried rice several times a week, although the amount of oil may need to be reduced depending on the individual's condition. Other plant oils may be used instead of sesame. Cancer patients may need to restrict their oil and may use 2 to 3 tablespoons of water to replace the oil. Check dietary recommendations carefully.

VARIATION: Use scallions, parsley, or a combination of vegetables such as carrots and onion, cabbage and mushroom, and daikon and daikon leaves.

RICE WITH BEANS

1 cup brown rice   *1½ to 2 cups spring water*
⅒ to ⅛ cup beans per cup of rice   *pinch of sea salt*

Wash rice and beans. Cook beans 30 minutes beforehand following basic recipes in bean section on page 478. Allow beans to cool. Add with cooking water and sea salt to rice. Bean water counts as part of the total water in the recipe. Pressure-cook for 45 to 50 minutes and serve as with plain rice.

Note: Cancer patients should generally use smaller beans such as aduki, chickpeas, or lentils. Those in good health may use a wider variety of other beans as well. Grains and beans cooked together make a substantial meal and save the time and fuel needed for cooking each dish separately.

RICE AND VEGETABLES

1 cup brown rice
1/4 cup dried daikon
1/2 cup carrots, finely diced or small
    matchsticks

1/8 cup green peas
1 1/2 to 2 cups spring water per cup
    of rice
pinch of sea salt per cup of rice

Place washed rice in heavy pot and mix with vegetables. Add water and salt, cover, and cook as for plain rice.

VARIATION: A small amount of shoyu may be added with salt before cooking. Other vegetables that go well with rice are sweet rice, green beans, and carrots. Soft vegetables such as onion and green leafy vegetables tend to become mushy and should be avoided for this dish. Rice and vegetables may also be cooked with sesame seeds, walnuts, or lotus seeds, as well as with aduki beans or black soybeans.

RICE BALLS WITH NORI SEA VEGETABLE

1 sheet toasted nori
pinch of sea salt
dish of spring water

1 cup cooked brown rice
1/2 to 1 umeboshi plum

Roast a thin sheet of nori by holding the shiny side over a burner about 10 to 12 inches from the flame. Rotate for 3 to 5 seconds until color changes from black to green. Fold nori in half and tear into two pieces. Fold and tear again. You should now have four pieces that are about 3 inches to a side. Add salt to dish of water and wet your hands. Form a handful of rice into a solid ball. Press a hole in the center with your thumb and place a small piece of umeboshi inside. Then close hole and compact ball again until solid. Cover rice ball with nori, one piece at a time, until it sticks. Wet hands occasionally to prevent rice and nori from sticking to them, but do not use too much water.

Note: Rice balls make a tasty, convenient lunch or snack because they can be eaten without utensils. They are great to take along when traveling and keep fresh for a few days. Use less or no umeboshi when making rice balls for children.

VARIATION: Rice can be made into triangles instead of balls by cupping your hands into a V shape. Balls or triangles can be rolled in toasted sesame seeds and eaten with nori. Small pieces of salt or bran pickles, vegetables, pickled fish, or other condiments can be inserted inside instead of umeboshi. Instead of nori sheets, use roasted crushed sesame seeds, shiso leaves, pickled rice leaves, dried wakame sheets, or green leafy vegetable leaves.

WHOLE OATS

1 cup whole oats   *pinch of sea salt*
5 to 6 cups spring water

Wash oats and place in pot. Add water and salt. Cover and bring to a boil. Reduce flame and simmer for several hours or overnight, until water is absorbed. Use a flame deflector to prevent burning. Makes an excellent cereal.

Note: Whole oats are very strengthening for cancer patients and are to be preferred, although steel-cut oats or rolled oats may be used occasionally.

VARIATION: Cooking time can be reduced by pressure-cooking following the basic brown rice recipe. For a very nourishing and peaceful dish, combine 1½ cups barley, 1 cup whole oats, and ½ cup partially cooked beans. Add 3 pinches of sea salt and about 4 cups of water, and pressure-cook as usual.

SWEET RICE

1 cup sweet rice   *pinch of sea salt*
1½ to 2 cups spring water

Wash rice, add water and salt, and cook following the basic rice recipe.

Note: Sweet rice is more glutinous than regular rice and should be used only occasionally. It may also be added in small volume to regular rice for a sweeter taste.

MOCHI

Mochi is sweet rice served in cakes or squares. They are made by pounding cooked sweet rice in a wooden bowl with a heavy wooden pestle. Pound until the grains are crushed and become very sticky. Wet pestle occasionally to prevent rice from sticking to it. Form rice into small balls or cakes, or spread on a baking sheet that has been oiled and dusted with flour, and allow to dry. Cut into pieces and roast in a dry skillet, bake, or deep-fry. For occasional use and special celebrations.

RYE

1 cup rye   pinch of sea salt
2 cups spring water

Cook the same as brown rice.

Note: Since rye is hard and requires a lot of chewing, it is usually mixed with other grains or consumed in flour form as rye bread. For a delicious chewy dish, add 1 part rye to 3 parts brown rice. Rye may be dry-roasted in a skillet for a few minutes prior to cooking to make it more digestible.

CORN

Prepare fresh corn on the cob by steaming or boiling in a saucepan for 10 minutes or until done. Instead of butter or margarine, season with a little bit of umeboshi plum.

WHEAT

1 cup wheat berries   pinch of sea salt
2 cups spring water

Cook following the basic brown rice recipe. Boiled wheat usually takes longer to cook than rice.

Note: Wheat is difficult to digest in whole form and must be thoroughly chewed. It also requires longer cooking time. Soaking wheat berries 3 to 5 hours beforehand reduces cooking time and makes a softer, more digestible dish. For a tasty combination, combine 1 part wheat berries and 3 parts rice or other grain.

NOODLES AND BROTH

Spring water   2 dried shiitake mushrooms
1 package udon or soba noodles   2 to 3 tablespoons shoyu
1 piece of kombu, 2 to 3 inches long

Boil 4 cups spring water. Asian noodles already contain salt, so no salt needs to be added. Add noodles to water and boil. After about 10 minutes, check to see if they are done by breaking the end of a noodle. Buckwheat cooks faster than whole wheat, and thinner noodles cook faster than thicker ones. If the inside and outside are the same color, noodles are ready. Remove noodles from pot, strain, and rinse with cold water to stop them from cooking and prevent clumping. To make the broth, place kombu in pot, add 4 cups spring water and mushrooms that have been soaked, their stems cut off, and sliced. Bring to boil. Lower flame and simmer for 3 to 5 minutes. Remove kombu and mushrooms. Add shoyu to taste and simmer for 3 to 5 minutes. Place cooked noodles in the broth to warm up. Do not boil. When hot, remove and serve immediately. Garnish with scallions, chives, or toasted nori.

Note: Soba buckwheat noodles are strengthening. In summer they can be cooked and enjoyed cold. Udon wheat noodles are much lighter. Western-style whole grain noodles and pasta may also be used regularly. These include whole wheat spaghetti, shells, spirals, elbows, flat noodles, lasagna, etc. Use a pinch of salt in water when cooking. Those with a yang condition may need to avoid or limit soba because it is too contracting.

FRIED NOODLES

1 package udon or soba noodles
1 tablespoon sesame oil
2 cups cabbage

1 tablespoon shoyu
1/2 cup sliced scallions

Cook noodles as in previous recipe, rinse under cold water, and drain. Oil skillet and add cabbage. Place noodles on top of cabbage. Cover and cook over low flame for several minutes, until noodles become warm. Add shoyu and mix noodles and cabbage well. At the very end of cooking, add scallions. Serve hot or cold.

Note: If you cannot take oil, use 2 tablespoons of water for sautéing.

VARIATION: Many combinations of vegetables may be used, including carrots and onions, scallions and mushrooms, and cabbage and tofu.

WHOLE WHEAT BREAD

8 cups whole wheat flour
1/4 to 1/2 teaspoon sea salt

spring water
2 tablespoons sesame oil (optional)

Mix flour and salt, add oil, and sift thoroughly together by hand. Form a ball of dough by adding just enough water and knead 300 to 350 times. Oil two bread pans with sesame oil and place dough in pans. Place damp cloth over pans and let sit for 8 to 12 hours in a warm place. After dough has risen, bake at 300°F for 15 minutes and then 1¼ hours longer at 350°F.

Note: Flour products, including bread, may need to be avoided or limited by cancer patients.

VARIATION: A delicious sourdough starter for bread can be made by combining 1 cup flour and enough water to make a thick batter. Cover with damp cloth and allow to ferment for 3 to 4 days in a warm place. After starter has soured, add 1 to 1½ cups starter to bread dough, knead, and proceed as above. For rye bread use 3 cups rye flour to 5 cups whole wheat flour.

RICE KAYU BREAD

2 cups brown rice   *8 cups spring water*

Pressure-cook rice in water for 1 hour or more. Remove rice and allow to cool in a large bowl. While still slightly warm, add to rice:

2 teaspoons sesame oil (optional)   *enough whole wheat flour to form*
½ teaspoon sea salt   *a ball of dough*

Add oil and salt to rice and mix well. Add enough flour to make a soft ball of dough. Knead 300 to 350 times, adding flour to ball from time to time to keep from getting too sticky. Place dough in two oiled bread pans, shape into loaves, cover with a damp cloth, set in a warm place, and let rise 8 to 12 hours. Bake at 300°F for 30 minutes and 350°F for another hour, or until golden brown.

Note: This bread is better for cancer patients than whole wheat bread but should still be used moderately.

BULGUR

1 cup bulgur   *pinch of sea salt*
water

Rinse bulgur in cold water several times. Place in saucepan and add 3–4 cups water, and salt. Bring to a boil, lower flame, cover, and simmer about 20 to 30 minutes.

VARIATION: Add diced onions, carrots, celery, or other vegetables when cooking.

COUSCOUS

1 cup couscous
water   *pinch of sea salt*

Rinse couscous in cold water several times. Place in saucepan. Add 3–4 cups water and salt. Bring to a boil, lower flame, cover, and simmer about 20 to 30 minutes.

SOUPS

BASIC VEGETABLE MISO SOUP

3-inch piece of dry wakame sea   *1¼ teaspoons miso*
  vegetable   *scallions, parsley, ginger, or*
1 cup thinly sliced onions   *watercress*
1 quart spring water

Rinse wakame quickly in cold water, soak for 3 to 5 minutes, and slice into ½-inch pieces. Place wakame and onions in pot and add water. Bring to a boil, cover flame, and simmer for 10 to 20 minutes or until tender. Reduce flame to very low, not boiling or bubbling. Place miso in a bowl or suribachi. Add ¼ cup broth and puree until miso is completely dissolved in liquid. Add pureed miso to soup. Simmer for 3 to 5 minutes. Serve garnished with scallions, parsley, ginger, or watercress.

Note: Be careful to reduce the flame while the miso is cooking in order to preserve the beneficial enzymes in miso. As a general rule, use about ½ teaspoon miso for each cup of water in the broth. Soup shouldn't taste too salty or too bland.

VARIATION: Barley or brown rice miso is highly recommended. Hatcho (100 percent soybean) miso is strong but not salty and also may be used to help restore health. Other misos may be used occasionally. In terms of aging, select miso that has fermented 2 years or more. All types of miso may be eaten year-round and slightly modified in proportion according to the season or condition of health. Vegetables may be varied often. Other basic combinations include wakame, onions, tofu; onions and squash; cabbage and carrots; and daikon and daikon greens. If your health allows for oil, you may brush 1 teaspoon or less of unrefined vegetable oil, especially dark sesame oil, sauté the vegetables first, and then add to the wakame in the pot.

MISO SOUP WITH DAIKON AND WAKAME

1½ cups daikon
1 quart spring water
3-inch piece of wakame

3 teaspoons miso
chopped scallion

Wash and slice daikon into ½-inch slices and add to water. Cook for 5 minutes. Meanwhile, soak wakame for 3 to 5 minutes and chop into small pieces. Add wakame to pot and cook over low flame until vegetables are soft. Dilute and add miso to stock. Simmer for 3 minutes. Garnish with chopped scallion.

Note: Daikon is particularly helpful to eliminate excess mucus, fat, protein, and water from the body. Cooking time of wakame depends on how soft or hard it is.

MILLET AND SWEET VEGETABLE SOUP

1 cup millet
½ cup finely chopped butternut or
   buttercup squash
½ cup finely chopped carrots
½ cup finely chopped cabbage

½ onion, finely chopped
1-inch piece of wakame
small piece of shiitake mushroom
miso (½ teaspoon per person) or
   shoyu (several drops)

Combine ingredients except miso or shoyu with 3 times as much water. Bring to a boil, lower heat, and let simmer about 30 minutes or until done. Toward the end of cooking, season lightly with miso or shoyu and simmer another 3 to 4 minutes.

SHOYU BROTH

2 shiitake mushrooms
3-inch piece of kombu
   sea vegetable
4 cups spring water

2 cakes tofu, cubed
2 to 3 tablespoons shoyu
¼ cup sliced scallions or nori

Soak shiitake 10 to 20 minutes. Place kombu and shiitake in water (including soaking water) and boil for 3 to 4 minutes. Remove kombu and shiitake and save for another recipe. Add tofu and boil until it comes to the surface. Do not boil tofu too long, or it will become too hard. Tofu in soup is best enjoyed soft. Add shoyu and simmer for 2 to 3 minutes. Garnish with scallions and nori.

VARIATION: This clear broth soup can be made with chopped watercress and other vegetables instead of tofu. The shiitake, too, is optional but very good for cancer patients.

LENTIL SOUP

1 cup lentils   *1 quart spring water*
2 onions, diced   *¼ to ½ teaspoon sea salt*
1 carrot, diced   *1 tablespoon chopped parsley*
1 small burdock root, diced

Wash lentils. Layer vegetables starting with onions, then carrot, burdock, and lentils on top. Add water and pinch of salt. Bring to a boil. Reduce flame to low, cover, and simmer for 45 minutes. Add parsley and remaining salt. Simmer 20 more minutes and serve. Shoyu may be added for flavor.

VARIATION: For those who can use oil, vegetables may first be sautéed and then cooked with lentils as above.

ADUKI BEAN SOUP

1-inch square of dried kombu   *½ cup sliced carrots*
1 cup aduki beans   *¼ to ½ teaspoon sea salt*
1 quart spring water   *shoyu to taste (optional)*
1 medium onion, sliced   *scallions or parsley*

Soak kombu 5 minutes and slice. Wash beans, place in pot, and add water. Bring to a boil. Reduce the flame and simmer for 1¼ hours or until beans are 80 percent done. Remove cooked beans or use other pot. Put onion on the bottom, then carrots, then aduki beans, and kombu on top. Add salt. Cook 20 to 25 minutes more until vegetables are soft. At the very end, add shoyu to taste. Garnish with scallions or parsley and serve.

VARIATION: Instead of carrots and onion, winter squash may be used. This is particularly recommended for kidney, spleen, pancreas, and liver troubles.

CHICKPEA SOUP

3-inch piece of kombu
1 cup chickpeas soaked overnight
4 to 5 cups spring water
1 onion, diced

1 carrot, diced
1 burdock stalk, quartered
¼ to ½ teaspoon sea salt
scallions, parsley, or bread crumbs

Place kombu, chickpeas, and water in pressure cooker and cook for 1 to 1½ hours. Bring pressure down. Place beans in another pot. Add vegetables and salt. Cook for 20 to 25 minutes on medium-low flame. Garnish with scallions, parsley, or bread crumbs.

BARLEY SOUP

½ cup barley
¼ cup lentils
1 celery stalk
3 onions, diced

1 carrot
5 to 6 cups spring water
¼ to ½ teaspoon sea salt

Wash barley and lentils. Layer vegetables in pot starting with celery on bottom, then onions, carrot, lentils, and barley on top. Add water just enough to cover and bring to a boil. Add sea salt just before boiling. Lower flame and simmer until barley becomes soft and milky. Check taste. You may add a drop of shoyu for flavor and garnish with nori or parsley.

Note: Barley broth is very nourishing for cancer patients. The amount of barley may be increased, and other variations of vegetables may be used.

VARIATION: You may cook barley before using it for soup by adding ½ cup barley to 1½ cups water. Cook 20 to 30 minutes and then follow recipe.

BROWN RICE SOUP

3 shiitake mushrooms
3-inch piece kombu
1 quart spring water
2 cups cooked brown rice

¼ cup diced celery
1 to 2 tablespoons shoyu
scallions, sliced

Boil mushrooms and kombu in water for 2 to 3 minutes. Remove and slice into thin strips or pieces. Place them back in the water, add rice, and bring to a boil. Lower flame and cook for 30 to 40 minutes. Add celery and simmer for 5 minutes. Add shoyu to taste and simmer for final 5 minutes, garnish with scallion, and serve.

VARIATION: You may also add miso for a wonderful warming soup.

CORN SOUP

4 ears fresh corn
1 celery stalk, diced
2 onions, diced
5 to 6 cups spring water or
    kombu stock

¼ teaspoon sea salt
shoyu to taste
chopped parsley, watercress, or
    scallions and nori

Strip kernels from corn with a knife. Place celery, onions, and corn in pot. Add water and pinch of salt. Bring to a boil, lower flame, cover, and simmer until celery and corn are soft. Add rest of salt and shoyu to taste if desired. Serve with chopped parsley, watercress, or scallions and nori.

KOMBU SEA VEGETABLE STOCK

Wipe kombu with a dried brush quickly to remove dust. Minerals are lost by wiping, so if not dusty, place immediately in pot containing cold spring water. Boil 3 to 5 minutes. Remove kombu and use in other dishes or dry out and use as a condiment or side dish. Use stock for miso, grain, bean, or vegetable soups.

SHIITAKE MUSHROOM STOCK

Soak 5 to 6 shiitakes in water for 30 minutes. Add shiitakes and their soaking water to 1 to 2 quarts spring water and bring to a boil. Boil 5 to 10 minutes. Remove shiitakes and save for soup (in which case be sure to remove stems) or use in another recipe. Kombu may also be combined with shiitakes to make a stock.

FRESH VEGETABLE STOCK

Save vegetable roots, stems, tops, and leaves for a nutritious soup stock. Boil in 1 to 2 quarts spring water for 5 to 10 minutes. Remove vegetable pieces and discard.

VEGETABLES

Vegetables may be prepared in a variety of other styles, including baking, broiling, and tempuraing (deep-frying). However, these are not generally recommended for cancer patients.

NISHIME DISH (WATERLESS COOKING)

Use a heavy pot with a heavy lid or cookware specifically designed for waterless cooking. Soak a 3-inch piece of kombu until soft and cut into 1-inch-square pieces. Place in pot and cover with water (about 1 to 2 inches). Add sliced vegetables. For nishime preparations, vegetables are cut in a large size and are usually a combination of two or three, such as carrot, burdock, and kombu or burdock, lotus root, and kombu. Onions, hard winter squash, or cabbage may also be used. Layer the vegetables in the pot after cutting, on top of the kombu, or place in sections around the pot. Sprinkle on a few pinches of sea salt or shoyu. Cover and set flame on high until a lot of steam is generated. Lower flame and cook gently for 15 to 20 minutes. If the water should evaporate too quickly, add more water to the bottom of the pot. When each vegetable has become soft and edible, add a few drops of shoyu and gently shake the pot (rather than stirring). Remove cover, turn off flame, and let the vegetables sit about 2 minutes. You may serve the vegetable juice, which is delicious, along with the dish.

Nishime combination suggestions:
1. Carrot, burdock, and kombu
2. Burdock, lotus root, and kombu
3. Daikon, lotus root, and kombu
4. Carrot, parsnip, and kombu
5. Turnip, shiitake mushroom, and kombu
6. Squash, onion, and kombu

BOILED VEGETABLES

Place about ½ to 1 inch of cold spring water in pot; add a pinch of sea salt. Bring to a boil and add vegetables, which should be tender but crisp.

Note: In order to keep a green color, cook watercress, parsley, scallions, and other green leafy vegetables on a high flame for only 1 to 2 minutes. In order to preserve the taste, it is also better not to add salt after boiling. Shoyu may be added at the end of cooking for flavor.

VARIATION: For an especially sweet taste, place a 3-inch piece of kombu on bottom of pot when cooking round vegetables such as carrots or daikon. Vegetables may be seasoned with shoyu or miso instead of salt. Tasty combinations of boiled vegetables include broccoli and cauliflower; cabbage, corn, and tofu; and carrots, onions, and green peas.

ADUKI, KOMBU, AND SQUASH

1 cup aduki beans   *spring water*
two 3-inch strips of kombu   *sea salt*
1 hard winter squash

Wash and soak aduki beans with kombu. Remove from water after soaking. Chop kombu into 1-inch-square pieces and place at bottom of pot. Add chopped hard winter squash such as acorn, butternut, or hokaido. Add adukis on top of squash. Cover with water and cook over low flame until beans and squash are soft. Sprinkle lightly with sea salt. Cover and cook for 10 to 15 minutes. Turn off flame and let sit for several minutes before serving.

Note: This dish is helpful in regulating blood sugar levels, especially in those who are hypoglycemic or diabetic or have pancreatic or liver disorders. It is naturally sweet and delicious and will reduce the craving for sweets. May be prepared 1 to 2 times per week.

VARIATION: You may cook aduki beans 50 to 70 percent, place them on top of squash, and proceed as above.

DRIED DAIKON WITH KOMBU AND SHOYU

two 6-inch strips of kombu   *shoyu to taste*
½ cup dried daikon (long white radish)

Soak kombu, slice lengthwise into ¼-inch strips, and place in bottom of heavy pot with a heavy lid. Soak daikon until soft. If it is very dark in color, wash first. Place daikon on top of kombu in pot. Add enough kombu and daikon soaking water (and spring water if needed) to just cover top of daikon. Cover pot, bring to boil, lower flame, add shoyu, and simmer 30 to 40 minutes, until kombu is tender. Cook away excess liquid.

Note: This dish helps dissolve fat deposits throughout the body.

VARIATION: Fresh daikon has more power than dried. Slice fresh daikon and cook as above until very tender. If daikon is unavailable, red radish may be used, although the effect is not so strong.

DAIKON AND DAIKON LEAVES

Finely chop 1 daikon radish and the daikon leaves. Place in pot with a small amount of spring water. Cover and cook with high steam about 10 minutes. Toward the end of cooking, add a small pinch of sea salt or few drops of shoyu and simmer for 2 to 4 minutes.

Note: You may lightly cook the root part first and the leafy part later on.

VARIATION: Carrots and carrot tops, turnips and turnip greens, or dandelion roots and dandelion leaves may be cooked in the same way.

STEAMED VEGETABLES

Place ½ inch of spring water in pot. Insert a vegetable steamer inside pot or a wooden Japanese steamer on top of pot. Place sliced vegetables in steamer and sprinkle with a pinch of sea salt. Cover and bring water to a boil. Steam until tender but slightly crisp. Greens will take only 1 to 2 minutes, other vegetables 5 to 7 minutes depending on type, size, and thickness.

Note: Lightly steamed greens can be eaten every day. These include leafy tops of turnip, daikon, and carrot; watercress; kale; mustard greens; Chinese cabbage; and parsley.

VARIATION: If you don't have a steamer, place ½ inch of water in bottom of pot. Add vegetables and a pinch of sea salt. Bring to a boil, lower flame to medium, and steam until tender. Save vegetable water for soup stock or sauces.

STEAMED GREENS DISH

Wash and slice any of the following vegetables: turnip greens, daikon greens, carrot tops, kale, mustard greens, watercress, collard greens, Chinese cabbage, bok choy. Place the vegetables in a small amount of water, about ½ inch, or in a stainless steel steamer over 1 inch of boiling water. Cover and steam for 2 to 3 minutes, depending on the texture of the vegetables. At the end of cooking, lightly sprinkle shoyu over the vegetables. Transfer quickly to a serving dish. When served, the greens should still be fresh and bright.

SAUTÉED VEGETABLES

There are two basic ways to sauté: with oil and with water. In the first, cut the vegetables into small pieces. Lightly brush skillet with dark or light sesame oil. Heat oil, but before it begins to smoke, add vegetables and a pinch of sea salt to bring out their natural sweetness. Turn over or move vegetables occasionally with chopsticks or wooden spoon to ensure even cooking. However, do not stir. Sauté for 5 minutes on medium flame, followed by 10 minutes on low flame. Gently mix from time to time to avoid burning. Season to taste with sea salt or shoyu and cook 2 to 3 minutes longer. You may also quick sauté vegetables cut into matchsticks for 3 to 5 minutes.

The second method combines water and oil. Vegetables may be prepared either in small pieces or in large, thick pieces. Sauté as above in lightly oiled skillet about 5 minutes. Then add enough cold water to cover vegetables halfway or to cover surface of skillet. Add a pinch of sea salt, cover, and cook until almost tender. When 80 percent done, season with sea salt or shoyu and cook 3 to 4 minutes more. Remove cover and simmer until water evaporates.

Note: Sautéing with oil is not recommended for many cancer patients or others who need to avoid or reduce oil. However, for those in good health, sautéed vegetables may be prepared daily. For those who cannot use oil, use 1 to 2 tablespoons water instead. Leftover bean juice—the delicious liquid remaining after cooking beans—may also be used from time to time.

VARIATION: Delicious combinations include burdock and carrots; onion and carrots; cabbage, onion, and carrots; parsnips and onions; mushrooms and celery; broccoli and cauliflower; Chinese cabbage, mushrooms and tofu; and kale and seitan. Soft vegetables take only 1 to 2 minutes to sauté, while cooking time for root vegetables is longer. Other unrefined vegetable oils may be used in this way; especially sesame and corn oil and occasionally olive oil.

KINPIRA

Lightly brush sesame oil in a skillet and heat up. Place equal amounts of burdock and carrots (cut into matchsticks or shaved) into a skillet and add a pinch of sea salt. Sauté for 2 to 3 minutes. Add spring water to lightly cover bottom of skillet. Cover and cook until vegetables are 80 percent done, about 30 minutes or more. Add several drops of shoyu, cover, and cook for several minutes, until remaining water has cooked down. At the end of cooking, add a few drops of ginger juice (squeezed from grated ginger).

Note: Onions, turnips, or lotus root can be substituted or used together with carrots and burdock.

DRIED TOFU, TOFU, OR TEMPEH WITH VEGETABLES (Stew)

Soak a 4-inch piece of kombu in 3 cups water. Bring to a boil and cook for 3 to 5 minutes. Add one of the following to the boiling water: soaked and sliced dried tofu *or* tempeh cubes along with sliced daikon, burdock, carrots, or lotus root. Cook about 15 minutes. Add a pinch of sea salt or a dash of shoyu. Add a combination (2 or 3) of the following vegetables: onions, cabbage, Chinese cabbage, squash, Brussels sprouts, scallions. Cook for 3 to 5 minutes. If you use fresh tofu, add it with the lighter green vegetables toward the end of cooking. Finely chop 2 or 3 scallions, cook for 1 minute, and serve.

Note: All vegetables should be boiled and cooked until soft, but the leafy greens should still be fresh. A small amount of ginger may be added at the very end of cooking. A mild seasoning of miso may be added at the end of cooking instead of shoyu.

VARIATION: Cooked seitan may be used instead of tofu or tempeh. If so, you may not need to add any additional salt or shoyu because seitan is usually salty.

BOILED SALAD

spring water　　　　　　　　*1/2 cup thinly sliced carrots*
sea salt　　　　　　　　　　*1/2 cup sliced celery*
1 cup sliced Chinese cabbage　*1 bunch watercress*
1/2 cup sliced onion

When making a boiled salad, boil each vegetable separately, but they may be boiled in the same water. Cook the mildest-tasting vegetables first so that each will retain its distinctive flavor. Place 1 inch of water and a pinch of sea salt in pot and bring to a boil. Drop Chinese cabbage slices into water and boil 1 to 2 minutes. All vegetables should be slightly crisp but not raw. To remove vegetables from water, pour into a strainer that has been placed inside a bowl so as to retain the cooking water. Put the cooking water back into pot, reboil, and then boil the sliced onion. Drain as above, retaining water and returning to boil. Next boil sliced carrots followed by sliced celery. Finally, add water-cress to boiling water for just a few seconds. In order for vegetables to keep their bright color, each vegetable should be allowed to cool off. Sometimes you can run under cold water while in the strainer, but it is not ideal. Mix vegetables together after boiling. A dressing of 1 umeboshi plum or 1 teaspoon umeboshi paste may be added to ½ cup water (vegetable stock from boiling may be used) and pureed in a bowl or suribachi for seasoning.

Note: This refreshing way to prepare vegetables instead of raw salad is especially recommended for cancer patients who cannot have uncooked foods. This method removes the raw taste and preserves the crispy freshness.

PRESSED SALAD

Wash and slice desired vegetables into very thin pieces, such as ½ cabbage (may be shredded), 1 cucumber, 1 stalk celery, 2 red radishes, 1 onion. Place in a pickle press or large bowl, sprinkle with ½ teaspoon sea salt, and mix. Apply pressure to the press. If you use a bowl in place of a press, put a small plate on top of the vegetables and place a stone or weight on top. Leave for at least 30 to 45 minutes or up to 3 to 4 days. The longer you press the vegetables, the more they will resemble light pickles.

Note: This method is used to remove excess liquid from raw vegetables. For cancer patients a boiled salad is preferable.

VARIATION: A press is not necessary when using soft vegetables. Just mix with salt and serve after 30 minutes.

FRESH SALAD

A variety of fresh uncooked vegetables may be used in this preparation. In addition to lettuce, these include cabbage, grated carrots, radishes, cucumbers, celery, and watercress.

VARIATION: Rice, bulgur, couscous, or other grain placed on a bed of lettuce with some of these vegetables makes a tasty meal in the spring or summer.

SALAD DRESSING SUGGESTIONS

Use homemade rather than store-bought dressings, which are usually high in oil, as well as herbs and spices.

1. One umeboshi plum or 1 teaspoon umeboshi paste may be added to ½ cup spring water and pureed in a suribachi.
2. Dilute a few teaspoons of miso in warm water and heat for several minutes. Add a few drops of rice vinegar.
3. Use condiments such as gomashio or shiso leaf powder.
4. Sprinkle on a few drops of umeboshi vinegar.
5. Add a few drops of shoyu and lemon juice.

PRESSED SALT PICKLES

2 large daikon and their leaves   *¼ to ½ cup sea salt*

Wash daikon and their leaves 2 to 3 times with cold water, making sure all dirt is removed, especially from the leaves. Set aside and let dry about 24 hours. Slice the daikon into small rounds. Sprinkle sea salt on the bottom of a heavy ceramic or wooden crock or keg. Layer some of the daikon leaves, followed by a layer of daikon rounds. Sprinkle with sea salt again. Repeat until the daikon is used up or the crock is filled. Place a lid or plate that will fit inside the crock on top of the daikon, daikon leaves, and salt. Place a heavy rock or brick on top of the lid or plate. Cover with a thin layer of cheesecloth to keep out dust. Water will soon begin to be squeezed out and rise to the surface of the plate. When this happens, replace the heavy weight with a lighter one. Store in a cool, dark place for 1 to 2 weeks or longer. If water is not entirely squeezed out, add more salt. Make sure water is always covered, or contents will spoil. When ready, remove a portion, wash under cold water, slice, and serve.

Note: Pickles are a naturally fermented food and aid in digestion. A small amount may be eaten daily. However, commercial pickles such as dill pickles that have been made with vinegar and spices should be strictly avoided.

VARIATION: Pickles may also be made in this manner from Chinese cabbage, carrots, cauliflower, and other vegetables.

SHOYU PICKLES

Mix equal parts spring water and shoyu in a bowl or glass jar. Slice vegetables such as turnips or rutabaga and place in this liquid. Soak for 4 hours or up to 2 weeks, depending on the strength desired.

RICE BRAN PICKLES (NUKA)

Long Time (ready in 3 to 5 months)   *Short Time (ready in 1 to 2 weeks)*
10 to 12 cups nuka (rice bran) or   *10 to 12 cups nuka*
  wheat bran   *⅛ to ¼ cup sea salt*
1½ to 2 cups sea salt   *3 to 5 cups spring water*
3 to 5 cups spring water

Roast nuka or wheat bran in a dry skillet until it gives off a nutty aroma. Allow to cool. Combine roasted nuka or wheat bran with salt and mix well. Place a layer of bran mixture on the bottom of a wooden keg or ceramic crock. A single vegetable such as daikon, turnips, rutabaga, onion, or Chinese cabbage may be used. Slice vegetables into 2- to 3-inch pieces and layer on top of the nuka. If more than one type of vegetable is used, layer one on top of the other. Sprinkle a layer of nuka on top of the vegetables. Repeat this layering until the nuka mixture is used up or the crock is filled. Always make sure that the nuka mixture is the top layer. Place a wooden disk or plate that fits inside the crock on top of the vegetables and nuka. Place a heavy weight, such as a rock or brick, on top of the plate. Soon water will begin to be squeezed out and rise to the surface of the plate. When this happens, replace heavy weight with a lighter one. Cover with a thin layer of cheesecloth and store in a cool room. To serve, remove pickled vegetables as needed and rinse under cold water to remove excess bran and salt. The same nuka paste may be used; just keep adding vegetables and a little more bran and salt.

BEANS AND BEAN PRODUCTS

ADUKI BEANS

1 cup aduki beans   *¼ teaspoon sea salt per cup of beans*
2 ½ cups spring water per cup of beans

Wash beans and place in pressure cooker. Add water, cover, and bring to pressure. Reduce flame to medium-low and cook for 45 minutes. Remove pressure cooker from burner and rinse with cold water to bring pressure down quickly. Open, add salt, and cook uncovered until liquid evaporates.

Note: Most other types of beans can be pressure-cooked in this way. Chickpeas and yellow soybeans should first be soaked. Black soybeans should not be pressure-cooked because they clog up the gauge. Lentils cook quickly and need only be boiled.

VARIATION: Beans may also be boiled by putting them in a pot, adding 3½ to 4 cups water per cup of beans, and cooking about 1 hour and 45 minutes. When 80 percent cooked, add salt and cook another 15 to 20 minutes, until liquid is evaporated. To reduce cooking time, add flavor, and make beans more digestible, lay a 3-inch piece of kombu under beans at the beginning. A small amount of vegetables may also be cooked along with beans, such as chopped squash, onions, or carrots.

LENTILS

2 cups brown lentils   ¼ teaspoon sea salt
2 ½ cups spring water

Wash lentils and place in pot. Add water, cover, and bring to a boil. Reduce flame to medium-low. After 30 minutes, add salt and cook another 15 to 20 minutes. Remove cover and allow liquid to cook off.

VARIATION: Chopped onions and celery go well with lentils and may be cooked together. Red lentils make a nice variation occasionally. They cook up more quickly than green or brown lentils and are softer.

CHICKPEAS

1 cup chickpeas   ½ teaspoon sea salt
3 cups spring water

Wash chickpeas and soak overnight. Place in soaking water in pressure cooker. Add more water if necessary. Bring to pressure, reduce flame to medium-low, and cook 1 to 1½ hours. Remove from burner and allow pressure to come down. Take off lid, add salt, and return to burner. Cook uncovered for another 45 to 60 minutes.

VARIATION: Diced onion and carrots may be added to beans during last hour of cooking.

COLORFUL SOYBEAN CASSEROLE

2 cups yellow soybeans	1 burdock, sliced
two 3-inch pieces kombu	1 stalk of celery, sliced
1 shiitake mushroom	1 dried daikon, shredded
5 large pieces dried lotus root	soaking water
6 dried tofu	1½ tablespoons shoyu
1 carrot, sliced	1 teaspoon kuzu

Soak soybeans overnight in 2½ cups cold water per cup of soybeans. The next day, place beans and soaking water in a pressure cooker and bring to pressure. Soak kombu, mushroom, lotus root, and dried tofu for 10 minutes. After beans have cooked 70 to 80 percent (approximately 15 minutes), reduce pressure, open, and layer kombu, mushroom, lotus root, and dried tofu on top. Bring back to pressure and cook 10 minutes more. Reduce pressure, open, skim off hulls from beans, remove vegetables, and put on separate plates. Meanwhile, cut up carrot, burdock, celery, and dried daikon. Slice cooked kombu and put in bottom of a large saucepan in a little water. On top of kombu add soft vegetables: celery, mushroom, daikon, and tofu; then root vegetables: carrots, burdock, and lotus root. Finally, add soybeans and water remaining in pressure cooker. Add 1½ tablespoons shoyu, cover, and cook 30 minutes. Add 1 teaspoon kuzu to make creamy and a little grated ginger for flavoring. Soybeans should be very tender and sweet.

Note: This dish is extremely nourishing and highly recommended for cancer patients. However, those with yin cancer should be careful not to use more than one shiitake mushroom. Those with yang cancer or healthy persons may use 5 to 6 shiitakes.

VARIATION: Depending on availability, some vegetables may be omitted or added. Also, seitan makes this dish especially delicious.

BLACK SOYBEANS

2 cups black soybeans	spring water
1 teaspoon sea salt	shoyu

Wash beans quickly and soak overnight in cold water, adding ¼ to ½ teaspoon sea salt per cup of beans. The salt will prevent the skins from peeling. In the morning, place beans and soaking water in pot. If necessary, add additional water to cover beans. Bring to a boil, reduce heat, and simmer uncovered. When a dark foam rises to the surface, skim and discard. Continue in this way until no more foam rises. Cover beans and cook for 2½ to 3 hours. Add water to cover surface of beans if necessary. Toward end of cooking, uncover and add a little shoyu to give the skins a shiny black color. Cook away excess liquid. Shake pot up and down to coat beans with remaining juice, then serve.

Note: This dish is particularly beneficial for the sexual organs and to relieve an overly yang condition caused by excess meat or fish. Avoid pressure-cooking black beans since they may clog the valve.

MISO

Miso (fermented soybean paste) is highly recommended for daily use. There are now many types of miso available. For daily miso soup, we recommend using traditionally made organic or natural miso that has fermented 2 to 3 years. Barley miso, brown rice miso, or hatcho miso (all soybean) may be used. Short-time misos, including red miso and white and yellow misos, may be used occasionally for sauces, dressings, and special dishes. Instant miso is suitable for traveling but not for daily home use. As a rule of thumb, about ½ to 1 teaspoon of miso is used per cup of soup. Also, because miso contains beneficial enzymes that can be destroyed by very high heat, it is usually recommended that soup not be boiled, but after adding the miso, let it simmer for 3 to 4 minutes over a low flame.

TOFU

Tofu is soybean curd made from cooked soybeans and nigari (crystallized salt). It is high in protein and is used in soups, vegetable dishes, dressings, and other dishes. It can be made at home (see *Aveline Kushi's Complete Guide to Macrobiotic Cooking* for a recipe) or purchased inexpensively at natural foods stores and most supermarkets. Obtain an organic-quality tofu if available. Firm tofu usually holds up better than silken in most dishes. Avoid the spicy ones.

TEMPEH

Tempeh is a traditional fermented soy food originating in Indonesia. In the last decade it has become increasingly popular in the Far East and the West and is now available in many natural foods stores and supermarkets. Tempeh is crisp, delicious, and nourishing, and may be steamed, boiled, baked, or sautéed. It is enjoyed with a wide variety of grains, vegetables, and noodles, and may be used in soups, salads, or sandwiches. Tempeh should always be cooked before eating. Tempeh may also be made at home. A special culture is available in many natural foods stores or may be obtained through mail order.

CABBAGE-ROLL TEMPEH

2 strips kombu
several outer layers of cabbage

8 ounces tempeh
2 onions

Soak kombu 1 hour or more. Steam cabbage until soft. Cut the tempeh into 2-inch rectangles and steam or boil. Place on cabbage leaves and roll up. Thinly slice soaked kombu and onions. Layer kombu and onions on bottom of pot. Add water and cabbage rolls. Add sea salt to taste if desired. Cook until very soft.

Note: Avoid cooking with salt or shoyu when serving tempeh to children. Tempeh is very energizing, and salt could make them overactive.

NATTO

Natto is a fermented soy product that aids digestion and strengthens the intestines. It looks like baked beans connected by long slippery strands and has a unique odor. Natto is available in macrobiotic specialty stores or can be made at home (see *Aveline Kushi's Complete Guide to Macrobiotic Cooking* for a recipe). Natto is usually eaten with a little shoyu, mixed with rice, or served on top of buckwheat noodles.

SEA VEGETABLES

WAKAME

2 cups soaked wakame
1 medium onion, sliced

soaking water
2 teaspoons shoyu

Rinse wakame quickly under cold water and soak 3 to 5 minutes. Slice into 1-inch pieces. Put onion in pot and wakame on top. Add soaking water to cover vegetables. Bring to a boil, lower the flame, and simmer for 30 minutes or until wakame is soft. Add shoyu to taste and simmer 10 to 15 more minutes.

Note: Wakame is the chief vegetable added to miso soup. It also makes a tasty side dish and can be used as an alternative in most recipes calling for kombu.

KOMBU

one 12-inch strip kombu
1 onion, quartered
1 carrot, cut in triangular pieces

spring water
1 tablespoon shoyu

Soak kombu 3 to 5 minutes, slice in half, and then slice diagonally into 1-inch pieces. Place in pot and add vegetables and enough soaking water to cover vegetables halfway. Add 1 tablespoon shoyu and bring to a boil. Reduce the flame to low and simmer for 30 minutes. Add additional shoyu to taste if desired and cook for 5 to 10 more minutes.

Note: Kombu is delicious as a side dish and can be used as a stock for soups. Adding a 3-inch piece of kombu beneath the beans will speed up cooking, add flavor, and make beans more digestible. When cooking with kombu, oil is usually not used. Kombu may be too strong for those with yang cancers such as those of the prostate and ovary.

HIJIKI AND ARAME

2 cups soaked hijiki or arame
spring water
1 medium onion, sliced

1 carrot, sliced in matchsticks
3 to 4 tablespoons shoyu

Wash hijiki quickly under cold water. Place in a bowl, cover with water, and soak 5–10 minutes. Drain water and save. Slice hijiki in 1- to 2-inch pieces. Place hijiki on top of other vegetables in pot. Add enough soaking water to cover hijiki. Bring to a boil, cover, and reduce flame to low. Add 1 tablespoon shoyu. Cook on low flame for 45 to 60 minutes. Season with additional shoyu to taste and simmer 20 minutes more, until the liquid evaporates. Mix the vegetables only at the end and serve.

Note: Hijiki is thicker and coarser in texture than arame. Arame is milder, softer, has less of a briny taste, takes less time to cook, and is usually the sea vegetable preferred by those new to macrobiotic cooking.

VARIATION: Both hijiki and arame can be cooked with lotus root, daikon, and other vegetables. They can be combined with grains or tofu, added to a salad, or put into a pie crust and baked as a roll. For those who can use oil, a strong, rich dish can be created by adding a little oil at the beginning of cooking.

NORI

Nori comes in thin sheets and can be used for wrapping rice balls (see recipe in grain section). It is also used to make vegetable sushi and serves as an attractive garnish for soups, noodles, and salads. Toast lightly by holding nori, shiny side up, 10 to 12 inches from the flame and rotating 3 to 5 seconds until the nori changes from black to green.

DULSE

Dulse may be eaten dry as a snack or dry-roasted and ground into a powder in a suribachi to make a condiment. Dulse can also be used to season soups at the very end of cooking, salad, and main dishes.

AGAR

This whitish sea vegetable forms into gelatin when cooked and is used to make vegetable aspics and delicious fruit desserts. See recipe for kanten in dessert section.

SAUCES, DRESSINGS, AND SPREADS

KUZU SAUCE

1 tablespoon kuzu   *1½ cups vegetable stock or water*

Dilute kuzu (a white starch) in a small amount of cold water and add to pot containing stock or water. Bring to a boil, lower flame, and simmer 10 to 15 minutes. Stir constantly. Add shoyu to taste. Serve over vegetables, tofu, noodles, grains, or beans.

VARIATION: Arrowroot powder may be used instead of kuzu. Avoid thickeners such as corn starch.

BÉCHAMEL SAUCE

1 medium onion, diced
1 teaspoon sesame oil
½ cup whole wheat pastry flour

3 cups spring water, kombu stock,
or vegetable soup stock
1 tablespoon shoyu

Sauté onion in lightly oiled skillet until transparent. Stir in flour and sauté 2 to 3 minutes, until each piece is coated. Gradually add water or stock and stir continually to prevent lumping. Bring to a boil, lower flame, and simmer 2 to 3 minutes. Add shoyu to taste and cook 10 to 12 minutes more, until thick and brown. Serve over millet, buckwheat, or seitan.

Note: This savory sauce can be mucus-producing and should be used only occasionally by those in good health. Cancer patients should avoid it altogether.

UMEBOSHI DRESSING

2 umeboshi plums
¼ to ½ teaspoon grated onion

½ teaspoon sesame oil
½ cup spring water

Puree umeboshi and onion in a suribachi. Add slightly heated oil and mix. Add water and mix to smooth consistency. Serve on salad.

Note: Cancer patients can make this dressing without oil by adding a little bit more water.

VARIATION: Umeboshi paste may be used instead of plums. Use 1 teaspoon paste per plum. Also, chives and scallions may be substituted for onions and the mixture used as a dip for crackers or chips.

TOFU DRESSING

½ teaspoon pureed umeboshi plum
¼ onion, grated or diced
2 teaspoons spring water

8 ounces tofu
chopped scallions or parsley

Puree umeboshi, onion, and water in a suribachi. Add tofu and puree until creamy. Add water to increase creaminess if desired. Garnish with scallions or parsley. Serve with salad.

TAHINI DRESSING

2 umeboshi plums   *2 tablespoons tahini*
½ small onion, grated or diced   *½ to ¾ cup spring water*

Puree umeboshi, onion, and tahini in a suribachi. Add water and puree until creamy. Serve with salad.

Note: Tahini is high in oil and generally not recommended for cancer patients.

MISO-TAHINI SPREAD

6 tablespoons tahini   *1 tablespoon barley or rice miso*

Dry-roast tahini in a skillet over medium-low flame until golden brown. Stir constantly to prevent burning. In a suribachi, stir tahini with miso. Delicious with bread or crackers.

VARIATION: Add chopped scallions.

Note: This spread is high in oil and should be avoided by most cancer patients.

CONDIMENTS

SHOYU

Shoyu refers to traditional, naturally made soy sauce as distinguished from the commercial, chemically processed soy sauce found in many Oriental restaurants and supermarkets. Natural foods stores now offer a wheat-free soy sauce known as tamari. It is stronger in flavor. Shoyu, however, is recommended for regular use and should be used primarily in cooking and not added to rice or vegetables at the table. Tamari may be used occasionally for special dishes.

GOMASHIO (Sesame Salt)

Dry-roast 1 part sea salt. Wash and dry-roast 16 to 18 parts sesame seeds. Add seeds to sea salt and grind in a suribachi (mortar) until about two-thirds of the seeds are crushed. Used to season grains, noodles, vegetables, salad, or soup at the table. Use about 1 teaspoon per day.

ROASTED SEA VEGETABLE POWDER

Use either wakame, kombu, dulse, or kelp. Roast sea vegetable in oven until nearly charred (10 to 15 minutes at 350°F) and crush in a suribachi (mortar).

Note: For yin cancer, this powder can be used more frequently in larger amounts (up to 1 teaspoon per day). For yang cancer, slightly less is advisable (about ½ teaspoon per day). For cancers caused by a combination of both, a moderate amount is recommended.

UMEBOSHI PLUMS

Umeboshi are special plums (imported from Japan and now also grown in the United States) that have been dried and pickled with sea salt and aged from one to three years. They usually come with shiso (beefsteak) leaves, which contribute to their distinctive red color. Umeboshi plums may be eaten by themselves or used to enhance grains and vegetables. They may also be pureed to make a tart, tangy dressing, sauce, or tea. The umeboshi contains a harmonious balance of more yin factors, such as the natural sourness of the plum, and more yang factors created by the salt, pressure, and aging used in their preparation. Umeboshi plums are excellent for strengthening the intestines and may be used occasionally by persons with all types of cancer. Some natural foods stores also sell umeboshi paste without the pits. The paste is not as strong or balanced, and cancer patients are advised to use the whole plums.

TEKKA (Root Vegetable Condiment)

⅓ cup finely minced burdock	*½ teaspoon grated ginger*
⅓ cup finely minced carrot	*¼ cup sesame oil*
⅓ cup finely minced lotus root	*⅔ cup hatcho miso*

Prepare vegetables, mincing as finely as possible. Heat oil in a skillet and sauté vegetables. Add miso. Reduce flame to low and cook for 3 to 4 hours. Stir frequently until liquid evaporates and a dry black mixture is left.

Note: Tekka is very strengthening for the blood but should be used sparingly because of its strong contractive nature. For many yin cancers it can be used daily (about ½ teaspoon). For many yang cancers or cancer caused by a combination of yin and yang, use a small amount only on occasion.

SHOYU-NORI CONDIMENT

Place dried nori or several sheets of fresh nori in ½ to 1 cup spring water and simmer until most of the water cooks down to a thick paste. Add shoyu several minutes before the end of cooking for a light to moderate taste.

Note: This special condiment helps the body recover its ability to discharge toxins. It may be eaten by persons with all types of cancer. For yang cancer, use a slightly smaller volume (approximately ½ teaspoon per day). For yin cancer, use up to 1 teaspoon daily. Those with cancers caused by a combination of both may eat a moderate amount.

SHIO-KOMBU CONDIMENT

1 cup sliced kombu   *½ cup shoyu*
½ cup spring water

Soak kombu until soft and cut into 1-inch-square pieces. Add to water with shoyu. Bring to a boil and simmer until the liquid evaporates. Let cool and place in a covered jar to keep for several days.

Note: This condiment is very high in minerals and aids in the discharge of toxins. Cancer patients may eat several pieces daily. If it is too salty, reduce the amount of shoyu.

SAUERKRAUT

A small amount of sauerkraut made from organic cabbage and sea salt may be used as a condiment occasionally.

VINEGAR

Brown rice vinegar, sweet brown rice vinegar, and umeboshi vinegar may be used moderately. Avoid red-wine and apple-cider vinegars.

GINGER

Fresh grated gingerroot may be used occasionally in a small amount as a garnish or flavoring in vegetable dishes, soups, pickled vegetables, and especially fish and seafood.

HORSERADISH

Horseradish may be used occasionally by those in good health to aid digestion, especially on fish and seafood.

CARP AND BURDOCK SOUP (Koi Koku)

1 fresh carp	*miso to taste*
burdock in weight at least equal to that of fish	*1 tablespoon grated ginger*
½ to 1 cup used bancha tea leaves and stems	*spring water and bancha (kukicha) tea*
	chopped scallions

Select a live carp and express your gratitude for taking its life. Ask a fishmonger to carefully remove gallbladder and yellow bitter bone (thyroid) and leave the rest of the fish intact. This includes all scales, bones, head, and fins. At home, cut entire fish into 1- to 2-inch slices. Remove eyes if you wish. Also cut burdock (ideally at least equal to weight of fish) into thinly shaved slices or matchsticks. This quantity of burdock may take a while to prepare. When everything is chopped up, place burdock and fish in pressure cooker. Tie old bancha (kukicha) tea leaves and stems from your teapot in cheesecloth. It should be the size of a small ball. Place this ball in pressure cooker on top or nestled inside fish. The tea stems will help soften the bones while cooking. Add enough liquid to cover fish and burdock, approximately ⅓ bancha tea and ⅔ spring water. Pressure-cook for 1 hour. Bring down pressure and take off lid. Add miso to taste (½ to 1 teaspoon per cup of soup) and ginger. Simmer for 5 minutes. Garnish with scallions and serve hot.

Note: This delicious, invigorating soup is excellent for restoring strength and vitality and opening the electromagnetic channel of energy in the body. It may be eaten occasionally by all cancer patients, even those who otherwise shouldn't eat animal products. It is also good for mothers who have just given birth or who are breast-feeding. In cold weather it is particularly warming. Be careful, however, to eat only a small amount (1 cup or less) at a time. Otherwise you will become too yang and be attracted to liquids, fruits, sweets, and other strong yin. Soup will keep for a week in the refrigerator or several months in the freezer where it can be taken out as needed.

VARIATION: For those whose oil isn't restricted, the burdock may be sautéed for a few minutes in sesame oil at the start, prior to cooking with the fish. Soup may also be made by boiling in lidded pot for 4 to 6 hours or until all bones are soft and dissolved. As liquid evaporates, more water or bancha tea should be added. If carp is unavailable, substitute another more yin fish such as perch, red snapper, or trout. If burdock is scarce, use carrots instead, or use half burdock and half carrots.

VEGETARIAN OPTION: For those who are vegetarian or vegan, a strengthening alternative is Kinpira Soup (below).

KINPIRA SOUP

This strengthening soup should be like a hearty stew. It is similar in use and texture to Koi Koku (Carp and Burdock Soup) in the above recipe.

Chop very finely equal amounts of burdock root, carrot, and lotus root. (If using lotus root, either fresh or dried and soaked.) Lightly brush sesame oil in the bottom of pan (or add a small amount of water if not using oil) and heat over a medium high flame. When oil or water is hot, sauté burdock for 2 to 3 minutes, adding a pinch of sea salt if desired.

Layer the lotus root (optional) and carrots on top of the burdock. Cover all vegetables with spring water, bring to a boil, lower the flame, cover, and simmer for 30 to 40 minutes, until all vegetables are very soft. Water may need to be added from time to time.

Add very finely chopped onion and sweet winter squash, and cook until they become very soft. Mix equal amounts of sweet young white miso and dark aged barley miso, and add in some soup broth. Slowly add mixture, for a nice taste, stir gently, and simmer another 5 minutes.

DESSERTS AND SNACKS

COOKED APPLES

Wash apples and peel, unless organically grown, in which case skins may be eaten. Slice and place in pot with a small amount of water (about ¼ to ½ cup) to keep from burning. Add a pinch of sea salt and simmer for 10 minutes, or until soft.

Note: Those with yin cancer should avoid or limit desserts almost completely. Those with yang cancer may have a small amount of cooked fruit on occasion if craved.

VARIATION: Puree in a food mill to make applesauce. Other fruits may be cooked in this way.

ROASTED SEEDS

Dry-roast sesame, sunflower, pumpkin, or squash seeds by placing several cups of seeds in a skillet over medium-low flame. Stir gently with wooden roasting paddle or spoon for 10 to 15 minutes. When done, seeds should be darker in color and crisp, and give off a fragrant aroma.

Note: Cancer patients may occasionally have roasted seeds in a small amount. Those in good health may season the seeds lightly with shoyu while roasting.

KANTEN (Gelatin)

3 apples, sliced   *pinch of sea salt*
2 cups spring water   *agar flakes*
2 cups apple juice

Wash and slice apples and place in pot with water, juice, and salt. Add agar flakes in amount according to package directions (varies from several teaspoons to several tablespoons). Stir well and bring to a boil. Reduce flame to low and simmer 2 to 3 minutes. Place in a shallow dish or mold and put in refrigerator to harden.

Note: This delicious natural gelatin is not recommended for some cancer patients because of the high fruit and fruit juice content. In that case, just plain kanten can be made without the fruit or juice. It is very soothing and good for the intestines.

VARIATION: Kanten may also be made with other temperate-climate fruits, including strawberries, blueberries, peaches, or melon. Nuts and raisins may be added to the fruit. Vegetable aspics may be made in this same way with vegetable soup stock instead of fruit juice and vegetable pieces instead of fruit. Aduki beans and raisins are a delicious combination.

AMASAKE (Sweet Rice Beverage)

4 cups sweet brown rice   *½ cup koji*
8 cups spring water

Wash rice, drain, and then soak in water overnight. Place rice in pressure cooker and bring to pressure. Reduce flame and cook for 45 minutes. Turn off heat and allow to sit in pressure cooker for 45 minutes. When cool enough, mix koji (polished or semi-polished rice inoculated with bacteria) as a starter into rice by hand and allow to ferment 4 to 8 hours. During fermentation, place mixture in a glass bowl, cover with wet cloth or towel, and place near oven, radiator, or other warm place. During the fermentation period, stir the mixture occasionally to melt the koji. After fermenting, place ingredients in pot and bring to a boil. When bubbles appear, turn off flame. Allow to cool. Refrigerate in a glass bowl or jar.

Notes: Amasake may be served hot or cold as a nourishing beverage or used as a natural sweetener for making cookies, pies, puddings, or other desserts. As a beverage, first blend the amasake and place in saucepan with a pinch of sea salt and enough spring water for desired consistency. Bring to a boil and serve hot or allow to cool.

Cancer patients may have amasake occasionally as a beverage, especially to satisfy craving for a sweet taste.

RICE PUDDING

½ cup almonds   *1½ cups apple juice*
3 to 4 tablespoons tahini   *¼ teaspoon sea salt*
¾ cup spring water   *⅓ to ½ cup spring water*
3½ cups cooked brown rice

Boil almonds and tahini in ¾ cup water and puree in a blender. Place mixture and other ingredients in pressure cooker and cook for 45 minutes. After pressure has come down, remove mixture and place in a baking dish or covered casserole. Bake at 350°F for 45 to 60 minutes.

Note: This is a tasty dessert for those in good health but best avoided by cancer patients.

SWEET VEGETABLE JAM

Finely cut an equally large amount of onions, cabbage, carrots, and hard winter squash such as butternut or buttercup. Place the cut vegetables in large pot and add 1½ times water. Bring to a boil, then reduce the flame to low. Cook for 4 to 5 hours, or until the vegetables cook down into a jam. Add a pinch of sea salt and cook another 20 minutes. Remove sweet vegetable jam and put in a jar. This jar may be refrigerated for about a week. Sweet vegetable jam can be used as a spread to satisfy sweet cravings, such as on rice cakes and steamed sourdough bread.

HOMEMADE TAHINI

Roast black sesame seeds in a dry skillet. Grind them in a suribachi with a little salt until about half crushed. Use as a spread on rice cakes and steamed sourdough bread.

WAKAME SNACK

Take a small piece (2 to 3 inches) of wakame and chew it raw. It is a little salty, so don't eat every day. Occasional use is fine or just a few days in a row.

KUZU WITH BARLEY MALT

For a sweet taste, mix 1 teaspoon kuzu in cold water, heat in a pan with 1 cup spring water, and stir until dissolved, about 5 minutes. Add a few drops of barley malt and simmer another minute.

BEVERAGES

BANCHA TWIG TEA (Kukicha)

Bancha twig tea is the usual daily beverage in most macrobiotic households. The organic or natural bancha twig tea in natural foods stores has usually been dry-roasted. To make tea, add 2 tablespoons roasted twigs to 1½ quarts spring water and bring to a boil. Lower flame and simmer for several minutes. Place tea strainer in cup and pour out tea. Twigs in strainer may be returned to teapot and used several times, adding a few fresh twigs each time.

BROWN RICE TEA

Dry-roast uncooked brown rice over medium flame for 10 minutes or until a fragrant aroma develops. Stir and shake pan occasionally to prevent burning. Add 2 to 3 tablespoons roasted rice to 1½ quarts spring water. Bring to a boil, reduce flame, and simmer 10 to 15 minutes.

VARIATION: Teas may be made from other whole grains in this way.

ROASTED BARLEY TEA

Prepare the same way as roasted brown rice tea above. This tea is especially good for melting animal fat from the body. Roasted barley tea also makes a very nice summer drink and may aid in the reduction of fever.

MU TEA

Mu tea is a medicinal tea made with a variety of herbs, including ginseng. Mu #9 is excellent for strengthening the female sex organs and for stomach troubles, and it may also be used therapeutically by men. Mu tea is sold prepackaged in most natural foods stores. Stir package into 1 quart water and simmer for 10 minutes. Except for medicinal purposes, macrobiotic cooking does not recommend ginseng, which is extremely yang, and fragrant and aromatic herbs, which are too yin for ordinary daily consumption.

34

Menus

The following weekly menu is a sample of the kinds of meals that might be prepared by an individual or family in relatively good health. It is set for the end of the summer and early autumn, so seasonal adjustments are recommended for other times of the year.

Breakfast	Lunch	Dinner
	Sunday	
Miso Soup	Udon and Broth	Boiled Brown Rice
Soft Brown Rice	Steamed Brussels	Colorful Soybean
with Kombu and	Sprouts	Casserole
Shiitake	Garden Salad	Steamed Mustard
Mushrooms	Bancha Tea	Greens
Steamed Cabbage		Cooked Peaches
Bancha Tea		Bancha Tea
	Monday	
Miso Soup	Tofu Stew	Pressure-Cooked Brown Rice with Millet

(continued)

Breakfast	Lunch	Dinner

Monday *(continued)*

Breakfast	Lunch	Dinner
Soft Barley with Shiitake Mushrooms Steamed Collards Bancha Tea	Couscous Boiled Peas and Mushrooms Grain Coffee	Aduki Beans with Kombu and Winter Squash Corn Soup Arame with Carrots, Lotus Root, and Onions Bancha Tea

Tuesday

Breakfast	Lunch	Dinner
Miso Soup with Millet Whole Oatmeal Steamed Greens Bancha Tea	Corn on the Cob with Umeboshi Paste Pressed Salad Arame Bancha Tea	Boiled Brown Rice with Barley Lentil Soup Boiled Kale, Broccoli, and Carrots Watermelon Bancha Tea

Wednesday

Breakfast	Lunch	Dinner
Soft Brown Rice with Winter Squash Rice Kayu Bread Steamed Bok Choy Bancha Tea	Fried Rice with Scallions and Chinese Cabbage Navy Beans with Kombu Bancha Tea	Boiled Brown Rice Whole Wheat Lasagna with Tofu Filling Boiled String Beans and Onions Steamed Watercress Bancha Tea

Thursday

Breakfast	Lunch	Dinner
Miso with Daikon and Wakame Soft Millet Steamed Broccoli Bancha Tea	Bulgur Salad with Carrots, Onions, and Celery Steamed Kale Fresh Cantaloupe Grain Coffee	Pressure-Cooked Brown Rice with Aduki Beans Squash Soup Boiled Mustard Greens Cabbage Roll Tempeh Amasake Pudding Bancha Tea

Breakfast	Lunch	Dinner
	Friday	
Barley Miso Soup	Fried Soba	Steamed Scrod with
Steamed Rye Bread	Boiled Celery	Ginger Sauce
Boiled Cauliflower	Natto	Boiled Brown Rice
Bancha Tea	Bancha Tea	Steamed Carrots and
		Onions
		Boiled Kale
		Fresh Salad
		Roasted Barley Tea
	Saturday	
Shoyu Broth	Rice Ball with Nori	Boiled Brown Rice
Whole Oatmeal	Boiled Salad	with Rye
Steamed Kale	Bancha Tea	Millet Soup with
Bancha Tea		Sweet Vegetables
		Kidney Beans with
		Kombu
		Steamed Cabbage
		Blueberry Pie
		Bancha Tea

MENU FOR CANCER PATIENTS

The following is an example of a weekly meal plan for someone with cancer. It does not include pickles, condiments, and special drinks and side dishes, which should also be prepared. It does not include oil, which may be used in some cases or may be used after the first month in others. Also, the use of whole oats, seitan, soba, fruit, and desserts may be limited in some cases. These foods are indicated with an asterisk (*). Please check the dietary recommendations for each illness and make adjustments before implementing this general meal plan.

Breakfast	Lunch	Dinner
	Sunday	
Miso Soup	Udon Noodles	Boiled Brown Rice
Mochi	Millet Soup with	Aduki-Squash-Kombu
	Sweet Vegetables	

(continued)

Breakfast	Lunch	Dinner

Sunday (continued)

Breakfast	Lunch	Dinner
Steamed Kale Bancha Tea	Boiled Salad Brown Rice Tea	Carrots and Carrot Tops Kinpira Bancha Tea

Monday

Breakfast	Lunch	Dinner

Miso Soup
Soft Rice
Dried Daikon
  with Kombu
Bancha Tea
	Corn on the Cob
	*Seitan Stew
	Arame
	Boiled Salad
	Bancha Tea
		Pressure-Cooked
		  Brown Rice with
		  Millet
		Lentil Soup
		Nishime-Style Vegeta-
		  bles with Tempeh
		Steamed Watercress
		*Amasake Pudding
		Bancha Tea

Tuesday

Breakfast	Lunch	Dinner

Miso Soup
Soft Rice with Millet
Steamed Rice
*Kayu Bread
Steamed Cauliflower
Bancha Tea
	Rice Balls with Nori
	Tofu with Water-
	  Sautéed Vegetables
	Daikon and Daikon
	  Tops
	Barley Tea
		Boiled Brown Rice
		  with Barley
		Shoyu Broth
		Aduki-Squash-Kombu
		Steamed Collard
		  Greens
		Boiled Salad
		Bancha Tea

Wednesday

Breakfast	Lunch	Dinner

Miso Soup
Soft Rice with Barley
Dried Daikon with
  Kombu
Boiled Kale
Bancha Tea
	*Soba Noodles
	Millet Soup with
	  Sweet Vegetables
	Kinpira
	Bancha Tea
		Boiled Brown Rice
		  with Chickpeas
		Nishime-Style
		  Vegetables
		Steamed Bok Choy
		               Pressed Salad
		*Apple Kanten
		Bancha Tea

Breakfast	Lunch	Dinner

Thursday

Breakfast	Lunch	Dinner
Miso Soup	Corn on the Cob	Pressure-Cooked
Soft Rice with	Leftover Rice	Brown Rice
Chickpeas	Hijiki	Shoyu Broth
Steamed Cabbage	Steamed Broccoli	Aduki-Squash-Kombu
Bancha Tea	and Cauliflower	Boiled Salad
	Bancha Tea	Bancha Tea

Friday

Breakfast	Lunch	Dinner
Miso Soup	Rice Ball with Nori	Boiled Brown Rice
Soft Rice	Corn Chowder	with Millet
Steamed Chinese	Nishime-Style	Colorful Soybean
Cabbage	Vegetables	Casserole
Hato Mugi (Pearl	Bancha Tea	Carrots and
Barley) Tea		Carrot Tops
		Pressed Salad
		Bancha Tea

Saturday

Breakfast	Lunch	Dinner
Miso Soup	Whole Rye	Boiled Brown Rice
*Whole Oatmeal	Dried Tofu with	with Barley
*Steamed Sourdough	Vegetables	Aduki Bean Soup
Bread	Pressed Salad	Water-Sautéed
Steamed Kale	Bancha Tea	Vegetables
Bancha Tea		Boiled Salad
		Bancha Tea

35

Kitchen Utensils

Pressure Cooker

A pressure cooker is used occasionally for many whole grains and beans. Stainless steel or ceramic is recommended.

Cooking Pots

Stainless steel and cast iron are recommended, although Pyrex, stoneware, or unchipped enamelware may also be used. Avoid aluminum or Teflon-coated pans.

Metal Flame Deflectors

These are especially helpful when cooking rice and other grains because they help distribute heat more evenly and prevent burning. Avoid asbestos pads.

Suribachi (Grinding Bowl)

A suribachi is a ceramic bowl with grooves set into its surface. It is used with a wooden pestle and is needed in preparing condiments, pureed foods, salad dressings, and other items. A 6-inch size is generally fine for regular use.

Flat Grater

A small enamel or steel hand-style grater that will grate finely is recommended.

Pickle Press

Several pickle presses or heavy crocks with a plate and weight should be available for regular use in the preparation of pickles and pressed salads.

Steamer Basket

The small stainless steel steamers are suitable. Bamboo steamers are also fine for regular use.

Wire-Mesh Strainer

A large strainer is useful for washing grains, beans, sea vegetables, and some other vegetables, and for draining noodles. A small, fine-mesh strainer is good for washing smaller items such as millet or sesame seeds.

Vegetable Knife

A sharp, high-quality Asian knife with a wide rectangular blade allows for a more even, attractive, and quick cutting of vegetables. Stainless steel and carbon steel varieties are recommended.

Cutting Board

It is important to cut vegetables on a clean, flat surface. Wooden cutting boards are ideal for this purpose. They should be wiped clean after each use.

A separate board should be used for the preparation of dishes containing animal foods.

Foley Hand Food Mill

This utensil is useful for pureeing, especially when preparing baby foods or dishes requiring a creamy texture.

Glass Jars

Large glass jars are useful for storing grains, seeds, nuts, beans, or dried foods. Wood or ceramic containers, which allow air to circulate, are better but may be difficult to locate.

Shoyu Dispenser

This small glass bottle with a spout is very helpful in controlling the quantity of shoyu used in cooking.

Tea Strainer

Small, inexpensive bamboo strainers are ideal, but small mesh strainers may also be used.

Vegetable Brush

A natural-bristle vegetable brush is recommended for cleaning most vegetables.

Small Utensils

Wooden utensils such as spoons, rice paddles, and cooking chopsticks are recommended since they will not scratch pots and pans or leave a metallic taste in food.

Bamboo Mats

Small bamboo mats or the mats used to roll sushi may be used in covering food. They are designed to allow heat to escape and air to enter so that food does not spoil quickly if unrefrigerated.

Electrical Appliances

Those who are ill should avoid all electrical appliances as much as possible when preparing foods or cooking. Gas gives stronger energy. Instead of toasting bread, steam or bake it. Instead of using an electric blender, use a suribachi to puree sauces and dressings. An automatic blender may be used occasionally, to grind the soybeans for making tofu when cooking for those in good health, or for a party or a large number of people. Use common sense. If you use electric equipment, such as juicers, let the vibration settle for 5 to 10 minutes before eating or drinking.

36

Home Remedies and Care

The following home remedies are based on traditional Oriental medicine, folk medicine, and contemporary macrobiotic practice modified and adjusted for more practical use in modern society. Similar remedies have been used for thousands of years to help alleviate various imbalances caused by a faulty diet or unhealthy lifestyle activities. They should be followed only after acquiring a complete understanding of their uses. If there is any doubt as to whether these remedies should be used, please seek an experienced macrobiotic counselor or medical professional for proper guidance. After a stipulated period of time, these remedies are generally stopped or used only half as often (e.g., every other day instead of daily). After the second round of use, they should be stopped altogether. Many of these are powerful and are not suitable for daily use, so once they have served their purpose, they should be discontinued except for very occasional use as needed for a specific purpose.

For convenience the remedies are divided into Special Drinks and Dishes (taken internally) and Compresses, Plasters, and Other External Applications.

SPECIAL DRINKS AND DISHES

ADUKI BEAN TEA

Place 1 cup aduki beans in a pot with a 2-inch strip of kombu. Soak 4 hours or overnight, then finely chop the kombu. Add 4 cups water and bring to a boil. Lower the flame, cover, and simmer for 20 to 30 minutes. Strain to remove the beans and drink the liquid while hot. You may continue cooking the beans longer with additional water until soft and edible for regular consumption.

BAKED KOMBU-SHIITAKE-SESAME CONDIMENT

Bake kombu in a dry skillet, crush into powder, and set aside. This will constitute 50 percent of the condiment. Bake dried shiitake mushroom, by volume about 25 percent of the total mixture, place on a dry surface, chop, and set aside. Roast black sesame seeds, about 25 percent by volume, and crush in a suribachi. Mix all the ingredients together and crush once more. Take 1 teaspoon every day for 10 days.

BEET JUICE

Extract the juice from red beets and drink it either at room temperature or heated. If in good health, an electric juicer may be used, provided the juice is allowed to sit for 3 minutes after juicing to allow the electric charge to disperse. If not in good health, it is better to finely grate or finely mince the beets, and then mash in a suribachi. The juice is squeezed out using a cheesecloth. Depending on the condition, the juice can be drunk lightly salted or unseasoned.

If there are liver conditions, add a little lemon in case of liver stagnation.

VARIATION: Another drink can be made from grated daikon (1 part), grated beets (2 parts), dried shiitake mushroom (1 part), and 3 times as much water. Bring to a boil and simmer. Add 3–4 drops of lemon juice at the end of cooking.

BROWN RICE AND BARLEY PORRIDGE
WITH GRATED DAIKON

Wash ½ cup brown rice and ½ cup barley. Place in a heavy pot and add 5 cups spring water. Soak 4 hours or overnight for more digestible porridge.

Add a pinch of sea salt, turn the flame to medium-high, and bring to a boil. Lower the flame and cook about 1 hour. Remove 1 cup of the porridge and put it in a small saucepan. Grate 1 tablespoon fresh daikon and add to the saucepan. Bring to a boil and simmer 2 to 3 minutes, until the daikon becomes sweet. Serve in a rice bowl.

This porridge can be pressure-cooked about 50 minutes, using 3 to 4 cups water.

BROWN RICE AND CORN PORRIDGE

Wash ½ cup brown rice. Add ½ cup fresh corn that has been cut off the cob. Place in a heavy pot and add 5 cups spring water. Soak 4 hours or overnight for more digestible porridge. Add a pinch of sea salt, place over an initially low flame, bring to a boil slowly, and then cook about 1 hour. Remove 1 cup porridge, and put in a small saucepan. Grate about 1 tablespoon fresh daikon and add to the saucepan. Bring to a boil, and simmer 2 to 3 minutes, until the daikon becomes sweet. Serve in a rice bowl.

For stronger effects:

- This porridge can be pressure-cooked about 50 minutes, using 3–4 cups of water.
- The corn can be added after the rice has cooked alone.
- Cook 1 cup leftover brown rice with 1½ cups water for 15 minutes, until soft. Add the fresh corn and simmer about 5 minutes, until the corn is soft and sweet.

BROWN RICE CREAM

Follow the recipe for Genuine Brown Rice Cream in the recipe section. You may boil for 2 hours or pressure-cook for 1 hour. Let the rice cool sufficiently to be handled. Place the rice in a cheesecloth or clean unbleached muslin cloth, tie, and squeeze out the creamy liquid.

Sweeten it at the end with a little brown rice syrup, barley malt, amasake, or apple juice.

BROWN RICE LIQUID WITH DAIKON, UMEBOSHI, AND SHISO

Brown rice liquid is the liquid that rises to the surface after cooking soft brown rice. (See Brown Rice in the recipe section.) In Japanese it is known as *omoyu*. Add a little grated daikon, a small piece of an umeboshi plum, and several small shiso leaves. Take 1 to 2 small cups daily for a couple of weeks for male-related cancers, then occasionally for another few weeks, and stop.

BROWN RICE MILK (SWEETENED)

This beverage is made from grains, beans, vegetables, and sea vegetables. In a big pot, mix the following ingredients: brown rice (40 percent); sweet brown rice (10 percent); beans (10 percent) selecting among aduki beans, soybeans, and others; other grains (10 percent), which can include barley, millet, corn, and others; chopped vegetables (15 percent), selecting among winter squash or pumpkin, onion, daikon, carrot, cabbage, daikon leaves or turnip leaves; seaweed (10 percent), selecting among nori, wakame, arame, and others; and apple (5 percent).

Then add 5 to 7 times the total volume of water, bring to a boil, lower the flame, and cook a long time, on a flame deflector, to make a porridge-like cream. Shut off the flame, and allow the mixture to cool to a moderate temperature.

Wrap in gauze or cheesecloth and squeeze out the sticky cream. Add water to the cream and cook it for 2 to 3 minutes. Then sweeten the grain milk with amasake, brown rice syrup, or barley malt to taste, and drink it.

BROWN RICE PORRIDGE WITH GRATED DAIKON

Make Brown Rice Porridge (see recipe section), season lightly with sea salt or miso, and add 20 to 30 percent grated daikon. Simmer about 2 minutes.

BROWN RICE PORRIDGE WITH GRATED DAIKON AND LEMON

Make Brown Rice Porridge (see recipe section) and add 20 to 30 percent grated daikon. Simmer about 2 minutes. Season with a pinch of sea salt or shoyu, squeeze in a few drops of lemon juice, and then mix well.

BROWN RICE PORRIDGE WITH GRATED DAIKON AND UMEBOSHI

Make Brown Rice Porridge (see recipe section) and mix in grated daikon and chopped umeboshi plum (from which the pit has been removed). Simmer for 3 minutes.

BROWN RICE PORRIDGE WITH GRATED LOTUS ROOT

Add 20 to 30 percent grated lotus root to thin brown rice porridge (see recipe section) and stir well. Simmer on a low flame for 2 to 3 minutes.

BROWN RICE WITH MARINATED DRIED DAIKON

Finely chop dried shredded daikon and marinate it for 1 hour in shoyu that has been diluted with 2 times the amount of water. Pressure-cook it together with brown rice, making it softer. The amount of dried daikon should be 5 to 10 percent of the volume of the brown rice.

BROWN RICE WITH WATER-SAUTÉED DAIKON AND DAIKON LEAVES

Finely chop dried shredded daikon and daikon leaves. Sauté with water. Season lightly with shoyu. Mix vegetables into already-cooked brown rice and set aside for 3 to 4 minutes before eating.

BROWN RICE, MILLET, BUCKWHEAT, AND VEGETABLE PORRIDGE

Make Brown Rice Porridge (see recipe section) with the following ingredients: lightly roasted brown rice (3 parts), lightly roasted millet (2 parts), lightly roasted buckwheat groats (1 part), and chopped vegetables (3 parts, combining chopped burdock, carrot, daikon, cabbage, and onion), along with a small piece of kombu and water.

Caution: For cases of yang lymphoma, omit the buckwheat and burdock and substitute barley for the millet.

CABBAGE JUICE

In case of abdominal pain, make raw Cabbage Juice. Very finely chop or grate raw cabbage. Mash it in a suribachi, wrap in cheesecloth, and squeeze out the raw juice. Simmer juice slightly, about 3 minutes.

CABBAGE AND CARROT JUICE

For medicinal purposes it is preferable to juice vegetables by hand rather than by an electric juicer, which destroys much of their vitamin C. Very finely chop or grate the cabbage and carrot. Then squeeze out the juice by wringing out the gratings wrapped in cheesecloth. If the cabbage is still not fine enough, it may have to be mashed in a suribachi.

Combine fresh cabbage juice (2 parts) with fresh carrot juice (1 part), stir gently, and drink.

VARIATION: Add a small amount of water and cook for 2 to 3 minutes before drinking.

CABBAGE TEA

Finely chop cabbage leaves. Place in pot, cover with spring water, bring to a boil, then lower the flame and simmer until the cabbage becomes soft and sweet. Strain off the cooking liquid as Cabbage Tea.

FOR LYMPHOMA (SWEATING): Cool the tea to room temperature before drinking.

CARBONIZED UMEBOSHI AND CARBONIZED UMEBOSHI SEEDS

Place several umeboshi plums in the oven under the broiler until their outer surface turns black. Crush the baked umeboshi meat to a powder. Take this powder with 1 tablespoon hot water or bancha twig tea. For Carbonized Umeboshi Seeds, roast the seeds inside the pit in the oven at a very high temperature. Crush them into a black powder and store in a jar. It is a very yang preparation. Take 1 teaspoon bancha twig tea for stomach or intestinal troubles. It can also be sprinkled on rice or other grains as a condiment.

CARROT-DAIKON DRINK

This drink was first developed for liver troubles, to help discharge eggs, cheese, and beef fat. But it is helpful in dissolving fat deposits anywhere in the body and quickly reducing high cholesterol. It also helps dissolve calcified stones in kidneys and the gallbladder. It is now recommended for many chronic conditions, including many forms of heart disease and tumors.

Daikon is relatively yin and gives a dissolving effect, while the carrot is relatively yang and is added to strengthen and help move energy down in the body. If continuously taken together, however, they tend to weaken. By adding umeboshi and nori, this drink can be taken every day for 10 days or every other day for 3 weeks.

Finely grate ½ cup each of carrots and daikon. Place in a saucepan. Do not let the gratings sit for a long time. Add 2 cups water and bring to a gentle boil. Add ⅓ of a nori sheet and half of an umeboshi plum. Cook together with the grated vegetables. Simmer about 3 minutes and add a few drops of shoyu toward the end. Eat and drink the vegetables and broth.

VARIATIONS:

- Add ⅓ cup grated lotus root, especially for lung or lymphatic conditions.
- A little scallion or ginger may be added to the basic recipe if desired.
- This drink may also be used to eliminate fat and oil that accompanies stagnated conditions.

CARROT JUICE

Carrot juice may be drunk by most people 2 to 3 times a week if desired. Juicing in an electric juicer destroys some vitamins. For those who are healing, juicing by hand is recommended, although organic store-bought juice is fine.

Wash 1 to 3 fresh carrots and finely grate them. Place the gratings in cheesecloth and wring to squeeze out the juice. Collect the liquid; it may be drunk heated, cold, or at room temperature. The gratings can be added to soups, stews, salads, and other dishes.

CORN SOUP WITH LOTUS SEEDS

Combine 50 percent corn, 10 percent onion, 10 percent daikon, 10 percent soaked lotus seeds, 15 percent daikon leaves, and 5 percent shiitake mushroom or nori. Add 3 times the total amount of water, bring to a boil, and simmer until soft. Season with miso, shoyu, or sea salt.

DAIKON AND DAIKON LEAVES

Follow the recipe for Pressed Salad, using finely sliced daikon, daikon leaves, and sea salt. After pressing for half a day or longer, rinse the salad with water to remove the excess salt before serving. Eat a small amount of this preparation with your meals.

DAIKON LEAVES QUICK PICKLES

Eat light Daikon Leaf Pickles. These are pickled briefly in sea salt the same as a Pressed Salad or brine pickles. See the recipe section. If they are salty, rinse off the excess salt before eating.

DRIED DAIKON AND SHIITAKE TEA

Soak and finely chop dried, shredded daikon (3 parts) and dried shiitake mushroom (1 part). Place in a pot and add 3 times the total amount of water. Bring to a boil, lower the flame, and simmer for 20 to 25 minutes. Strain and save the tea in a thermos or a refrigerator.

DRIED DAIKON, DAIKON LEAVES, AND SHIITAKE TEA

After soaking, finely chop and combine dried, shredded daikon (3 parts), daikon leaves (2 parts), and dried shiitake mushroom (1 part). Add 3 times the total amount of water, bring to a boil, and simmer about 25 minutes. Strain and keep this broth in a thermos.

DRIED DAIKON, DAIKON LEAVES, ROASTED BROWN RICE, AND SHIITAKE TEA

Combine dried, shredded daikon (3 parts), daikon leaves (3 parts), lightly roasted brown rice (2 parts), and dried shiitake mushroom (1 part). Add 3 times the total amount of water, bring to a boil, and simmer on a low flame for 20 to 25 minutes. Strain the liquid and save this broth in a thermos.

DRIED DAIKON, DRIED DAIKON LEAVES, AND BURDOCK TEA

Finely chop soaked, dried, shredded daikon (3 parts), soaked, dried daikon leaves (2 parts), and burdock (1 part). Add 3 times the total amount of water, bring to a boil, and simmer for 25 minutes over a low flame. Strain and put this tea in a thermos.

DRIED DAIKON, DRIED DAIKON LEAVES, BURDOCK, SHIITAKE MUSHROOM, AND CABBAGE TEA

Finely chop soaked, dried, shredded daikon (3 parts), burdock (1 part), dried shiitake mushroom (1 part), cabbage (1 part), and soaked, dried daikon leaves (2 parts). Add 3 times the total amount of water, bring to a boil, and simmer about 25 minutes. Put this tea in a thermos.

DRIED DAIKON, DRIED DAIKON LEAVES, SHIITAKE MUSHROOM, DRIED LOTUS ROOT, AND ROASTED BROWN RICE TEA

Soak dried daikon (2 parts), dried daikon leaves (2 parts), dried shiitake mushroom (1 part), and dried lotus root (1 part). Finely chop all ingredients. Mix with 2 parts lightly roasted brown rice. Add 3 times the total amount of water, bring to a boil, and simmer 25 to 30 minutes. Strain and store in a thermos or refrigerator.

DRIED DAIKON, SHIITAKE MUSHROOM, AND CABBAGE TEA

Finely chop soaked, dried, shredded daikon (3 parts), dried shiitake mushroom (1 part), and fresh cabbage (2 parts). Mix in pot and add 3 times the total amount of water. Bring to a boil and simmer on a low flame for 20 to 25 minutes. Strain and save this broth in a thermos.

DRIED DAIKON, SHIITAKE MUSHROOM, AND KOMBU TEA

Soak dried, shredded daikon (3 parts), dried shiitake mushroom (1 part), and kombu (1 part). Finely chop and mix in pot. Add 4 times the total amount of water and simmer on a low flame for 20 to 25 minutes. Strain and drink the liquid.

FOR SKIN CANCER: Add 3 times the total amount of water.

DRIED DAIKON, SHIITAKE MUSHROOM, AND ONION TEA

Finely chop and combine soaked, dried, shredded daikon (3 parts), soaked, dried shiitake mushroom (1 part), and fresh onion (2 parts). Add 3 times the total amount of water, bring to a boil, and simmer for 20 to 25 minutes. Strain and keep this broth in a thermos or refrigerator.

DRIED DAIKON, SHIITAKE MUSHROOM, CABBAGE, BURDOCK, AND ROASTED RICE TEA

Combine soaked, dried, shredded daikon (3 parts), soaked, dried shiitake mushroom (1 part), burdock or carrot (2 parts), and roasted brown rice (2 parts). Add 3 times the total amount of water, bring to a boil, and simmer about 25 minutes. Strain and save this liquid in a thermos or a refrigerator.

DRIED DAIKON, SHIITAKE MUSHROOM, DRIED LOTUS ROOT, AND CARROT LEAF TEA

Finely chop and combine soaked, dried, shredded daikon (3 parts), soaked, dried shiitake mushroom (1 part), soaked, dried lotus root (2 parts), and carrot leaves (2 parts). Add 3 times the total amount of water, bring to a boil, and simmer on a low flame for 20 to 30 minutes. Strain and save the broth in a thermos or refrigerator.

FRESH APPLE JUICE AND SWEET VEGETABLE DRINK

Combine equal amounts of fresh apple juice and sweet vegetable drink. Simmer about 2 minutes.

GRATED CARROT AND DAIKON

Finely grate ½ cup each of daikon and carrot and mix well. Add a few drops of shoyu, mix well again, and then eat. If daikon is too pungent, you may also add a small amount of water and simmer for 2 to 3 minutes, adding shoyu near the end of cooking.

FOR FATIGUE: A teaspoon of squeezed lemon juice may be added.

GRATED DAIKON

Fresh grated daikon is used in small amounts as a garnish for tempura, deep-fried, and other oily foods, for fish and other seafood, mochi, and other rich styles of cooking.

Finely grate a small amount of fresh daikon with a hand grater, using gentle circular motions. Grated daikon is customarily eaten with a few drops of shoyu. It is used in many medicinal preparations, as described below.

GRATED DAIKON AND CARROT
WITH SCALLIONS AND SHOYU

Grate the same amount each of daikon and carrot, and mix well. Add 1 teaspoon finely chopped scallions and then mix well. Simmer quickly with just enough water to cover the ingredients in pan and add a few drops of shoyu.

GRATED DAIKON AND CARROT WITH SHIITAKE TEA

Combine finely grated daikon (3 parts), finely grated carrot (1 part), and soaked and finely chopped dried shiitake mushroom (1 part). Add 2 times the total amount of water and simmer on a low flame about 3 to 4 minutes.

GRATED DAIKON AND CARROT WITH UMEBOSHI,
SHISO, LEMON, AND SHOYU

Combine finely grated daikon (3 parts) and finely grated carrot (1 part) to make 1 small cup of this mixture. Add half of a umeboshi plum and 1 teaspoonful shiso leaves (the red leaves pickled with umeboshi), finely chopped and with the surface salt washed off. Add 1 teaspoon lemon juice and mix well. Add a few drops of shoyu.

GRATED DAIKON AND POTATO JUICE

Prepare grated daikon and squeeze the juice from it. Peel and finely grate a potato and squeeze the juice from it. Mix together equal amounts of the daikon and potato juice. Add a pinch of sea salt for seasoning if desired, but be careful not to use too much because an excess can lead to weakness.

GRATED DAIKON WITH CARROT AND SHOYU

In a saucepan combine finely grated daikon (2 parts) and finely grated carrot (1 part). Add a small amount of water and simmer about 2 minutes. Add a pinch of sea salt or a few drops of shoyu.

GRATED SOUR APPLE

This remedy is recommended to help reduce fever, liver troubles, and swelling of the feet and legs. Peel and grate a sour green apple (Granny Smith). Put in a small saucepan, add a small amount of water, and simmer about 2 minutes.

HIJIKI WITH DRIED DAIKON AND SHIITAKE MUSHROOM

Soak and chop hijiki (4 parts), dried shredded daikon (1 part), and dried shiitake mushroom (1 part). A few drops of sesame oil can be added to fry pan. Layer shiitake on bottom, then daikon, and hijiki on top. Add a small amount of water to just cover the daikon. Bring to a boil, turn the heat to low, and add a small amount of shoyu. Cover and simmer for 40 to 60 minutes, until the bitter taste of the hijiki disappears. Add a little more shoyu to taste. (Be careful not to make it too salty.) Simmer another 5 to 10 minutes on a low flame, stirring well until the liquid evaporates.

HOTO

Hoto is a special noodle stew made with udon or other whole wheat noodles, squash (included when available), and about a half dozen other fall and winter season vegetables. Hoto is traditionally prepared in a ceramic dish, which gives a more peaceful, stable vibration than metal, especially for healing. It is very strong and energizing, especially for those with weak, more yin conditions.

Prepare by making homemade noodles or boiling a quart of water and cooking an 8-ounce package of ready-made udon. Set the noodles aside to be added with the vegetables later. Select among such vegetables as daikon, carrots, onions, and lotus root. Slice equal amounts of 5 or 6 vegetables and layer with the more yang (denser, harder, or firmer) on the bottom (e.g., carrot) in a ceramic pot on the stovetop. Half-cover with water and cook for 20 to 30 minutes, or until done. When the vegetables are almost done, add the noodles and, if desired, small pieces of mochi for further strength. To season, add miso (especially young sweet miso) to taste and several pinches of sea salt to firm up the noodles and make the vegetables sweeter. Watch the water level carefully, especially after adding the noodles, and add more when needed. Serve when done. The dish should have sufficient broth to be enjoyed as a stew or soup.

Note: Dried tofu may be added to this dish, but usually not fresh tofu.

KIDNEY DRINK

Prepare a special drink consisting of soaked aduki beans (1 part), dried, shredded daikon (1 part), dried shiitake mushroom (1 part), and kombu (1 part). Add 5 times as much water, boil, and then simmer about 25 minutes. Drink 1 cup every day for 10 days. Don't eat the kombu.

KINPIRA-STYLE BURDOCK, CARROT, AND KOMBU

This dish may be water-sautéed or oil-sautéed using a few drops of sesame oil. Prepare following the recipe for Kinpira, using burdock (2 parts), carrot (2 parts), and kombu (1 part). The kombu, sliced into matchsticks, may be sautéed in the beginning along with the burdock, and the carrots layered on top. Cook as in the recipe. At the end of cooking, season with a pinch of sea salt or a few drops of shoyu.

KOMBU-LOTUS-SHIITAKE DRINK

Combine chopped kombu (20 percent), lotus root (40 percent), and shiitake (40 percent). Add 4 to 5 times as much water, cook 20 minutes or longer. Add several drops of shoyu at the end of cooking and a pinch of grated ginger, and let simmer several minutes. Take 1 small cup for 3 weeks, then twice a week for 1 month, and then occasionally as needed.

KUMQUAT JAM

Finely slice kumquats. Do not peel them. Remove all seeds and stems. Add a small amount of water and a pinch of sea salt, and then simmer to make a jam.

KUMQUAT TEA

Dissolve Kumquat Jam in bancha twig tea or hot water and drink.

KUZU DRINK WITH GRATED DAIKON

Dissolve 1 teaspoon kuzu powder in 1 cup hot water and cook briefly with 2 teaspoons grated daikon or radish and a little shoyu for taste. Take frequently.

LARGE INTESTINE DRINK

Prepare the following special drink: lotus root (2 parts), daikon root (1 part), daikon greens (1 part), carrot (1 part), carrot tops (1 part), and dried shiitake mushroom (1 part). Add 4 to 5 times as much water, bring to a boil, and then let simmer for 15 to 20 minutes. Drink 1 cup for 3 to 5 days.

LEAFY GREENS JUICE

This special drink was originally devised to treat liver disorders, especially yang conditions resulting from eating eggs. It helps dissolve heavy, stagnated protein, animal fat, and cholesterol deposits. To obtain counterbalancing, light, upward energy from leafy greens, it is easier for many people to take the juice of young barley plants (sold under the name Green Magma in the natural foods store) or another preparation, but this is not as effective. This drink may be taken daily.

Very finely chop 2 or 3 kinds of large leafy green vegetables (kale, collards, dandelion, daikon or turnip leaves, or Chinese cabbage). Add twice the amount of cold water. Bring to a gentle boil and simmer for 3 to 5 minutes. Strain out the solid vegetables. Add a pinch of sea salt or a few drops of shoyu toward the end of simmering and stir. Drink hot or at room temperature.

Note: If you wish, you may reuse the leafy green vegetables.

VARIATION: Heat 1 cup fresh celery or leafy green vegetable juice, add a small pinch of sea salt, and simmer for 3 to 5 minutes. Drink hot, warm, or at room temperature.

LIVER DRINK

Finely chop and mix the following ingredients in the proportions given: unroasted buckwheat groats (2 parts), daikon (1 part), daikon greens, turnip greens, radish greens, or other large greens (2 parts), scallions (1 part), sprouts of any kind, such as alfalfa, mung bean, soy (2 parts), and, shiitake mushroom (1 part). Add 5 times the total amount of water, bring to a boil, lower the flame, and simmer about 30 minutes. Strain out the contents and save the liquid.

LOTUS-DAIKON-CABBAGE JUICE

Mix ½ cup raw juice squeezed from grated lotus root, ¼ cup juice squeezed from grated daikon, and ¼ cup juice squeezed from finely chopped and mashed cabbage leaves. Add a small amount of water and simmer for 2 minutes.

LOTUS ROOT-CARROT-KOMBU-ADUKI CONDIMENT

Chop ½ cup lotus root. Add ⅓ cup kombu, ⅓ cup carrots, and ⅓ cup cooked aduki beans. Combine with 5 times as much water. Cook for 30 minutes and add a little salt at the end.

LOTUS ROOT JUICE TEA

In case of a wet or mucousy cough, grate fresh lotus root. Wrap the grated pulp in cheesecloth and then squeeze out the juice by hand. (The pulp may be saved and added to other dishes such as Brown Rice Porridge, Miso Soup, or croquettes.) Drink ½ to ⅔ small cup of juice.

You may also place the juice in a saucepan with a small amount of water. Add a pinch of sea salt or a few drops of shoyu, bring to a boil, and let simmer gently on a low flame for 2 to 3 minutes. This tea should be thick and creamy, and it should be drunk while hot. If your condition permits, you may also add a few drops of grated ginger juice toward the end.

It is best to drink this preparation from evening time to night when you cough.

LOTUS SEEDS

Lotus seeds are traditionally said to contribute to vitality and longevity. They are the seeds of the lotus plant, and they fall from pods into the bottom of the pond. There they sprout upward shoots that become lotus leaves and sideways shoots that become lotus roots—the long, many-chambered, pale roots of the lotus plant. Lotus seeds are delicious cooked with aduki beans and kombu, brown rice, roasted brown rice, or deep-fried seitan with carrots and scallion roots.

LOTUS SEED, SEAWEED AND ONION TEA

Place soaked lotus seeds in a pot, add 10 percent of the total volume of soaked and chopped wakame or arame and 20 percent of the total amount of finely chopped scallion or onion. Bring to a boil and simmer together in water to make a tea.

LUNG DRINK

This special drink consists of lotus root (2 parts), daikon root (1 part), daikon greens (1 part), carrot (1 part), carrot greens (1 part), and dried shiitake mushroom (1 part). Add 4 to 5 times as much water, boil, and simmer for 15 to 20 minutes. Drink 1 cup for 3 to 5 days.

MARINATED DAIKON AND CARROT

Slice 1 cup daikon and ½ cup carrots into matchsticks and mix them together. Prepare a marinade of either 1 tablespoon brown rice vinegar and a small amount of shoyu or 1 tablespoon umeboshi vinegar and 1 tablespoon spring water. Pour on the liquid and marinate for 30 minutes or longer.

MILLET AND SWEET VEGETABLE PORRIDGE

1 cup millet (regular or sweet millet)
1 to 1½ cups sweet vegetables cut into small chunks: winter squash (the sweetest is
    from a cold region such as Hokkaido pumpkin, kabocha, buttercup, butternut,
    sweet dumpling, delicata, etc.), cabbage, carrot, onion, sweet corn, parsnip, etc.
pinch of sea salt
3 to 4 cups water

Wash millet in cold water. Add chunks of sweet vegetables to the bottom of a large saucepan or pressure cooker. For the sweetest porridge, layer the vegetables with the most yin on the bottom and the most yang on top: (the bottom has onion, sweet corn, cabbage; the middle has squash; the top has carrot or parsnip, etc.). Place the millet on top and gently pour fresh cooking water down the sides so not to disturb the layering. Bring to a boil slowly, scooping off any foam that rises to the top. Lower the flame and add the seasoning. Cover and bring to pressure if using a pressure cooker. Place a flame deflector underneath and let it simmer about 20 to

25 minutes or pressure-cook for 15 to 20 minutes. Remove from the heat and let the pressure reduce naturally if necessary. Place in serving bowls and garnish with chopped scallions, parsley, gomashio, or other condiment. This makes a sweet, delicious morning porridge and is also very strengthening.

VARIATION: Pressure-cooking gives the porridge a creamier texture.

Note: If this is difficult to eat, you may add miso and a little water and make Millet and Sweet Vegetable Soup.

MISO-SCALLION CONDIMENT

The pungent taste of scallions goes very well with miso, creating a warm energy. Use on rice, other grains, noodles, boiled vegetables, or as a spread on bread.

Wash 2 to 3 scallions with scallion roots very well. Soak the roots in cold water, if necessary, to loosen any soil. Finely slice the scallions and roots and measure the amount. Pour an equal amount of sesame oil into a frying pan. Layer the roots and then the scallions in the pan. Form a little hollow in the center of the scallions. Measure out 3 times the amount of miso as scallions or oil and puree it in a very small amount of spring water. Pour this mixture into the hollow. Cover and simmer about 3 minutes. Mix very well when done and serve.

MISO SOUP WITH OKARA AND VEGETABLES

Okara is the coarse soybean pulp left over when tofu is made fresh at home. It is delicious in soups but should not be cooked too long in order to preserve its taste.

Make mild miso soup with 1 part each of chopped onion, winter squash or pumpkin, cabbage, carrot, daikon, and daikon leaves, as well as a small amount of washed, soaked, and chopped wakame seaweed. Cook until all the vegetables are soft. Reduce the heat to very low and add the okara and pureed miso to the soup stock. Simmer 2 to 3 minutes more and serve hot.

MISO-ZOSUI (OJIYA)

Also called Brown Rice Zosui (Ojiya), this porridge consists of soft-cooked brown rice with seaweed, root vegetables, leafy greens, round sweet vegetables, and miso.

Cook brown rice in 3 times the amount of water until it becomes soft-ened and has an almost kayu-like cream texture. Add some chopped veg-etables, such as winter squash, pumpkin, onion, daikon, carrot, and cabbage. Simmer until every ingredient becomes soft, and it is smooth and creamy. Add a moderate amount of miso, which has been fermented for a long time, and gently stir. Simmer another 2 to 3 minutes on a low flame and then remove pot from flame. Set aside for 5 minutes or more before eating.

VARIATION: If you use rice that has already been cooked, simmer the cooked rice in pot with 2 times the amount of water and follow the above directions.

MISO-ZOSUI BROWN RICE AND MILLET

Wash and finely chop cabbage (1 part), soaked dried shiitake mushroom (1 part), daikon (1 part), daikon leaves (1 part), and onion (1 part). Wash and drain 3 parts brown rice and 1 part millet. Layer onion, shiitake, daikon leaves, daikon, and cabbage in pot and then place millet and brown rice on top. Gently pour in 2½ to 3 times the total amount of water. Bring to a boil, lower the flame, and simmer for 1 hour or more with a heavy lid covering pot. Season lightly with pureed miso.

NABE-STYLE VEGETABLES WITH DIPPING SAUCE

Nabe (pronounced "na-bay") style is a quick, light, summer style of boil-ing that is done on a portable burner at the table, usually in a large open ce-ramic or metal nabe pot. If a special earthenware nabe pot and portable burner are not available, this dish may be prepared quickly on the stovetop in a large stainless steel skillet. It differs from nishime style since it uses more leafy greens than root vegetables, more water, no lid, no seasoning, a higher flame, and much less cooking time.

Select among green upward-growing vegetables and slice several of the following: kale, collard greens, cabbage, Chinese cabbage, red cabbage, leeks, mustard greens, carrot tops, daikon tops, radish tops, turnip tops, scallions, dandelion greens, broccoli, broc-coli rabe, fresh or dried shiitake and other mushrooms, string beans, celery, chives, snap peas, snowpeas, sprouts, brussels sprouts, bamboo shoots, fresh green shiso leaves, onion, etc.

Select among daikon, carrot, lotus root, and other root vegetables, in smaller amounts (optional).

Select among fresh or dried tofu, precooked udon noodles, fu, mochi, and white meat fish (optional).
Strip of kombu (about 2 inches by 3 inches for 4 cups vegetables)
Spring or well water.

Slice as many types of vegetables as desired and place in sections on a large platter. Pour 1 to 2 inches of water into the nabe pot with a strip of kombu (may be omitted if necessary) and with soaked and chopped dried shiitake mushrooms if desired. Bring to a rapid boil on a high flame and cook until the kombu and/or mushrooms soften. You need not add any other seasonings to this dish. Begin to add the sliced vegetables in separate sections to the rapidly boiling broth, starting with the harder vegetables that require the longest cooking time. Slowly add all the vegetables. Most should require only 1 to 2 minutes of boiling. End with those that require only several seconds of cooking, such as sprouts, scallions, and fresh green shiso leaves. Occasionally, for variety, fresh or dried tofu, precooked udon noodles, soaked fu, mochi, or white-meat fish may be added. It may be necessary to add more water during cooking as the bubbling broth evaporates.

When finished, this dish should yield a large sectioned pot of fresh, light, bright green vegetables. It should be served immediately. If cooked on the table, vegetables may be eaten continuously and new ones added to the pot. Cook a sufficient quantity to be eaten by a family at one meal to get the maximum freshness and lightness. It should be the main dish at this particular meal, two-thirds or more of the total meal and with grains one-third or less of the total meal.

Dipping broth:

Nabe cooking broth
Grated ginger (optional)
Toasted nori (optional)

Miso, shoyu, or umeboshi paste
Chopped scallions

The cooking broth is delicious and refreshing to drink, and it may be used to make a dipping sauce as follows: Heat a small amount of the broth and add miso, shoyu, or umeboshi paste to taste. Simmer about 3 minutes. Grate a small amount of ginger and squeeze in a few drops of juice if desired. Add freshly chopped scallions and small pieces of toasted nori. Pour into a small dipping cup and dip in vegetables while eating at the table.

For cervical cancer: Nabe-style vegetables are also nice to eat often, but do not use udon noodles. Cook shiso leaves, Chinese cabbage, cabbage, and other leafy greens together. It is all right to add tofu or yuba.

Rather than ginger, use nori and chopped scallions for the dipping sauce. It is all right to add a squeeze of yuzu (a kind of lemon) or lemon juice to the dipping sauce.

NISHIME-STYLE ROOT VEGETABLES

Nishime-style is a method of cooking root vegetables that have been cut in large chunks. They are cooked a long time in their own juices, and only a small amount of water is added. Seasoning may be at the beginning or at the end. The cooked vegetables are very juicy and are served along with the cooking liquid. See Nishime-Style Vegetables in the recipe section.

Suggested combinations of vegetables include the following (all cooked with kombu): carrot, burdock, onions; carrot, parsnip, cabbage; turnip, shiitake mushroom, cabbage; burdock, leeks, lotus root; daikon or lotus root, carrot, corn; carrot, onion, cabbage; squash, onion, daikon; daikon, squash, cabbage; cabbage, onion. Carrot and daikon or carrot and turnip do not go together very well. Do not use oil or sweeteners in this recipe.

For leukemia: Nishime-style burdock, carrot, daikon, lotus, jinenjo (mountain potato), and kombu, cooked over a low flame, is particularly good.

OHAGI

Ohagis are soft, dumpling-size balls of brown rice and sweet brown rice filled with or coated with other ingredients. They are a traditional festive dish in the Far East and may be used medicinally as well as for special occasions. Popular types include ohagis with aduki beans cooked with barley malt or brown rice syrup, ohagis cooked and mashed with winter squash or pumpkin, and ohagis with mashed chestnut.

Cook 2 cups sweet rice with 1½ cups water per cup of rice and a pinch of sea salt, as in the recipe for Pressure-Cooked Brown Rice. Pound the rice in a wooden bowl with a heavy pestle or mallet until all the grains are half crushed and sticky. Wet the pestle occasionally to prevent the rice from sticking to it. This takes about 20 minutes or more of pounding. Form the dough into small balls and roll in various coatings.

For ohagis with aduki beans, soak the beans overnight and cook them the next morning. Add barley malt or salt several minutes before putting out the flame and mix well. Mash well with a suribachi. Cover the small rice balls with the aduki paste when the aduki mixture has cooled. Aduki paste may be ¼ inch thick.

For ohagis with squash or pumpkin, peel the skin of a medium-sized squash or pumpkin and cut it in pieces. Place in saucepan with a lid and add water to a level of about one-third of the vegetable pieces. Cook over a high flame, reduce when it starts to boil, and cook until tender. Add a pinch of salt and cook another 2 or 3 minutes. Mash the pieces in a suribachi. When they are cool, cover the rice balls with the paste to make it about ¼ inch thick.

For ohagis with chestnut, remove the shells from 1 cup or more of chestnuts and place them in a saucepan with a lid. Add water to a level of about one-third of the chestnuts. Cook over a high flame, reduce when it starts to boil, and cook until the chestnuts become soft. Add a pinch of salt, cook another 3 or 4 minutes, and mash in suribachi. When the mixture has cooled, cover the rice balls with the paste to about ¼ inch thick. Note that dried chestnuts must be soaked overnight.

For leukemia: Ohagis made with black sesame seed gomashio are particularly recommended.

RICE JUICE

The liquid that rises to the surface after cooking brown rice may be drunk frequently to harmonize the kidney, bladder, and skeletal functions.

ROASTED BROWN RICE PORRIDGE WITH GRATED DAIKON AND SHOYU

Roast washed brown rice in dry skillet without oil. Place in a large pot and add 3 to 4 times the amount of water. Bring to a boil and then simmer to make a thin porridge (gruel). Add 1 tablespoon grated daikon for 1 cup porridge. Simmer another 2 to 3 minutes and then add a little shoyu.

ROASTED BUCKWHEAT AND SCALLION TEA

Make a tea by mixing lightly roasted buckwheat grouts (3 parts) with chopped raw scallions (2 parts) and 5 times the total amount of water.

SHIITAKE-DAIKON TEA

This tea is good for body and mouth odor, bone and joint disorders, kidney and bladder problems, and muscle problems. This tea also helps to eliminate the accumulation of fat and to lower fever.

Soak 2 shiitake mushrooms for 30 minutes. Add ¼ cup grated daikon and 2 cups water. Bring to a boil and then simmer for 20 to 30 minutes. Take only half of this preparation at one time.

SHIO-KOMBU

Shio-kombu means salty kombu and is a popular condiment in Japan. It is traditionally made by rinsing the dust off kombu strips, cutting them with scissors into small squares, and soaking in shoyu for 1 to 2 days. After soaking, the kombu is put in a pot with just enough shoyu to cover and cooked over low heat without a cover. It is cooked until nearly all the juice has evaporated, 1 to 2 hours, and care is taken to prevent burning. At the end, each piece of kombu is mixed very slowly to coat it with the remaining juice and a few roasted sesame seeds are mixed in. The salty kombu will keep for over a year unrefrigerated. Only 1 or 2 small pieces are eaten at a time.

For a faster method, soak 5 to 6 strips of kombu, 8 to 12 inches long, for several minutes or until they are soft enough to cut. Slice into 1-inch squares. Place in saucepan and cover with a mixture of ½ cup shoyu and ½ cup water. Simmer until all the liquid evaporates, 30 to 40 minutes. Let cool and then store in a glass jar.

For an even faster method, wash and soak 1 ounce of dried kombu for 3 to 5 minutes. Cut with scissors into ½-inch squares. Put the kombu in a pressure cooker and add 3 tablespoons shoyu and ½ cup water. Bring up to pressure and cook for 10 minutes. Let the pressure come down naturally, uncover, and simmer until all the liquid has evaporated.

SWEET VEGETABLE DRINK

This drink was developed to help offset the effects of chicken, egg, and cheese consumption, leading to hypoglycemia, or chronic low blood sugar, a condition that affects about 75 percent or 80 percent of everyone in modern society.

Sweet vegetable drink is good for softening tightness caused by heavy animal food consumption and for relaxing the body and muscles. It is especially beneficial for softening the pancreas and helping to stabilize blood sugar levels. A small cup may be had daily or every other day, especially in mid- to late afternoon. It will satisfy the desire for a sweet taste and help reduce cravings for simple sugars and other stronger sweets.

Finely chop equal amounts of 4 sweet vegetables: onions, carrots, cabbage, and sweet winter squash. Boil 3 to 4 times the amount of water, add the vegetables, and allow to boil uncovered for 3 minutes. Reduce the flame to low, cover, and let simmer for 20 minutes.

Strain the vegetables, reserving the broth. (You may occasionally use the vegetables in soups and stews.) Drink the broth, either hot or at room temperature.

Notes: No seasoning is used in this recipe.

Sweet vegetable drink may be kept in the refrigerator up to 2 days but should be warmed again or allowed to return to room temperature before drinking.

VARIATION: Substitute daikon and lotus root for carrots and squash. Substitute sweet potato for carrot if your condition is too yang.

TANGERINE JAM

Finely slice tangerines. (Do not peel them.) Add a small amount of water and a pinch of sea salt, and bring to a boil. Lower the flame and then simmer to make a jam.

TANGERINE TEA

Dissolve tangerine jam in bancha twig tea or hot water and drink.

THYROID DRINK

Prepare the following special drink: carrots (2 parts), burdock (2 parts), daikon (2 parts), lotus root (2 parts), kombu (1 part), and daikon greens or other hard leafy greens (4 parts). Finely chop, add 4 times as much water, bring to a boil, and then simmer 15 to 20 minutes. Add a pinch of sea salt at the end of cooking or 3 or 4 drops of shoyu. Drink and eat the residue of 1 cup every day for 10 to 14 days, then every other day for an equal period.

TOMATO-MISO SAUCE WITH SCALLIONS AND CHINESE CABBAGE

Combine mashed tomatoes (7 parts), chopped scallion (1 part), and chopped Chinese cabbage (1 part). Bring to a boil and then simmer. Add 10 percent (1 part) of the total amount of miso and simmer for a long time. Take 1 tablespoonful at dinnertime.

UME-KUZU DRINK

Dissolve 1 teaspoon kuzu in 2 to 3 teaspoons cold water. Add 1 cup cold water to the dissolved kuzu. Bring to a boil in a saucepan over a medium flame, stirring constantly with a wooden spoon or wooden chopsticks to avoid lumping, until the liquid becomes translucent. Reduce the flame as low as possible. Add the pulp of ½ to 1 umeboshi plum that has had the pit removed and been chopped or ground to a paste. Do not add shoyu for Ume-Kuzu (this is called Ume-Sho-Kuzu). Simmer for a short time longer and then drink it hot.

UME-SHISO-BANCHA

Slightly rinse an umeboshi plum and ume-shiso leaves (that have been pickled with the plum) to remove the surface salt. Chop them and place them in a cup. Pour over the plum and leaves 7 to 8 times the total amount of either bancha twig tea or bancha stem tea.

UME-SHO-KUZU

This drink strengthens the blood, promotes good digestion, and restores energy. Dissolve 1 teaspoon pure kuzu in 2 or 3 tablespoons cold water. Add 1 cup cold water to the dissolved kuzu. Bring to a boil over a very low flame, stirring constantly with a wooden spoon or wooden chopsticks to avoid lumping, until the liquid becomes translucent, 2 to 3 minutes. Add the pulp of ½ to 1 umeboshi plum that has been pitted, chopped, and ground to a paste. Reduce the flame as low as possible. Add several drops to ½ teaspoon shoyu and stir gently. Simmer for 2 to 3 minutes. Drink and eat while hot.

WATER-SAUTÉED DAIKON AND DAIKON LEAVES

Chop daikon and daikon leaves, and water-sauté as in Sautéed Vegetables in the recipe section. Season with a little miso or shoyu for colon cancer and a few drops of shoyu for uterine cancer.

ZOSUI WITH SWEET VEGETABLES AND NORI

Cook a porridge using 70 percent brown rice (barley, millet, or other grains can be mixed 20 to 30 percent) and 30 percent cabbage, onion, winter squash or pumpkin, carrot, daikon, and nori (the same amount for each). Season with a small amount of miso, shoyu, or sea salt. See Miso-Zosui.

Note: Seasoning is not necessary for 10 days if a person has no appetite for salt.

COMPRESSES, PLASTERS, AND OTHER EXTERNAL APPLICATIONS

Body Scrub

A body scrub will help activate blood circulation and promote the physical and mental energy flow of the whole body. It will also help clear and clean the skin, discharge fat accumulated under the skin, and open pores to promote smooth and regular elimination of any excess fat and toxins to the surface of the body. A scrub is usually recommended every morning and every evening, twice a day, before or after a shower or bath, but apart from it.

Dip a small cotton towel or cloth in hot water. Wring out the excess water. Scrub the whole body, dipping the towel or cloth into hot water again when cool. Include the hands and feet, each finger and toe. The skin should become pink or slightly red. This result may take a few days to achieve if the skin is clogged with accumulated fats.

Buckwheat Plaster

This traditional Far Eastern remedy helps draw out water or other excess fluids that are retained by the body. It may be applied to swollen areas on the legs, arms, abdomen, etc. Buckwheat, which is a very yang, grain-like plant, attracts and draws out the more yin water or liquid. It is more effective to make fresh flour from whole buckwheat groats than to use packaged buckwheat flour. The energy is much stronger. However, if groats are not available, you may use store-bought flour.

First apply a hot towel compress or ginger compress to the affected region to make the area hot before applying the buckwheat plaster. The plaster should be as stiff, hot, and dry as possible.

Mix buckwheat flour with a little sesame oil and enough hot water to form a stiff, hard dough. Spread the dough on a cotton cloth about ½ inch thick. Apply the dough side (not the cloth side) directly to the swollen area. Remove after one to two hours. As the plaster draws out the fluid, the dough will become soft and watery. When this happens, replace the plaster with a new stiff dough.

Cabbage Leaf Compress

The leaves of large, leafy green vegetables are very helpful in cooling down fevers, neutralizing inflammations, and relieving burns and bruises. Sometimes just putting leaves (either big ones or ones that grow upward) such as cabbage leaves on the head, chest, or arms will provide immediate relief. Cabbage is particularly good because it is a more yang vegetable and has drawing, or contractive, power. This compress is used to cool down quickly, and it can be recycled by dipping the used leaves in cold water and reusing. The Cabbage Leaf Plaster, on the other hand, is used for a longer time to dissolve lumps and facilitate healing.

Carefully remove whole leaves from a head of cabbage or Chinese cabbage. Flatten them slightly by scoring the spine horizontally with a vegetable knife. Apply the leaves 2 layers thick on the hot or inflamed area. They may be held on for a short time by wrapping with a piece of cheesecloth. As the leaves become heated, they may be cooled in cold water and reused.

For a brain tumor: Ice cubes cannot be used. Keep changing the leaves to cool down the affected area of the brain and reduce swelling.

Cabbage Leaf Plaster

The Cabbage Leaf Compress above is used short-term to cool down, and it can be recycled by dipping the used leaves in cold water and reusing. The Cabbage Leaf Plaster, on the other hand, is used for a longer time to dissolve lumps and facilitate healing.

Carefully remove whole leaves from a head of cabbage or Chinese cabbage. Flatten them slightly by scoring the spine horizontally with a vegetable knife. Apply the leaves 2 layers thick on the affected area. They may be held on for 2 to 3 hours by wrapping with a piece of cheesecloth. They are generally not reusable.

For breast cancer arm swelling: Wrap the entire swollen arm area in cabbage leaves.

For thyroid and throat cancer: Raw cabbage leaf can be applied directly to the throat.

Cabbage Plaster

This differs from Cabbage Leaf Plaster in that the leaves are chopped and mashed and made into a paste with white flour. It has a more concentrated effect and may be used at once or after whole leaves have absorbed the initial heat.

Finely chop and mash fresh raw cabbage; add 10 to 20 percent white flour to it to make a paste. Spread it 1 inch thick on a piece of cotton linen and apply it directly to the affected area.

Cold Towel Compress

Cold towels can be used to relieve tension and reduce pain caused by too much sugar, sweets, soft drinks, fruit, ice cream, and other more extreme yin foods. For example, a headache in the front of the head is usually caused by these types of foods, and applying this compress will help ease the ache. In some cases, hot and cold towels may be alternated every few minutes. For example, leg cramps (usually caused by extreme yin foods but characterized by yang cramping) can be treated in this way. First massage toward and immediately above the cramping region (but not on it directly). Then apply towels drenched alternately in hot and cold water.

To do a cold towel compress, dip plain cotton towels in cold water, wring out, and apply to affected areas. Remove towels as they lose their strength, replacing them with fresh towels for up to 7 minutes or until the area becomes pink. See also Hot Towel Compress.

For a brain tumor: If a seizure occurs or consciousness is lost, similar to epilepsy, cover the whole head, including the forehead, with a cold towel compress. Massage the toes well (especially the first toe).

Daikon Hip Bath

This treatment warms the body and is good for women's reproductive organs, skin problems, drawing out excess fat and oil from the body, and discharging body odors arising from the consumption of animal foods.

Dry fresh daikon leaves in a shady place until they are brown and brittle. If daikon leaves are not available, use turnip leaves or a handful of arame sea vegetable. Place about 4 or 5 bunches of dried leaves or a handful of arame in a large pot. Add 4 or 5 quarts of water and bring to a boil. Reduce to a medium flame and simmer until the water is brown. Add approximately 1 cup of any kind of sea salt to pot and stir well to dissolve. Pour the hot liquid into a small tub or bath. Add water until the bath level is waist-high when sitting in the tub. Keep the temperature as hot as possible and cover your upper body with a large towel to induce perspiration. Stay in the bath for 10 to 20 minutes or until the hip becomes very red and hot. Keep the hip area warm after coming out of the bath. This bath is best and most effective just before bedtime but at least an hour after eating.

VARIATION: If daikon or other leaves or arame is not available, do a Salt Hip Bath, following the process outlined above and using a handful of any kind of sea salt in the hot bathwater.

Dried Daikon Leaves

These are used to warm the body and to treat various disorders of the skin and female sex organs. They are also helpful in drawing odors and excessive oils from the body. Dry fresh daikon leaves in the shade, away from direct sunlight, until they turn brown and brittle. (If daikon leaves are unavailable, turnip greens may be substituted.) Boil 4 to 5 bunches of leaves in 4 to 5 quarts of water until the water turns brown. Stir in a handful of sea salt and use in one of the following ways: (1) Dip cotton linen into the hot liquid and wring lightly. Apply to the affected area repeatedly, until the skin becomes completely red. (2) Women experiencing problems in their sexual organs should sit in a hot bath to which the daikon leaves liquid described above has been added along with a handful of sea salt. The water should come to waist level, with the upper portion of the body covered with a towel. Remain in the water until the whole body becomes warm and perspiration begins. This generally takes about 10 minutes. Repeat as needed, up to 10 days. Following this bath, douche with warm bancha tea, ⅛ teaspoon sea salt, and juice of half a lemon or similar amount of brown rice vinegar.

Fasting

It is helpful to practice fasting, but it is ideally limited to 1 meal or 1 day at a time. Take water or tea at that time. Otherwise, one can become too contracted and start overeating or bingeing.

Ginger Compress

Limited use: cancer (see important note below).

Contraindicated: The Ginger Compress is not recommended for use on the brain or on the head when high fever is present, on the lower abdominal area during pregnancy, for appendicitis, or for a baby or an older person.

The purpose of the hot Ginger Compress is to dissolve stagnation and tension, melt blockages, and stimulate blood circulation and energy flow.

Bring about 1 gallon of water to a boil. Meanwhile, grate enough gingerroot to equal the size of a baseball. When the water comes to a boil, reduce the heat to low and place the ginger in a double layer of cheesecloth tied with string long enough so that the other end hangs out of the pot for easy retrieval. The water at this point should be just below the boiling point. Place the sack in the pot and allow it to steep in the water without boiling for 5 minutes. Dip a towel in the ginger water, wring out tightly (using a long wooden cooking spoon or stick), and apply it to the desired area on the body. Cover with a second towel to hold in the heat. Change the towel every 2 to 3 minutes, replacing it with a fresh hot towel. This can be done by using 2 towels and alternating them so that the skin does not cool off between applications. Continue the applications 10 to 15 minutes, until the area becomes pink.

Important note: For people with cancer, this remedy is sometimes used preceding a Hato Mugi Plaster or other compress. But do not use a ginger compress more than once or twice and for no more than 3 to 5 minutes each time.

Be sure to keep the towels even on the back, not turned up at one or both ends. It is better to keep the pot on the flame in between the applications of towel, so that the water remains consistently hot; this is better than turning off the flame or placing the pot on the floor next to the person.

Hato Mugi–Cabbage Plaster

Hato mugi, also called pearl barley or Job's Tears, is a grass, not a grain. It is used in macrobiotic cooking as an occasional supplemental grain. Do not confuse pearl barley with pearled barley or polished barley. In Far Eastern medicine, hato mugi has traditionally been used to melt excess animal protein and fat and to beautify the skin. In this plaster it is good for harmonizing body energy and drawing out and softening excess fat and protein. The cabbage in the plaster is very helpful in cooling down fever and neutralizing inflammation. Cabbage is particularly good because it is a more yang vegetable and has drawing, or contractive, power. It tends to keep tumors from spreading.

Cook hato mugi following the basic recipe for Pressure-Cooked Brown Rice or Boiled Brown Rice, using slightly more water. While it is still warm, mash it in a suribachi. Let it cool to room temperature and then very finely chop and mash the same amount of fresh cabbage as pearl barley and combine them. Mix 10 to 20 percent of the total amount of white flour into the barley mixture to make it less watery and to make a paste for the plaster.

Spread the mixture about 1 inch thick on a cotton cloth. Apply the mixture directly on the breast and tie with a cotton strip or a bolt of cheesecloth. Cover if necessary with a cotton brassiere and a large cotton towel, pinned together.

Leave the plaster on for 4 hours or more. Repeat once or twice every day. You may leave the plaster on overnight while you are sleeping.

Hato Mugi with Cabbage Plaster

Follow the recipe for Hato Mugi–Cabbage Plaster but change the ratio of hato mugi and cabbage from equal amounts to two-thirds and one-third. Combine with 10 to 20 percent of white flour if necessary. Spread it about 1 inch thick on a cotton cloth and apply it directly to the painful part for 3 to 4 hours, twice a day. You may also sleep with it overnight.

Hato Mugi–Potato Plaster

Cook hato mugi following the basic recipe for Pressure-Cooked Brown Rice or Boiled Brown Rice, using slightly more water. While still warm, mash it in a suribachi. Let it cool to room temperature. Peel and finely grate potatoes. Combine equal amounts of mashed hato mugi and potato. Add 10 to 20 percent white flour to make a paste. Spread the plaster about 1 inch thick on a cotton cloth. Apply the plaster directly on the affected part of the ovary area. Leave the plaster on for 4 hours or longer. Repeat twice a day or leave the plaster on overnight if possible. Continue every day for about 3 weeks.

Hato Mugi–Potato–Cabbage Plaster

Cook hato mugi following the basic recipe for Pressure-Cooked Brown Rice or Boiled Brown Rice, using slightly more water. While still warm, mash it in a suribachi. Let it cool to room temperature. Meanwhile, peel and finely grate potatoes in the same amount as the hato mugi. Finally, very finely chop and mash the same amount of fresh cabbage as the pearl barley and potato. Combine the pearl barley, potato, and cabbage, one-third each. Mix 10 to 20 percent of the total amount of white flour to make it less watery and to make a paste for the plaster.

Spread this about 1 inch thick on a cotton linen and apply it directly to the affected area. Keep it on for 3 to 4 hours twice a day or leave it on overnight. Do this for 2 to 3 weeks.

Hot Foot Soak

Contraindicated: ovarian cancer.

Soak your feet in somewhat hot water for 3 to 5 minutes to promote better circulation.

Hot Towel Compress

Hot towels can be used to relieve tension and reduce pain, especially on areas of the body that are tight from overconsumption of animal food, salt, or other more contractive foods. For example, a headache in the back of the head is usually caused by these foods, and applying a hot towel will ease the ache. In some cases, hot and cold towels may be alternated every few minutes. For example, leg cramps (usually caused by extreme yin foods but characterized by yang cramping) can be treated in this way. First massage toward and immediately above the cramping region (but not on it directly). Then alternately apply towels drenched in hot and cold water.

To prepare this compress, dip plain cotton towels in hot water, wring out, and apply to affected areas. Remove towels as they lose their strength, replacing them with fresh towels for up to 7 minutes, or until the area becomes pink. See also Cold Towel Compress.

Kombu Plaster

Soften strips of kombu by soaking in hot water for 10 to 15 minutes. Cut 2 pieces to a proper size, large enough to cover the affected part. Apply the soaked kombu, 2 layers thick, directly on the skin. Hold in place with a cotton towel, cotton linen, or cotton cheesecloth. The cloth or towels help soften the kombu prior to removing it. Keep it on 2 to 3 hours a couple of times a day or overnight.

Kombu-Cabbage Plaster

A kombu plaster is good for burns from radiation (such as medical X-rays), skin lesions, and scars. It is also good to help relieve stagnation and tumors caused by dairy consumption. The cabbage is particularly good because it is a more yang vegetable and has a drawing, or contractive, power. It helps cool down fever, neutralize inflammation, and relieve burns and bruises.

Soften strips of kombu by soaking in hot water for 10 to 15 minutes. Cut 2 pieces to a proper size, large enough to cover the affected area. Apply the soaked kombu, 2 layers thick, directly on the skin. Then carefully separate cabbage leaves from a large cabbage and score the spine with a vegetable knife so that the leaf flattens slightly. Apply a layer of cabbage leaves on top of the kombu. Hold in place with a cotton towel, cotton linen, or cheesecloth. The cloth or towels help soften the kombu prior to removing it.

For breast cancer: After surgery, a lump of fat sometimes grows on the scar. To prevent a lump from growing, do a Kombu and Cabbage Plaster. Leave on for about 4 hours or overnight.

For lymphoma: Apply this plaster directly on the swollen area. Wrap it with bleached cotton and keep it on about 4 hours. Do this twice a day or, if possible, keep it on overnight. This can be continued until the swelling disappears.

For prostate cancer: If the lymph nodes are swollen, apply and leave on for 6 hours or more. You may leave it on overnight. Repeat once or twice every day for 2 to 3 weeks.

Leafy Greens Plaster (Chlorophyll Plaster)

The leaves of large, leafy green vegetables are very helpful in cooling down fever, neutralizing inflammation, and relieving burns and bruises. Sometimes just putting leaves (either big ones or ones that grow upward) such as cabbage leaves, collard greens, turnip tops, or daikon tops on the head, chest, or arms will provide immediate relief. This plaster has a more concentrated effect than just the leaves and may be used at once or after whole leaves have absorbed the initial heat.

Finely chop several green leafy vegetables such as daikon leaves, kale, collards, cabbage, or Chinese cabbage. Place in a suribachi and mash well. Add 10 to 20 percent unbleached white flour and mix into a paste. Spread the mixture about ½ inch thick on a towel or cloth and apply the greens directly to the skin (not the cloth side). Leave on for 2 to 3 hours.

Lotus Root Plaster

Lotus root—the long, many-chambered, pale root of the lotus plant—is known traditionally for helping to dissolve excess mucus in the lungs, bronchi, throat, and sinuses. This is often caused by dairy food consumption, but lotus is good to release any kind of stagnation, including chicken and egg fat. This remedy is traditionally known for its effectiveness in dispersing and moving stagnated mucus in the respiratory system.

Activate the area to be treated first with a Hot Towel Compress or Ginger Compress for 5 minutes. Generally, stagnation begins to loosen up and mucus starts to drain within 3 applications of this plaster. Calcified stones in the sinuses sometimes are loosened and come out with sneezing. Stubborn ones can take 3 weeks to discharge.

Grate enough lotus root to cover the area about ½ inch thick. Mix thoroughly with 5 percent grated ginger, if using ginger, and 10 to 15 percent unbleached white flour. Spread the mixture on a cloth or paper towel and apply directly to the skin (not the cloth side). Leave on for 20 minutes to 1 hour.

Note: To dissolve mucus deposits in the sinuses, you may leave the plaster on for several hours or overnight. In this case, sew a gauze mask with holes for the nose and eyes. The lotus plaster should cover the area around the eyes and above the nose. This application should be repeated for 7 to 10 days, and may sometimes take up to 2 to 3 weeks to clear the sinuses. Watery or thick mucus may start to be discharged from the eyes and nose.

Massage

Massage of the fingers and toes helps stimulate various organs, systems, and functions by activating energy flow through the meridians that begin or end in the extremities. Basic books on massage are *Beginner's Guide to Shiatsu* by Patrick McCarty and *Basic Shiatsu* by Michio Kushi. More comprehensive books are *Shiatsu Handbook* by Shizuko Yamamoto and Patrick McCarty, and *Barefoot Shiatsu* by the same authors. For self-massage please see *The Book of Do-In* by Michio Kushi.

Miso Plaster

Contraindication: This should not be used for puncture wounds.
Soybeans have a cooling effect on the body. Raw soybeans soaked in

water, crushed, and applied to the affected area can remove fever. Miso—the fermented soybean paste used daily in macrobiotic cooking for soup, condiments, and seasoning—also has many medicinal applications. A miso plaster consists of raw miso applied directly on the body. The enzymes in miso neutralize bacteria and help prevent infection. In the kitchen, nicks and cuts when cutting vegetables can be treated with a dab of miso. It is also good for burns from radiation or other medical procedures.

A miso plaster can also draw out bee stingers, help relieve itchy skin diseases, and reduce any kind of swelling. It is an essential ingredient in a home first-aid kit. Use regular barley, rice, or hatcho miso for this purpose. It is all right if the miso has been pasteurized. It will still be effective.

Place raw miso on the affected area, about ¼ to ½ inch thick. Wrap with a single layer of cheesecloth.

Note: When putting miso directly on the skin, do not pack it down firmly because this can cause scarring.

Moxabustion

Moxabustion (or moxa) is a traditional Far Eastern healing method that employs heat along the meridians and points to activate and supply energy to specific regions, organs, systems, and functions of the body. Moxa can be used for general strengthening, such as on Stomach Meridian Point 36 on the leg for health and longevity; to help relieve specific symptoms such as constipation or facial problems, such as Large Intestine Point 4 on the hand; or for chronic conditions, such as multiple sclerosis, on certain points along the spine. It has also been used for helping someone who is dying recover strength, energy, or consciousness.

Traditionally, dried mugwort is used, and long sticks of moxa or small moxa cones are available in acupuncture clinics, Oriental markets, or, occasionally, natural foods stores.

To apply, light the moxa stick and approach the point in a slow, gentle clockwise spiral. Hold the moxa stick above the point (not touching the skin) for several seconds until the person feels strong heat. Then pull back the stick and after a few seconds apply again in the same way. Usually five times is enough for most applications, although emergency treatments may take more time.

Notes: Locations of the points are different for everyone, so you can't just mechanically follow an acupuncture chart or diagram in a book. A thorough understanding of Far Eastern philosophy and medicine, including the meridian system, is recommended before use of this method. Moxa is generally not used for yang conditions or symptoms characterized by excess energy.

Please consult a text on moxabustion for further information.

VARIATION: If a moxa stick is not available, an ordinary cigarette may be used.

Mustard Plaster

The mustard plaster, a traditional Far Eastern remedy, dissolves stagnation and stimulates circulation, especially in the lungs. It can help relieve mucus accumulation or coughing and is good for muscle stiffness.

While preparing the plaster, warm two towels. Crush enough mustard seeds to obtain a handful of mustard powder. As a substitute, mustard powder or mustard spread from a jar may be used. Bring some water to a boil and add enough to the mustard to make a moist paste. The consistency should be light and soft, something like mustard from a jar. Spread the paste on half of a triple layer of paper towels or one layer of waxed paper. (The area should be large enough to cover the chest if it is being used for the lungs or upper back.) Fold in half to cover the paste on both sides. Spread a towel on the area to be treated. Place the mixture in this wrapper of paper towels or waxed paper on top of the towel and cover with the second towel. Leave the plaster on until the heat starts to feel uncomfortable, usually 10 to 15 minutes.

Notes: The skin will become red, which is normal. The effects will last as long as the red color remains.

Do not apply mustard directly on the skin because it will burn!

When using this plaster on children, mix in an equal amount of flour.

If some mustard inadvertently leaks and burns the skin, spread a small amount of olive oil or other light vegetable-quality oil on the affected area.

For lung troubles you may apply the plaster on the chest, back, or both.

In case of an acute condition, you may apply the plaster two or three times a day but refrain from too frequent use because it may burn the skin if repeated too often.

Palm Healing

Palm healing involves the use of the palms and hands to channel energy to different parts of the body. It is also known as *laying on of hands* and *therapeutic touch*. Simple techniques allow the energies of heaven and earth to circulate through the giver's palms and hands to the head, neck, shoulders, chest, or other region of the recipient. Palm healing is a very powerful type of healing and may succeed in difficult cases where dietary and lifestyle methods are not effective. The standard reference, *Macrobiotic Palm Healing* by Michio Kushi with Olivia Oredsen, presents the principles of palm healing along with hundreds of practical applications and exercises.

Potato Plaster

Peel, grate, and mash an ordinary potato. Add 20 to 30 percent white flour and make into a paste, adding a little water if necessary. Spread the mixture about 1 inch thick on a cotton cloth. Before applying, apply a Hot Towel Compress on the affected area about 3 minutes to promote better circulation. Then apply the plaster directly on the skin. Tie it with a cotton strip, bolt of cheesecloth, or cotton towel. Leave it on overnight so the plaster does not move. Leave the plaster on for 4 hours or the whole night. Repeat every day for 2 weeks or more.

Potato-Cabbage Plaster

This plaster has a softening and drawing effect on tumors. Grate potato. If the potato is too watery, place it in a double layer of cheesecloth and squeeze out the excess water before combining it with the other ingredients. In a suribachi, mash an equal amount of finely chopped raw cabbage leaves. Combine potato (1 part) and cabbage (1 part). Make a plaster by mashing them together. Twenty to 30 percent white flour may be added to make a paste. Spread the mixture about 1 inch thick on a cotton cloth. Before applying, place a Hot Towel Compress on the affected area about 3 minutes to promote better circulation. Then apply the plaster directly on the skin. Tie it with a cotton strip, bolt of cheesecloth, or cotton towel. Leave it on overnight so the plaster does not move. Leave the plaster on for 4 hours or the whole night. Repeat every day for 2 weeks or more.

Potato-Cabbage-Hato Mugi Plaster

Follow the instructions for making a Potato-Cabbage Plaster above, adding 1 part cooked hato mugi.

Rice Bran (Nuka) Plaster

Generally, commercial soaps, creams, and lotions clog the meridians, holes, and sweat glands, impeding ki energy flow. People who eat dairy food are especially attracted to these products. Dry skin comes from a layer of oil and fat blocking the skin, not from a lack of oil. Rice bran is very helpful for this and many other skin conditions. It is soothing for broken bones and may also be put on the toes for frostbite lesions.

Traditionally, rice bran (known as *nuka* in the East) has been used thousands of years. Rice was traditionally kept unpolished until eaten, and then the polishings, or bran, were kept for pickling and soap. Nuka will make the skin very clean and shiny. It has strong healing power.

To a handful of rice bran add about one-third as much flour and mix. Use rice flour, if available, or hato mugi flour. Otherwise, use wheat or white flour. Add cold water as needed to make a thick paste. Put the mixture in cheesecloth, dip in hot water, and apply to the skin. Rinse the plaster off and apply a fresh one when it becomes warm.

Note: Nuka water can be applied around the vagina, but do not use as a douche because the bran texture may be irritating in this region. Nuka may also be added to the bath.

VARIATION: Use wheat or oat bran if rice bran is not available.

Salt Pack

This is used to warm any part of the body. For the relief of diarrhea, for example, apply the pack to the abdominal region. Roast salt in a dry pan until hot and then wrap in a thick cotton linen pillowcase or towel and tie with string or cord like a package. Apply to the troubled area and change when the pack begins to cool.

Salt Water

Cold salt water will contract the skin in the case of burns, while warm salt water can be used to clean the rectum, colon, and vagina. When the skin is damaged by fire, immediately soak the burned area in cold salt water until the irritation disappears. Then apply vegetable oil to seal the wound from the air. For constipation or mucus or fat accumulation in the rectum, colon, and vaginal regions, use warm water (body temperature) as an enema or douche.

Sesame Oil–Ginger Rub

In the Far East, sesame seeds are considered medicine for longevity. By adding a little ginger oil to the sesame, its effectiveness can be increased. This remedy is good for bone cancer, especially stiffness after radiation treatment, as well as arthritis, rheumatism, pain in the joints, and to activate blood circulation. It is also good for dandruff and for hair falling out. It can be put in the ear or eye (see note below). Use toasted dark sesame oil if available. Otherwise, light sesame is suitable.

Mix raw sesame oil (1 part) with the juice squeezed from freshly grated ginger (1 part). Shake well before using and soak a cotton linen in the mixture. Rub the stiff area with the cloth to make the muscles relax.

Notes: If a burning sensation results, reduce the ginger. If put in the eye, heat the oil, let it cool, and then strain through a handkerchief.

For radiation stiffness: After radiotherapy, sometimes the muscles get stiff and pain occurs when moving. After 10 minutes, clean the skin with a warm towel. Do it twice a day.

For rheumatism and arthritis: To improve circulation, rub on the stiff area for 10 to 15 minutes and wipe off the oil with a warm towel. This may be repeated every day or every other day for 2 to 3 weeks.

Shiatsu

Shiatsu is a form of acupressure massage that stimulates energy flow in the body through pressure on points, meridians, and other parts of the body. It can be very effective in treating a wide range of conditions and disorders. It is easy to learn and can be done among family members and friends. For serious conditions a qualified practitioner is recommended. Please consult with a qualified specialist or refer to some of the numerous books about doing shiatsu at home: *Beginner's Guide to Shiatsu* by Patrick McCarty; *Basic Shiatsu* by Michio Kushi; *Barefoot Shiatsu* by Shizuko Yamamoto and Patrick McCarty; or *Shiatsu Handbook* by Shizuko Yamamoto and Patrick McCarty.

Tofu Plaster

Contraindication: high fever from chickenpox or measles (see note below).

The tofu plaster helps relieve inflammations, swellings, fevers, burns, dental abscesses, and bruises. The tofu is cold and therefore leads to contraction (a yang effect), serving to neutralize heat or inflammation. It is more effective than ice. The soft, yin quality of the tofu, meanwhile, absorbs fevers far more effectively than ice (which is hard or yang) and does not produce any side effects such as a secondary increase in fever. It extinguishes inflammatory processes and prevents swelling or decreases existing swelling.

This remedy has been successfully used in some cases of paralysis, such as those resulting from a stroke, or for a concussion resulting from a motorcycle accident in which the person is left unconscious. In cases such as these, after seeking medical attention and going to the hospital, immediately apply crushed cold tofu to the affected part of the head and continuously make and apply tofu plasters. They will help heal and repair the damage quickly. Apply as soon as possible. Four hours later may be too late.

Squeeze out the liquid from a block of tofu and mash the tofu in a suribachi. Mix well to take out all lumps. Add 10 to 20 percent unbleached white flour and 5 percent grated ginger. Mix well. (It is better to peel the ginger before grating for cool plasters because ginger can irritate the skin.) Apply the mixture (which should be moist) directly to the skin and cover with a towel. You may want to secure it in place with a bandage or tie it with a cotton strip. Change the plaster every 2 to 3 hours or when it becomes hot.

VARIATIONS: Tofu Plaster may be combined with mashed leafy greens (as in the Leafy Greens Plaster), especially for hemorrhages. (See Tofu and Leafy Greens Plaster.)

A Tofu and Grain Plaster may be used as an alternative, especially if the tofu plaster feels too cold. Make by mixing 50 percent cooked and mashed whole grain (rice or barley) that has cooled to room temperature with 50 percent squeezed and mashed tofu.

For high fevers: Apply the tofu plaster to the head, including the brain area, if affected.

For inflammatory processes: For acute pneumonia or bronchitis when the inflammation is located deeper in the body. First apply a Ginger Compress.

For contusion, concussion, or sprain: Apply immediately afterward to prevent the formation of large intra-tissular bleeding and swelling.

For bleeding within tissue, including brain hemorrhage: Tofu plasters will prevent the clotting and hardening of the blood and will accelerate the reabsorption of the blood.

Counterindication: Do not apply tofu plasters when fever is caused by measles or chickenpox unless really high (105°F or 40°C, or higher). The temperature should only be kept within a safe range.

Visualization

Visualization is a type of meditation in which the person sits quietly for a few minutes, focusing on a visual image or sound. It is commonly used for healing purposes, and some people are encouraged to visualize red blood cells fighting cancer cells or other diseased parts of the body. From the macrobiotic view, this type of violent, combative visualization is counterproductive and should be avoided. Disease is not an attack on the body but the result of living in disharmony with nature. It is actually a beneficial mechanism. Therefore, visualization should be entirely peaceful and harmonious. Visualizing oneself getting better as a result of wholesome food, natural environmental influences, and healthy relationships is strongly encouraged.

Yoga

Yoga is a traditional system of unifying mind, body, and spirit that originated in India. It is now practiced all around the world. There are many types and styles of yoga. You may acquaint yourself with yoga by reading books or attending a class with a qualified teacher. It is recommended that you study with a yoga teacher who is eating macrobiotically or understands the energetics of food. Avoid complicated and inverted postures as a general practice.

37

Prayers, Meditations, and Visualizations

PRAYERS

Daily Dedication for One Peaceful World

When we eat, let us reflect that we have come from food, which has come from nature by the order of the infinite universe, and let us be grateful for all that we have been given.

When we meet people, let us see them as brothers and sisters and remember that we have all come from the infinite universe through our parents and ancestors, and let us pray as One with all of humanity for universal love and peace on earth.

When we see the sun and moon, the sky and stars, mountains and rivers, seas and forests, fields and valleys, birds and animals, and all the wonders of nature, let us remember that we have come with them all from the infinite universe. Let us be thankful for our environment on earth, and live in harmony with all that surrounds us.

When we see farms and villages, towns and cities, arts and cultures, societies and civilizations, and all the works of humanity, let us recall that our creativity has come from the infinite universe and has passed from generation to generation and spread over the entire earth. Let us be grateful for our birth on this planet with intelligence and wisdom, and let us vow with all to realize endlessly our eternal dream of One Peaceful World through health, freedom, love, and justice.

Meditation and Prayer at the Meal

I am grateful to the meal now being offered to me.
I am grateful to people, nature, and the universe for having made this meal available
    to me.
I now reflect whether I truly deserve to have this meal.
I now pray that, through this meal, I may achieve a healthy body and peaceful mind.
I now resolve that, through this meal, I will continue to realize my dream of love and
    peace in our eternal journey of endless life.

VISUALIZATION

Positive visualization reduces stress and inspires hope for the future. Your daily life can then become the process through which you actualize this positive, healthy image of yourself. Here are several simple visualization exercises.

Visualization to Change Sickness to Health

Relax, close your eyes, and stabilize your breathing.

In your mind, create an image of the infinite universe. See the heavens filled with billions and billions of galaxies and stars, solar systems and planets, cycling in perfect harmony.

Imagine the earth bathed in the gentle, peaceful energy from all these celestial bodies.

Imagine this energy coming down and into our planet in centripetal spiral waves and making it spin on its axis, coming up again from the center of the earth in centrifugal waves that spiral in a complementary, outward, upward direction.

Imagine this energy of heaven and earth making the plants and animals grow, the grains blowing gently in the wind, the vegetables, beans, and other seeds pushing up from below ground, the seaweed swaying peacefully in the oceans, the salt and other minerals collecting in the sea, absorbing and gathering this vital energy.

Imagine eating a delicious, balanced meal made from these foods and that strong nourishing energy flowing through your body, from the digestive system, to the circulatory system, to the nervous system, to all organs, functions, tissues, and cells.

Imagine this energy creating fresh, new blood and lymph and gently melting away hardness, stagnation, and blockages that may have developed in the past.

Imagine your tumor or growth gradually shrinking and dissolving as this peaceful, harmonious energy is received.

Imagine yourself restored to health, surrounded by the love of family and friends.

Imagine yourself now completely well, guiding and helping other people with serious illness rediscover the laws of nature and the healing power of their own minds and bodies.

Imagine yourself five, ten, fifteen, twenty years or more from now, experiencing ever greater realms of self-realization. Hold this image for a few minutes, let it subside naturally, and resume normal consciousness.

Visualization for Healing Planet Earth

Sit quietly in any comfortable position and hold your hands on your lap or in the prayer position with palms touching. Stabilize your breathing.

Visualize the earth as a bright tiny ball in the vastness of space. Visualize that blue-green ball temporarily covered with a heavy, dark aura.

Visualize the way of life and health spreading from kitchen to kitchen, home to home, family to family, beginning with you.

Visualize people gradually recovering their health as they eat and live in a more natural direction.

Visualize more and more of the land devoted to growing grains and vegetables and less and less to raising cattle and other livestock.

Visualize the rivers and streams becoming cleaner and cleaner as natural farming and organic gardening spread.

Visualize the air becoming purer and purer as less industrial pollutants are released into the atmosphere.

Visualize the plants and animals thriving and returning to forests and woodlands, oceans and lakes.

Visualize human beings living peacefully on the planet, with no more war, crime, or violence; no more cancer, heart disease, or major sickness; no more poverty and injustice.

Visualize people of all colors, sexes, ages, and backgrounds living harmoniously in a world of enduring peace, playing from morning till night, traveling freely, and respecting one another's customs, traditions, and ways of life.

Visualize the stagnated energy of the earth from sickness, crime, war, climate change, and other sources melting into the general circulation of the energy as a whole.

Visualize the earth becoming lighter and more energized.

Visualize the dark aura of global warming around the earth gradually dissolving, the temperature declining, and the earth's aura—the ozone layer,

Van Allen belt, aurora borealis—becoming brighter and brighter, lighter and lighter.

Visualize the earth as a tiny ball in outer space surrounded by a radiant halo of energy spiraling through the Milky Way.

Visualize yourself as being at one with the earth and all of life. Hold this image for a few minutes, let it subside naturally, and allow your consciousness to return to normal.

APPENDIX I

Dietary Guidelines for Tropical and Semitropical Regions and for Polar and Semipolar Regions

TROPICAL AND SEMITROPICAL REGIONS

Traditionally, in South Asia, Southeast Asia, Africa, Central and South America, and other tropical and semitropical regions, people have been eating cooked whole cereal grains as principal food. The grain, including long-grain rice, basmati rice, sorghum, and others, is complemented with vegetables as well as soup and broth, beans and sea vegetables, and other categories of food in the standard macrobiotic diet.

Proportions of foods, cooking styles, seasoning, and other factors may differ from standard cooking in temperate regions. For example, the amount of vegetables, fresh raw salad, and fruit may be slightly higher; steaming, stir-frying, braising, and other lighter cooking methods may be used more frequently, including the boiling of grain rather than pressure-cooking; and less salt, miso, and soy sauce or lighter miso and other seasonings may be used. However, in a hot and humid climate, a salty taste may be required more often than in a temperate climate.

In addition to whole grains, some cultures and island societies such as Hawaii and the Caribbean islands have traditionally consumed cassava, taro, yams, sweet potatoes, and other roots and tubers as staple food. In such cases, these may be included in the grain category as the principal source of complex carbohydrates. Couscous, bulgur, and other light processed grains are also consumed more in hotter and warmer climates.

In addition to fish and seafood, a small amount of wild animals, birds, and insects may be eaten if traditionally and commonly consumed. Also, a small amount of spices, herbs, and aromatic, fragrant beverages may be consumed on occasion to help offset the high heat and humidity. Typical foods in tropical and semitropical regions include the following:

Whole Grains and Staple Roots and Tubers

Amaranth

Barley

Bulgur

Cassava (yucca, manioc, tapioca)

Corn

Couscous

Medium, long-grain, and
  basmati rice

Quinoa

Sorghum

Sweet potato

Taro (albi, poi)

Teff

Yam

Other grains, grain products, staple roots, and tubers that have traditionally been consumed in tropical and semitropical regions

Vegetables from Land and Sea

Artichoke

Asparagus

Avocado

Bamboo shoots

Curly dock

Eggplant

Fennel

Green pepper

Jicama

Okra

Plantain

Potato (traditionally processed)

Purslane

Sea vegetables, water moss,
  river and lake moss

Spinach

Swiss chard

Zucchini

Other vegetables that have traditionally been consumed in tropical and semitropical regions

Fruit, Nuts, and Seeds

All seeds and nuts

Banana

Breadfruit

Coconut

Date

Fig

Grapefruit

Guava

Kiwi

Mango

Orange

Papaya

Pineapple

Plantain

Quince

Tangerine

Other fruits that have traditionally been consumed in tropical and semitropical regions

POLAR AND SEMIPOLAR REGIONS

Traditionally, in Alaska, northern Canada, Greenland, Iceland, Scandinavia, northern Russia, Siberia, Mongolia, Tibet, the Andes, and other cold climates and regions, the standard diet has included proportionately more animal food than in temperate latitudes. Because of the short growing season, grains and vegetables are in shorter supply, although traditional hardy strains of buckwheat, mountain barley, and other grains were harvested, as well as a wide variety of wild plants (including wild burdock, milkweed, dandelion, mugwort, wild leek, water lily root, wild ginger, and wild beans), sea vegetables and mosses, fruits (including chokeberry, wild cherry, currants, cranberries, blueberries, wild strawberries, and grapes), seeds and nuts (such as acorns), and roots, stems, leaves, and flowers of many kinds.

In addition to slightly more fish and seafood (on average from 20 to 30 percent of the daily diet, especially in colder seasons), people in polar and semipolar regions ate a small amount of whale, caribou, wild game, and dairy food. Because of the cold weather and hard physical activity, they were able to digest small amounts of these foods without ill effects, as is the case in other climates and environments and among people observing a more sedentary lifestyle. Further, pressure-cooking, longtime boiling, broiling, baking, roasting, and other stronger cooking methods may be used more frequently; and more salt, miso, shoyu, and other seasonings as well as darker miso may be used.

Illness in the Kushi Family

by Michio Kushi

The macrobiotic dietary and lifestyle approach has been shown to be highly effective in the prevention and reversal of cancer. However, no one is immune from cancer in the modern world, not even longtime macrobiotic teachers, friends, and families. The primary reason for this is that the accelerating speed of life today, the advent of new technology, the decline in soil and food quality, and rapid climate change make it more and more challenging to practice macrobiotics in an optimal manner.

My own family is a case in point. Since the last edition of this book, my wife, Aveline, my daughter, Lily, and myself all experienced cancer. Many people who hear of illness in our family assume that macrobiotics doesn't work. Let's look briefly at these three cases and determine if this conclusion is warranted.

AVELINE KUSHI

For over thirty years Aveline led a heroically purposeful and hectic life. She created and managed up to a dozen macrobiotic study houses in the Boston area with two hundred students; founded Erewhon, America's pioneer natural foods company; persuaded farmers in California to start growing the first organic rice in the United States; and taught thousands of cooking classes—all the while bringing up five children, tending later to many grandchildren, and traveling around the world with her globe-trotting husband.

Naturally, she couldn't eat well during much of this time, especially when traveling internationally. Also, in keeping with a more strict Japanese style of macrobiotics that she learned when studying with George Ohsawa after World War II, she tended to avoid fresh salad, fruits, and other lighter fare. As a result, she became more and more contracted, or what we call yang. She loved fried kombu, the strongest sea vegetable, and she enjoyed deep-fried sourdough bread. Baking and deep-frying are each very yang and in combination are extremely tightening. The end result over time was cervical cancer, a very yang tumor, in the contracted lower part of her body.

After Aveline became sick, in the mid-1990s, she immediately changed her way of eating, balanced her macrobiotic diet, and began to get well. The tumor began to shrink. But because it was so hard and contracted, she agreed to strong medical treatment to help eliminate it when compresses reached their limit. She underwent radiation therapy, a relatively mild dose, and within about one and a half months her cancer was gone.

While I was away traveling, Aveline received medical advice to undergo experimental internal radiation. Without my advice, she agreed, and it took place one entire night at the hospital. Within a few weeks pain began in her spine and other bones, and it spread through the Governing Vessel, one of the major meridians. In macrobiotics, radiation is classified as more expansive or yin. In a mild dose, it originally helped, along with diet, to melt her tumor. In the strong experimental internal dose, it led to excessive expansion of her skeletal frame and pain. I was away teaching at the time and would have strongly discouraged Aveline from taking this second round of radiation had I known.

After that, Aveline suffered from chronic pain over the next several years. She had to use a cane or walker to get around. She was well taken care of at home, eating as healthfully as possible. She consumed good-quality sweets and amasake, a fermented rice beverage, but she couldn't offset the effects of the radiation. She passed away in 2001, in my view from iatrogenesis, or a medically caused disease.

LILY KUSHI

Lily Kushi, my daughter, also suffered from cervical cancer. Actually, her case began a little before Aveline's. She was an excellent musician and composer and lived for seven years in Los Angeles writing music for the movies. Her social life revolved around the film industry, and she often stayed up late and went out to parties to keep up her social contacts. She avoided eating many foods that weren't good for her, but not completely. She especially liked salmon, in the form of sandwiches, sashimi, and smoked salmon. She never ate meat, very rarely eggs, and ate a little sugar on social occasions. She developed cervical cancer from indulging primarily in this extreme diet. Salmon is a red-meat fish and extremely yangizing. Her cancer appeared in the cervix, a very yang, constricted organ.

Returning from California, she went to the Kushi Institute, our educational center in Becket, Massachusetts, and for a while lived in a rented house in Becket. Cooking for herself, she improved, but her condition continued to fluctuate. Following a checkup at Massachusetts General Hospital in Boston, she received a moderate dose of radiation and was completely free of cancer after that.

Again, however, the same doctor who recommended internal radiation for Aveline suggested it for Lily. Actually, they received it at the same time, while I was away teaching. After that treatment, the radiation spread through Lily's liver meridian, and the liver became very swollen. At home she continued to receive good food and home care, but the radiation was so strong that her leg started to swell. Returning to the hospital, the liver pain continued, and she eventually passed away one evening toward sunset. She survived about one and a half years after her diagnosis. Aveline lived about five years. Both lived much longer than normal for patients with similar conditions. They were both such wonderful, loving women. Aveline (whose name was coined by her teacher, George Ohsawa, from Ave Maria, representing the Virgin Mary) selflessly devoted her life to compassionately serving humanity, and Lily brought her family much joy and touched the hearts of all who knew her.

MICHIO KUSHI

In my case, I also led an extremely hectic life, traveling constantly and giving macrobiotic seminars around the world. For three to four months every year for many years I stayed at hotels, flew on commercial jetliners, and followed a very unnatural lifestyle in order to spread the macrobiotic philosophy and lifestyle.

My illness came primarily after a decade of intensive teaching in Japan in the 1990s and early 2000s. The organizers would make very beautiful macrobiotic dishes for me to enjoy. But almost every night after my lectures I was obliged to meet with students, businessmen, journalists, and friends and colleagues who lined up at mealtime for advice, to sign a book, ask a question, or present me their business cards. Naturally, I couldn't eat or drink in such an environment. At 10 p.m. I would return to my hotel and order something to eat. I avoided beef, pork, and other extreme foods, of course, but I enjoyed pancakes, sandwiches, and other baked flour products. And I violated one of the cardinal macrobiotic guidelines: Don't eat late at night right before sleep. In the United States I also developed a habit of snacking on doughnuts and baked goods to relax, as I took breaks at coffee shops in between classes and consultations.

The end result was that I developed cancer in the large intestine, specifically the transverse colon. This is the central part of the colon. Usually, cancer in the descending colon (and rectum) are caused by beef and other strong animal foods. Malignancy in the ascending colon is caused by sugar, oil, and more yin, expansive foods. In my case, the transverse colon was affected primarily by my baked white flour consumption and the in-between combination of strong yin and yang.

I noticed pain from time to time while traveling and eventually had it checked out medically. Following the diagnosis, I immediately stopped all traveling, returned to a more orderly and balanced way of eating, and widened my diet to consume more salad, fruits, and lighter macrobiotic dishes. Meanwhile, the tumor grew and almost completely blocked the transverse colon. I was advised to have an operation immediately. Since I couldn't eat and compresses were unable to open the blockage, I agreed to the surgery. After the operation, the doctors studied the part they had removed and found it unlike any tumor they had ever seen (because I was not eating any meat or dairy). Altogether, about forty cancer specialists, medical students, and M.D.s gathered to discuss my case. They eventually recommended an experimental chemotherapy, but I declined.

I went home, ate well, and rested. I used no particular compresses. Midori, a young woman from Japan studying macrobiotics, helped me in the hospital and at home until I could get up and manage myself, about three months after the operation. After that, I slowly grew stronger. I returned to Japan intermittently over the next couple of years and to Europe to give seminars, but it took a toll on my recovery. For the last several years I have curtailed my teaching and adopted a more comfortable schedule. Recently, Midori and I were married, and we look forward to many happy years together while continuing to spread the macrobiotic way of life.

In many cases of cancer, if not most, medical treatment, especially extreme methods such as radiation therapy and chemotherapy, are not needed. As my family's cases show, however, medical treatment and macrobiotics can be successfully—or unsuccessfully—combined. I very much appreciate the benefits of modern medicine, including radiation and chemotherapy, in difficult cases such as ours. But high doses should be very carefully controlled and monitored. Lower and more moderate doses are recommended, especially for those observing a macrobiotic, vegetarian, or more plant-quality diet.

There were other indirect factors in our illnesses. It has been shown that cancer often develops after a trauma such as an injury. In Aveline and Lily's cases, both had accidents prior to their sicknesses. In the Berkshires, Aveline was in a car accident in which the vehicle turned upside down. She suffered no severe injury and walked away from the mishap. She also fell down a staircase at home and recovered several days later. In Lily's case, she was hit by a train while walking along the tracks on a visit to Japan. She was rendered unconscious and carried to the hospital where she recovered in about a month. Accidents such as these show that a person's life is out of balance and needs to change. There may also have been emotional factors. Both Lily and Aveline developed the same kind of cancer at the same time even though they were living apart and eating differently. This suggests a deep emotional or spiritual bond between them in which they shared each other's pain and suffering.

Friends and colleagues have suggested several other possible factors in our illnesses. First, they wondered if exposure to atomic radiation after the bombing of Hiroshima and Nagasaki could have influenced the development of cancer in Aveline and me and created susceptibility in our daughter. At the time of the atomic bombing of Japan, Aveline lived in Yokota, a small mountain village several hours away from Hiroshima by railroad, and she had relatives in the area. In my case, after I was discharged from the Japanese army and about a month after the bombing, I visited Hiroshima and saw the ruined city for myself. It is doubtful Aveline was affected by the radiation. Possibly I was more influenced by direct exposure to lingering radioactivity. But as Dr. Akizuki in Nagasaki showed, survivors eating a macrobiotic diet protected themselves from radiation sickness through eating miso soup, brown rice balls, kombu, and other strengthening foods. Practically speaking, atomic radiation was not a contributing factor.

It is also well known that when a healer/medical practitioner is working day and night with people who are ill, there is a transmission of energy from the patient to the healer/environment. Sick people were constantly in our home. Aveline cooked and cared for many cancer patients over the years who came to us as a last resort. While cancer itself is not contagious, the energetic and psychic vibrations of weakened and sick persons, especially those who have taken great quantities of chemotherapy or radiation, can produce a vibrational effect and influence the mind and emotions of the caretaker. We preserved a calm, clear mind and spirit as best we could over the years. Whether or not this was a significant factor, we were happy to help others and never regarded it as an excuse for our own illness.

From our experiences, can it be concluded that macrobiotics doesn't work? I don't think so. If anything, our cases attest to the power of macrobiotics to help heal after one has lost his or her balance and become seriously ill. By returning to sound, healthful dietary and lifestyle practices, Aveline, Lily, and I all improved and initially recovered. Modern medicine helped us, but in the first two cases it also did harm. Modern medicine has moved dramatically toward complementary and holistic medicine in recent years, including toward macrobiotics. In the same way, macrobiotics is moving toward modern medicine. The world as a whole faces multiple crises today related to the environment, energy, food quality and sustain-ability, war and peace, the proper use of technology, and financial and eco-nomic security. We need to be flexible, open, and grateful for all approaches as we find our own balance and contribute to planetary health and peace.

We all live in two worlds today—the natural world and the modern world. It is extremely challenging to lead a completely natural or macrobiotic way of life and keep one's health. It is hoped that the next generation will learn from our mistakes and discover the way that is appropriate for their personal growth and development and for their era.

APPENDIX III

Cancer in Animals

Cancer appears in dogs and cats for pretty much the same reason it appears in people. In modern society we feed our pets low-quality, highly processed foods high in meat and other animal protein and fat, low in complex carbohydrates, deficient in many vitamins and minerals, and abundant with chemical additives. But another reason, as Dr. Norman Ralston pointed out, is that we commonly feed our pets some of the same food we eat as leftovers. Ralston, a pioneer macrobiotic veterinarian from Texas, said he often observed the same kind of diseases in people as in their animals.

In his book, *Raising Healthy Pets,* Dr. Ralston said that the first step to improving your pet's health is to stop feeding it canned foods, dog or cat chow, or other commercial products. Ralston lived before organic pet food was widely introduced on the market. While organic is definitely of higher quality, he would probably continue to recommend that animals receive home-cooked fare or share the same natural foods as their owners.

For dogs, he suggested that the ideal diet consisted of about 50 percent whole grains, 25 percent vegetables, and 25 percent meat or other fresh animal food. He believed that, as canines, dogs and cats could digest significantly more animal protein than humans. In addition to beef for dogs, he recommended rabbit, squirrel, and other small animals that their ancestors caught in the wild. Cats thrive on a similar regimen, but in their case fish is preferred.

The grains could be brown rice, millet, barley, or any of the other grains we normally eat. Generally, adding some pieces of the meat or fish to a broth and putting it over the grain will promote its consumption. As they frequently are for humans, vegetables are often an acquired taste, with dogs and cats usually relishing some and avoiding others.

In addition to whole foods, Dr. Ralston used herbs, which his grandmother taught him when growing up on a farm, homeopathic treatments, and as a last resort conventional medicine to relieve disease and disorders.

Unfortunately, Dr. Ralston passed away before completing his second book with specific remedies for different kinds of cancer and other diseases. However, Alex Jack, who collaborated on the first book with him, has his notes. For further information, please see TheCancerPreventionDiet.com.

NOTES

CHAPTER 1: CANCER, DIET, AND MACROBIOTICS

1. *The American Medical Association Family Medical Guide* (New York: Random House, 1987).
2. Miriam S. Wetzel et al., "Courses Involving Complementary and Alternative Medicine at U.S. Medical Schools," *Journal of the American Medical Association* 280:784–87, 1998.

CHAPTER 5: THE MACROBIOTIC CANCER PREVENTION DIET

1. L. Chatenoud et al., "Whole Grain Food Intake and Cancer Risk," *International Journal of Cancer* 77(1):24–28, 1998.
2. D. T. Verhoeven et al., "Epidemiological Studies on Brassica Vegetables and Cancer Risk," *Cancer Epidemiology Biomarkers Prevention* 5(9): 733–48, 1996.
3. T. Itoh et al., "Potential Ability of Hot Water Adzuki (Vigna angularis) Extracts to Inhibit the Adhesion, Invasion, and Metastasis of Murine B16 Melanoma Cells," *Bioscience, Biotechnology, and Biochemistry* 69(3):448–54, 2005.
4. B. R. Goldin et al., "Effect of Diet on Excretion of Estrogens in Pre- and Postmenopausal Incidence of Breast Cancer in Vegetarian Women," *Cancer Research* 41:3771–73, 1981.
5. Anthony J. Satillaro, M.D., *Recalled by Life: The Story of My Recovery from Cancer* with Tom Monte (Boston: Houghton-Mifflin, 1982).
6. Office of Technology Assessment (OTA), *Unconventional Cancer Treatments* (Washington, D.C.: Government Printing Office, 1990).

7. James P. Carter et al., "Hypothesis: Dietary Management May Improve Survival from Nutritionally Linked Cancers Based on Analysis of Representative Cases," *Journal of the American College of Nutrition* 12:209–26, 1993.

8. Rik Vermutten, *MacroMuse,* Fall/Metal 1984, p. 39.

9. Alex Jack, *Let Food Be Thy Medicine* (One Peaceful World, 1999).

10. Franco Berrino et al., "Reducing Bioavailable Sex Hormones Through a Comprehensive Change in Diet: The Diet and Androgens (DIANA) Randomized Trial," *Cancer Epidemiology, Biomarkers, and Prevention* 10:25–33, January 2001.

11. University of South Carolina, Prevention Research Center, 2002.

12. *Minutes of the Fifth Meeting, Cancer Advisory Panel for Complementary and Alternative Medicine* (CAPCAM), Bethesda, Maryland, February 25, 2002; Ralph Moss, Ph.D., "The Olive Branch Bears Fruit," *The Moss Reports,* February 27, 2002; www.cancerdecisions.com/022702.html.

13. "Macrobiotic Research Project," Jane Teas, Ph.D., principal investigator; Joan Cunningham, Ph.D., co-principal investigator, sponsored by the Centers for Disease Control, October 2000 to September 2002, University of South Carolina, Prevention Research Center, School of Public Health, Charleston, S.C.; www.macrobiotics.sph.sc.edu/project.htm. Personal correspondence from Jane Teas, November 1, 2003.

14. "Nutrition and Special Diet: Macrobiotics," M. D. Anderson Cancer Center, the University of Texas, www.mdanderson.org/departments/cimer, 2003–2006.

15. R. Kaaks, "Effects of Dietary Intervention on IGF-Binding Proteins, and Related Alterations in Sex Steroid Metabolism: The Diet and Androgens (DIANA) Randomized Trial," *European Journal of Clinical Nutrition* 57(9):1079–88, 2003.

16. C. Colombo et al., "Plant-Based Diet, Serum Fatty Acid Profile, and Free Radicals in Postmenopausal Women: The Diet and Androgens (DIANA) Randomized Trial," *International Journal of Biological Markers* 20(3):169–76, 2005.

17. G. A. Saxe et al., "Potential Attenuation of Disease Progression in Recurrent Prostate Cancer with Plant-Based Diet and Stress Reduction," *Integrative Cancer Therapies* 5(3)206–13, 2006.

18. J. Y. Nguyen et al., "Adoption of a Plant-Based Diet by Patients with Recurrent Prostate Cancer," *Integrative Cancer Therapies* 5(3):214–23, 2006.

CHAPTER 14: BONE CANCER

1. G. Chihara et al., "Fractionation and Purification of the Polysaccharides with Marked Antitumor Activity, Especially Lentinan, from *Lentinus edodes* (Berk.) Sing. (an Edible Mushroom)," *Cancer Research* 30:2776–81, November 1, 1970.

2. I. Yamamoto et al., "Antitumor Effect of Seaweeds," *Japanese Journal of Experimental Medicine* 44(6):543–46, 1974.

3. "A Mother Heals Breast Cancer: Change in Diet Aids Remission of Tumors and Metastases to the Bone," *One Peaceful World Newsletter,* Spring 1990.

CHAPTER 15: BRAIN CANCER

1. H. Chen et al., "Diet and Risk of Adult Glioma in Eastern Nebraska, U.S." *Cancer Causes Control* 13(7):647–55, 2002.

2. "Chemists Learn Why Vegetables Are Good for You," *New York Times,* April 13, 1993.

3. Jeanne M. Wallace, "The Healing Power of a Wholesome Diet for Brain Tumor Patients," www.tbts.org, 2004.
4. Mona Sanders, "Healing a Terminal Brain Tumor," *One Peaceful World Newsletter,* Autumn/Winter, 1990.

CHAPTER 16: BREAST CANCER

1. Quoted in *Cancer and Civilization* 1:215–17, 1924.
2. A. Tannenbaum, "The Genesis and Growth of Tumors II: Effects of Caloric Restriction Per Se," *Cancer Research* 2:460–67.
3. Marian Tompson, President, La Leche League International, *The People's Doctor: A Medical Newsletter* 4, no. 4:8, 1980.
4. R. L. Phillips, "Role of Life-Style and Dietary Habits in Risk of Cancer Among Seventh-Day Adventists," *Cancer Research* 35:3513–22.
5. G. Hems, "The Contributions of Diet and Childbearing to Breast-Cancer Rates," *British Journal of Cancer* 37:974–82.
6. B. R. Goldin et al., "Effect of Diet on Excretion of Estrogens in Pre- and Postmenopausal Incidence of Breast Cancer in Vegetarian Women," *Cancer Research* 41:3771–73.
7. D. M. Ingram, "Trends in Diet and Breast Cancer Mortality in England and Wales, 1928–1977," *Nutrition and Cancer,* no. 2:75–80, 1982.
8. J. Teas, M. L. Harbison, and R. S. Gelman, "Dietary Seaweed" *[Laminaria]* and Mammary Carcinogenesis in Rats," *Cancer Research* 44:2758–61.
9. Ichiro Yamamoto et al., "The Effect of Dietary Seaweeds on 7, 12-Dimethyl-Benz[a]Anthracene-Induced Mammary Tumorigenesis in Rats," *Cancer Letters* 35:109–18.
10. L. A. Cohen et al., "Modulation of N-Nitrosomethylurea-Induced Mammary Tumor Promotion by Dietary Fiber and Fat," *Journal of the National Cancer Institute* 83:496–500, and "Fiber Is Linked to Reduced Breast Cancer Risk," *Boston Globe,* April 3, 1991.
11. "Chemists Learn Why Vegetables Are Good for You," *New York Times,* April 13, 1993.
12. Shoichiro Tsugane, "Soy, Isoflavones, and Breast Cancer Risk in Japan," *Journal of the National Cancer Institute* 95:906–913, 2003.
13. Maria Cone, "Common Chemicals Are Linked to Breast Cancer," *New York Times,* May 14, 2007.
14. Phyllis W. Crabtree, "A Grandmother Heals Herself," *East West Journal,* 74–81, November 1978.
15. East West Foundation with Ann Fawcett and Cynthia Smith, *Cancer-Free: 30 Who Triumphed over Cancer Naturally* (New York and Tokyo: Japan Publications, 1991).
16. "Macrobiotics for Breast Cancer," *Breathe Magazine,* December 2002.
17. Meg Wolff, "Healing Breast Cancer with Diet," *Amberwaves* 8, 2003; Meg Wolff, *Becoming Whole,* Lulu.com, 2006.
18. Gayle Stolove, "My Story," www.whollymacrobiotics.com.

CHAPTER 17: CHILDREN'S CANCER

1. J. Hergenrather et al., "Pollutants in Breast Milk of Vegetarians" (letter), *New England Journal of Medicine* 304:792, 1976.

CHAPTER 18: COLON AND RECTAL CANCER

1. Denis P. Burkitt, M.D., *Eat Right—to Stay Healthy and Enjoy Life More,* 11, 66–71 (New York: Arco, 1979).
2. F. M. Sacks et al., "Effects of Ingestion of Meat on Plasma Cholesterol of Vegetarians," *Journal of the American Medical Association,* 246:640–44.
3. M. L. Slattery, "Plant Foods and Colon Cancer: An Assessment of Specific Foods and Their Related Nutrients," *Cancer Causes Control* 8(4):575–90, 1997.
4. Y. Ohuchi et al., "Decrease in Size of Azoxymethane Induced Colon Carcinoma in F344 Rats by 180-Day Fermented Miso," *Oncology Reports* 14(6):1559–64, 2005.
5. A. Strohle et al., "Nutrition and Colorectal Cancer," *Med Monatsschr Pharm* 30(1):25–32, 2007.
6. East West Foundation with Ann Fawcett and Cynthia Smith, *Cancer-Free: 30 Who Triumphed over Cancer Naturally* (New York and Tokyo: Japan Publications, 1991).
7. Ibid.

CHAPTER 19: FEMALE REPRODUCTIVE CANCERS: OVARY, UTERUS, CERVIX, AND VAGINA

1. Frederick Hoffman, *Cancer and Diet,* 6 (Baltimore: Williams & Wilkins, 1937).
2. Robert Bell, M.D., *Ten Years' Record of the Treatment of Cancer Without Operation,* 6, 14–15 (London: Dean & Son, 1906).
3. R. L. Phillips, "Role of Life-styles and Dietary Habits in Risk of Cancer Among Seventh-Day Adventists," *Cancer Research* 35:3513–22.
4. Samuel S. Epstein, M.D., *The Politics of Cancer,* 222 (New York: Doubleday, 1979).
5. Gloria Swanson, "I'm Still a Woman," *East West Journal,* 34–35, March 1977.
6. Elaine Nussbaum, *Recovery From Cancer to Health Through Macrobiotics* (Garden City Park, NY: Avery Publishing Group, 1991).
7. Liliane Papin, Ph.D., "Life Is a Phoenix: A Yugoslavian Family's Triumph over Cancer," *One Peaceful World Newsletter,* Spring 1989. Milenka Dobic, *My Beautiful Life* (Forres, Scotland: Findhorn Press, 1999).
8. Gerry DeMello, "Healing Ovarian Cancer with Diet," *Amberwaves* 12, 2005.

CHAPTER 20: KIDNEY AND BLADDER CANCER

1. Albert Schweitzer, M.D., *Briefe aus dem Lambarenespital,* Box 27, Albert Schweitzer, Fellowship Records, Syracuse University, Syracuse, NY, 1954.
2. R. L. Phillips, "Role of Life-Styles and Dietary Habits in Risk of Cancer Among Seventh-Day Adventists," *Cancer Research* 35:3513–22.
3. T. Kuno et al., "Chemoprevention of Mouse Urinary Bladder Carcinogenesis by Fermented Brown Rice and Rice Bran," *Oncology Reports* 15(3):533–38, 2006.
4. Sheldon Rice, "Embracing Health," *Planetary Health* 2, Summer, 2000.

CHAPTER 21: LEUKEMIA

1. J. A. Saxton, Jr., et al., "Observations on the Inhibition of Development of Spontaneous Leukemias in Mice by Underfeeding," *Cancer Research* 4:401–9, 1944.
2. K. Morishita, M.D., *The Hidden Truth of Cancer* (San Francisco: George Ohsawa Macrobiotic Foundation, 1972).
3. R. L. Phillips, "Role of Life-Style and Dietary Habits in Risk of Cancer Among Seventh-Day Adventists," *Cancer Research* 35:3513–22.
4. F. M. Uckun et al., "Biotherapy of B-Cell Precursors Leukemia by Targeting Genistein to CD19-Associated Tyrosine Kinases," *Science* 267(5199):886–91, 1995.
5. H. F. Liao et al., "Rice (Oryza sativa L.) Inhibits Growth and Induces Differentiation of Human Leukemia U937 Cells Through Activation of Peripheral Blood Mononuclear Cells," *Food Chemistry and Toxicology* 44(10):1724–29, 2006.
6. Christina Pirello, "Macrobiotics: Getting Started," *MacroNews,* January/February 1990.
7. East West Foundation with Ann Fawcett and Cynthia Smith, *Cancer-Free: 30 Who Triumphed over Cancer Naturally* (Tokyo and New York: Japan Publications, 1991).
8. T. Akizuki, M.D., *Documentary of A-Bombed Nagasaki* (Nagasaki: Nagasaki Printing Company, 1977); Ida Honoroff, "A Report to the Consumer," May 1978; and Hideo Ohmori, "Report from Japan," *A Nutritional Approach to Cancer* (Boston: East West Foundation, 1977), 28–32.
9. Sawako Hiraga, "How I Survived the Atomic Bomb," *Macrobiotic,* November/December 1979.
10. Hiroko Furo, Ph.D., foreword by George W. Yu, M.D., *Healing with Miso: Dietary Practice of Atomic Bomb Survivors in Hiroshima and Nagasaki* (Amberwaves, 2007).
11. Alex Jack, "Soviets Embrace Macrobiotics," *One Peaceful World Newsletter,* Autumn/Winter 1990; personal communication to Alex Jack, April 1991; and personal communication to Michio Kushi, May 4, 1992.

CHAPTER 22: LIVER CANCER

1. L. J. Rather, *The Genesis of Cancer: A Study in the History of Ideas,* 17 (Baltimore: Johns Hopkins University Press, 1978).
2. A. Tannenbaum, "The Dependence of Tumor Formation on the Composition of the Calorie-Restricted Diet as Well as on the Degree of Restriction," *Cancer Research* 5:616–25.
3. N. Iritani and S. Nogi, "Effects of Spinach and Wakame on Cholesterol Turnover in the Rat," *Atherosclerosis* 15:87–92, 1972.
4. J. E. Engstrom, "Health and Dietary Practices and Cancer Mortality Among California Mormons," in *Cancer Incidence in Defined Populations, Banbury Report 4* edited by J. Cairns et al., 69–90 (Cold Spring Harbor, NY: Cold Spring Harbor Laboratory, 1980).
5. Shigehiro Kataoka, "Functional Effects of Japanese Style Fermented Soy Sauce (Shoyu) and Its Components," *Journal of Bioscience and Bioengineering* 200:227–34, 2005.
6. Personal communication from Hilda Sorhagen, and Alex Jack and Karin Stephan, "Whole-Grain Ashram," *East West Journal,* 8–9, July 1982.

CHAPTER 23: LUNG CANCER

1. B. Peyrilhe, M.D., *A Dissertation on Cancerous Diseases* (London, 1777); and Michael Shimkin, *Contrary to Nature,* 183 (Washington, D.C.: National Institutes of Health, 1977).
2. J. L. Bulkley, M.D., "Cancer Among Primitive Tribes," *Cancer* 4:289–95, 1927.
3. Wayne Martin, *Medical Heroes and Heretics,* 84 (Old Greenwich, CT: Devin-Adair, 1977).
4. "Tobacco: Is There a 'Cure' for Cancer?" *Medical World News,* 17–19, March 16, 1973.
5. Y. Kagawa, "Impact of Westernization on the Nutrition of Japan," *Preventive Medicine* 7:205–17.
6. P. Knekt et al., "Dietary Antioxidants and the Risk of Lung Cancer," *American Journal of Epidemiology* 134:471–79.
7. Emanuela Taioli et al., "Possible Role of Diet as a Host Factor in the Aetiology of Tobacco-Induced Lung Cancer," *International Journal of Epidemiology* 20:611–14, 1991.
8. R. Rylander et al., "Lung Cancer, Smoking and Diet Among Swedish Men," *Lung Cancer* 14 (Supplement 1):S75–83, 1996.
9. D. T. Verhoeven et al., "Epidemiological Studies on Brassica Vegetables and Cancer Risk," *Cancer Epidemiology Biomarkers Prevention* 5(9):733–48, 1996.
10. E. De Stefani et al., "Dietary Sugar and Lung Cancer: A Case-Control Study in Uruguay," *Nutrition and Cancer* 31(2):132–37, 1998.
11. K. Shiraki et al., "Inhibition by Long-Term Fermented Miso of Induction of Pulmonary Adenocarcinoma by Dilsopropanolnitrosamine in Wistar Rats," *Hiroshima Journal of Medical Science* 52(1):9–13, 2003.
12. T. Itoh et al., "Potential Ability of Hot Water Adzuki (*Vigna angularis*) Extracts to Inhibit the Adhesion, Invasion, and Metastasis of Murine B_{16} Melanoma Cells," *Bioscience Biotechnology and Biochemistry* 69(3):448–54, 2005.
13. Gale Jack, "Given Two Weeks to Live—Seven Years Ago: Elizabeth Masters's Story," *One Peaceful World Newsletter,* Autumn/Winter 1991.
14. Janet E. Vitt, R.N., "Healing Metastatic Cancer with Diet," *One Peaceful World Journal* 37:1–10, 1999.

CHAPTER 24: LYMPHATIC CANCER: LYMPHOMA AND HODGKIN'S DISEASE

1. A. S. Cunningham, "Lymphomas and Animal-Protein Consumption," *Lancet* 2:1184–86, 1976.
2. Samuel S. Epstein, M.D., *The Politics of Cancer,* 18687 (New York: Doubleday, 1979).
3. A. Tavani et al., "Diet and Risk of Lymphoid Neoplasms and Soft Tissue Sarcomas," *Nutrition and Cancer* 27(3):25660, 1997.
4. C. I. Gill et al., "Watercress Supplementation in Diet Reduces Lymphocyte DNA Damage and Alters Blood Antioxidant Status in Healthy Adults," *American Journal of Clinical Nutrition* 85(2):504–10, 2007.
5. *Case History Reports,* vol. 1, no. 3, 5–7 (Boston: East West Foundation, 1976).
6. East West Foundation with Ann Fawcett and Cynthia Smith, *Cancer-Free: 30 Who Triumphed over Cancer Naturally* (New York and Tokyo: Japan Publications, 1991).

7. Judy MacKenney, "Healing Lymphoma with Macrobiotics," *One Peaceful World Journal* 33:1–6, 1998.

CHAPTER 25: MALE REPRODUCTIVE CANCERS: PROSTATE AND TESTES

1. M. A. Howell, "Factor Analysis of International Cancer Mortality Data and Per Capita Food Consumption," *British Journal of Cancer* 29:328–36.
2. R. L. Phillips, "Role of Life-Styles and Dietary Habits in Risk of Cancer Among Seventh-Day Adventists," *Cancer Research* 35:3513–22.
3. J. L. Colli and A. Colli, "International Comparisons of Prostate Cancer Mortality Rates with Dietary Practices and Sunlight Levels," *Urologic Oncology* 24(3):184–94, 2006.
4. A. Stang et al., "Adolescent Milk Fat and Galactose Consumption and Testicular Germ Cell Cancer," *Cancer Epidemiology Biomarkers and Prevention* 15(11):2189–2195, 2006.
5. East West Foundation with Ann Fawcett and Cynthia Smith, *Cancer-Free: 30 Who Triumphed over Cancer Naturally* (New York and Tokyo: Japan Publications, 1991).
6. Ibid.
7. March Scholz, M.D., and Ralph Blum, "Can Diet Really Control Prostate Cancer?" *Prostate Cancer Research Institute Insights* 9(1), 2006.

CHAPTER 26: ORAL AND UPPER DIGESTIVE CANCERS: MOUTH, LARYNX, PHARYNX, AND ESOPHAGUS

1. H. Hormozdiari et al., "Dietary Factors and Esophageal Cancer in the Caspian Littoral of Iran," *Cancer Research* 35:3493–98.
2. J. E. Engstrom, "Health and Dietary Practices and Cancer Mortality Among California Mormons," in *Cancer Incidence in Defined Populations, Banbury Report 4* edited by J. Cairns et al., 69–90 (Cold Spring Harbor, NY: Cold Spring Harbor Laboratory, 1980).
3. J. M. Wang et al., "Diet Habits, Alcohol Drinking, Tobacco Smoking, Green Tea Drinking, and the Risk of Esophageal Squamous Cell Carcinoma in the Chinese Population," *European Journal of Gastroenterology and Hepatology* 19(2):171–76, 2007.
4. "Granular Myoblastoma on the Vocal Cord," *The Cancer Prevention Diet,* 87–89 (Brookline, MA: East West Foundation, 1981).

CHAPTER 27: PANCREATIC CANCER

1. J. E. Engstrom, "Health and Dietary Practices and Cancer Mortality Among California Mormons," in *Cancer Incidence in Defined Populations, Banbury Report 4* edited by J. Cairns et al., 69–90 (Cold Spring Harbor, NY: Cold Spring Harbor Laboratory).
2. Gordon Saxe, "A Retrospective Study of Diet and Cancer of the Pancreas," in *Cancer-Free: 30 Who Triumphed Naturally over Cancer* by East West Foundation with Ann Fawcett and Cynthia Smith (Tokyo and New York: Japan Publications, 1991).

3. S. Ohba et al., "Eating Habits and Pancreas Cancer," *International Journal of Pancreatology* 20(1):37–42, 1996.
4. Susanna C. Larsson et al., "Consumption of Sugar and Sugar-Sweetened Foods and the Risk of Pancreatic Cancer in a Prospective Study," *American Journal of Clinical Nutrition,* November 2006.
5. "Whole Grains and Risk of Pancreatic Cancer in a Large Population–Based Case-Control Study in San Francisco Bay Area, California," *American Journal of Epidemiology* 166:10, 1174–85, November 2007.
6. Jean and Mary Alice Kohler, *Healing Miracles from Macrobiotics* (West Nyack, NY: Parker, 1979), and Tom Monte, "The Legacy of Jean Kohler," *East West Journal,* 14–18, March 1981.
7. Letters from Norman Arnold to Congressman Claude Pepper, Chairman of the U.S. House Subcommittee on Health and Long-Term Care, January 18, 1984.

CHAPTER 28: SKIN CANCER AND MELANOMA

1. H. B. Demopoulos, "Effects of Reducing the Phenylalanine-Tyrosine Intake of Patients with Advanced Malignant Melanoma," *Cancer* 19:657–64, 1966.
2. *Carcinogens, Job Health Hazards Series,* 7–8 (Washington, D.C.: Occupational Safety and Health Administration, 1975).
3. W. Troll, "Blocking of Tumor Promotion by Protease Inhibitors," in *Cancer: Achievement, Challenges, and Prospects for the 1980s* edited by J. H. Burchenal and H. F. Oettgen, 1:549–55 (New York: Grune and Stratton, 1985).
4. T. Itoh et al., "Potential Ability of Hot Water Adzuki (*Vigna angularis*) Extracts to Inhibit the Adhesion, Invasion, and Metastasis of Murine B_{16} Melanoma Cells," *Bioscience, Biotechnology, and Biochemistry* 69(3):448–54, 2005.
5. P. Thejass and G. Kuttan, "Antimetastatic Activity of Sulforaphne," *Life Sciences* 78(26):3043–50, 2006.
6. *Case History Reports,* vol. 1, no. 3, 1–2 (Boston: East West Foundation, 1976).
7. "Malignant Melanoma, Stage IV," *Cancer and Diet,* 69–70 (Brookline, MA: East West Foundation, 1980), and interview with Alex Jack, September 30, 1982.
8. *One Peaceful World Newsletter,* Autumn 1989.

CHAPTER 29: STOMACH CANCER

1. Robert McCarrison, M.D., "Faulty Food in Relation to Gastro-Intestinal Disorder," *Journal of the American Medical Association* 78, 1–8, 1922, and G. T. Wrench, M.D., *The Wheel of Health* (London: O. W. Daniel, 1938).
2. T. Hirayama, "Epidemiology of Stomach Cancer," in *Early Gastric Cancer, Gann Monograph on Cancer Research* edited by T. Murakami (Tokyo: University of Tokyo Press) 1:3–19.
3. T. Hirayama, "Relationship of Soybean Paste Soup Intake to Gastric Cancer Risk," *Nutrition and Cancer* 3:223–33.
4. J. Raloff, "A Soy Sauce Surprise," *Science News* 139:357, 1991.
5. Paul Talalay, *Proceedings of the National Academy of Sciences,* March 16, 1992, and "Broccoli Contains Powerful Cancer Fighter, Study Shows," *Cleveland Plain Dealer,* March 15, 1992.

6. M. Ohara et al., "Inhibition by Long-Term Fermented Miso of Induction of Gastric Tumors by N-Methyl-N-Nitro-N-Nitrosoguanidine in CD (SD) Rats," *Oncology Reports* 9(3):613–16, 2002.
7. Michio Kushi with Alex Jack, *One Peaceful World* (New York: St. Martin's Press, 1987).

CHAPTER 30: THYROID CANCER

1. S. Franceschi et al., "Diet and Thyroid Cancer: A Pooled Analysis of Four European Case-Control Studies," *International Journal of Cancer* 48(3):395–98, May 30, 1991.
2. M. R. Galanti et al., "Diet and the Risk of Papillary and Follicular Thyroid Carcinoma: A Population-Based Case-Control Study in Sweden and Norway," *Cancer Causes Control* 8(2):205–14, March 1997.
3. L. Chatenoud et al., "Refined-Cereal Intake and Risk of Selected Cancers in Italy," *American Journal of Clinical Nutrition* 70(6):1107–10, December 1999.
4. P. L. Horn-Ross et al., "Phytoestrogens and Thyroid Cancer Risk: The San Francisco Bay Area Thyroid Cancer Study," *Cancer Epidemiology Biomarkers Prevention* 11(1):43–49, January 2002.
5. S. Memon et al., "Benign Thyroid Disease and Dietary Factors in Thyroid Cancer: A Case-Control Study in Kuwait," *British Journal of Cancer* 86(11):1745–50, June 5, 2002.
6. Rosemary Traill, Report for Cancer Research, UK, 2002.

RESOURCES AND COUNSELING

PERSONAL COUNSELING

Michio Kushi is no longer counseling on a regular basis. He occasionally gives individual or group counseling during seminars.

Alex Jack offers counseling in person, on the telephone, and by email. For further information or to download his counseling forms, please see TheCancerPreventionDiet.com or MacrobioticPath.com. See Internet Resources on page 572 for additional counseling services.

RECOMMENDED READING

The following books are suggested for further reading and study. The ones marked with an asterisk (*) are particularly recommended. Some of them are out of print and have been reissued by the Kushi Institute of Europe (macrobiotics.nl). Deshima, the KIE's mail-order store, also carries a large selection of books in French, German, Spanish, Italian, and other languages. Other hard-to-find books may be available on Amazon.com.

Akizuki, Tatsuichiro, M.D. *Nagasaki 1945* (Quartet Books, U.K., 1981, distributed by Charles River Books in the U.S.). An absorbing account of how a macrobiotic doctor saved his patients after the atomic bomb of Nagasaki.

Benedict, Dirk. *Confessions of a Kamikaze Cowboy* (Avery, 1991). An actor's recovery from prostate cancer.

Briscoe, David, and Charlotte Mahoney-Briscoe. *A Personal Peace* (Japan Publications, 1989). A mother helps her son recover from schizophrenia with the help of macrobiotics.

Brown, Virginia, with Susan Stayman. *Macrobiotic Miracle: How a Vermont Family Overcame Cancer* (Japan Publications, 1985). A nurse heals herself of malignant melanoma.

Campbell, Don. *The Mozart Effect* (Avon, 1997). The healing power of music. Written with Alex Jack.

*Dobic, Milenka. *My Beautiful Life* (Square One, 2007). The story of a Serbian journalist and mother who healed herself of incurable ovarian cancer with macrobiotics.

Dufty, William. *Sugar Blues* (Warner Books, 1975). Classic critique of the devastating role that sugar played historically, including financing the slave trade and its corrosive effects on society and personal health.

Esko, Edward. *Healing Planet Earth* (One Peaceful World Press, 1995). The macrobiotic approach to ecology.

———. *Contemporary Macrobiotics* (1stbooks.com, 2000). Essays on health and healing by a leading macrobiotic teacher and counselor.

Esko, Edward, and Wendy Esko. *Macrobiotic Cooking for Everyone* (Japan Publications, 1980). General all-purpose cookbook.

Esko, Wendy. *Aveline Kushi's Introducing Macrobiotic Cooking* (Japan Publications, 1987). Excellent general cookbook.

———. *Eat Your Veggies* (One Peaceful World Press, 1996). One hundred delicious easy-to-make recipes.

———. *Rice Is Nice* (Amberwaves, 2001). One hundred and eight delicious brown rice recipes.

———. *Soup du Jour* (One Peaceful World Press, 1995). Over one hundred hearty soups, stews, and broths.

Jack, Gale, and Wendy Esko. ed. *Women's Health Guide* (One Peaceful World Press, 1997). The macrobiotic approach to women's health and concerns.

Jack, Gale, and Alex Jack. *Promenade Home: Macrobiotics and Women's Health* (Japan Publications, 1988). Autobiography of a Texas schoolteacher.

Jack, Alex. *Imagine a World Without Monarch Butterflies* (One Peaceful World Press, 2000). Awakening to the hazards of genetically altered foods.

———. *Let Food Be Thy Medicine* (One Peaceful World Press, third edition, 1999). Summary of 750 scientific and medical studies related to macrobiotics and holistic health.

———. *Profiles in Oriental Diagnosis.* Vol. 1: *The Renaissance;* Vol. 2: *Vegetarian Bride of Frankenstein;* Vol. 3: *Evolution at the Dinner Table* (One Peaceful World Press, 1995–2000). Case histories of famous artists, explorers, and poets, including Leonardo da Vinci, Shakespeare, Descartes, Newton, Darwin, and Pasteur.

Jack, Alex, and Edward Esko, eds. *Saving Organic Rice* (Amberwaves, 2001). Passionate critique of genetically engineered rice featuring essays by Vandana Shiva, Mae-Wan Ho, Amory and Hunter Lovins, and other scientists and environmentalists.

Kushi, Aveline, and Wendy Esko. *Aveline Kushi's Wonderful World of Salads* (Japan Publications, 1989). Complete guide to salads and an in-depth introduction to the art of cutting.

———. *The Changing Seasons Macrobiotic Cookbook* (Avery, 1985). Cooking with the four seasons.

———. *The Complete Whole Grain Cookbook* (Japan Publications, 1997). Two hundred and fifty grain-based recipes for all occasions.

Kushi, Aveline, Wendy Esko, and Maya Tiwari. *Diet for Natural Beauty* (Japan Publications, 1991). Encyclopedia of using food internally and externally for beautiful skin and radiance.

Kushi, Aveline, and Alex Jack. *Aveline: The Life and Dream of the Woman Behind Macrobiotics Today* (Japan Publications, 1988). Aveline's autobiography and history of macrobiotics in America.

*———. *Aveline Kushi's Complete Guide to Macrobiotic Cooking for Health, Harmony, and Peace* (Warner Books, 1985). The standard all-purpose macrobiotic cookbook.

Kushi, Michio. *Basic Home Remedies* (One Peaceful World Press, 1994). Guide to the fifty most common macrobiotic home care treatments.

*———. *The Do-In Way* (Square One, 2007). The traditional art of self-massage, including hundreds of exercises to strengthen different organs, meridians, and systems.

———. *The Macrobiotic Way* (Avery, 1993). An excellent general introduction to macrobiotics, including recipes and exercises.

———. *Standard Macrobiotic Diet* (One Peaceful World Press, 1996, rev. ed.). Basic description of the macrobiotic way of eating and a dozen recipes.

*———. *Your Body Never Lies* (Square One, 2007). Basic text on physiognomy and visual diagnosis.

Kushi, Michio, and Edward Esko. *Basic Shiatsu* (One Peaceful World Press, 1995). How to give a simple home-style massage.

———. *Dream Diagnosis* (One Peaceful World Press, 1995). How diet affects our dreams, including a dictionary of symbols.

———. *Macrobiotic Seminars of Michio Kushi* (One Peaceful World Press, 1998). Classic lectures on health, diet, and the order of the universe.

*Kushi, Michio, and Alex Jack. *The Book of Macrobiotics* (Japan Publications, 1986). Standard text on macrobiotic principles and practice.

———. *Diet for a Strong Heart* (St. Martin's Press, 1985). Standard text on all aspects of cardiovascular health.

———. *The Gospel of Peace: Jesus's Teachings of Eternal Truth* (Japan Publications, 1992). Commentary on the lost Gospel of Thomas and Jesus's macrobiotic approach.

———. *Humanity at the Crossroads* (One Peaceful World Press, 1997). Dietary and lifestyle guidelines for the age of cloning, EMFs, AIDS, mad cow disease, and global warming.

*———. *The Macrobiotic Path to Total Health* (Ballantine Books, 2003). A complete guide to naturally preventing and relieving more than two hundred chronic conditions and disorders.

———. *One Peaceful World* (St. Martin's Press, 1986). Michio Kushi's autobiography and standard text on world peace and a macrobiotic approach to social change.

Kushi, Michio, and Aveline and Alex Jack. *Food Governs Your Destiny: The Teachings of Mizuno Namboku* (Japan Publications, 1986). Insightful observations of an eighteenth-century physiognomist.

*———. *Macrobiotic Diet* (Japan Publications, 1993). Standard text on nutrition and food energy.

*Kushi, Michio, and Olivia Oredson Saunders, *Macrobiotic Palm Healing: Energy at Your Fingertips* (Japan Publications, 1988). Standard text on healing directly with heaven and earth's forces.

*McKenna, Marlene, with Tom Monte. *When Hope Never Dies* (Kensington Press, 2000). The story of a stockbroker and mother who healed herself of incurable malignant melanoma with the help of macrobiotics.

Monte, Tom. *The Way of Hope: Michio Kushi's Anti-AIDS Program* (Warner Books, 1989). The story of ten men with AIDS-related symptoms who followed a macrobiotic approach.

*Nussbaum, Elaine. *Recovery: From Cancer to Health Through Macrobiotics* (Avery, 1992). A mother heals herself of inoperable uterine cancer.

Ohsawa, George. *The Art of Peace* (G.O.M.F., 1990). A meditation on how to achieve universal peace, freedom, and justice.

Pirello, Christina. *Cooking the Whole Foods Way* (Putnam Berkley Group, 1997). Five hundred natural foods recipes from a noted macrobiotic teacher and host of the PBS show *Christina Cooks!*

Porter, Jessica. *The Hip Chick's Guide to Macrobiotics* (Avery, 2004). A wry approach by a comedienne and macrobiotic cook.

Ralston, Norman, D.V.M., with Gale Jack. *Raising Healthy Pets* (One Peaceful World Press, 1996). Keeping dogs and cats healthy by a macrobiotic vet.

Rogers, Sherry A., M.D. *The Cure Is in the Kitchen* (Prestige, 1991). The story of a macrobiotic physician who healed herself of environmental illness (E.I.).

*Sattilaro, Anthony, M.D., and Tom Monte. *Recalled by Life* (Houghton-Mifflin, 1982). A medical doctor and president of a large hospital in Philadelphia overcomes terminal cancer.

Spear, William. *Feng Shui Made Easy* (Harper Collins, 1995). The art of household siting and arrangement.

Stanchich, Lino. *Power Eating Program* (Healthy Products, 1989). A macrobiotic self-development program emphasizing thorough chewing.

Todd, Alexandra. *Double Vision* (University Press of New England, 1994). A mother helps her son overcome a brain tumor with macrobiotics and modern medicine.

Waxman, Denny. *The Great Life Diet* (Pegasus, 2007). A ten-step program to better health by an experienced macrobiotics teacher and counselor.

*Wolff, Meg. *Becoming Whole: My Recovery from Breast Cancer* (Lulu.com, 2007). A mother's inspiring story of recovering from breast cancer.

Yamamoto, Shizuko, and Patrick McCarty. *The Shiatsu Handbook* (Avery, 1996). A comprehensive collection of acupressure techniques.

INTERNET RESOURCES

Amberwaves.org. A macrobiotic-oriented network of friends and families protecting the environment and food supply from genetic engineering, climate change, and other threats.

Annabohm.com. Web site of psychologist Anna Böhm, offering research and information on the role of the emotions in health and well-being.

Macrobiotics.nl. Web site of the Kushi Institute of Europe, offering year-round programs in Amsterdam and an International Macrobiotic Summer Conference with hundreds of participants from across Europe, Africa, the Middle East, Asia, and North America.

Absolutelymacro.com. Web site of macrobiotic and wellness counselor and cooking teacher Jane Steinberg, MPH, based in Santa Fe, New Mexico.

Andreabeaman.com. Web site of macrobiotic and holistic health counselor Andream Beaman, based in New York City.

Atlantamacrobioltics.com. Web site of Marsha Rueff, a macrobiotic teacher and counselor, based in Atlanta, Georgia.

Cybermacro.com. An online macrobiotic community offering mail-order food, books, kitchenware, and forums with offices in Hooksett, New Hampshire.

Davidsnieckus.com. Web site of macrobiotic teacher, counselor, chef, and author David Snieckus, based in Boston.

http://users.stargate.net/~rncjr/eastwest.htm East West Center of Cleveland. A macrobiotic educational center directed by Robert N. Carr, Jr., offering classes and counseling services.

Edenfoods.com. The largest macrobiotic food manufacturer and distributor in America, offering a comprehensive online macrobiotic mail-order service featuring Muso high quality Japanese products and their own lines of food.

Goldminenaturalfoods.com. A San Diego, California, based macrobiotic mail-order company offering a wide selection of organic grains, beans, sea vegetables, and other staples, as well as cookware, books, and other products.

Greatlifeglobal.com. Web site of Lino Stanchich and Jane Quincannon-Stanchich, senior teachers and counselors who instruct internationally and offer mountain retreats in Asheville, North Carolina.

Healingcuisine.com. Web site of Meredith McCarty, macrobiotic consultant, author, and lecturer based in Northern California.

Kijapan.jp/English. Web site of the Kushi Institute of Japan, offering a variety of programs and activities.

Macrobiotic.com. Web site of John Kozinski, a teacher and counselor at the Kushi Institute.

Macrobioticcenter.com. Web site of Margaret Lawson, longtime macrobiotic cook, teacher, and counselor in Dallas.

Macrobioticsnewengland.com. Web site of Warren Kramer, a macrobiotic cook, counselor, and teacher based in Boston.

Macrobioticsonline.com. Web site of the Kushi Institute in western Massachusetts offering instruction and guidance.

Makropedia.com. A forthcoming new Wikipedia-style macrobiotic site, organized by Alex Jack and Adelbert Nelissen, offering comprehensive information on diet and health.

Megwolff.com. Web site of a macrobiotic breast cancer survivor, author, lecturer, and counselor.

Michaelrossoff.com. Web site of a longtime macrobiotic counselor and teacher and acupuncturist based in Asheville, North Carolina, who served as dean of Atlantic University of Chinese Medicine.

Minadobic.org. Web site of Mina Dobic, a twenty-year, macrobiotic cancer survivor who is an international teacher and counselor based in San Diego.

Nadinebarner.com. Web site of Nadine Barner, a macrobiotic cook, teacher, and counselor based in Los Angeles.

Naturalepicurean.com. Web site of the Natural Epicurean Academy of Culinary Arts, a macrobiotic cooking school founded by Dawn Pallavi in Austin, Texas.

Naturalimport.com. Offers a large mail-order selection of traditional Japanese macrobiotic products from Mitoku at discount prices. The company is based in Asheville, North Carolina.

Natural-lifestyle.com. A family-operated macrobiotic mail-order company in Asheville, North Carolina, offering a wide variety of organic foods, cookware, books, and other natural-living products by mail order.

Quantumrabbit.com. An alternative energy site presenting research on new energy sources based on macrobiotic principles.

Strengtheninghealth.org. Web site of the Strengthening Health Institute, a macrobiotic training center in Philadelphia founded by Denny Waxman, offering year-round classes and activities and an organic café.

Susankriegerhealth.com. Web site of Susan Krieger, Lic. Ac. MS, a macrobiotic teacher, acupunturist, and shiatsu practitioner based in New York City.

Whollymacrobiotics.com. Web site of Gayle Stolove, a macrobiotic breast cancer survivor, who offers classes and counseling in South Florida.

PERIODICALS

Amberwaves/Macrobiotic Path, Becket, Massachusetts
Christina Cooks, Philadelphia, Pennsylvania
Macrobiotics Today, Oroville, California

ABOUT THE AUTHORS

Michio Kushi, leader of the international macrobiotic community, was born in Japan in 1926, studied international law at Tokyo University, and came to America in 1949. Influenced by the devastation of World War II, he decided to dedicate his life to the achievement of world peace and the development of humanity. Sponsored by Norman Cousins, he came to New York and furthered his studies at Columbia University and in personal meetings with Albert Einstein, Thomas Mann, Upton Sinclair, Pitirim Sorokin, and other prominent scientists, authors, and statesmen.

With the help of his wife, Aveline, who came to the United States in 1951, Michio Kushi introduced modern macrobiotics and founded Erewhon, the pioneer natural foods company in Boston in the early 1960s. The Kushis went on to found the East West Foundation, the *East West Journal,* the Kushi Foundation, and other organizations to spread macrobiotics worldwide. Over the last fifty years Michio Kushi has guided thousands of individuals and families to greater health and happiness, lectured to physicians and scientists, advised governments, inspired medical research, and served as a consultant to natural foods businesses and industries.

The author of many books, Michio Kushi received the Award of Excellence from the United Nations Writers Society. In recognition of his role in launching the modern health and diet revolution, the Smithsonian Institution opened a permanent Kushi Family Collection on Macrobiotics and Alternative Health Care in 1999. In Washington, D.C., he made a presentation on macrobiotics to the White House Commission on Complementary and Alternative Medicine, and in New York he was a featured speaker at the first Asian Therapies for Cancer Conference.

Michio Kushi lives in Brookline, Massachusetts. He has four children and many grandchildren. His wife, Aveline, died in 2001, and he recently married Midori Hiyashi.

Alex Jack was born in Chicago in 1945, grew up in Evanston, Illinois, and Scarsdale, New York, and received a degree in philosophy from Oberlin College. He served as a reporter in Vietnam and has written for many magazines and publications. Over the last thirty years he has been active in the macrobiotic and holistic community as an author, teacher, and dietary counselor. He has served as editor-in-chief of the *East West Journal,* general manager of the Kushi Institute, and director of the One Peaceful World Society. He is founder and president of Amberwaves, a grassroots network devoted to promoting whole grains and protecting rice, wheat, and other essential foods from the threat of genetic engineering.

He is the author, coauthor, or editor of many books, including *The Cancer Prevention Diet* and *Diet for a Strong Heart* with Michio Kushi (both published by St. Martin's Press), *Aveline Kushi's Complete Guide to Macrobiotic Cooking* (Warner Books), *The Book of Macrobiotics* with Michio Kushi (Japan Publications), *Let Food Be Thy Medicine* (One Peaceful World Press), *The Mozart Effect* with Don Campbell (Avon Books), *Imagine a World Without Monarch Butterflies* (One Peaceful World Press), and *Saving Organic Rice* (Amberwaves).

Alex has traveled and helped introduce macrobiotics in Russia, China, and other countries, and is on the visiting faculty of the Kushi Institute of Europe and the Nippon C.I. (Ohsawa Center) in Japan.

He is a founder and vice president of Quantum Rabbit, an alternative energy company, editor of *Macrobiotic Path*, and cofounder of Makropedia .com. A student of Elizabethan literature, he is the editor of *The 400th Anniversary Edition of Hamlet* by Christopher Marlowe and William Shakespeare that he introduced at the new Globe Theatre in London in 2005. He divides his time between America and Europe. Contact Alex Jack at shenwa26@yahoo.com.

Anna Böhm, was born in Germany in 1983, grew up in a pioneer macrobiotic community in France, and has two masters degrees in psychology. For one she specialized in clinical psychology and in psychoanalysis for the other. She now lives in Vienna, where she is practicing as a psychologist. If you would like to know more about her research, visit her Web site, annabohm.com, or contact her at anna-bohm@live.com.

INDEX